Lippincott's
Illustrated Reviews:
Pharmacology

4th edition

Lippincott's Illustrated Reviews: Pharmacology

Richard Finkel, Pharm.D.

Department of Pharmaceutical and Administrative Sciences
Nova Southeastern University
College of Pharmacy
Fort Lauderdale, Florida

Michelle A. Clark, Ph.D.

Department of Pharmaceutical and Administrative Sciences
Nova Southeastern University
College of Pharmacy
Fort Lauderdale, Florida

Luigi X. Cubeddu, M.D., Ph.D.

Department of Pharmaceutical and Administrative Sciences
Nova Southeastern University
College of Pharmacy
Fort Lauderdale, Florida

Series Editors

Richard A. Harvey, Ph.D.

Department of Biochemistry
University of Medicine and Dentistry of New Jersey–
Robert Wood Johnson Medical School
Piscataway, New Jersey

Pamela C. Champe, Ph.D.

Department of Biochemistry
University of Medicine and Dentistry of New Jersey–
Robert Wood Johnson Medical School
Piscataway, New Jersey

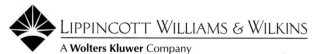

LIPPINCOTT WILLIAMS & WILKINS
A **Wolters Kluwer** Company
Philadelphia · Baltimore · New York · London
Buenos Aires · Hong Kong · Sydney · Tokyo

Kathy Fuller, Pharm.D., BCNSP
Department of Pharmaceutical and Administrative
Sciences
Nova Southeastern University
College of Pharmacy
Fort Lauderdale, Florida

David Gazze, Ph.D.
Department of Pharmaceutical and Administrative
Sciences
Nova Southeastern University
College of Pharmacy
Fort Lauderdale, Florida

Kathleen K. Graham, Pharm.D.
Children's Diagnostic & Treatment Center
and Nova Southeastern University
College of Pharmacy
Ft. Lauderdale, Florida

Katherine Heller, Pharm.D.
Palm Beach Atlantic University
Lloyd L. Gregory School of Pharmacy
West Palm Beach, Florida

Sharon S. Kelley, B.S., PMD
Associates in Emergency Medical Education, Inc.
Tampa, Florida

Deborah J. Larison, Pharm.D.
Lakeland Regional Medical Center
Lakeland, Florida

Ruth E. Nemire, Pharm.D.
Touro College of Pharmacy
New York, New York

Appu Rathinavelu, Ph.D.
Department of Pharmaceutical and Administrative
Sciences
Nova Southeastern University
College of Pharmacy
Fort Lauderdale, Florida

Jose Rey, Pharm.D.
Department of Pharmaceutical and Administrative
Sciences
Nova Southeastern University
College of Pharmacy
Fort Lauderdale, Florida

Devada Singh-Franco, Pharm.D.
Department of Pharmacy Practice
Nova Southeastern University
College of Pharmacy
Fort Lauderdale, Florida

Lester G. Sultatos, Ph.D.
Department of Pharmacology,
New Jersey Medical School
Newark, New Jersey

Sony Tuteja, Pharm.D., BCPS
Division of Clinical and Administrative Pharmacy
University of Iowa
College of Pharmacy
Iowa City, Iowa

Karen Whalen, Pharm.D., BCPS
Department of Pharmacy Practice
Nova Southeastern University
College of Pharmacy
Fort Lauderdale, Florida

Illustration and Graphic Design

Michael Cooper
Cooper Graphic
www.cooper247.com

Christopher T. Flatt
Department of Visual Communications
Ivy Tech Community College
Sellersburg, Indiana

Acknowledgments

We are grateful to the many friends and colleagues who generously contributed their time and effort to help us make this book as accurate and as useful as possible. The editors and production staff of Lippincott William & Wilkins were a constant source of encouragement and discipline. We particularly want to acknowledge the tremendously helpful, supportive, creative contributions of our editors, Betty Sun, Donna Balado, and Kelly Horvath, whose imagination and positive attitude helped us out of the valleys. Final editing and assembly of the book has been greatly enhanced through the efforts of Kathleen Scogna and Jennifer Glazer.

Acquisitions Editor: Donna Balado
Managing Editor: Kelly Horvath
Marketing Manager: Jennifer Kuklinski
Production Editor: Kevin Johnson
Designer: Holly McLaughlin

First edition, 1992
Second edition, 1997
Millennium edition, 2000
Third edition, 2006

To purchase additional copies of this book, call our customer service department at (800) 638-3030 or fax orders to (301) 223-2320. International customers should call (301) 223-2300.

To send comments to the authors, e-mail: **richardaharvey@gmail.com**

Visit Lippincott Williams & Wilkins on the Internet: http://www.LWW.com. Lippincott Williams & Wilkins customer service representatives are available from 8:30 am to 6:00 pm, EST.

Library of Congress Cataloging-in-Publication Data

Finkel, Richard, PharmD.
  Pharmacology / Richard Finkel, Michelle A. Clark, Luigi X. Cubeddu ; editors, Richard A. Harvey, Pamela C. Champe. -- 4th ed.
     p. ; cm. -- (Lippincott's illustrated reviews)
  Includes index.
  ISBN-13: 978-0-7817-7155-9
  ISBN-10: 0-7817-7155-2
1. Pharmacology--Outlines, syllabi, etc. 2. Pharmacology--Examinations, questions, etc. I. Clark, Michelle. II. Cubeddu, Luigi X. III. Title. IV. Series.
  [DNLM: 1. Pharmacology--Examination Questions. 2. Pharmacology--Outlines. QV 18.2 F499pa 2009]
  RM301.14.F56 2009
  615'.1076--dc22
                        2008011182

Contents

Lippincott's Illustrated Reviews: Pharmacology

4th edition

Pharmacokinetics

1

I. OVERVIEW

The goal of drug therapy is to prevent, cure, or control various disease states. To achieve this goal, adequate drug doses must be delivered to the target tissues so that therapeutic yet nontoxic levels are obtained. Pharmacokinetics examines the movement of a drug over time through the body. Pharmacological as well as toxicological actions of drugs are primarily related to the plasma concentrations of drugs. Thus, the clinician must recognize that the speed of onset of drug action, the intensity of the drug's effect, and the duration of drug action are controlled by four fundamental pathways of drug movement and modification in the body (Figure 1.1). First, drug absorption from the site of administration (Absorption) permits entry of the therapeutic agent (either directly or indirectly) into plasma. Second, the drug may then reversibly leave the bloodstream and distribute into the interstitial and intracellular fluids (Distribution). Third, the drug may be metabolized by the liver, kidney, or other tissues (Metabolism). Finally, the drug and its metabolites are removed from the body in urine, bile, or feces (Elimination). This chapter describes how knowledge of these four processes (Absorption, Distribution, Metabolism, and Elimination) influences the clinician's decision of the route of administration for a specific drug, the amount and frequency of each dose, and the dosing intervals.

II. ROUTES OF DRUG ADMINISTRATION

The route of administration is determined primarily by the properties of the drug (for example, water or lipid solubility, ionization, etc.) and by the therapeutic objectives (for example, the desirability of a rapid onset of action or the need for long-term administration or restriction to a local site). There are two major routes of drug administration, enteral and parenteral. (Figure 1.2 illustrates the subcategories of these routes as well as other methods of drug administration.)

A. Enteral

Enteral administration, or administering a drug by mouth, is the simplest and most common means of administering drugs. When the drug is given in the mouth, it may be swallowed, allowing oral delivery, or it may be placed under the tongue, facilitating direct absorption into the bloodstream.

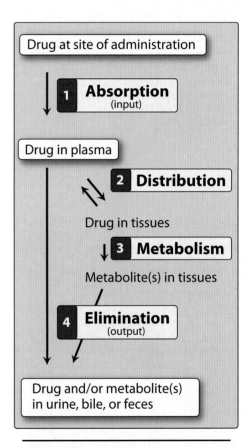

Figure 1.1
Schematic representation of drug absorption, distribution, metabolism, and elimination.

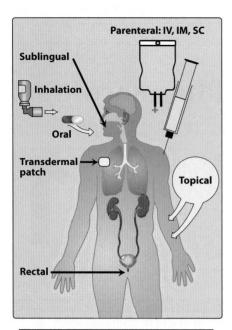

Figure 1.2
Commonly used routes of drug administration. IV = intravenous; IM = intramuscular; SC = subcutaneous.

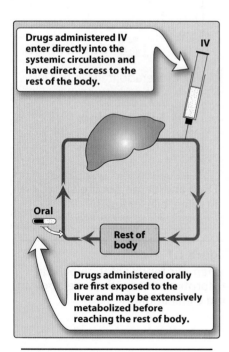

Figure 1.3
First-pass metabolism can occur with orally administered drugs. IV = intravenous.

1. Oral: Giving a drug by mouth provides many advantages to the patient; oral drugs are easily self-administered and limit the number of systemic infections that could complicate treatment. Moreover, toxicities or overdose by the oral route may be overcome with antidotes such as activated charcoal. On the other hand, the pathways involved in drug absorption are the most complicated, and the drug is exposed to harsh gastrointestinal (GI) environments that may limit its absorption. Some drugs are absorbed from the stomach; however, the duodenum is a major site of entry to the systemic circulation because of its larger absorptive surface. Most drugs absorbed from the GI tract enter the portal circulation and encounter the liver before they are distributed into the general circulation. These drugs undergo first-pass metabolism in the liver, where they may be extensively metabolized before entering the systemic circulation (Figure 1.3). [Note: First-pass metabolism by the intestine or liver limits the efficacy of many drugs when taken orally. For example, more than ninety percent of *nitroglycerin* is cleared during a single passage through the liver, which is the primary reason why this agent is not administered orally.] Drugs that exhibit high first-pass metabolism should be given in sufficient quantities to ensure that enough of the active drug reaches the target organ. Ingestion of drugs with food, or in combination with other drugs, can influence absorption. The presence of food in the stomach delays gastric emptying, so drugs that are destroyed by acid (for example, *penicillin*) become unavailable for absorption (see p. 364). [Note: Enteric coating of a drug protects it from the acidic environment; the coating may prevent gastric irritation, and depending on the formulation, the release of the drug may be prolonged, producing a sustained-release effect.]

2. Sublingual: Placement under the tongue allows a drug to diffuse into the capillary network and, therefore, to enter the systemic circulation directly. Administration of an agent, sublingually, has several advantages including rapid absorption, convenience of administration, low incidence of infection, avoidance of the harsh GI environment, and avoidance of first-pass metabolism.

B. Parenteral

The parenteral route introduces drugs directly across the body's barrier defenses into the systemic circulation or other vascular tissue. Parenteral administration is used for drugs that are poorly absorbed from the GI tract (for example *heparin*) and for agents that are unstable in the GI tract (for example, *insulin*). Parenteral administration is also used for treatment of unconscious patients and under circumstances that require a rapid onset of action. In addition, these routes have the highest bioavailability and are not subject to first-pass metabolism or harsh GI environments. Parenteral administration provides the most control over the actual dose of drug delivered to the body. However, these routes are irreversible and may cause pain, fear, and infections. The three major parenteral routes are intravascular (intravenous or intra-arterial), intramuscular, and subcutaneous (see Figure 1.2). Each route has advantages and drawbacks.

1. Intravenous (IV): Injection is the most common parenteral route. For drugs that are not absorbed orally, such as the neuromuscular blocker *atracurium*, there is often no other choice. With IV administration, the drug avoids the GI tract and therefore, first-pass metabolism by the liver. Intravenous delivery permits a rapid effect and a maximal degree of control over the circulating levels of the drug. However, unlike drugs in the GI tract, those that are injected cannot be recalled by strategies such as emesis or by binding to activated charcoal. Intravenous injection may inadvertently introduce bacteria through contamination at the site of injection. IV injection may also induce hemolysis or cause other adverse reactions by the too-rapid delivery of high concentrations of drug to the plasma and tissues. Therefore, the rate of infusion must be carefully controlled. Similar concerns apply to intra-arterially injected drugs.

2. **Intramuscular (IM):** Drugs administered IM can be aqueous solutions or specialized depot preparations—often a suspension of drug in a nonaqueous vehicle such as polyethylene glycol. Absorption of drugs in an aqueous solution is fast, whereas that from depot preparations is slow. As the vehicle diffuses out of the muscle, the drug precipitates at the site of injection. The drug then dissolves slowly, providing a sustained dose over an extended period of time. An example is sustained-release *haloperidol decanoate* (see p. 155), which slowly diffuses from the muscle and produces an extended neuroleptic effect.

3. **Subcutaneous (SC):** This route of administration, like that of IM injection, requires absorption and is somewhat slower than the IV route. Subcutaneous injection minimizes the risks associated with intravascular injection. [Note: Minute amounts of *epinephrine* are sometimes combined with a drug to restrict its area of action. *Epinephrine* acts as a local vasoconstrictor and decreases removal of a drug, such as *lidocaine*, from the site of administration.] Other examples of drugs utilizing SC administration include solids, such as a single rod containing the contraceptive *etonogestrel* that is implanted for long-term activity (see p. 306), and also programmable mechanical pumps that can be implanted to deliver *insulin* in diabetic patients.

C. Other

1. **Inhalation:** Inhalation provides the rapid delivery of a drug across the large surface area of the mucous membranes of the respiratory tract and pulmonary epithelium, producing an effect almost as rapidly as with IV injection. This route of administration is used for drugs that are gases (for example, some anesthetics) or those that can be dispersed in an aerosol. This route is particularly effective and convenient for patients with respiratory complaints (such as asthma, or chronic obstructive pulmonary disease) because the drug is delivered directly to the site of action and systemic side effects are minimized. Examples of drugs administered via this route include *albuterol*, and corticosteroids, such as *fluticasone*.

2. **Intranasal:** This route involves administration of drugs directly into the nose. Agents include nasal decongestants such as the anti-inflammatory corticosteroid *mometasone furoate*. *Desmopressin* is administered intranasally in the treatment of diabetes insipidus; salmon *calcitonin*, a peptide hormone used in the treatment of osteoporosis, is also available as a nasal spray. The abused drug, *cocaine*, is generally taken by intranasal sniffing.

3. **Intrathecal/intraventricular:** It is sometimes necessary to introduce drugs directly into the cerebrospinal fluid. For example, *amphotericin B* is used in treating cryptococcal meningitis (see p. 408).

4. **Topical:** Topical application is used when a local effect of the drug is desired. For example, *clotrimazole* is applied as a cream directly to the skin in the treatment of dermatophytosis, and *tropicamide* or *cyclopentolate* are instilled (administered drop by drop) directly into the eye to dilate the pupil and permit measurement of refractive errors.

5. **Transdermal:** This route of administration achieves systemic effects by application of drugs to the skin, usually via a transdermal patch. The rate of absorption can vary markedly, depending on the physical characteristics of the skin at the site of application. This route is most often used for the sustained delivery of drugs, such as the antianginal drug *nitroglycerin*, the antiemetic *scopolamine*, and the once-a-week contraceptive patch (Ortho Evra) that has an efficacy similar to oral birth control pills.

6. **Rectal:** Fifty percent of the drainage of the rectal region bypasses the portal circulation; thus, the biotransformation of drugs by the liver is minimized. Like the sublingual route of administration, the rectal route of administration has the additional advantage of preventing the destruction of the drug by intestinal enzymes or by low pH in the stomach. The rectal route is also useful if the drug induces vomiting when given orally, if the patient is already vomiting, or if the patient is unconscious. [Note: The rectal route is commonly used to administer antiemetic agents.] On the other hand, rectal absorption is often erratic and incomplete, and many drugs irritate the rectal mucosa.

III. ABSORPTION OF DRUGS

Absorption is the transfer of a drug from its site of administration to the bloodstream. The rate and efficiency of absorption depend on the route of administration. For IV delivery, absorption is complete; that is, the total dose of drug reaches the systemic circulation. Drug delivery by other routes may result in only partial absorption and, thus, lower bioavailability. For example, the oral route requires that a drug dissolve in the GI fluid and then penetrate the epithelial cells of the intestinal mucosa, yet disease states or the presence of food may affect this process.

A. Transport of a drug from the GI tract

Depending on their chemical properties, drugs may be absorbed from the GI tract by either passive diffusion or active transport.

1. **Passive diffusion:** The driving force for passive absorption of a drug is the concentration gradient across a membrane separating two body compartments; that is, the drug moves from a region of high concentration to one of lower concentration. Passive diffusion does not involve a carrier, is not saturable, and shows a low structural specificity. The vast majority of drugs gain access to the body by this mechanism. Lipid-soluble drugs readily move across most biologic membranes due to their solubility in the membrane bilayers. Water-soluble drugs penetrate the cell membrane through aque-

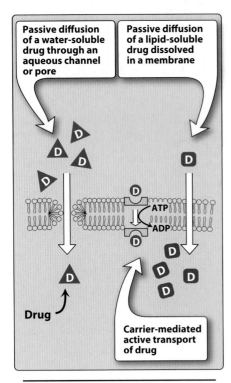

Passive diffusion of a water-soluble drug through an aqueous channel or pore

Passive diffusion of a lipid-soluble drug dissolved in a membrane

ATP

ADP

Drug

Carrier-mediated active transport of drug

Figure 1.4
Schematic representation of drugs crossing a cell membrane of an epithelial cell of the gastrointestinal tract. ATP = adenosine triphosphate; ADP = adenosine diphosphate.

ous channels or pores (Figure 1.4). Other agents can enter the cell through specialized transmembrane carrier proteins that facilitate the passage of large molecules. These carrier proteins undergo conformational changes allowing the passage of drugs or endogenous molecules into the interior of cells, moving them from an area of high concentration to an area of low concentration. This process is known as facilitated diffusion. This type of diffusion does not require energy, can be saturated, and may be inhibited.

2. **Active transport:** This mode of drug entry also involves specific carrier proteins that span the membrane. A few drugs that closely resemble the structure of naturally occurring metabolites are actively transported across cell membranes using these specific carrier proteins. Active transport is energy-dependent and is driven by the hydrolysis of adenosine triphosphate (see Figure 1.4). It is capable of moving drugs against a concentration gradient—that is, from a region of low drug concentration to one of higher drug concentration. The process shows saturation kinetics for the carrier, much in the same way that an enzyme-catalyzed reaction shows a maximal velocity at high substrate levels where all the active sites are filled with substrate.[1]

3. **Endocytosis and exocytosis:** This type of drug delivery transports drugs of exceptionally large size across the cell membrane. Endocytosis involves engulfment of a drug molecule by the cell membrane and transport into the cell by pinching off the drug-filled vesicle. Exocytosis is the reverse of endocytosis and is used by cells to secrete many substances by a similar vesicle formation process. For example, vitamin B_{12} is transported across the gut wall by endocytosis. Certain neurotransmitters (for example, norepinephrine) are stored in membrane-bound vesicles in the nerve terminal and are released by exocytosis.

B. Effect of pH on drug absorption

Most drugs are either weak acids or weak bases. Acidic drugs (HA) release an H^+ causing a charged anion (A^-) to form:[2]

$$HA \rightleftarrows H^+ + A^-$$

Weak bases (BH^+) can also release an H^+. However, the protonated form of basic drugs is usually charged, and loss of a proton produces the uncharged base (B):

$$BH^+ \rightleftarrows B + H^+$$

1. **Passage of an uncharged drug through a membrane:** A drug passes through membranes more readily if it is uncharged (Figure 1.5). Thus, for a weak acid, the uncharged HA can permeate through membranes, and A^- cannot. For a weak base, the uncharged form, B, penetrates through the cell membrane, but BH^+ does not. Therefore, the effective concentration of the permeable form of each drug at its absorption site is determined by the relative concentrations of the charged and uncharged forms. The ratio between the two forms is, in turn, determined by the pH at the site of absorption and by the

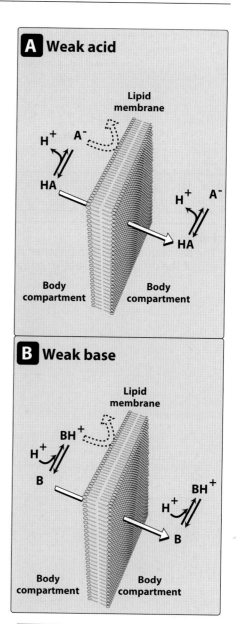

Figure 1.5
A. Diffusion of the non-ionized form of a weak acid through a lipid membrane. B. Diffusion of the non-ionized form of a weak base through a lipid membrane.

[1] See p. 58 in **Lippincott's Illustrated Reviews: Biochemistry** (4th ed.) for a discussion of enzyme kinetics.
[2] See p. 5 in **Lippincott's Illustrated Reviews: Biochemistry** (4th ed.) for a discussion of acid-base chemistry.

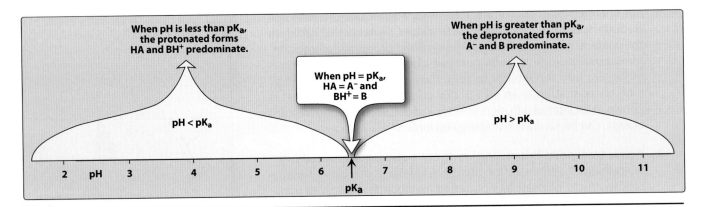

Figure 1.6
The distribution of a drug between its ionized and non-ionized forms depends on the ambient pH and pKa of the drug. For illustrative purposes, the drug has been assigned a pKa of 6.5.

strength of the weak acid or base, which is represented by the pK_a (Figure 1.6). [Note: The pK_a is a measure of the strength of the interaction of a compound with a proton. The lower the pK_a of a drug, the more acidic it is. Conversely, the higher the pK_a, the more basic is the drug.] Distribution equilibrium is achieved when the permeable form of a drug achieves an equal concentration in all body water spaces. [Note: Highly lipid-soluble drugs rapidly cross membranes and often enter tissues at a rate determined by blood flow.]

2. **Determination of how much drug will be found on either side of a membrane:** The relationship of pK_a and the ratio of acid-base concentrations to pH is expressed by the Henderson-Hasselbalch equation:[3]

$$pH = pK_a + \log \frac{[\text{nonprotonated species}]}{[\text{protonated species}]}$$

$$\text{For acids: } pH = pK_a + \log \frac{[A^-]}{[HA]}$$

$$\text{For bases: } pH = pK_a + \log \frac{[B]}{[BH^+]}$$

This equation is useful in determining how much drug will be found on either side of a membrane that separates two compartments that differ in pH—for example, stomach (pH 1.0–1.5) and blood plasma (pH 7.4). [Note: The lipid solubility of the non-ionized drug directly determines its rate of equilibration.]

C. **Physical factors influencing absorption**

1. **Blood flow to the absorption site:** Blood flow to the intestine is much greater than the flow to the stomach; thus, absorption from the intestine is favored over that from the stomach. [Note: Shock severely reduces blood flow to cutaneous tissues, thus minimizing the absorption from SC administration.]

 [3]See p. 6 in *Lippincott's Illustrated Reviews: Biochemistry* (4th ed.) for a discussion of the Henderson-Hasselbalch equation.

2. **Total surface area available for absorption:** Because the intestine has a surface rich in microvilli, it has a surface area about 1000-fold that of the stomach; thus, absorption of the drug across the intestine is more efficient.

3. **Contact time at the absorption surface:** If a drug moves through the GI tract very quickly, as in severe diarrhea, it is not well absorbed. Conversely, anything that delays the transport of the drug from the stomach to the intestine delays the rate of absorption of the drug. [Note: Parasympathetic input increases the rate of gastric emptying, whereas sympathetic input (prompted, for example, by exercise or stressful emotions), as well as anticholinergics (for example, *dicyclomine*), prolongs gastric emptying. Also, the presence of food in the stomach both dilutes the drug and slows gastric emptying. Therefore, a drug taken with a meal is generally absorbed more slowly.]

IV. BIOAVAILABILITY

Bioavailability is the fraction of administered drug that reaches the systemic circulation. Bioavailability is expressed as the fraction of administered drug that gains access to the systemic circulation in a chemically unchanged form. For example, if 100 mg of a drug are administered orally and 70 mg of this drug are absorbed unchanged, the bioavailability is 0.7 or seventy percent.

A. Determination of bioavailability

Bioavailability is determined by comparing plasma levels of a drug after a particular route of administration (for example, oral administration) with plasma drug levels achieved by IV injection—in which all of the agent rapidly enters the circulation. When the drug is given orally, only part of the administered dose appears in the plasma. By plotting plasma concentrations of the drug versus time, one can measure the area under the curve (AUC). This curve reflects the extent of absorption of the drug. [Note: By definition, this is 100 percent for drugs delivered IV.] Bioavailability of a drug administered orally is the ratio of the area calculated for oral administration compared with the area calculated for IV injection (Figure 1.7).

B. Factors that influence bioavailability

1. **First-pass hepatic metabolism:** When a drug is absorbed across the GI tract, it enters the portal circulation before entering the systemic circulation (see Figure 1.3). If the drug is rapidly metabolized by the liver, the amount of unchanged drug that gains access to the systemic circulation is decreased. Many drugs, such as *propranolol* or *lidocaine*, undergo significant biotransformation during a single passage through the liver.

2. **Solubility of the drug:** Very hydrophilic drugs are poorly absorbed because of their inability to cross the lipid-rich cell membranes. Paradoxically, drugs that are extremely hydrophobic are also poorly absorbed, because they are totally insoluble in aqueous body fluids and, therefore, cannot gain access to the surface of cells. For a drug to be readily absorbed, it must be largely hydrophobic, yet have some solubility in aqueous solutions. This is one reason why many drugs are weak acids or weak bases. There are some drugs that are highly lipid-soluble, and they are transported in the aqueous solutions of the body on carrier proteins such as albumin.

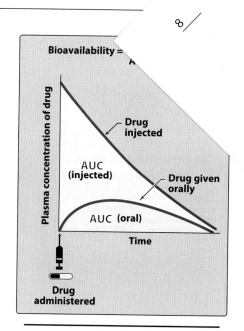

Figure 1.7
Determination of the bioavailability of a drug. (AUC = area under curve.)

3. **Chemical instability:** Some drugs, such as *penicillin G*, are unstable in the pH of the gastric contents. Others, such as *insulin*, are destroyed in the GI tract by degradative enzymes.

4. **Nature of the drug formulation:** Drug absorption may be altered by factors unrelated to the chemistry of the drug. For example, particle size, salt form, crystal polymorphism, enteric coatings and the presence of excipients (such as binders and dispersing agents) can influence the ease of dissolution and, therefore, alter the rate of absorption.

C. Bioequivalence

Two related drugs are bioequivalent if they show comparable bioavailability and similar times to achieve peak blood concentrations. Two related drugs with a significant difference in bioavailability are said to be bioinequivalent.

D. Therapeutic equivalence

Two similar drugs are therapeutically equivalent if they have comparable efficacy and safety. [Note: Clinical effectiveness often depends on both the maximum serum drug concentrations and on the time required (after administration) to reach peak concentration. Therefore, two drugs that are bioequivalent may not be therapeutically equivalent.]

V. DRUG DISTRIBUTION

Drug distribution is the process by which a drug reversibly leaves the bloodstream and enters the interstitium (extracellular fluid) and/or the cells of the tissues. The delivery of a drug from the plasma to the interstitium primarily depends on blood flow, capillary permeability, the degree of binding of the drug to plasma and tissue proteins, and the relative hydrophobicity of the drug.

A. Blood flow

The rate of blood flow to the tissue capillaries varies widely as a result of the unequal distribution of cardiac output to the various organs. Blood flow to the brain, liver, and kidney is greater than that to the skeletal muscles; adipose tissue has a still lower rate of blood flow. This differential blood flow partly explains the short duration of hypnosis produced by a bolus IV injection of *thiopental* (see p. 135). The high blood flow, together with the superior lipid solubility of *thiopental,* permit it to rapidly move into the central nervous system (CNS) and produce anesthesia. Slower distribution to skeletal muscle and adipose tissue lowers the plasma concentration sufficiently so that the higher concentrations within the CNS decrease, and consciousness is regained. Although this phenomenon occurs with all drugs to some extent, redistribution accounts for the extremely short duration of action of *thiopental* and compounds of similar chemical and pharmacologic properties.

B. Capillary permeability

Capillary permeability is determined by capillary structure and by the chemical nature of the drug.

1. **Capillary structure:** Capillary structure varies widely in terms of the fraction of the basement membrane that is exposed by slit junctions between endothelial cells. In the brain, the capillary structure is continuous, and there are no slit junctions (Figure 1.8). This contrasts

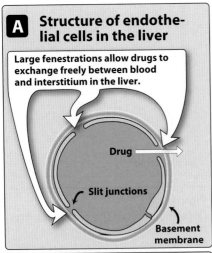

A Structure of endothelial cells in the liver

Large fenestrations allow drugs to exchange freely between blood and interstitium in the liver.

Drug

Slit junctions

Basement membrane

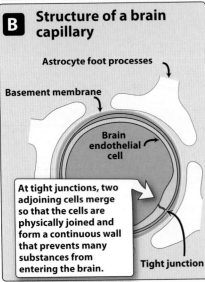

B Structure of a brain capillary

Astrocyte foot processes

Basement membrane

Brain endothelial cell

At tight junctions, two adjoining cells merge so that the cells are physically joined and form a continuous wall that prevents many substances from entering the brain.

Tight junction

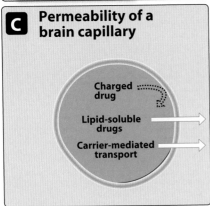

C Permeability of a brain capillary

Charged drug

Lipid-soluble drugs

Carrier-mediated transport

Figure 1.8
Cross-section of liver and brain capillaries.

with the liver and spleen, where a large part of the basement membrane is exposed due to large, discontinuous capillaries through which large plasma proteins can pass.

a. Blood-brain barrier: To enter the brain, drugs must pass through the endothelial cells of the capillaries of the CNS or be actively transported. For example, a specific transporter for the large neutral amino acid transporter carries *levodopa* into the brain. By contrast, lipid-soluble drugs readily penetrate into the CNS because they can dissolve in the membrane of the endothelial cells. Ionized or polar drugs generally fail to enter the CNS because they are unable to pass through the endothelial cells of the CNS, which have no slit junctions. These tightly juxtaposed cells form tight junctions that constitute the so-called blood-brain barrier.

2. Drug structure: The chemical nature of a drug strongly influences its ability to cross cell membranes. Hydrophobic drugs, which have a uniform distribution of electrons and no net charge, readily move across most biologic membranes. These drugs can dissolve in the lipid membranes and, therefore, permeate the entire cell's surface. The major factor influencing the hydrophobic drug's distribution is the blood flow to the area. By contrast, hydrophilic drugs, which have either a nonuniform distribution of electrons or a positive or negative charge, do not readily penetrate cell membranes, and therefore, must go through the slit junctions.

C. Binding of drugs to plasma proteins

Reversible binding to plasma proteins sequesters drugs in a nondiffusible form and slows their transfer out of the vascular compartment. Binding is relatively nonselective as to chemical structure and takes place at sites on the protein to which endogenous compounds, such as bilirubin, normally attach. Plasma albumin is the major drug-binding protein and may act as a drug reservoir; that is, as the concentration of the free drug decreases due to elimination by metabolism or excretion, the bound drug dissociates from the protein. This maintains the free-drug concentration as a constant fraction of the total drug in the plasma.

VI. VOLUME OF DISTRIBUTION

The volume of distribution is a hypothetical volume of fluid into which a drug is dispersed. Although the volume of distribution has no physiologic or physical basis, it is sometimes useful to compare the distribution of a drug with the volumes of the water compartments in the body (Figure 1.9).

A. Water compartments in the body

Once a drug enters the body, from whatever route of administration, it has the potential to distribute into any one of three functionally distinct compartments of body water or to become sequestered in a cellular site.

1. Plasma compartment: If a drug has a very large molecular weight or binds extensively to plasma proteins, it is too large to move out through the endothelial slit junctions of the capillaries and, thus, is effectively trapped within the plasma (vascular) compartment. As a consequence, the drug distributes in a volume (the plasma) that is about six percent of the body weight or, in a 70-kg individual, about 4 L of body fluid. *Heparin* (see p. 236) shows this type of distribution.

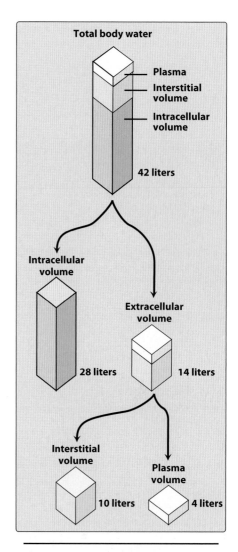

Figure 1.9
Relative size of various distribution volumes within a 70-kg individual.

2. **Extracellular fluid:** If a drug has a low molecular weight but is hydrophilic, it can move through the endothelial slit junctions of the capillaries into the interstitial fluid. However, hydrophilic drugs cannot move across the lipid membranes of cells to enter the water phase inside the cell. Therefore, these drugs distribute into a volume that is the sum of the plasma water and the interstitial fluid, which together constitute the extracellular fluid. This is about twenty percent of the body weight, or about 14 L in a 70-kg individual. Aminoglycoside antibiotics (see p. 377) show this type of distribution.

3. **Total body water:** If a drug has a low molecular weight and is hydrophobic, not only can it move into the interstitium through the slit junctions, but it can also move through the cell membranes into the intracellular fluid. The drug, therefore, distributes into a volume of about sixty percent of body weight, or about 42 L in a 70-kg individual. *Ethanol* exhibits this apparent volume of distribution (see below).

4. **Other sites:** In pregnancy, the fetus may take up drugs and thus increase the volume of distribution. Drugs that are extremely lipid-soluble, such as *thiopental* (see p. 135), may also have unusually high volumes of distribution.

B. Apparent volume of distribution

A drug rarely associates exclusively with only one of the water compartments of the body. Instead, the vast majority of drugs distribute into several compartments, often avidly binding cellular components—for example, lipids (abundant in adipocytes and cell membranes), proteins (abundant in plasma and within cells), or nucleic acids (abundant in the nuclei of cells). Therefore, the volume into which drugs distribute is called the apparent volume of distribution, or V_d. Another useful way to think of this constant is as the partition coefficient of a drug between the plasma and the rest of the body.

1. **Determination of V_d**

   a. **Distribution of drug in the absence of elimination:** The apparent volume into which a drug distributes, V_d, is determined by injection of a standard dose of drug, which is initially contained entirely in the vascular system. The agent may then move from the plasma into the interstitium and into cells, causing the plasma concentration to decrease with time. Assume for simplicity that the drug is not eliminated from the body; the drug then achieves a uniform concentration that is sustained with time (Figure 1.10). The concentration within the vascular compartment is the total amount of drug administered, divided by the volume into which it distributes, V_d:

   $$C = D/V_d \text{ or } V_d = D/C$$

   where C = the plasma concentration of the drug and D = the total amount of drug in the body. For example, if 25 mg of a drug (D = 25 mg) are administered and the plasma concentration is 1 mg/L, then V_d = 25 mg/1 mg/L = 25 L.

   b. **Distribution of drug when elimination is present:** In reality, drugs are eliminated from the body, and a plot of plasma

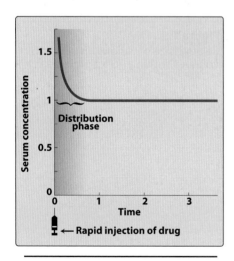

Figure 1.10
Drug concentrations in serum after a single injection of drug at time = 0. Assume that the drug distributes but is not eliminated.

concentration versus time shows two phases. The initial decrease in plasma concentration is due to a rapid distribution phase in which the drug is transferred from the plasma into the interstitium and the intracellular water. This is followed by a slower elimination phase during which the drug leaves the plasma compartment and is lost from the body—for example, by renal or biliary excretion or by hepatic biotransformation (Figure 1.11). The rate at which the drug is eliminated is usually proportional to the concentration of drug, C; that is, the rate for most drugs is first-order and shows a linear relationship with time—if $\ln C$ (where $\ln C$ is the natural log of C, rather than C) is plotted versus time (Figure 1.12). This is because the elimination processes are not saturated.

c. **Calculation of drug concentration if distribution is instantaneous:** Assume that the elimination process began at the time of injection and continued throughout the distribution phase. Then, the concentration of drug in the plasma, C, can be extrapolated back to time zero (the time of injection) to determine C_0, which is the concentration of drug that would have been achieved if the distribution phase had occurred instantly. For example, if 10 mg of drug are injected into a patient and the plasma concentration is extrapolated to time zero, the concentration is $C_0 = 1$ mg/L (from the graph shown in Figure 1.12), and then $V_d = 10$ mg/1 mg/L = 10 L.

d. **Uneven drug distribution between compartments:** The apparent volume of distribution assumes that the drug distributes uniformly, in a single compartment. However, most drugs distribute unevenly, in several compartments, and the volume of distribution does not describe a real, physical volume, but rather, reflects the ratio of drug in the extraplasmic spaces relative to the plasma space. Nonetheless, V_d is useful because it can be used to calculate the amount of drug needed to achieve a desired plasma concentration. For example, assume the arrhythmia of a cardiac patient is not well controlled due to inadequate plasma levels of *digitalis*. Suppose the concentration of the drug in the plasma is C_1 and the desired level of *digitalis* (known from clinical studies) is a higher concentration, C_2. The clinician needs to know how much additional drug should be administered to bring the circulating level of the drug from C_1 to C_2:

$(V_d)(C_1)$ = amount of drug initially in the body

$(V_d)(C_2)$ = amount of drug in the body needed to achieve the desired plasma concentration

The difference between the two values is the additional dosage needed, which equals $V_d(C_2 - C_1)$.

2. **Effect of a large V_d on the half-life of a drug**

A large V_d has an important influence on the half-life of a drug, because drug elimination depends on the amount of drug delivered to the liver or kidney (or other organs where metabolism occurs) per unit of time. Delivery of drug to the organs of elimination depends not only on blood flow, but also on the fraction of the drug in the plasma. If the V_d for a drug is large, most of the drug is in the extraplasmic space and is unavailable to the excretory organs. Therefore,

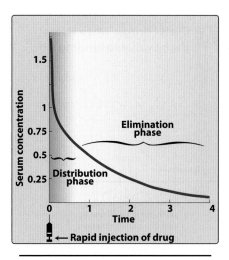

Figure 1.11
Drug concentrations in serum after a single injection of drug at time = 0. Assume that the drug distributes and is subsequently eliminated.

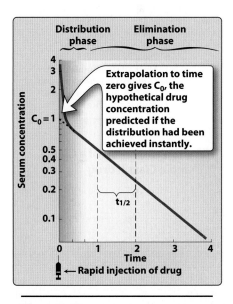

Figure 1.12
Drug concentrations in serum after a single injection of drug at time = 0. Data are plotted on a log scale.

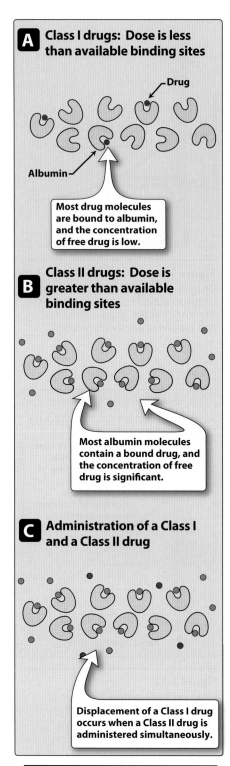

A **Class I drugs: Dose is less than available binding sites**

Albumin

Drug

> Most drug molecules are bound to albumin, and the concentration of free drug is low.

B **Class II drugs: Dose is greater than available binding sites**

> Most albumin molecules contain a bound drug, and the concentration of free drug is significant.

C **Administration of a Class I and a Class II drug**

> Displacement of a Class I drug occurs when a Class II drug is administered simultaneously.

Figure 1.13
Binding of Class I and Class II drugs to albumin when drugs are administered alone (A and B) or together (C).

any factor that increases the volume of distribution can lead to an increase in the half-life and extend the duration of action of the drug. [Note: An exceptionally large V_d indicates considerable sequestration of the drug in some organ or compartment.]

VII. BINDING OF DRUGS TO PLASMA PROTEINS

Drug molecules may bind to plasma proteins (usually albumin). Bound drugs are pharmacologically inactive; only the free, unbound drug can act on target sites in the tissues, elicit a biologic response, and be available to the processes of elimination. [Note: Hypoalbuminemia may alter the level of free drug.]

A. Binding capacity of albumin

The binding of drugs to albumin is reversible and may show low capacity (one drug molecule per albumin molecule) or high capacity (a number of drug molecules binding to a single albumin molecule). Drugs can also bind with varying affinities. Albumin has the strongest affinities for anionic drugs (weak acids) and hydrophobic drugs. Most hydrophilic drugs and neutral drugs do not bind to albumin. [Note: Many drugs are hydrophobic by design, because this property permits absorption after oral administration.]

B. Competition for binding between drugs

When two drugs are given, each with high affinity for albumin, they compete for the available binding sites. The drugs with high affinity for albumin can be divided into two classes, depending on whether the dose of drug (the amount of drug found in the body under conditions used clinically) is greater than, or less than, the binding capacity of albumin (quantified as the number of millimoles of albumin multiplied by the number of binding sites; Figure 1.13).

1. **Class I drugs:** If the dose of drug is less than the binding capacity of albumin, then the dose/capacity ratio is low. The binding sites are in excess of the available drug, and the bound-drug fraction is high. This is the case for Class I drugs, which include the majority of clinically useful agents.

2. **Class II drugs:** These drugs are given in doses that greatly exceed the number of albumin binding sites. The dose/capacity ratio is high, and a relatively high proportion of the drug exists in the free state, not bound to albumin.

3. **Clinical importance of drug displacement:** This assignment of drug classification assumes importance when a patient taking a Class I drug, such as *warfarin*, is given a Class II drug, such as a *sulfonamide antibiotic*. *Warfarin* is highly bound to albumin, and only a small fraction is free. This means that most of the drug is sequestered on albumin and is inert in terms of exerting pharmacologic actions. If a *sulfonamide* is administered, it displaces *warfarin* from albumin, leading to a rapid increase in the concentration of free *warfarin* in plasma, because almost 100 percent is now free, compared with the initial small percentage. [Note: The increase in *warfarin* concentration may lead to increased therapeutic effects, as well as increased toxic effects, such as bleeding.]

C. Relationship of drug displacement to V_d

The impact of drug displacement from albumin depends on both the V_d and the therapeutic index (see p. 33) of the drug. If the V_d is large, the drug displaced from the albumin distributes to the periphery, and the change in free-drug concentration in the plasma is not significant. If the V_d is small, the newly displaced drug does not move into the tissues as much, and the increase in free drug in the plasma is more profound. If the therapeutic index of the drug is small, this increase in drug concentration may have significant clinical consequences. [Note: Clinically, drug displacement from albumin is one of the most significant sources of drug interactions.]

VIII. DRUG METABOLISM

Drugs are most often eliminated by biotransformation and/or excretion into the urine or bile. The process of metabolism transforms lipophilic drugs into more polar readily excretable products. The liver is the major site for drug metabolism, but specific drugs may undergo biotransformation in other tissues, such as the kidney and the intestines. [Note: Some agents are initially administered as inactive compounds (pro-drugs) and must be metabolized to their active forms.]

A. Kinetics of metabolism

1. **First-order kinetics:** The metabolic transformation of drugs is catalyzed by enzymes, and most of the reactions obey Michaelis-Menten kinetics:[4]

$$v = \text{rate of drug metabolism} = \frac{V_{max}\,[C]}{K_m + [C]}$$

In most clinical situations, the concentration of the drug, [C], is much less than the Michaelis constant, K_m, and the Michaelis-Menten equation reduces to,

$$v = \text{rate of drug metabolism} = \frac{V_{max}\,[C]}{K_m}$$

That is, the rate of drug metabolism is directly proportional to the concentration of free drug, and first-order kinetics are observed (Figure 1.14). This means that a constant fraction of drug is metabolized per unit of time.

2. **Zero-order kinetics:** With a few drugs, such as *aspirin*, *ethanol*, and *phenytoin*, the doses are very large. Therefore [C] is much greater than K_m, and the velocity equation becomes

$$v = \text{rate of drug metabolism} = \frac{V_{max}\,[C]}{[C]} = V_{max}$$

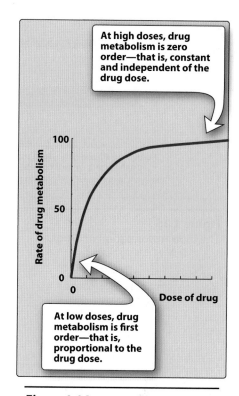

At high doses, drug metabolism is zero order—that is, constant and independent of the drug dose.

At low doses, drug metabolism is first order—that is, proportional to the drug dose.

Figure 1.14
Effect of drug dose on the rate of metabolism.

[4]See p. 58 in *Lippincott's Illustrated Reviews: Biochemistry* (4th ed.) for a discussion of Michaelis-Menten kinetics.

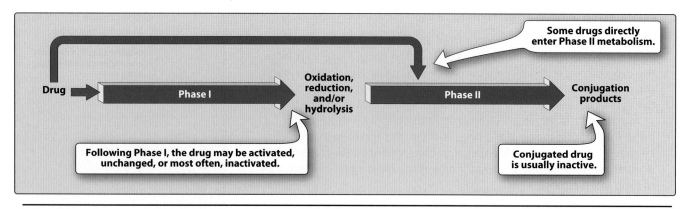

Figure 1.15
The biotransformation of drugs.

The enzyme is saturated by a high free-drug concentration, and the rate of metabolism remains constant over time. This is called zero-order kinetics (sometimes referred to clinically as nonlinear kinetics). A constant amount of drug is metabolized per unit of time.

B. Reactions of drug metabolism

The kidney cannot efficiently eliminate lipophilic drugs that readily cross cell membranes and are reabsorbed in the distal tubules. Therefore, lipid-soluble agents must first be metabolized in the liver using two general sets of reactions, called Phase I and Phase II (Figure 1.15).

1. **Phase I:** Phase I reactions function to convert lipophilic molecules into more polar molecules by introducing or unmasking a polar functional group, such as –OH or $-NH_2$. Phase I metabolism may increase, decrease, or leave unaltered the drug's pharmacologic activity.

   a. **Phase I reactions utilizing the P450 system:** The Phase I reactions most frequently involved in drug metabolism are catalyzed by the cytochrome P450 system (also called microsomal mixed function oxidase):

   $$Drug + O_2 + NADPH + H^+ \rightarrow Drug_{modified} + H_2O + NADP^+$$

   The oxidation proceeds by the drug binding to the oxidized form of cytochrome P450, and then oxygen is introduced through a reductive step, coupled to NADPH:cytochrome P450 oxidoreductase.

   b. **Summary of the P450 system:** The P450 system is important for the metabolism of many endogenous compounds (steroids, lipids, etc.) and for the biotransformation of exogenous substances (xenobiotics). Cytochrome P450, designated as CYP, is composed of many families of heme-containing isozymes that are located in most cells but are primarily found in the liver and GI tract. The family name is indicated by an arabic number followed by a capital letter for the subfamily (for example, CYP3A). Another number is added to indicate the specific isozyme (CYP3A4). There are many different genes, and many different enzymes; thus, the various P450s are known as isoforms. Six isozymes are responsible for the vast majority of P450-catalyzed reactions: CYP3A4, CYP2D6, CYP2C9/10, CYP2C19, CYP2E1, and CYP1A2. The percentages of currently available drugs that are substrates for these isozymes are

60, 25, 15, 15, 2, and 2 percent, respectively. [Note: An individual drug may be a substrate for more than one isozyme.] Considerable amounts of CYP3A4 are found in intestinal mucosa, accounting for first-pass metabolism of drugs such as *chlorpromazine* and *clonazepam*. As might be expected, these enzymes exhibit considerable genetic variability, which has implications for individual dosing regimens, and even more importantly, as determinants of therapeutic responsiveness and the risk of adverse events. CYP2D6, in particular, has been shown to exhibit genetic polymorphism.[5] Mutations result in very low capacities to metabolize substrates. Some individuals, for example, obtain no benefit from the opioid analgesic *codeine* because they lack the enzyme that O-demethylates and activates the drug. This reaction is CYP2D6-dependent. The frequency of this polymorphism is in part racially determined, with a prevalence of five to ten percent in European Caucasians as compared to less than two percent of Southeast Asians. Similar polymorphisms have been characterized for the CYP2C subfamily of isozymes. Although CYP3A4 exhibits a greater than ten-fold interindividual variability, no polymorphisms have been identified for this P450 isozyme.

c. **Inducers:** The cytochrome P450–dependent enzymes are an important target for pharmacokinetic drug interactions. One such interaction is the induction of selected CYP isozymes. Certain drugs, most notably *phenobarbital*, *rifampin*, and *carbamazepine*, are capable of increasing the synthesis of one or more CYP isozymes. This results in increased biotransformations of drugs and can lead to significant decreases in plasma concentrations of drugs metabolized by these CYP isozymes, as measured by AUC, with concurrent loss of pharmacologic effect. For example, *rifampin*, an antituberculosis drug (see p. 402), significantly decreases the plasma concentrations of human immunodeficiency virus (HIV) protease inhibitors,[6] diminishing their ability to suppress HIV virion maturation. Figure 1.16 lists some of the more important inducers for representative CYP isozymes. Consequences of increased drug metabolism include: 1) decreased plasma drug concentrations, 2) decreased drug activity if metabolite is inactive, 3) increased drug activity if metabolite is active, and 4) decreased therapeutic drug effect. In addition to drugs, natural substances and pollutants can also induce CYP isozymes. For example, polycyclic aromatic hydrocarbons (found as air pollutants) can induce CYP1A. This has implications for certain drugs; for example, *amitriptyline* and *warfarin* are metabolized by P4501A2. Polycyclic hydrocarbons induce P4501A2, which decreases the therapeutic concentrations of these agents.

d. **Inhibitors:** Inhibition of CYP isozyme activity is an important source of drug interactions that leads to serious adverse events. The most common form of inhibition is through competition for the same isozyme. Some drugs, however, are capable of inhibiting reactions for which they are not substrates (for

Isozyme: CYP2C9/10	
COMMON SUBSTRATES	**INDUCERS**
Warfarin *Phenytoin* *Ibuprofen* *Tolbutamide*	*Phenobarbital* *Rifampin*

Isozyme: CYP2D6	
COMMON SUBSTRATES	**INDUCERS**
Desipramine *Imipramine* *Haloperidol* *Propranolol*	

Isozyme: CYP3A4/5	
COMMON SUBSTRATES	**INDUCERS**
Carbamazepine *Cyclosporine* *Erythromycin* *Nifedipine* *Verapamil*	*Carbamazepine* *Dexamethasone* *Phenobarbital* *Phenytoin* *Rifampin*

Figure 1.16
Some representative P450 isozymes.

---

[5]See p. 473 in *Lippincott's Illustrated Reviews: Biochemistry* (4th ed.) for a discussion of genetic polymorphism.
[6]See p. 303 in *Lippincott's Illustrated Reviews: Microbiology* (2nd ed.) for a discussion of HIV protease inhibitors.

example, *ketoconazole*), leading to drug interactions. Numerous drugs have been shown to inhibit one or more of the CYP-dependent biotransformation pathways of *warfarin*. For example, *omeprazole* is a potent inhibitor of three of the CYP isozymes responsible for *warfarin* metabolism. If the two drugs are taken together, plasma concentrations of *warfarin* increase, which leads to greater inhibition of coagulation and risk of hemorrhage and other serious bleeding reactions. [Note: The more important CYP inhibitors are *erythromycin*, *ketoconazole*, and *ritonavir*, because they each inhibit several CYP isozymes.] *Cimetidine* blocks the metabolism of *theophylline*, *clozapine,* and *warfarin*. Natural substances such as grapefruit juice may inhibit drug metabolism. Grapefruit juice inhibits CYP3A4 and, thus, drugs such as *amlodipine*, *clarithromycin*, and *indinavir,* which are metabolized by this system, have greater amounts in the systemic circulation—leading to higher blood levels and the potential to increase therapeutic and/or toxic effects of the drugs. Inhibition of drug metabolism may lead to increased plasma levels over time with long-term medications, prolonged pharmacological drug effect, and increased drug-induced toxicities.

   e. Phase I reactions not involving the P450 system: These include amine oxidation (for example, oxidation of catecholamines or histamine), alcohol dehydrogenation (for example, ethanol oxidation), esterases (for example, metabolism of *pravastatin* in liver), and hydrolysis (for example, of *procaine*).

2. **Phase II:** This phase consists of conjugation reactions. If the metabolite from Phase I metabolism is sufficiently polar, it can be excreted by the kidneys. However, many Phase I metabolites are too lipophilic to be retained in the kidney tubules. A subsequent conjugation reaction with an endogenous substrate, such as glucuronic acid, sulfuric acid, acetic acid, or an amino acid, results in polar, usually more water-soluble compounds that are most often therapeutically inactive. A notable exception is *morphine-6-glucuronide*, which is more potent than *morphine*. Glucuronidation is the most common and the most important conjugation reaction. Neonates are deficient in this conjugating system, making them particularly vulnerable to drugs such as *chloramphenicol,* which is inactivated by the addition of glucuronic acid (see p. 382). [Note: Drugs already possessing an –OH, –HN$_2$, or –COOH group may enter Phase II directly and become conjugated without prior Phase I metabolism.] The highly polar drug conjugates may then be excreted by the kidney or bile.

3. **Reversal of order of the phases:** Not all drugs undergo Phase I and II reactions in that order. For example, *isoniazid* is first acetylated (a Phase II reaction) and then hydrolyzed to isonicotinic acid (a Phase I reaction).

IX. DRUG ELIMINATION

Removal of a drug from the body occurs via a number of routes, the most important being through the kidney into the urine. Other routes include the bile, intestine, lung, or milk in nursing mothers. A patient in renal failure may undergo extracorporeal dialysis, which removes small molecules such as drugs.

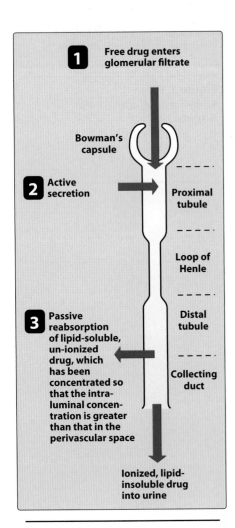

Figure 1.17
Drug elimination by the kidney.

A. Renal elimination of a drug

1. **Glomerular filtration:** Drugs enter the kidney through renal arteries, which divide to form a glomerular capillary plexus. Free drug (not bound to albumin) flows through the capillary slits into Bowman's space as part of the glomerular filtrate (Figure 1.17). The glomerular filtration rate (125 mL/min) is normally about twenty percent of the renal plasma flow (600 mL/min). [Note: Lipid solubility and pH do not influence the passage of drugs into the glomerular filtrate]

2. **Proximal tubular secretion:** Drugs that were not transferred into the glomerular filtrate leave the glomeruli through efferent arterioles, which divide to form a capillary plexus surrounding the nephric lumen in the proximal tubule. Secretion primarily occurs in the proximal tubules by two energy-requiring active transport (carrier-requiring) systems, one for anions (for example, deprotonated forms of weak acids) and one for cations (for example, protonated forms of weak bases). Each of these transport systems shows low specificity and can transport many compounds; thus, competition between drugs for these carriers can occur within each transport system (for example, see *probenecid*, p. 513). [Note: Premature infants and neonates have an incompletely developed tubular secretory mechanism and, thus, may retain certain drugs in the glomerular filtrate.]

3. **Distal tubular reabsorption:** As a drug moves toward the distal convoluted tubule, its concentration increases, and exceeds that of the perivascular space. The drug, if uncharged, may diffuse out of the nephric lumen, back into the systemic circulation. Manipulating the pH of the urine to increase the ionized form of the drug in the lumen may be used to minimize the amount of back-diffusion, and hence, increase the clearance of an undesirable drug. As a general rule, weak acids can be eliminated by alkalinization of the urine, whereas elimination of weak bases may be increased by acidification of the urine. This process is called "ion trapping." For example, a patient presenting with *phenobarbital* (weak acid) overdose can be given *bicarbonate*, which alkalinizes the urine and keeps the drug ionized, thereby decreasing its reabsorption. If overdose is with a weak base, such as *cocaine*, acidification of the urine with NH_4Cl leads to protonation of the drug and an increase in its clearance.

4. **Role of drug metabolism:** Most drugs are lipid soluble and without chemical modification would diffuse out of the kidney's tubular lumen when the drug concentration in the filtrate becomes greater than that in the perivascular space. To minimize this reabsorption, drugs are modified primarily in the liver into more polar substances using two types of reactions: Phase I reactions (see p. 14) that involve either the addition of hydroxyl groups or the removal of blocking groups from hydroxyl, carboxyl, or amino groups, and Phase II reactions (see p. 16) that use conjugation with sulfate, glycine, or glucuronic acid to increase drug polarity. The conjugates are ionized, and the charged molecules cannot back-diffuse out of the kidney lumen (Figure 1.18).

B. Quantitative aspects of renal drug elimination

Plasma clearance is expressed as the volume of plasma from which all drug appears to be removed in a given time—for example, as mL/min. Clearance equals the amount of renal plasma flow multiplied by the

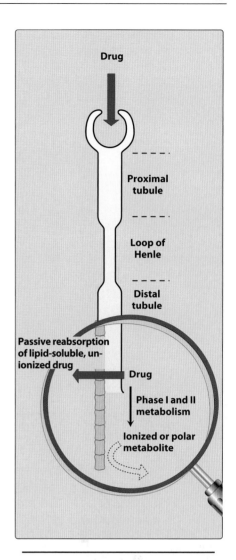

Figure 1.18
Effect of drug metabolism on reabsorption in the distal tubule.

extraction ratio, and because these are normally invariant over time, clearance is constant.

1. **Extraction ratio:** This ratio is the decline of drug concentration in the plasma from the arterial to the venous side of the kidney. The drugs enter the kidneys at concentration C_1 and exit the kidneys at concentration C_2. The extraction ratio = C_2/C_1.

2. **Excretion rate:** The excretion ratio is determined the equation:

$$\text{Excretion rate} = (\text{clearance})(\text{plasma concentration})$$

$$\text{mg/min} \qquad \text{mL/min} \qquad \text{mg/mL}$$

The elimination of a drug usually follows first-order kinetics, and the concentration of drug in plasma drops exponentially with time. This can be used to determine the half-life, $\frac{1}{2}$, of the drug (the time during which the concentration of a drug at equilibrium decreases from C to $\frac{1}{2}$C):

$$t_{1/2} = \ln 0.5/k_e = 0.693 \, V_d/CL$$

where k_e = the first-order rate constant for drug elimination from the total body and CL = clearance.

C. **Total body clearance**

The total body (systemic) clearance, CL_{total} or CL_t, is the sum of the clearances from the various drug-metabolizing and drug-eliminating organs. The kidney is often the major organ of excretion; however, the liver also contributes to drug loss through metabolism and/or excretion into the bile. A patient in renal failure may sometimes benefit from a drug that is excreted by this pathway, into the intestine and feces, rather than through the kidney. Some drugs may also be reabsorbed through the enterohepatic circulation, thus prolonging their half-life. Total clearance can be calculated by using the following equation:

$$CL_{total} = CL_{hepatic} + CL_{renal} + CL_{pulmonary} + CL_{other}$$

It is not possible to measure and sum these individual clearances. However, total clearance can be derived from the steady-state equation:

$$CL_{total} = k_e V_d$$

D. **Clinical situations resulting in changes in drug half-life**

When a patient has an abnormality that alters the half-life of a drug, adjustment in dosage is required. It is important to be able to predict in which patients a drug is likely to have a change in half-life. The half-life of a drug is increased by 1) diminished renal plasma flow or hepatic blood flow—for example, in cardiogenic shock, heart failure, or hemorrhage; 2) decreased extraction ratio—for example, as seen in renal disease; and 3) decreased metabolism—for example, when another drug inhibits its biotransformation or in hepatic insufficiency, as with cirrhosis. On the other hand, the half-life of a drug may decrease by 1) increased hepatic blood flow, 2) decreased protein binding, and 3) increased metabolism.

X. KINETICS OF CONTINUOUS ADMINISTRATION

The preceding discussion describes the pharmacokinetic processes that determine the rates of absorption, distribution, and elimination of a drug.

Pharmacokinetics also describes the quantitative, time-dependent changes of both the plasma drug concentration and the total amount of drug in the body, following the drug's administration by various routes, with the two most common being IV infusion and oral fixed-dose/fixed-time interval regimens (for example, "one tablet every 4 hours"). The interactions of the processes previously described determine the pharmacokinetics profile of a drug. The significance of identifying the pharmacokinetics of a drug lies not only in defining the factors that influence its levels and persistence in the body, but also in tailoring the therapeutic use of drugs that have a high toxic potential. [Note: The following discussion assumes that the administered drug distributes into a single body compartment. In actuality, most drugs equilibrate between two or three compartments and, thus, display complex kinetic behavior. However, the simpler model suffices to demonstrate the concepts.]

A. Kinetics of IV infusion

With continuous IV infusion, the rate of drug entry into the body is constant. In the majority of cases, the elimination of a drug is first order; that is, a constant fraction of the agent is cleared per unit of time. Therefore, the rate of drug exit from the body increases proportionately as the plasma concentration increases, and at every point in time, it is proportional to the plasma concentration of the drug.

1. **Steady-state drug levels in blood:** Following the initiation of an IV infusion, the plasma concentration of drug rises until the rate of drug eliminated from the body precisely balances the input rate. Thus, a steady-state is achieved in which the plasma concentration of drug remains constant. [Note: The rate of drug elimination from the body = $(CL_t)(C)$, where CL_t = total body clearance (see p. 18) and C = the plasma concentration of drug.] Two questions can be asked about achieving the steady-state. First, what is the relationship between the rate of drug infusion and the plasma concentration of drug achieved at the plateau, or steady state? Second, what length of time is required to reach the steady state drug concentration?

2. **Influence of the rate of drug infusion on the steady state:** A steady-state plasma concentration of a drug occurs when the rate of drug elimination is equal to the rate of administration (Figure 1.19), as described by the following equation:

$$C_{ss} = R_o/k_e V_d = R_o/CL_t$$

where C_{ss} = the steady-state concentration of the drug, R_o = the infusion rate (for example, mg/min), k_e is the first-order elimination rate constant, and V_d = the volume of distribution. Because k_e, CL_t, and V_d are constant for most drugs showing first-order kinetics, C_{ss} is directly proportional to R_o; that is, the steady-state plasma concentration is directly proportional to the infusion rate. For example, if the infusion rate is doubled, the plasma concentration ultimately achieved at the steady state is doubled (Figure 1.20). Furthermore, the steady-state concentration is inversely proportional to the clearance of the drug, CL_t. Thus, any factor that decreases clearance, such as liver or kidney disease, increases the steady-state concentration of an infused drug (assuming V_d remains constant). Factors that increase clearance of a drug, such as increased metabolism, decrease the steady-state concentrations of an infused drug.

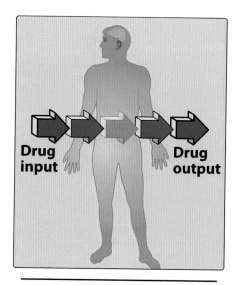

Figure 1.19
At steady state, input (rate of infusion) equals output (rate of elimination).

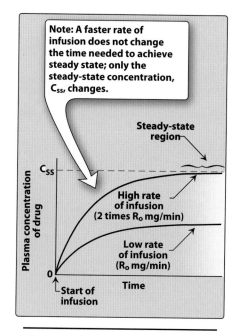

Note: A faster rate of infusion does not change the time needed to achieve steady state; only the steady-state concentration, C_{ss}, changes.

Steady-state region

C_{ss}

High rate of infusion (2 times R_o mg/min)

Low rate of infusion (R_o mg/min)

Plasma concentration of drug

Start of infusion

Time

Figure 1.20
Effect of infusion rate on the steady-state concentration of drug in the plasma. (R_o = rate of infusion of a drug.)

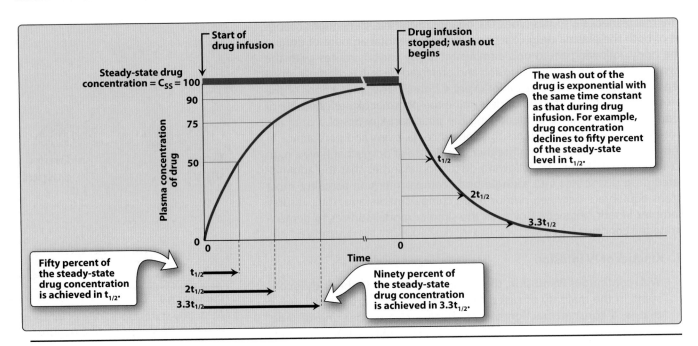

Figure 1.21
Rate of attainment of steady-state concentration of a drug in the plasma.

3. **Time required to reach the steady-state drug concentration:** The concentration of drug rises from zero at the start of the infusion to its ultimate steady-state level, C_{ss} (Figure 1.21). The fractional rate of approach to a steady state is achieved by a first-order process.

   a. **Exponential approach to steady state:** The rate constant for attainment of steady state is the rate constant for total body elimination of the drug, k_e. Thus, fifty percent of the final steady-state concentration of drug is observed after the time elapsed since the infusion, t, is equal to $t_{1/2}$, where $t_{1/2}$ (or half-life) is the time required for the drug concentration to change by fifty percent. Waiting another half-life allows the drug concentration to approach 75 percent of C_{ss} (see Figure 1.21). The drug concentration is ninety percent of the final steady-state concentration in 3.3 times $t_{1/2}$. For convenience, therefore, one can assume that a drug will reach steady-state in about four half-lives. The time required to reach a specific fraction of the steady-state is described by

   $$f = 1 - e^{-k_e t}$$

   where f = the fractional shift (for example, 0.9 if the time to reach ninety percent of the steady-state concentration was being calculated) and t = the time elapsed since the start of the infusion.

   b. **Effect of the rate of drug infusion:** The sole determinant of the rate that a drug approaches steady state is the $t_{1/2}$ or k_e, and this rate is influenced only by the factors that affect the half-life. The rate of approach to steady state is not affected by the rate of drug infusion. Although increasing the rate of infusion of a drug increases the rate at which any given concentration of drug in the plasma is achieved, it does not influence the time required to reach the ultimate steady-state concentration. This is because the steady-state concentration of drug rises directly with the infusion rate (see Figure 1.20).

c. Rate of drug decline when the infusion is stopped: When the infusion is stopped, the plasma concentration of a drug declines (washes out) to zero with the same time course observed in approaching the steady state (see Figure 1.21). This relationship is expressed as

$$C_t = C_0 - e^{-k_e t}$$

where C_t i = the plasma concentration at any time, C_0 = the starting plasma concentration, k_e = the first-order elimination rate constant, and t = the time elapsed.

d. Loading dose: A delay in achieving the desired plasma levels of drug may be clinically unacceptable. Therefore, a "loading dose" of drug can be injected as a single dose to achieve the desired plasma level rapidly, followed by an infusion to maintain the steady state (maintenance dose). In general, the loading dose can be calculated as

Loading dose = (V_d)(desired steady-state plasma concentration)

B. Kinetics of fixed-dose/fixed-time-interval regimens

Administration of a drug by fixed doses rather than by continuous infusion is often more convenient. However, fixed doses, given at fixed-time intervals, result in time-dependent fluctuations in the circulating level of drug.

1. Single IV injection: For simplicity, assume the injected drug rapidly distributes into a single compartment. Because the rate of elimination is usually first order in regard to drug concentration, the circulating level of drug decreases exponentially with time (Figure 1.22). [Note: The $t_{1/2}$ does not depend on the dose of drug administered.]

2. Multiple IV injections: When a drug is given repeatedly at regular intervals, the plasma concentration increases until a steady state is reached (Figure 1.23). Because most drugs are given at intervals shorter than five half-lives and are eliminated exponentially with time, some drug from the first dose remains in the body at the time that the second dose is administered, and some from the second dose remains at the time that the third dose is given, and so forth. Therefore, the drug accumulates until, within the dosing interval, the rate of drug loss (driven by an elevated plasma concentration) exactly balances the rate of drug administration—that is, until a steady state is achieved.

a. Effect of dosing frequency: The plasma concentration of a drug oscillates about a mean. Using smaller doses at shorter intervals reduces the amplitude of the swings in drug concentration. However, the steady-state concentration of the drug, and the rate at which the steady-state is approached, are not affected by the frequency of dosing.

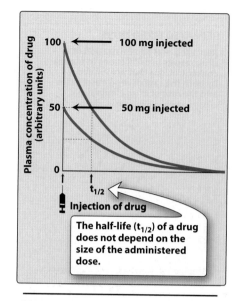

Figure 1.22
Effect of the dose of a single intra-venous injection of drug on plasma levels.

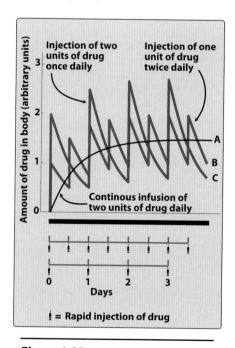

Figure 1.23
Predicted plasma concentrations of a drug given by infusion (A), twice-daily injection (B), or once-daily injection (C). Model assumes rapid mixing in a single body compartment and a half-life of twelve hours.

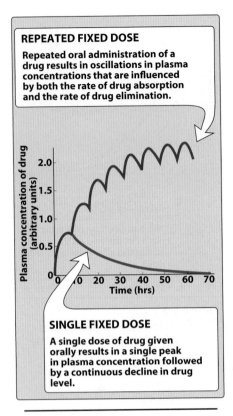

Figure 1.24
Predicted plasma concentrations of a drug given by repeated oral administrations.

b. Example of achievement of steady state using different dosage regimens: Curve B of Figure 1.23 shows the amount of drug in the body when 1 g of drug is administered IV to a patient and the dose is repeated at a time interval that corresponds to the half-life of the drug. At the end of the first dosing interval, 0.50 units of drug remain from the first dose when the second dose is administered. At the end of the second dosing interval, 0.75 units are present when the third dose is taken. The minimal amount of drug during the dosing interval progressively increases and approaches a value of 1.00 unit, whereas the maximal value immediately following drug administration progressively approaches 2.00 units. Therefore, at the steady state, 1.00 unit of drug is lost during the dosing interval, which is exactly matched by the rate at which the drug is administered—that is, the "rate in" equals the "rate out." As in the case for IV infusion, ninety percent of the steady-state value is achieved in 3.3 times $t_{1/2}$.

3. Orally administered drugs: Most drugs that are administered on an outpatient basis are taken orally on a fixed-dose/fixed-time-interval regimen—for example, a specific dose taken one, two, or three times daily. In contrast to IV injection, orally administered drugs may be absorbed slowly, and the plasma concentration of the drug is influenced by both the rate of absorption and the rate of drug elimination (Figure 1.24). This relationship can be expressed as:

$$C_{ss} = \frac{1}{(k_e)(V_d)} \frac{(D)(F)}{T}$$

where D = the dose, F = the fraction absorbed (bioavailability), T = dosage interval, C_{ss} = the steady-state concentration of the drug, k_e = the first-order rate constant for drug elimination from the total body, and V_d = the volume of distribution.

23

Study Questions

Choose the ONE best answer.

1.1 Which one of the following statements is correct?

A. Weak bases are absorbed efficiently across the epithelial cells of the stomach.
B. Coadministration of atropine speeds the absorption of a second drug.
C. Drugs showing a large V_d can be efficiently removed by dialysis of the plasma.
D. Stressful emotions can lead to a slowing of drug absorption.
E. If the V_d for a drug is small, most of the drug is in the extraplasmic space.

1.2 Which one of the following is true for a drug whose elimination from plasma shows first-order kinetics?

A. The half-life of the drug is proportional to the drug concentration in plasma.
B. The amount eliminated per unit of time is constant.
C. The rate of elimination is proportional to the plasma concentration.
D. Elimination involves a rate-limiting enzymic reaction operating at its maximal velocity (V_m).
E. A plot of drug concentration versus time is a straight line.

1.3 A patient is treated with drug A, which has a high affinity for albumin and is administered in amounts that do not exceed the binding capacity of albumin. A second drug, B, is added to the treatment regimen. Drug B also has a high affinity for albumin but is administered in amounts that are 100 times the binding capacity of albumin. Which of the following occurs after administration of drug B?

A. An increase in the tissue concentrations of drug A.
B. A decrease in the tissue concentrations of drug A.
C. A decrease in the volume of distribution of drug A.
D. A decrease in the half-life of drug A.
E. Addition of more drug A significantly alters the serum concentration of unbound drug B.

1.4 The addition of glucuronic acid to a drug:

A. Decreases its water solubility.
B. Usually leads to inactivation of the drug.
C. Is an example of a Phase I reaction.
D. Occurs at the same rate in adults and newborns.
E. Involves cytochrome P450.

Correct answer = D. Both exercise and strong emotions prompt sympathetic output, which slows gastric emptying. In the stomach, a weak base is primarily in the protonated, charged form, which does not readily cross the epithelial cells of the stomach. *Atropine* is a parasympathetic blocker and slows gastric emptying. This delays the rate of drug absorption. A large V_d indicates that most of the drug is outside the plasma space, and dialysis would not be effective. A small V_d indicates extensive binding to plasma proteins.

Correct answer = C. The direct proportionality between concentration and rate is the definition of first order. The half-life of a drug is a constant. For first-order reactions, the fraction of the drug eliminated, not the amount of drug, is constant. A rate limiting reaction operating at V_m would show zero-order kinetics. First-order kinetics shows a linear plot of log [drug concentration] versus time.

Correct answer = A. Drug A is largely bound to albumin, and only a small fraction is free. Most of drug A is sequestered on albumin and is inert in terms of exerting pharmacologic actions. If drug B is administered, it displaces drug A from albumin, leading to a rapid increase in the concentration of free drug A in plasma, because almost 100 percent is now free. Drug A moves out of the plasma into the interstitial water and the tissues. The V_d of drug A increases, providing less drug to the organ of excretion and prolonging the overall lifetime of the drug. Because drug B is already 100-fold in excess of its albumin-binding capacity, dislodging some of drug B from albumin does not significantly affect its serum concentration.

Correct answer = B. The addition of glucuronic acid prevents recognition of the drug by its receptor. Glucuronic acid is charged, and the drug conjugate has increased water solubility. Conjugation is a Phase II reaction. Neonates are deficient in the conjugating enzymes. Cytochrome P450 is involved in Phase I reactions.

1.5 Drugs showing zero-order kinetics of elimination:

A. Are more common than those showing first-order kinetics.
B. Decrease in concentration exponentially with time.
C. Have a half-life independent of dose.
D. Show a plot of drug concentration versus time that is linear.
E. Show a constant fraction of the drug eliminated per unit of time.

Correct answer = D. Drugs with zero-order kinetics of elimination show a linear relationship between drug concentration and time. In most clinical situations, the concentration of a drug is much less than the Michaelis constant (K_m). A decrease in drug concentration is linear with time. The half-life of the drug increases with dose. A constant amount of drug is eliminated per unit of time.

1.6 A drug, given as a 100-mg single dose, results in a peak plasma concentration of 20 μg/mL. The apparent volume of distribution is (assume a rapid distribution and negligible elimination prior to measuring the peak plasma level):

A. 0.5 L.
B. 1 L.
C. 2 L.
D. 5 L.
E. 10 L.

Correct answer = D. $V_d = D/C$, where D = the total amount of drug in the body, and C = the plasma concentration of drug. Thus, V_d = 100 mg/20 mg/mL = 100 mg/20 mg/L = 5 L.

1.7 A drug with a half-life of 12 hours is administered by continuous IV infusion. How long will it take for the drug to reach ninety percent of its final steady-state level?

A. 18 hours.
B. 24 hours.
C. 30 hours.
D. 40 hours.
E. 90 hours.

Correct answer = D. One approaches ninety percent of the final steady state in $(3.3)(t_{1/2}) = (3.3)(12) = {\sim}40$ hours.

1.8 Which of the following results in a doubling of the steady-state concentration of a drug?

A. Doubling the rate of infusion.
B. Maintaining the rate of infusion but doubling the loading dose.
C. Doubling the rate of infusion and doubling the concentration of the infused drug.
D. Tripling the rate of infusion.
E. Quadrupling the rate of infusion.

Correct answer = A. The steady-state concentration of a drug is directly proportional to the infusion rate. Increasing the loading dose provides a transient increase in drug level, but the steady-state level remains unchanged. Doubling both the rate of infusion and the concentration of infused drug leads to a four-fold increase in the steady-state drug concentration. Tripling or quadrupling the rate of infusion leads to either a three- or four-fold increase in the steady-state drug concentration.

Drug–Receptor Interactions and Pharmacodynamics

2

I. OVERVIEW

Most drugs exert their effects, both beneficial and harmful, by interacting with receptors—that is, specialized target macromolecules—present on the cell surface or intracellularly. Receptors bind drugs and initiate events leading to alterations in biochemical and/or biophysical activity of a cell, and consequently, the function of an organ (Figure 2.1). Drugs may interact with receptors in many different ways. Drugs may bind to enzymes (for example, inhibition of dihydrofolate reductase by *trimethoprim,* see p. 394), nucleic acids (for example, blockade of transcription by *dactinomycin,* see p. 469), or membrane receptors (for example, alteration of membrane permeability by *pilocarpine,* see p. 49). In each case, the formation of the drug–receptor complex leads to a biologic response. Most receptors are named to indicate the type of drug/chemical that interacts best with it; for example, the receptor for histamine is called a histamine receptor. Cells may have tens of thousands of receptors for certain ligands (drugs). Cells may also have different types of receptors, each of which is specific for a particular ligand. On the heart, for example, there are β receptors for norepinephrine, and muscarinic receptors for acetylcholine. These receptors dynamically interact to control vital functions of the heart. The magnitude of the response is proportional to the number of drug–receptor complexes:

Drug + Receptor ⇌ Drug–receptor complex → Biologic effect

This concept is closely related to the formation of complexes between enzyme and substrate,[1] or antigen and antibody; these interactions have many common features, perhaps the most noteworthy being specificity of the receptor for a given ligand. However, the receptor not only has the ability to recognize a ligand, but can also couple or transduce this binding into a response by causing a conformational change or a biochemical effect. Although much of this chapter will be centered on the interaction of drugs with specific receptors, it is important to be aware that not all drugs exert their effects by interacting with a receptor; for example, *antacids* chemically neutralize excess gastric acid, reducing the symptoms of "heartburn." This chapter introduces the study of pharmacodynamics—the influence of drug concentrations on the magnitude of the response. It deals with the interaction of drugs with receptors, the molecular consequences of these interactions, and their effects in the patient.

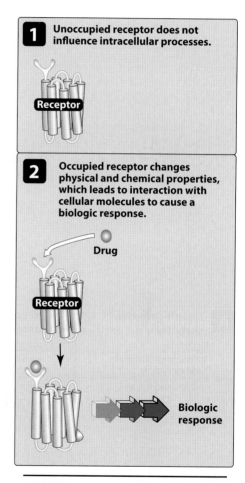

1 Unoccupied receptor does not influence intracellular processes.

Receptor

2 Occupied receptor changes physical and chemical properties, which leads to interaction with cellular molecules to cause a biologic response.

Drug

Receptor

Biologic response

Figure 2.1
The recognition of a drug by a receptor triggers a biologic response.

---

[1]See p. 58 in ***Lippincott's Illustrated Reviews: Biochemistry*** (4th ed.) for a discussion of the interaction of enzyme and substrate.

A fundamental principle of pharmacodynamics is that drugs only modify underlying biochemical and physiological processes; they do not create effects de novo.

II. CHEMISTRY OF RECEPTORS AND LIGANDS

Interaction of receptors with ligands involves the formation of chemical bonds, most commonly electrostatic and hydrogen bonds, as well as weak interactions involving van der Waals forces. These bonds are important in determining the selectivity of receptors, because the strength of these non-covalent bonds is related inversely to the distance between the interacting atoms. Therefore, the successful binding of a drug requires an exact fit of the ligand atoms with the complementary receptor atoms. The bonds are usually reversible, except for a handful of drugs (for example, the nonselective α-receptor blocker *phenoxybenzamine,* and acetylcholinesterase inhibitors in the organophosphate class) that covalently bond to their targets. The size, shape, and charge distribution of the drug molecule determines which of the myriad binding sites in the cells and tissues of the patient can interact with the ligand. The metaphor of the "lock and key" is a useful concept for understanding the interaction of receptors with their ligands. The precise fit required of the ligand echoes the characteristics of the "key," whereas the opening of the "lock" reflects the activation of the receptor. The interaction of the ligand with its receptor thus exhibits a high degree of specificity. The induced-fit model has largely replaced the lock-and-key concept as the preferred model describing the interaction of a receptor and a ligand. In the presence of a ligand, the receptor undergoes a conformational change to bind the ligand. The change in conformation of the receptor caused by binding of the agonist activates the receptor, which leads to the pharmacologic effect. This model suggests that the receptor is flexible, not rigid as implied by the lock-and-key model.

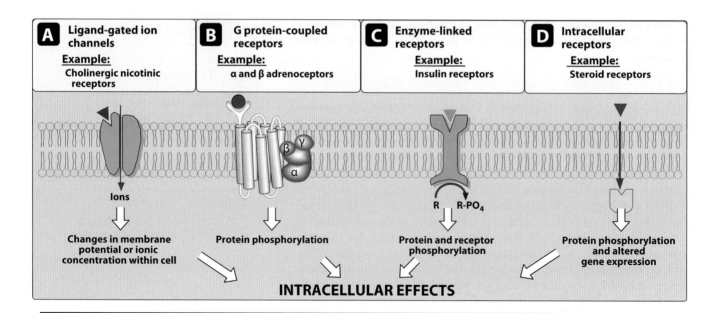

Figure 2.2
Transmembrane signaling mechanisms. A. Ligand binds to the extracellular domain of a ligand-gated channel. B. Ligand binds to a domain of a serpentine receptor, which is coupled to a G protein. C. Ligand binds to the extracellular domain of a receptor that activates a kinase enzyme. D. Lipid-soluble ligand diffuses across the membrane to interact with its intracellular receptor.

III. MAJOR RECEPTOR FAMILIES

Pharmacology defines a receptor as any biologic molecule to which a drug binds and produces a measurable response. Thus, enzymes and structural proteins can be considered to be pharmacologic receptors. However, the richest sources of therapeutically exploitable pharmacologic receptors are proteins that are responsible for transducing extracellular signals into intracellular responses. These receptors may be divided into four families: 1) ligand-gated ion channels, 2) G protein–coupled receptors, 3) enzyme-linked receptors, and 4) intracellular receptors (Figure 2.2). The type of receptor a ligand will interact with depends on the nature of the ligand. Hydrophobic ligands interact with receptors that are found on the cell surface (families 1, 2, and 3). In contrast, hydrophobic ligands can enter cells through the lipid bilayers of the cell membrane to interact with receptors found inside cells (family 4).

A. Ligand-gated ion channels

The first receptor family comprises ligand-gated ion channels that are responsible for regulation of the flow of ions across cell membranes (see Figure 2.2A). The activity of these channels is regulated by the binding of a ligand to the channel. Response to these receptors is very rapid, having durations of a few milliseconds. The nicotinic receptor and the γ-aminobutyric acid (GABA) receptor are important examples of ligand-gated receptors, the functions of which are modified by numerous drugs. Stimulation of the nicotinic receptor by *acetylcholine* results in sodium influx, generation of an action potential, and activation of contraction in skeletal muscle. *Benzodiazepines*, on the other hand, enhance the stimulation of the GABA receptor by GABA, resulting in increased chloride influx and hyperpolarization of the respective cell. Although not ligand-gated, ion channels, such as the voltage-gated sodium channel, are important drug receptors for several drug classes, including local anesthetics.

B. G protein–coupled receptors

A second family of receptors consists of G protein–coupled receptors. These receptors are comprised of a single peptide that has seven membrane-spanning regions, and these receptors are linked to a G protein (G_s and others) having three subunits, an α subunit that binds guanosine triphosphate (GTP) and a βγ subunit (Figure 2.3). Binding of the appropriate ligand to the extracellular region of the receptor activates the G protein so that GTP replaces guanosine diphosphate (GDP) on the α subunit. Dissociation of the G protein occurs, and both the α-GTP subunit and the βγ subunit subsequently interact with other cellular effectors, usually an enzyme or ion channel. These effectors then change the concentrations of second messengers that are responsible for further actions within the cell. Stimulation of these receptors results in responses that last several seconds to minutes.

1. **Second messengers:** These are essential in conducting and amplifying signals coming from G protein–coupled receptors. A common pathway turned on by G_s, and other types of G proteins, is the activation of adenylyl cyclase by α-GTP subunits, which results in the production of cyclic adenosine monophosphate (cAMP)—a second messenger that regulates protein phosphorylation. G proteins also activate phospholipase C, which is responsible for the generation of two other second messengers, namely inositol-1,4,5-trisphosphate and diacylglycerol. These effectors are responsible for the regulation of

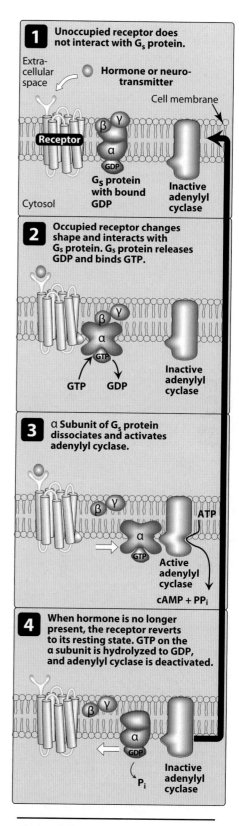

Figure 2.3
The recognition of chemical signals by G protein–coupled membrane receptors triggers an increase (or, less often, a decrease) in the activity of adenylyl cyclase.

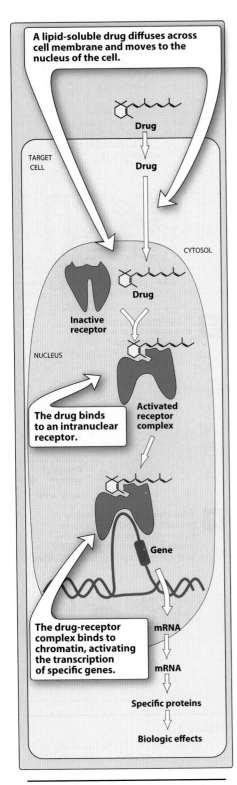

intracellular free calcium concentrations, and of other proteins as well. This family of receptors transduces signals derived from odors, light, and numerous neurotransmitters, including norepinephrine, dopamine, serotonin, and acetylcholine. G protein–coupled receptors also activate guanylyl cyclase, which converts (GTP) to cyclic guanosine monophosphate (cGMP), a fourth second messenger that stimulates cGMP-dependent protein kinase. cGMP signaling is important in only a few cells, for example, intestinal mucosa and vascular smooth muscle, where it causes relaxation of vascular smooth muscle cells. Some drugs such as *sildenafil* produce vasodilation by interfering with specific phosphodiesterases, the enzymes that metabolically break down cGMP.

C. Enzyme-linked receptors

A third major family of receptors consists of those having cytosolic enzyme activity as an integral component of their structure or function (see Figure 2.2C). Binding of a ligand to an extracellular domain activates or inhibits this cytosolic enzyme activity. Duration of responses to stimulation of these receptors is on the order of minutes to hours. The most common enzyme-linked receptors (epidermal growth factor, platelet-derived growth factor, *atrial natriuretic peptide, insulin,* and others) are those that have a tyrosine kinase activity as part of their structure. Typically, upon binding of the ligand to receptor subunits, the receptor undergoes conformational changes, converting from its inactive form to an active kinase form. The activated receptor autophosphorylates, and phosphorylates tyrosine residues on specific proteins. The addition of a phosphate group can substantially modify the three-dimensional structure of the target protein, thereby acting as a molecular switch. For example, when the peptide hormone *insulin* binds to two of its receptor subunits, their intrinsic tyrosine kinase activity causes autophosphorylation of the receptor itself. In turn, the phosphorylated receptor phosphorylates target molecules—insulin-receptor substrate peptides—that subsequently activate other important cellular signals such as IP3 and the mitogen-activated protein kinase system. This cascade of activations results in a multiplication of the initial signal, much like that which occurs with G protein–coupled receptors.

D. Intracellular receptors

The fourth family of receptors differs considerably from the other three in that the receptor is entirely intracellular and, therefore, the ligand must diffuse into the cell to interact with the receptor (Figure 2.4). This places constraints on the physical and chemical properties of the ligand in that it must have sufficient lipid solubility to be able to move across the target cell membrane. Because these receptor ligands are lipid soluble, they are transported in the body attached to plasma proteins, such as albumin. For example, *steroid hormones* exert their action on target cells via this receptor mechanism. Binding of the ligand with its receptor follows a general pattern in which the receptor becomes activated because of the dissociation of a small repressor peptide. The activated ligand–receptor complex migrates to the nucleus, where it binds to specific DNA sequences, resulting in the regulation of gene expression. The time course of activation and response of these receptors is much longer than that of the other mechanisms described above. Because gene expression and, therefore, protein synthesis is modified, cellular responses are not observed until considerable time has elapsed (thirty minutes or more), and the duration of the response (hours to days) is much greater than that of other receptor families.

Figure 2.4
Mechanism of intracellular receptors.

IV. SOME CHARACTERISTICS OF RECEPTORS

A. Spare receptors

A characteristic of many receptors, particularly those that respond to hormones, neurotransmitters, and peptides, is their ability to amplify signal duration and intensity. The family of G protein–linked receptors exemplifies many of the possible responses initiated by ligand binding to a receptor. Specifically, two phenomena account for the amplification of the ligand–receptor signal. First, a single ligand–receptor complex can interact with many G proteins, thereby multiplying the original signal many-fold. Second, the activated G proteins persist for a longer duration than the original ligand–receptor complex. The binding of *albuterol*, for example, may only exist for a few milliseconds, but the subsequent activated G proteins may last for hundreds of milliseconds. Further prolongation and amplification of the initial signal is mediated by the interaction between G proteins and their respective intracellular targets. Because of this amplification, only a fraction of the total receptors for a specific ligand may need to be occupied to elicit a maximal response from a cell. Systems that exhibit this behavior are said to have spare receptors. Spare receptors are exhibited by insulin receptors, where it has been estimated that 99 percent of the receptors are "spare." This constitutes an immense functional reserve that ensures adequate amounts of glucose enter the cell. On the other end of the scale is the human heart, in which about five to ten percent of the total β-adrenoceptors are spare. An important implication of this observation is that little functional reserve exists in the failing heart; most receptors must be occupied to obtain maximum contractility.

Figure 2.5
Desensitization of receptors.

B. Desensitization of receptors

Repeated or continuous administration of an agonist (or an antagonist) may lead to changes in the responsiveness of the receptor. To prevent potential damage to the cell (for example, high concentrations of calcium, initiating cell death), several mechanisms have evolved to protect a cell from excessive stimulation. When repeated administration of a drug results in a diminished effect, the phenomenon is called tachyphylaxis. The receptor becomes desensitized to the action of the drug (Figure 2.5). In this phenomenon, the receptors are still present on the cell surface but are unresponsive to the ligand. Other types of desensitization occur when receptors are down-regulated. Binding of the agonist results in molecular changes in the membrane-bound receptors, such that the receptor undergoes endocytosis and is sequestered from further agonist interaction. These receptors may be recycled to the cell surface, restoring sensitivity, or alternatively, may be further processed and degraded, decreasing the total number of receptors available. Some receptors, particularly voltage-gated channels, require a finite time (rest period) following stimulation before they can be activated again. During this recovery phase they are said to be "refractory" or "unresponsive."

→ action of arrestin

C. Importance of the receptor concept

It is important that we understand the roles and functions of receptors because most drugs interact with receptors that will determine selective therapeutic and toxic effects of the drug. Moreover, receptors largely determine the quantitative relations between dose of a drug and pharmacologic effect.

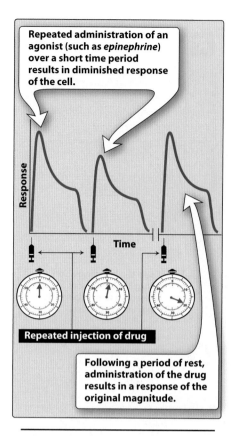

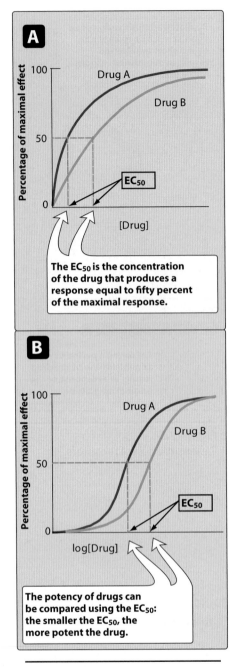

Figure 2.6
The effect of dose on the magnitude of pharmacologic response. Panel A is a linear graph. Panel B is a semilogarithmic plot of the same data. EC_{50} = drug dose that shows fifty percent of maximal response.

V. DOSE–RESPONSE RELATIONSHIPS

An agonist is defined as an agent that can bind to a receptor and elicit a biologic response. The magnitude of the drug effect depends on the drug concentration at the receptor site, which in turn is determined by the dose of drug administered and by factors characteristic of the drug pharmacokinetic profile, such as rate of absorption, distribution, and metabolism.

A. Graded dose–response relations

As the concentration of a drug increases, the magnitude of its pharmacologic effect also increases. The relationship between dose and response is a continuous one, and it can be mathematically described for many systems by application of the law of mass action, assuming the simplest model of drug binding:

$$[\text{Drug}] + [\text{Receptor}] \rightleftarrows [\text{Drug–receptor complex}]$$

The response is a graded effect, meaning that the response is continuous and gradual. This contrasts with a quantal response, which describes an all-or-nothing response. A graph of this relationship is known as a graded dose–response curve. Plotting the magnitude of the response against increasing doses of a drug produces a graph that has the general shape depicted in Figure 2.6A. The curve can be described as a rectangular hyperbola—a very familiar curve in biology, because it can be applied to diverse biological events, such as ligand binding, enzymatic activity, and responses to pharmacologic agents.

1. **Potency:** Two important properties of drugs can be determined by graded dose–response curves. The first is potency, a measure of the amount of drug necessary to produce an effect of a given magnitude. For a number of reasons, the concentration producing an effect that is fifty percent of the maximum is used to determine potency; it commonly designated as the EC_{50}. In Figure 2.6, the EC_{50} for Drugs A and B are indicated. Drug A is more potent than Drug B because less Drug A is needed to obtain 50 percent effect. Thus, therapeutic preparations of drugs will reflect the potency. For example, *candesartan* and *irbesartan* are angiotensin–receptor blockers that are used alone or in combination to treat hypertension. *Candesartan* is more potent than *irbesartan* because the dose range for *candesartan* is 4 to 32 mg, as compared to a dose range of 75 to 300 mg for *irbesartan*. *Candesartan* would be Drug A and *irbesartan* would be Drug B in Figure 2.6. An important contributing factor to the dimension of the EC_{50} is the affinity of the drug for the receptor. Semilogarithmic plots are often employed, because the range of doses (or concentrations) may span several orders of magnitude. By plotting the log of the concentration, the complete range of doses can be graphed. As shown in Figure 2.6B, the curves become sigmoidal in shape. It is also easier to visually estimate the EC_{50}.

2. **Efficacy [intrinsic activity]:** The second drug property that can be determined from graded dose–response plots is the efficacy of the drug. This is the ability of a drug to illicit a physiologic response when it interacts with a receptor. Efficacy is dependent on the number of drug–receptor complexes formed and the efficiency of the coupling of receptor activation to cellular responses. Analogous to the maximal velocity for enzyme-catalyzed reactions, the maximal response (E_{max}) or efficacy is more important than drug potency. A drug with

greater efficacy is more therapeutically beneficial than one that is more potent. Figure 2.7 shows the response to drugs of differing potency and efficacy.

3. **Drug–receptor binding:** The quantitative relationship between drug concentration and receptor occupancy applies the law of mass action to the kinetics of the binding of drug and receptor molecules. By making the assumption that the binding of one drug molecule does not alter the binding of subsequent molecules, we can mathematically express the relationship between the percentage (or fraction) of bound receptors and the drug concentration:

$$\frac{[DR]}{[R_t]} = \frac{[D]}{K_d + [D]} \qquad (1)$$

where [D] = the concentration of free drug; [DR] = the concentration of bound drug; [R_t] = the total concentration of receptors, and is equal to the sum of the concentrations of unbound (free) receptors and bound receptors and; K_d = [D][R]/[DR], and is the dissociation constant for the drug from the receptor. The value of K_d can be used to determine the affinity of a drug for its receptor. Affinity describes the strength of the interaction (binding) between a ligand and its receptor. The higher the K_d value, the weaker the interaction and the lower the affinity. The converse occurs when a drug has a low K_d. The binding of the ligand to the receptor is strong, and the affinity is high. Equation (1) defines a curve that has the shape of a rectangular hyperbola (Figure 2.8). As the concentration of free drug increases, the ratio of the concentrations of bound receptors to total receptors approaches unity. Doses are often plotted on a logarithmic scale, because the range from lowest to highest concentrations of doses often spans several orders of magnitude. It is important to note the similarity between these curves and those representing the relationship between dose and effect.

4. **Relationship of binding to effect:** The binding of the drug to its receptor initiates events that ultimately lead to a measurable biologic response. The mathematical model that describes drug concentration and receptor binding can be applied to dose (drug concentration) and response (or effect), providing the following assumptions are met: 1) The magnitude of the response is proportional to the amount of receptors bound or occupied, 2) the E_{max} occurs when all receptors are bound, and 3) binding of the drug to the receptor exhibits no cooperativity. In this case,

$$\frac{[E]}{[E_{max}]} = \frac{[D]}{K_d + [D]} \qquad (2)$$

where [E] = the effect of the drug at concentration [D] and [E_{max}] = the maximal effect of the drug.

5. **Agonists:** If a drug binds to a receptor and produces a biologic response that mimics the response to the endogenous ligand, it is known as an agonist. For example, *phenylephrine* is an agonist at α_1-adrenoceptors, because it produces effects that resemble the

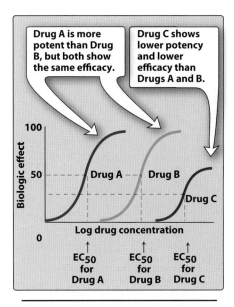

Figure 2.7
Typical dose-response curve for drugs showing differences in potency and efficacy. (EC_{50} = drug dose that shows fifty percent of maximal response.)

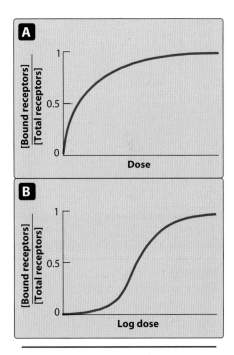

Figure 2.8
The effect of dose on the magnitude of drug binding.

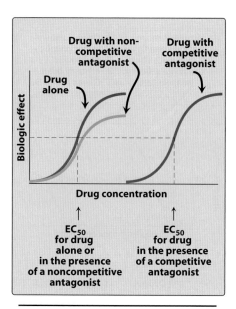

Figure 2.9
Effects of drug antagonists. EC_{50} = drug dose that shows fifty percent of maximal response.

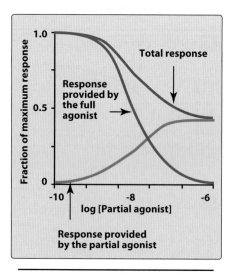

Figure 2.10
Effects of partial agonists.

action of the endogenous ligand, norepinephrine. Upon binding to α_1-adrenoceptors on the membranes of vascular smooth muscle, *phenylephrine* mobilizes intracellular Ca^{2+}, causing contraction of the actin and myosin filaments. The shortening of the muscle cells decreases the diameter of the arteriole, causing an increase in resistance to the flow of blood through the vessel. Blood pressure therefore rises to maintain the blood flow. As this brief description illustrates, an agonist may have many effects that can be measured, including actions on intracellular molecules, cells, tissues, and intact organisms. All of these actions are attributable to interaction of the drug molecule with the receptor molecule. In general, a full agonist has a strong affinity for its receptor and good efficacy.

6. **Antagonists:** Antagonists are drugs that decrease the actions of another drug or endogenous ligand. Antagonism may occur in several ways. Many antagonists act on the identical receptor macromolecule as the agonist. Antagonists, however, have no intrinsic activity and, therefore, produce no effect by themselves. Although antagonists have no intrinsic activity, they are able to bind avidly to target receptors because they possess strong affinity. If both the antagonist and the agonist bind to the same site on the receptor, they are said to be "competitive." For example, the antihypertensive drug *prazosin* competes with the endogenous ligand, norepinephrine, at α_1-adrenoceptors, decreasing vascular smooth muscle tone and reducing blood pressure. Plotting the effect of the competitive antagonist characteristically causes a shift of the agonist dose–response curve to the right. Competitive antagonists have no intrinsic activity. If the antagonist binds to a site other than where the agonist binds, the interaction is "noncompetitive" or "allosteric" (Figure 2.9). [Note: A drug may also act as a chemical antagonist by combining with another drug and rendering it inactive. For example, *protamine* ionically binds to *heparin*, rendering it inactive and antagonizing *heparin's* anticoagulant effect.]

7. **Functional antagonism:** An antagonist may act at a completely separate receptor, initiating effects that are functionally opposite those of the agonist. A classic example is the antagonism by *epinephrine* to histamine-induced bronchoconstriction. Histamine binds to H_1 histamine receptors on bronchial smooth muscle, causing contraction and narrowing of the bronchial tree. *Epinephrine* is an agonist at β_2-adrenoceptors on bronchial smooth muscle, which causes the muscles to actively relax. This functional antagonism is also known as "physiologic antagonism."

8. **Partial agonists:** Partial agonists have efficacies (intrinsic activities) greater than zero, but less than that of a full agonist. Even if all the receptors are occupied, partial agonists cannot produce an E_{max} of as great a magnitude as that of a full agonist. However, a partial agonist may have an affinity that is greater than, less than, or equivalent to that of a full agonist. A unique feature of these drugs is that, under appropriate conditions, a partial agonist may act as an antagonist of a full agonist. Consider what would happen to the E_{max} of an agonist in the presence of increasing concentrations of a partial agonist (Figure 2.10). As the number of receptors occupied by the partial agonist increases, the E_{max} would decrease until it reached the E_{max} of the partial agonist. This potential of partial agonists to act both agonistically and antagonistically may be therapeutically exploited.

For example, *aripiprazole*, an atypical neuroleptic agent, is a partial agonist at selected dopamine receptors. Dopaminergic pathways that were overactive would tend to be inhibited by the partial agonist, whereas pathways that were underactive may be stimulated. This might explain the ability of *aripiprazole* to improve many of the symptoms of schizophrenia, with a small risk of causing extrapyramidal adverse effects (see p. 33).

VI. QUANTAL DOSE–RESPONSE RELATIONSHIPS

Another important dose–response relationship is that of the influence of the magnitude of the dose on the proportion of a population that responds. These responses are known as quantal responses, because, for any individual, the effect either occurs or it does not. Even graded responses can be considered to be quantal if a predetermined level of the graded response is designated as the point at which a response occurs or not. For example, a quantal dose–response relationship can be determined in a population for the antihypertensive drug *atenolol*. A positive response is defined as at least a 5 mm Hg fall in diastolic blood pressure. Quantal dose–response curves are useful for determining doses to which most of the population responds.

A. Therapeutic index

The therapeutic index of a drug is the ratio of the dose that produces toxicity to the dose that produces a clinically desired or effective response in a population of individuals:

$$\text{Therapeutic index} = TD_{50}/ED_{50}$$

where TD_{50} = the drug dose that produces a toxic effect in half the population and ED_{50} = the drug dose that produces a therapeutic or desired response in half the population. The therapeutic index is a measure of a drug's safety, because a larger value indicates a wide margin between doses that are effective and doses that are toxic.

B. Determination of therapeutic index

The therapeutic index is determined by measuring the frequency of desired response, and toxic response, at various doses of drug. By convention, the doses that produce the therapeutic effect and the toxic effect in fifty percent of the population are employed; these are known as the ED_{50} and TD_{50}, respectively. In humans, the therapeutic index of a drug is determined using drug trials and accumulated clinical experience. These usually reveal a range of effective doses and a different (sometimes overlapping) range of toxic doses. Although some drugs have narrow therapeutic indices, they are routinely used to treat certain diseases. Several lethal diseases, such as Hodgkin's lymphoma, are treated with narrow therapeutic index drugs; however, treatment of a simple headache, for example, with a narrow therapeutic index drug would be unacceptable. Figure 2.11 shows the responses to *warfarin*, an oral anticoagulant with a narrow therapeutic index, and *penicillin*, an antimicrobial drug with a large therapeutic index.

1. **Warfarin (example of a drug with a small therapeutic index):** As the dose of *warfarin* is increased, a greater fraction of the patients respond (for this drug, the desired response is a two-fold increase in prothrombin time) until eventually, all patients respond (see Figure 2.11A). However, at higher doses of *warfarin*, a toxic response occurs,

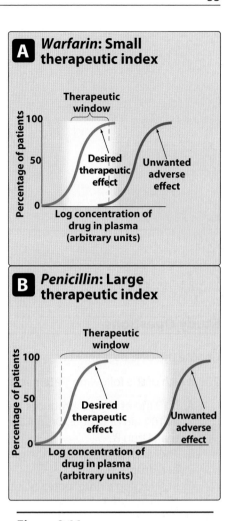

Figure 2.11
Cumulative percentage of patients responding to plasma levels of a drug.

namely a high degree of anticoagulation that results in hemorrhage. [Note: that when the therapeutic index is low, it is possible to have a range of concentrations where the effective and toxic responses overlap. That is, some patients hemorrhage, whereas others achieve the desired two-fold prolongation of prothrombin time. Variation in patient response is, therefore, most likely to occur with a drug showing a narrow therapeutic index, because the effective and toxic concentrations are similar. Agents with a low therapeutic index—that is, drugs for which dose is critically important—are those drugs for which bioavailability critically alters the therapeutic effects (see p. 7).

2. **Penicillin (example of a drug with a large therapeutic index):** For drugs such as *penicillin* (see Figure 2.11B), it is safe and common to give doses in excess (often about ten-fold excess) of that which is minimally required to achieve a desired response. In this case, bioavailability does not critically alter the therapeutic effects.

Study Questions

Choose the ONE best answer.

2.1. Which of the following statements is correct?

  A. If 10 mg of Drug A produces the same response as 100 mg of Drug B, Drug A is more efficacious than Drug B.
  B. The greater the efficacy, the greater the potency of a drug.
  C. In selecting a drug, potency is usually more important than efficacy.
  D. A competitive antagonist increases the ED_{50}.
  E. Variation in response to a drug among different individuals is most likely to occur with a drug showing a large therapeutic index.

Correct answer = D. In the presence of a competitive antagonist, a higher concentration of drug is required to elicit a given response. Efficacy and potency can vary independently, and the maximal response obtained is often more important than the amount of drug needed to achieve it. For example, in Choice A, no information is provided about the efficacy of Drug A, so all one can say is that Drug A is more potent than Drug B. Variability between patients in the pharmacokinetics of a drug is most important clinically when the effective and toxic doses are not very different, as is the case with a drug that shows a small therapeutic index.

2.2 Variation in the sensitivity of a population of individuals to increasing doses of a drug is best determined by which of the following?

  A. Efficacy.
  B. Potency.
  C. Therapeutic index.
  D. Graded dose–response curve.
  E. Quantal dose–response curve.

Correct answer = E. Only a quantal dose–response curve gives information about differences in the sensitivity of individuals to increasing doses of a drug.

2.3 Which of the following statements most accurately describes a system having spare receptors?

  A. The number of spare receptors determines the maximum effect.
  B. Spare receptors are sequestered in the cytosol.
  C. A single drug–receptor interaction results in many cellular response elements being activated.
  D. Spare receptors are active even in the absence of agonist.
  E. Agonist affinity for spare receptors is less than their affinity for nonspare receptors.

Correct answer = C. One explanation for the existence of spare receptors is that any one agonist–receptor binding event can lead to the activation of many more cellular response elements. Thus, only a small fraction of the total receptors need to be bound to elicit a maximum cellular response.

The Autonomic Nervous System

1

I. OVERVIEW

The autonomic nervous system, along with the endocrine system, coordinates the regulation and integration of bodily functions. The endocrine system sends signals to target tissues by varying the levels of blood-borne hormones. In contrast, the nervous system exerts its influence by the rapid transmission of electrical impulses over nerve fibers that terminate at effector cells, which specifically respond to the release of neuromediator substances. Drugs that produce their primary therapeutic effect by mimicking or altering the functions of the autonomic nervous system are called autonomic drugs and are discussed in the following four chapters. These autonomic agents act either by stimulating portions of the autonomic nervous system or by blocking the action of the autonomic nerves. This chapter outlines the fundamental physiology of the autonomic nervous system, and it describes the role of neurotransmitters in the communication between extracellular events and chemical changes within the cell.

II. INTRODUCTION TO THE NERVOUS SYSTEM

The nervous system is divided into two anatomical divisions: the central nervous system (CNS), which is composed of the brain and spinal cord, and the peripheral nervous system, which includes neurons located outside the brain and spinal cord—that is, any nerves that enter or leave the CNS (Figure 3.1). The peripheral nervous system is subdivided into the efferent division, the neurons of which carry signals away from the brain and spinal cord to the peripheral tissues, and the afferent division, the neurons of which bring information from the periphery to the CNS. Afferent neurons provide sensory input to modulate the function of the efferent division through reflex arcs, that is, neural pathways that mediate a reflex action.

A. Functional divisions within the nervous system

The efferent portion of the peripheral nervous system is further divided into two major functional subdivisions, the somatic and the autonomic systems (see Figure 3.1). The somatic efferent neurons are involved in the voluntary control of functions such as contraction of the skeletal muscles essential for locomotion. On the other hand, the autonomic system regulates the everyday requirements of vital bodily functions without the conscious participation of the mind. It is composed of efferent neurons that innervate smooth muscle of the vis-

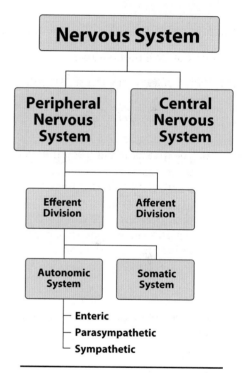

Figure 3.1
Organization of the nervous system.

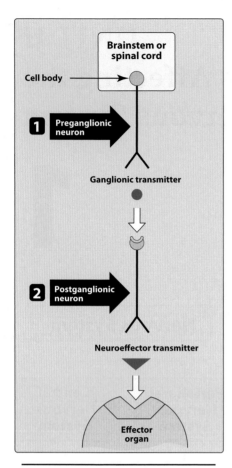

Figure 3.2
Efferent neurons of the
autonomic nervous system.

cera, cardiac muscle, vasculature, and the exocrine glands, thereby controlling digestion, cardiac output, blood flow, and glandular secretions.

B. Anatomy of the autonomic nervous system

1. **Efferent neurons:** The autonomic nervous system carries nerve impulses from the CNS to the effector organs by way of two types of efferent neurons (Figure 3.2). The first nerve cell is called a preganglionic neuron, and its cell body is located within the CNS. Preganglionic neurons emerge from the brainstem or spinal cord and make a synaptic connection in ganglia (an aggregation of nerve cell bodies located in the peripheral nervous system). These ganglia function as relay stations between a preganglionic neuron and a second nerve cell, the postganglionic neuron. The latter neuron has a cell body originating in the ganglion. It is generally nonmyelinated and terminates on effector organs, such as smooth muscles of the viscera, cardiac muscle, and the exocrine glands.

2. **Afferent neurons:** The afferent neurons (fibers) of the autonomic nervous system are important in the reflex regulation of this system (for example, by sensing pressure in the carotid sinus and aortic arch) and signaling the CNS to influence the efferent branch of the system to respond (see below).

3. **Sympathetic neurons:** The efferent autonomic nervous system is divided into the sympathetic and the parasympathetic nervous systems, as well as the enteric nervous system (see Figure 3.1). Anatomically, they originate in the CNS and emerge from two different spinal cord regions. The preganglionic neurons of the sympathetic system come from thoracic and lumbar regions of the spinal cord, and they synapse in two cord-like chains of ganglia that run in parallel on each side of the spinal cord. The preganglionic neurons are short in comparison to the postganglionic ones. Axons of the postganglionic neuron extend from these ganglia to the tissues that they innervate and regulate (see Chapter 6). [Note: The adrenal medulla, like the sympathetic ganglia, receives preganglionic fibers from the sympathetic system. Lacking axons, the adrenal medulla, in response to stimulation by the ganglionic neurotransmitter acetylcholine, influences other organs by secreting the hormone epinephrine, also known as adrenaline, and lesser amounts of norepinephrine into the blood.]

4. **Parasympathetic neurons:** The parasympathetic preganglionic fibers arise from the cranium (from cranial nerves III, VII, IX, and X) and from the sacral region of the spinal cord and synapse in ganglia near or on the effector organs. Thus, in contrast to the sympathetic system, the preganglionic fibers are long, and the postganglionic ones are short, with the ganglia close to or within the organ innervated. In most instances there is a one-to-one connection between the preganglionic and postganglionic neurons, enabling the discrete response of this division.

5. **Enteric neurons:** The enteric nervous system is the third division of the autonomic nervous system. It is a collection of nerve fibers that innervate the gastrointestinal tract, pancreas, and gallbladder, and it constitutes the "brain of the gut." This system functions independently of the CNS and controls the motility, exocrine and endocrine secretions, and microcirculation of the gastrointestinal tract. It is modulated by both the sympathetic and parasympathetic nervous systems.

C. Functions of the sympathetic nervous system

Although continually active to some degree (for example, in maintaining the tone of vascular beds), the sympathetic division has the property of adjusting in response to stressful situations, such as trauma, fear, hypoglycemia, cold, or exercise.

1. **Effects of stimulation of the sympathetic division:** The effect of sympathetic output is to increase heart rate and blood pressure, to mobilize energy stores of the body, and to increase blood flow to skeletal muscles and the heart while diverting flow from the skin and internal organs. Sympathetic stimulation results in dilation of the pupils and the bronchioles (Figure 3.3). It also affects gastrointestinal motility and the function of the bladder and sexual organs.

2. **Fight or flight response:** The changes experienced by the body during emergencies have been referred to as the "fight or flight" response (Figure 3.4). These reactions are triggered both by direct sympathetic activation of the effector organs and by stimulation of the adrenal medulla to release epinephrine and lesser amounts of norepinephrine. These hormones enter the bloodstream and promote responses in effector organs that contain adrenergic receptors (see Figure 6.6). The sympathetic nervous system tends to function as a unit, and it

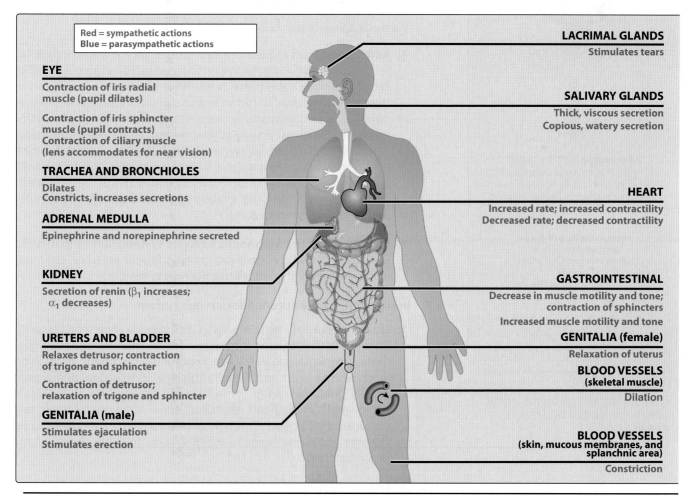

Figure 3.3
Action of sympathetic and parasympathetic nervous systems on effector organs.

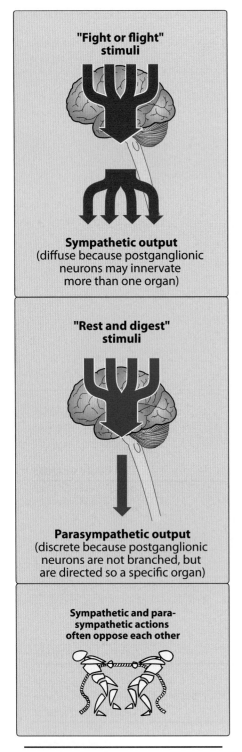

"Fight or flight" stimuli

Sympathetic output
(diffuse because postganglionic neurons may innervate more than one organ)

"Rest and digest" stimuli

Parasympathetic output
(discrete because postganglionic neurons are not branched, but are directed so a specific organ)

Sympathetic and parasympathetic actions often oppose each other

Figure 3.4
Sympathetic and parasympathetic actions are elicited by different stimuli.

often discharges as a complete system—for example, during severe exercise or in reactions to fear (see Figure 3.4). This system, with its diffuse distribution of postganglionic fibers, is involved in a wide array of physiologic activities, but it is not essential for life.

D. Functions of the parasympathetic nervous system

The parasympathetic division maintains essential bodily functions, such as digestive processes and elimination of wastes, and is required for life. It usually acts to oppose or balance the actions of the sympathetic division and is generally dominant over the sympathetic system in "rest and digest" situations. The parasympathetic system is not a functional entity as such, and it never discharges as a complete system. If it did, it would produce massive, undesirable, and unpleasant symptoms. Instead, discrete parasympathetic fibers are activated separately, and the system functions to affect specific organs, such as the stomach or eye.

E. Role of the CNS in autonomic control functions

Although the autonomic nervous system is a motor system, it does require sensory input from peripheral structures to provide information on the state of affairs in the body. This feedback is provided by streams of afferent impulses, originating in the viscera and other autonomically innervated structures, that travel to integrating centers in the CNS—that is, the hypothalamus, medulla oblongata, and spinal cord. These centers respond to the stimuli by sending out efferent reflex impulses via the autonomic nervous system (Figure 3.5).

1. **Reflex arcs:** Most of the afferent impulses are translated into reflex responses without involving consciousness. For example, a fall in blood pressure causes pressure-sensitive neurons (baroreceptors in the heart, vena cava, aortic arch, and carotid sinuses) to send fewer impulses to cardiovascular centers in the brain. This prompts a reflex response of increased sympathetic output to the heart and vasculature and decreased parasympathetic output to the heart, which results in a compensatory rise in blood pressure and tachycardia (see Figure 3.5). [Note: In each case, the reflex arcs of the autonomic nervsous system comprise a sensory (or afferent) arm, and a motor (or efferent, or effector) arm.]

2. **Emotions and the autonomic nervous system:** Stimuli that evoke feelings of strong emotion, such as rage, fear, or pleasure, can modify the activity of the autonomic nervous system.

F. Innervation by the autonomic nervous system

1. **Dual innervation:** Most organs in the body are innervated by both divisions of the autonomic nervous system. Thus, vagal parasympathetic innervation slows the heart rate, and sympathetic innervation increases the heart rate. Despite this dual innervation, one system usually predominates in controlling the activity of a given organ. For example, in the heart, the vagus nerve is the predominant factor for controlling rate. This type of antagonism is considered to be dynamic and is fine-tuned at any given time to control homeostatic organ functions.

2. **Organs receiving only sympathetic innervation:** Although most tissues receive dual innervation, some effector organs, such as the

adrenal medulla, kidney, pilomotor muscles, and sweat glands, receive innervation only from the sympathetic system. The control of blood pressure is also mainly a sympathetic activity, with essentially no participation by the parasympathetic system.

G. Somatic nervous system

The efferent somatic nervous system differs from the autonomic system in that a single myelinated motor neuron, originating in the CNS, travels directly to skeletal muscle without the mediation of ganglia. As noted earlier, the somatic nervous system is under voluntary control, whereas the autonomic is an involuntary system.

III. CHEMICAL SIGNALING BETWEEN CELLS

Neurotransmission in the autonomic nervous system is an example of the more general process of chemical signaling between cells. In addition to neurotransmission, other types of chemical signaling are the release of local mediators and the secretion of hormones.

A. Local mediators

Most cells in the body secrete chemicals that act locally—that is, on cells in their immediate environment. These chemical signals are rapidly destroyed or removed; therefore, they do not enter the blood and are not distributed throughout the body. Histamine (see p. 520) and the prostaglandins (see p. 519) are examples of local mediators.

B. Hormones

Specialized endocrine cells secrete hormones into the bloodstream, where they travel throughout the body exerting effects on broadly distributed target cells in the body. (Hormones are described in Chapters 23 through 26.)

C. Neurotransmitters

All neurons are distinct anatomic units, and no structural continuity exists between most neurons. Communication between nerve cells—and between nerve cells and effector organs—occurs through the release of specific chemical signals, called neurotransmitters, from the nerve terminals. This release is triggered by the arrival of the action potential at the nerve ending, leading to depolarization. Uptake of Ca^{2+} initiates fusion of the synaptic vesicles with the presynaptic membrane and release of their contents. The neurotransmitters rapidly diffuse across the synaptic cleft or space (synapse) between neurons and combine with specific receptors on the postsynaptic (target) cell (Figure 3.6 and see Chapter 2).

1. **Membrane receptors:** All neurotransmitters and most hormones and local mediators are too hydrophilic to penetrate the lipid bilayer of target-cell plasma membranes. Instead, their signal is mediated by binding to specific receptors on the cell surface of target organs. [Note: A receptor is defined as a recognition site for a substance. It has a binding specificity, and it is coupled to processes that eventually evoke a response. Most receptors are proteins. They need not be located in the membrane (see Chapter 2).]

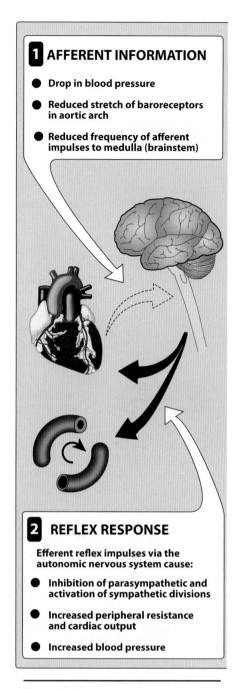

1 AFFERENT INFORMATION

- Drop in blood pressure
- Reduced stretch of baroreceptors in aortic arch
- Reduced frequency of afferent impulses to medulla (brainstem)

2 REFLEX RESPONSE

Efferent reflex impulses via the autonomic nervous system cause:

- Inhibition of parasympathetic and activation of sympathetic divisions
- Increased peripheral resistance and cardiac output
- Increased blood pressure

Figure 3.5
Baroreceptor reflex arc responds to a decrease in blood pressure.

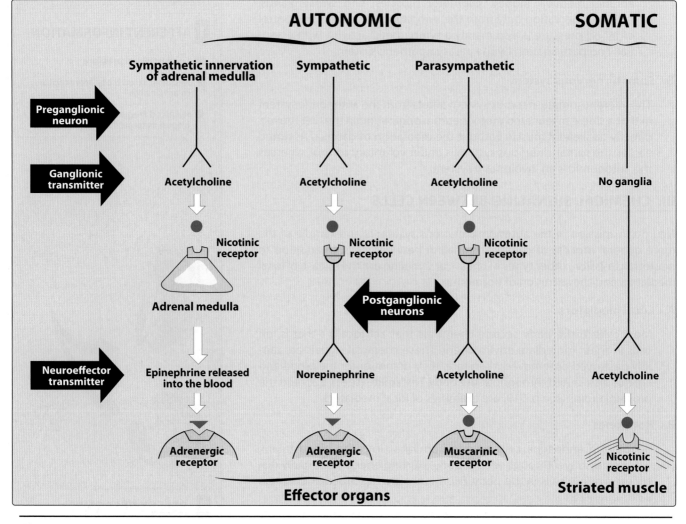

Figure 3.6
Summary of the neurotransmitters released and the types of receptors found within the autonomic and somatic nervous systems. [Note: This schematic diagram does not show that the parasympathetic ganglia are close to or on the surface of the effector organs and that the postganglionic fibers are usually shorter than the preganglionic fibers. By contrast, the ganglia of the sympathetic nervous system are close to the spinal cord. The postganglionic fibers are long, allowing extensive branching to innervate more than one organ system. This allows the sympathetic nervous system to discharge as a unit.]

2. **Types of neurotransmitters:** Although over fifty signal molecules in the nervous system have tentatively been identified, six signal compounds—norepinephrine (and the closely related epinephrine), acetylcholine, dopamine, serotonin, histamine, and γ-aminobutyric acid—are most commonly involved in the actions of therapeutically useful drugs. Each of these chemical signals binds to a specific family of receptors. Acetylcholine and norepinephrine are the primary chemical signals in the autonomic nervous system, whereas a wide variety of neurotransmitters function in the CNS. Not only are these neurotransmitters released on nerve stimulation, cotransmitters, such as adenosine, often accompany them and modulate the transmission process.

   a. **Acetylcholine:** The autonomic nerve fibers can be divided into two groups based on the chemical nature of the neurotransmitter released. If transmission is mediated by acetylcholine, the neuron is termed cholinergic (see Chapters 4 and 5). Acetylcholine mediates the transmission of nerve impulses across autonomic ganglia in both the sympathetic and parasympathetic nervous systems. It is the neurotransmitter at the adrenal medulla. Transmission from the autonomic postganglionic nerves to the effector organs in the parasympathetic system and a few sympathetic system organs also involves the release of acetylcholine. In the somatic nervous system, transmission at the neuromuscular junction (that is, between nerve fibers and voluntary muscles) is also cholinergic (see Figure 3.6).

b. Norepinephrine and epinephrine: When norepinephrine or epinephrine is the transmitter, the fiber is termed adrenergic (adrenaline being another name for epinephrine). In the sympathetic system, norepinephrine mediates the transmission of nerve impulses from autonomic postganglionic nerves to effector organs. Norepinephrine and adrenergic receptors are discussed in Chapters 6 and 7. A summary of the neuromediators released and the type of receptors within the peripheral nervous system is shown in Figure 3.6. [Note: A few sympathetic fibers, such as those involved in sweating, are cholinergic; for simplicity, they are not shown in the figure.]

IV. SECOND–MESSENGER SYSTEMS IN INTRACELLULAR RESPONSE

The binding of chemical signals to receptors activates enzymatic processes within the cell membrane that ultimately result in a cellular response, such as the phosphorylation of intracellular proteins or changes in the conductivity of ion channels. A neurotransmitter can be thought of as a signal and a receptor as a signal detector and transducer. Second-messenger molecules, produced in response to neurotransmitter binding to a receptor, translate the extracellular signal into a response that may be further propagated or amplified within the cell. Each component serves as a link in the communication between extracellular events and chemical changes within the cell (see Chapter 2).

A. Membrane receptors affecting ion permeability

Neurotransmitter receptors are membrane proteins that provide a binding site that recognizes and responds to neurotransmitter molecules. Some receptors, such as the postsynaptic receptors of nerve or muscle, are directly linked to membrane ion channels; thus, binding of the neurotransmitter occurs rapidly (within fractions of a millisecond) and directly affects ion permeability (Figure 3.7A). [Note: The effect of acetylcholine on these chemically gated ion channels is discussed on p. 27.]

B. Regulation involving second-messenger molecules

Many receptors are not directly coupled to ion gates. Rather, the receptor signals its recognition of a bound neurotransmitter by initiating a series of reactions, which ultimately results in a specific intracellular response. Second-messenger molecules—so named because they intervene between the original message (the neurotransmitter or hormone) and the ultimate effect on the cell—are part of the cascade of events that translates neurotransmitter binding into a cellular response, usually through the intervention of a G protein. The two most widely recognized

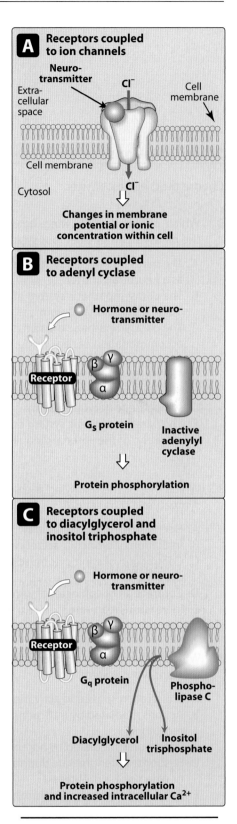

Figure 3.7
Three mechanisms whereby binding of a neurotransmitter leads to a cellular effect.

second messengers are the adenylyl cyclase system and the calcium/ phosphatidylinositol system (Figure 3.7B and C). [Note: G_s is the protein involved in the activation of adenylyl cyclase, and G_q is the subunit that activates phospholipase C to release diacylglycerol and inositol trisphosphate (see p. 27).]

Study Questions

Choose the ONE best answer.

3.1 Which one of the following statements concerning the parasympathetic nervous system is correct?

A. The parasympathetic system uses norepinephrine as a neurotransmitter.
B. The parasympathetic system often discharges as a single, functional system.
C. The parasympathetic division is involved in accommodation of near vision, movement of food, and urination.
D. The postganglionic fibers of the parasympathetic division are long compared to those of the sympathetic nervous system.
E. The parasympathetic system controls the secretion of the adrenal medulla.

Correct answer = C. The parasympathetic system maintains essential bodily functions, such as vision, movement of food, and urination. It uses acetylcholine, not norepinephrine, as a neurotransmitter, and it discharges as discrete fibers that are activated separately. The postganglionic fibers of the parasympathetic system are short compared to those of the sympathetic division. The adrenal medulla is under control of the sympathetic system.

3.2 Which one of the following is characteristic of parasympathetic stimulation?

A. Decrease in intestinal motility.
B. Inhibition of bronchial secretion.
C. Contraction of sphincter muscle in the iris of the eye (miosis).
D. Contraction of sphincter of urinary bladder.
E. Increase in heart rate.

Correct answer = C. The parasympathetic nervous system is essential in maintenance activities such as digestion and waste removal. Thus, one will see increase intestinal motility to facilitate peristalsis, relaxation of urinary bladder sphincters to cause urination and increase in bronchial secretions. Increase in heart rate is a function of the sympathetic nervous system.

3.3 Which of the following is characteristic of the sympathetic nervous system.

A A discrete response to activation
B. Actions mediated by muscarinic and nicotinic receptors
C. Effects only mediated by norepinephrine
D. Responses predominate during physical activity or when one is frightened
E. Subjected to voluntary control

Correct answer = D The sympathetic nervous system is activate by "fight or flight" stimuli. To achieve rapid activation of this system, the sympathetic nervous system often discharges as a unit. The receptors that mediate sympathetic nervous system effects on neuroeffector organs are alpha and beta receptors. Since the sympathetic nervous system is a division of the autonomic nervous system, it is not subject to voluntary control functioning below our conscious thoughts.

Cholinergic Agonists

4

I. OVERVIEW

Drugs affecting the autonomic nervous system are divided into two groups according to the type of neuron involved in their mechanism of action. The cholinergic drugs, which are described in this and the following chapter, act on receptors that are activated by acetylcholine. The second group—the adrenergic drugs (discussed in Chapters 6 and 7)—act on receptors that are stimulated by norepinephrine or epinephrine. Cholinergic and adrenergic drugs both act by either stimulating or blocking receptors of the autonomic nervous system. Figure 4.1 summarizes the cholinergic agonists discussed in this chapter.

II. THE CHOLINERGIC NEURON

The preganglionic fibers terminating in the adrenal medulla, the autonomic ganglia (both parasympathetic and sympathetic), and the postganglionic fibers of the parasympathetic division use acetylcholine as a neurotransmitter (Figure 4.2). In addition, cholinergic neurons innervate the muscles of the somatic system and also play an important role in the central nervous system (CNS). [Note: Patients with Alzheimer's disease have a significant loss of cholinergic neurons in the temporal lobe and entorhinal cortex. Most of the drugs available to treat the disease are acetylcholinesterase inhibitors (see p. 102).]

A. Neurotransmission at cholinergic neurons

Neurotransmission in cholinergic neurons involves sequential six steps. The first four—synthesis, storage, release, and binding of acetylcholine to a receptor—are followed by the fifth step, degradation of the neurotransmitter in the synaptic gap (that is, the space between the nerve endings and adjacent receptors located on nerves or effector organs), and the sixth step, the recycling of choline (Figure 4.3).

1. **Synthesis of acetylcholine:** Choline is transported from the extracellular fluid into the cytoplasm of the cholinergic neuron by an energy-dependent carrier system that cotransports sodium and that can be inhibited by the drug *hemicholinium*. [Note: Choline has a quaternary nitrogen and carries a permanent positive charge, and thus, cannot diffuse through the membrane.] The uptake of choline is the rate-limiting step in acetylcholine synthesis. Choline acetyltransferase catalyzes the reaction of choline with acetyl coenzyme A (CoA) to form acetylcholine—an ester—in the cytosol. Acetyl CoA is derived from the mitochondria and is produced by the Krebs cycle and fatty acid oxidation.

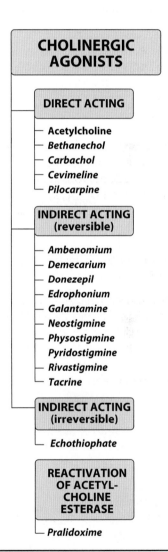

Figure 4.1
Summary of cholinergic agonists.

2. **Storage of acetylcholine in vesicles:** The acetylcholine is packaged into presynaptic vesicles by an active transport process coupled to the efflux of protons. The mature vesicle contains not only acetylcholine but also adenosine triphosphate (ATP) and proteoglycan. [Note: ATP has been suggested to be a cotransmitter acting at prejunctional purinergic receptors to inhibit the release of acetylcholine or norepinephrine.] Cotransmission from autonomic neurons is the rule rather than the exception. This means that most synaptic vesicles will contain the primary neurotransmitter, here acetylcholine, as well as a cotransmitter that will increase or decrease the effect of the primary neurotransmitter. The neurotransmitters in vesicles will appear as bead-like structures, known as varicosities, along the nerve terminal of the presynaptic neuron.

3. **Release of acetylcholine:** When an action potential propagated by the action of voltage-sensitive sodium channels arrives at a nerve ending, voltage-sensitive calcium channels on the presynaptic membrane open, causing an increase in the concentration of intracellular calcium. Elevated calcium levels promote the fusion of synaptic vesicles with the cell membrane and release of their contents into the synaptic space. This release can be blocked by botulinum toxin. In

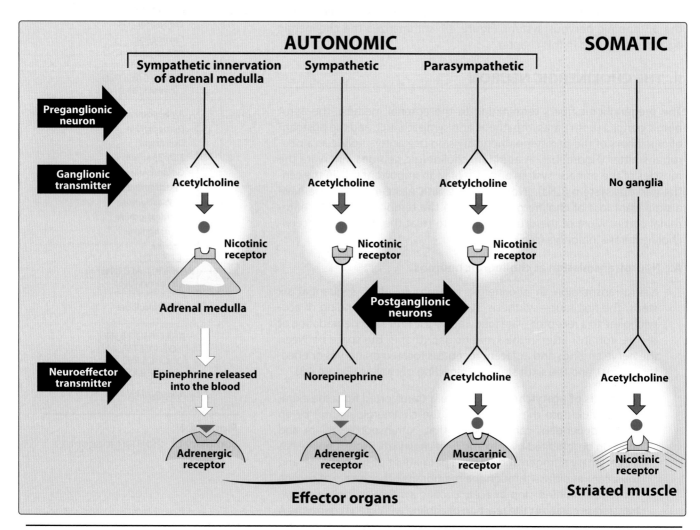

Figure 4.2
Sites of actions of cholinergic agonists in the autonomic and somatic nervous systems.

contrast, the toxin in black widow spider venom causes all the acetylcholine stored in synaptic vesicles to empty into the synaptic gap.

4. **Binding to the receptor:** Acetylcholine released from the synaptic vesicles diffuses across the synaptic space, and it binds to either of two postsynaptic receptors on the target cell or to presynaptic receptors in the membrane of the neuron that released the acetylcholine. The postsynaptic cholinergic receptors on the surface of the effector organs are divided into two classes—muscarinic and nicotinic. (see Figure 4.2 and p. 46). Binding to a receptor leads to a biologic response within the cell, such as the initiation of a nerve impulse in a postganglionic fiber or activation of specific enzymes in effector cells as mediated by second-messenger molecules (see p. 27 and below).

5. **Degradation of acetylcholine:** The signal at the postjunctional effector site is rapidly terminated, because acetylcholinesterase cleaves acetylcholine to choline and acetate in the synaptic cleft (see Figure 4.3). [Note: Butyrylcholinesterase, sometimes called pseudo-

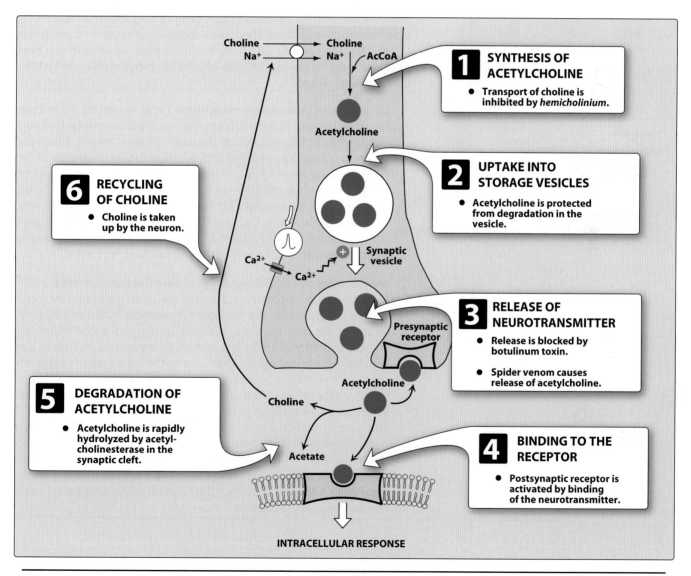

Figure 4.3
Synthesis and release of acetylcholine from the cholinergic neuron. AcCoA = acetyl coenzyme A.

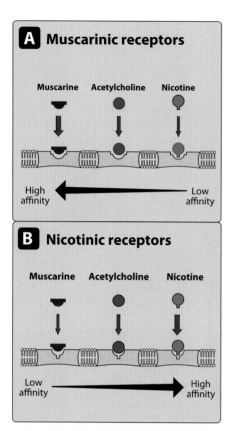

Figure 4.4
Types of cholinergic receptors.

cholinesterase, is found in the plasma, but it does not play a significant role in termination of acetylcholine's effect in the synapse.]

6. **Recycling of choline:** Choline may be recaptured by a sodium-coupled, high-affinity uptake system that transports the molecule back into the neuron, where it is acetylated into acetylcholine that is stored until released by a subsequent action potential.

III. CHOLINERGIC RECEPTORS (CHOLINOCEPTORS)

Two families of cholinoceptors, designated muscarinic and nicotinic receptors, can be distinguished from each other on the basis of their different affinities for agents that mimic the action of acetylcholine (cholinomimetic agents or parasympathomimetics).

A. Muscarinic receptors

These receptors, in addition to binding acetylcholine, also recognize muscarine, an alkaloid that is present in certain poisonous mushrooms. By contrast, the muscarinic receptors show only a weak affinity for nicotine (Figure 4.4A). Binding studies and specific inhibitors, as well as cDNA characterization, have distinguished five subclasses of muscarinic receptors: M_1, M_2, M_3, M_4, and M_5. Although five muscarinic receptors have been identified by gene cloning, only M_1, M_2 and M_3, receptors have been functionally characterized.

1. **Locations of muscarinic receptors:** These receptors have been found on ganglia of the peripheral nervous system and on the autonomic effector organs, such as the heart, smooth muscle, brain, and exocrine glands (see Figure 3.3, p. 37). Specifically, although all five subtypes have been found on neurons, M_1 receptors are also found on gastric parietal cells, M_2 receptors on cardiac cells and smooth muscle, and M_3 receptors on the bladder, exocrine glands, and smooth muscle. [Note: Drugs with muscarinic actions preferentially stimulate muscarinic receptors on these tissues, but at high concentration they may show some activity at nicotinic receptors.]

2. **Mechanisms of acetylcholine signal transduction:** A number of different molecular mechanisms transmit the signal generated by acetylcholine occupation of the receptor. For example, when the M_1 or M_3 receptors are activated, the receptor undergoes a conformational change and interacts with a G protein, designated G_q, which in turn activates phospholipase C.[1] This leads to the hydrolysis of phosphatidylinositol-(4,5)-bisphosphate-P_2 to yield diacylglycerol and inositol (1,4,5)-trisphosphate (formerly called inositol (1,4,5)-triphosphate), which cause an increase in intracellular Ca^{2+} (see Figure 3.7C, p. 41). This cation can then interact to stimulate or inhibit enzymes, or cause hyperpolarization, secretion, or contraction. In contrast, activation of the M_2 subtype on the cardiac muscle stimulates a G protein, designated G_i, that inhibits adenylyl cyclase[2] and increases K^+ conductance (see Figure 3.7B, p. 41), to which the heart responds with a decrease in rate and force of contraction.

[1]See p. 205 in *Lippincott's Illustrated Reviews: Biochemistry* (4th ed.) for a discussion of inositol trisphosphate and intracellular signaling.
[2]See p. 94 in *Lippincott's Illustrated Reviews: Biochemistry* (4th ed.) for a discussion of adenylyl cyclase and intracellular signaling.

3. **Muscarinic agonists and antagonists:** Attempts are currently underway to develop muscarinic agonists and antagonists that are directed against specific receptor subtypes. For example, *pirenzepine*, a tricyclic anticholinergic drug, has a greater selectivity for inhibiting M_1 muscarinic receptors, such as in the gastric mucosa. At therapeutic doses, *pirenzepine* does not cause many of the side effects seen with the non-subtype-specific drugs; however, it does produce a reflex tachycardia on rapid infusion due to blockade of M_2 receptors in the heart. Therefore, the usefulness of *pirenzepine* as an alternative to proton pump inhibitors in the treatment of gastric and duodenal ulcers is questionable. *Darifenacin* is a competitive muscarinic receptor antagonist with a greater affinity for the M_3 receptor than for the other muscarinic receptors. The drug is used in the treatment of overactive bladder. [Note: At present, no clinically important agents interact solely with the M_4 and M_5 receptors.]

4. **Nicotinic receptors:** These receptors, in addition to binding acetylcholine, also recognize nicotine but show only a weak affinity for muscarine (see Figure 4.4B). The nicotinic receptor is composed of five subunits, and it functions as a ligand-gated ion channel (see Figure 3.7A). Binding of two acetylcholine molecules elicits a conformational change that allows the entry of sodium ions, resulting in the depolarization of the effector cell. Nicotine (or acetylcholine) initially stimulates and then blocks the receptor. Nicotinic receptors are located in the CNS, adrenal medulla, autonomic ganglia, and the neuromuscular junction. Those at the neuromuscular junction are sometimes designated N_M and the others N_N. The nicotinic receptors of autonomic ganglia differ from those of the neuromuscular junction. For example, ganglionic receptors are selectively blocked by *hexamethonium*, whereas neuromuscular junction receptors are specifically blocked by *tubocurarine*.

IV. DIRECT-ACTING CHOLINERGIC AGONISTS

Cholinergic agonists (also known as parasympathomimetics) mimic the effects of acetylcholine by binding directly to cholinoceptors. These agents may be broadly classified into two groups: choline esters, which include acetylcholine and synthetic esters of choline, such as *carbachol* and *bethanechol*. Naturally occurring alkaloids, such as *pilocarpine* constiue the second group (Figure 4.5). All of the direct-acting cholinergic drugs have longer durations of action than acetylcholine. Some of the more therapeutically useful drugs (*pilocarpine* and *bethanechol*) preferentially bind to muscarinic receptors and are sometimes referred to as muscarinic agents. [Note: Muscarinic receptors are located primarily, but not exclusively, at the neuroeffector junction of the parasympathetic nervous system.] However, as a group, the direct-acting agonists show little specificity in their actions, which limits their clinical usefulness.

A. Acetylcholine

Acetylcholine [a-se-teel-KOE-leen] is a quaternary ammonium compound that cannot penetrate membranes. Although it is the neurotransmitter of parasympathetic and somatic nerves as well as autonomic ganglia, it is therapeutically of no importance because of its multiplicity of actions and its rapid inactivation by the cholinesterases. Acetylcholine has both muscarinic and nicotinic activity. Its actions include:

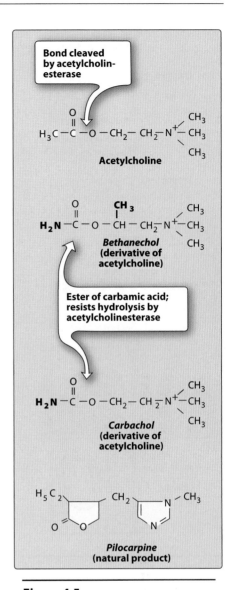

Figure 4.5
Comparison of the structures of some cholinergic agonists.

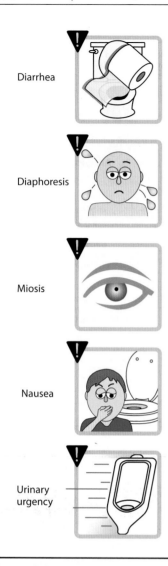

Diarrhea

Diaphoresis

Miosis

Nausea

Urinary urgency

Figure 4.6
Some adverse effects observed with cholinergic drugs.

1. **Decrease in heart rate and cardiac output:** The actions of acetylcholine on the heart mimic the effects of vagal stimulation. For example, acetylcholine, if injected intravenously, produces a brief decrease in cardiac rate (negative chronotropy) and stroke volume as a result of a reduction in the rate of firing at the sinoatrial (SA) node. [Note: It should be remembered that normal vagal activity regulates the heart by the release of acetylcholine at the SA node.]

2. **Decrease in blood pressure:** Injection of acetylcholine causes vasodilation and lowering of blood pressure by an indirect mechanism of action. Acetylcholine activates M_3 receptors found on endothelial cells lining the smooth muscles of blood vessels. This results in the production of nitric oxide from arginine.[3] [Note: nitric oxide is also known as endothelium-derived relaxing factor.] (See p. 341 for more detail on nitric oxide.) Nitric oxide then diffuses to vascular smooth muscle cells to stimulate protein kinase G production, leading to hyperpolarization and smooth muscle relaxation. In the absence of administered cholinergic agents, the vascular receptors have no known function, because acetylcholine is never released into the blood in any significant quantities. *Atropine* blocks these muscarinic receptors and prevents acetylcholine from producing vasodilation.

3. **Other actions:** In the gastrointestinal tract, acetylcholine increases salivary secretion and stimulates intestinal secretions and motility. Bronchiolar secretions are also enhanced. In the genitourinary tract, the tone of the detrusor urinae muscle is increased, causing expulsion of urine. In the eye, acetylcholine is involved in stimulating ciliary muscle contraction for near vision and in the constriction of the pupillae sphincter muscle, causing miosis (marked constriction of the pupil). Acetylcholine (1% solution) is instilled into the anterior chamber of the eye to produce miosis during ophthalmic surgery.

B. Bethanechol

Bethanechol [be-THAN-e-kole] is structurally related to acetylcholine, in which the acetate is replaced by carbamate and the choline is methylated (see Figure 4.5). Hence, it is not hydrolyzed by acetylcholinesterase (due to the addition of carbonic acid), although it is inactivated through hydrolysis by other esterases. It lacks nicotinic actions (due to the addition of the methyl group) but does have strong muscarinic activity. Its major actions are on the smooth musculature of the bladder and gastrointestinal tract. It has a duration of action of about 1 hour.

1. **Actions:** *Bethanechol* directly stimulates muscarinic receptors, causing increased intestinal motility and tone. It also stimulates the detrusor muscles of the bladder whereas the trigone and sphincter are relaxed, causing expulsion of urine.

2. **Therapeutic applications:** In urologic treatment, *bethanechol* is used to stimulate the atonic bladder, particularly in postpartum or postoperative, nonobstructive urinary retention. *Bethanechol* may also be used to treat neurogenic atony as well as megacolon.

 [3]See p. 150 in ***Lippincott's Illustrated Reviews: Biochemistry*** (4th ed.) for a discussion of the roles of nitric oxide.

3. **Adverse effects:** *Bethanechol* causes the effects of generalized cholinergic stimulation (Figure 4.6). These include sweating, salivation, flushing, decreased blood pressure, nausea, abdominal pain, diarrhea, and bronchospasm.

C. Carbachol (carbamylcholine)

Carbachol [KAR-ba-kole] has both muscarinic as well as nicotinic actions (lacks a methyl group present in *bethanechol*; see Figure 4.5). Like *bethanechol*, *carbachol* is an ester of carbamic acid and a poor substrate for acetylcholinesterase (see Figure 4.5). It is biotransformed by other esterases, but at a much slower rate. A single administration can last as long as 1 hour.

1. **Actions:** *Carbachol* has profound effects on both the cardiovascular system and the gastrointestinal system because of its ganglion-stimulating activity, and it may first stimulate and then depress these systems. It can cause release of epinephrine from the adrenal medulla by its nicotinic action. Locally instilled into the eye, it mimics the effects of acetylcholine, causing miosis and a spasm of accommodation in which the ciliary muscle of the eye remains in a constant state of contraction

2. **Therapeutic uses:** Because of its high potency, receptor nonselectivity, and relatively long duration of action, *carbachol* is rarely used therapeutically except in the eye as a miotic agent to treat glaucoma by causing pupillary contraction and a decrease in intraocular pressure.

3. **Adverse effects:** At doses used ophthalmologically, little or no side effects occur due to lack of systemic penetration (quaternary amine).

D. Pilocarpine

The alkaloid *pilocarpine* [pye-loe-KAR-peen] is a tertiary amine and is stable to hydrolysis by acetylcholinesterase (see Figure 4.5). Compared with acetylcholine and its derivatives, it is far less potent, but it is uncharged and will penetrate the CNS at therapeutic doses. *Pilocarpine* exhibits muscarinic activity and is used primarily in ophthalmology.

1. **Actions:** Applied topically to the cornea, *pilocarpine* produces a rapid miosis and contraction of the ciliary muscle. The eye undergoes miosis and a spasm of accommodation; the vision is fixed at some particular distance, making it impossible to focus (Figure 4.7). [Note the opposing effects of *atropine*, a muscarinic blocker, on the eye (see p. 57).] *Pilocarpine* is one of the most potent stimulators of secretions (secretagogue) such as sweat, tears, and saliva, but its use for producing these effects has been limited due to its lack of selectivity. The drug is beneficial in promoting salivation in patients with xerostomia resulting from irradiation of the head and neck. Sjögren's syndrome, which is characterized by dry mouth and lack of tears, is treated with oral *pilocarpime* tablets and *cevimeline*, a cholinergic drug that also has the drawback of being nonspecific.

2. **Therapeutic use in glaucoma:** *Pilocarpine* is the drug of choice in the emergency lowering of intraocular pressure of both narrow-angle (also called closed-angle) and wide-angle (also called open-angle) glaucoma. *Pilocarpine* is extremely effective in opening the trabecular meshwork around Schlemm's canal, causing an immediate drop

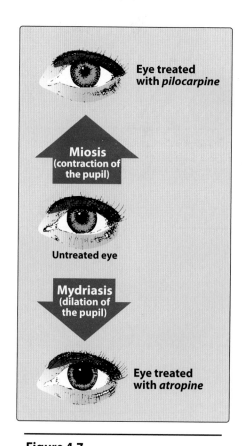

Figure 4.7
Actions of *pilocarpine* and *atropine* on the iris and ciliary muscle of the eye.

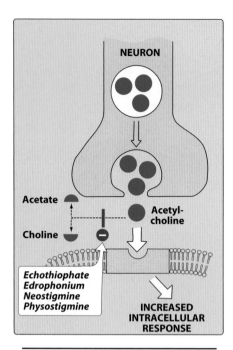

Figure 4.8
Mechanisms of action of indirect
(reversible) cholinergic agonists.

in intraocular pressure as a result of the increased drainage of aqueous humor. This action lasts up to 8 hours and can be repeated. The organophosphate *echothiophate* inhibits acetylcholinesterase and exerts the same effect for a longer duration. [Note: Carbonic anhydrase inhibitors, such as *acetazolamide*, as well as the β-adrenergic blocker *timolol*, are effective in treating glaucoma chronically but are not used for emergency lowering of intraocular pressure.]

3. **Adverse effects:** *Pilocarpine* can enter the brain and cause CNS disturbances. It stimulates profuse sweating and salivation.

V. INDIRECT-ACTING CHOLINERGIC AGONSISTS: ANTICHOLINESTERASES (REVERSIBLE)

Acetylcholinesterase is an enzyme that specifically cleaves acetylcholine to acetate and choline and, thus, terminates its actions. It is located both pre- and postsynaptically in the nerve terminal, where it is membrane bound. Inhibitors of acetylcholinesterase indirectly provide a cholinergic action by prolonging the lifetime of acetylcholine produced endogenously at the cholinergic nerve endings. This results in the accumulation of acetylcholine in the synaptic space (Figure 4.8). These drugs can thus provoke a response at all cholinoceptors in the body, including both muscarinic and nicotinic receptors of the autonomic nervous system, as well as at neuromuscular junctions and in the brain.

A. Physostigmine

Physostigmine [fi-zoe-STIG-meen] is a nitrogenous carbamic acid ester found naturally in plants and is a tertiary amine. It is a substrate for acetylcholinesterase, and it forms a relatively stable carbamoylated intermediate with the enzyme, which then becomes reversibly inactivated. The result is potentiation of cholinergic activity throughout the body.

1. **Actions:** *Physostigmine* has a wide range of effects as a result of its action, and not only the muscarinic and nicotinic sites of the autonomic nervous system but also the nicotinic receptors of the neuromuscular junction are stimulated. Its duration of action is about 2 to 4 hours, and it is considered to be an intermediate-acting agent. *Physostigmine* can enter and stimulate the cholinergic sites in the CNS.

2. **Therapeutic uses:** The drug increases intestinal and bladder motility, which serve as its therapeutic action in atony of either organ (Figure 4.9). Placed topically in the eye, it produces miosis and spasm of accommodation, as well as a lowering of intraocular pressure. It is used to treat glaucoma, but *pilocarpine* is more effective. *Physostigmine* is also used in the treatment of overdoses of drugs with anticholinergic actions, such as *atropine*, *phenothiazines*, and tricyclic antidepressants.

3. **Adverse effects:** The effects of *physostigmine* on the CNS may lead to convulsions when high doses are used. Bradycardia and a fall in cardiac output may also occur. Inhibition of acetylcholinesterase at the skeletal neuromuscular junction causes the accumulation of acetylcholine and, ultimately, results in paralysis of skeletal muscle. However, these effects are rarely seen with therapeutic doses.

B. Neostigmine

Neostigmine [nee-oh-STIG-meen] is a synthetic compound that is also a carbamic acid ester, and it reversibly inhibits acetylcholinesterase in a manner similar to that of *physostigmine*. Unlike *physostigmine*, *neostigmine* has a quaternary nitrogen; hence, it is more polar and does not enter the CNS. Its effect on skeletal muscle is greater than that of *physostigmine*, and it can stimulate contractility before it paralyzes. *Neostigmine* has a moderate duration of action, usually 30 minutes to 2 hours. It is used to stimulate the bladder and GI tract, and it is also used as an antidote for *tubocurarine* and other competitive neuromuscular blocking agents (see p. 60). *Neostigmine* has found use in symptomatic treatment of myasthenia gravis, an autoimmune disease caused by antibodies to the nicotinic receptor at neuromuscular junctions. This causes their degradation and, thus, makes fewer receptors available for interaction with the neurotransmitter. Adverse effects of *neostigmine* include those of generalized cholinergic stimulation, such as salivation, flushing, decreased blood pressure, nausea, abdominal pain, diarrhea, and bronchospasm. *Neostigmine* does not cause CNS side effects and is not used to overcome toxicity of central-acting antimuscarinic agents such as atropine.

C. Pyridostigmine and ambenomium

Pyridostigmine [peer-id-oh-STIG-meen] and *ambenomium* [am-be-NOE-mee-um] are other cholinesterase inhibitors that are used in the chronic management of myasthenia gravis. Their durations of action are intermediate (3 to 6 hours and 4 to 8 hours, respectively), but longer than that of *neostigmine*. Adverse effects of these agents are similar to those of *neostigmine*.

D. Demecarium

Demecarium [dem-e-KARE-ee-um] is another cholinesterase inhibitor used to treat chronic open-angle glaucoma (primarily in patients refractory to other agents) closed-angle glaucoma after irredectomy. It is also used for the diagnosis and treatment of accommodative esotropia. *Demecarium* is a quaternary amine that is structurally related to *neostigmine*. Mechanisms of actions and side effects are similar to those of *neostigmine*.

E. Edrophonium

The actions of *edrophonium* [ed-row-FOE-nee-um] are similar to those of *neostigmine*, except that it is more rapidly absorbed and has a short duration of action of 10 to 20 minutes (prototype short-acting agent). *Edrophonium* is a quaternary amine and is used in the diagnosis of myasthenia gravis. Intravenous injection of *edrophonium* leads to a rapid increase in muscle strength. Care must be taken, because excess drug may provoke a cholinergic crisis. *Atropine* is the antidote.

F. Tacrine, donepezil, rivastigmine, and galantamine

As mentioned above, patients with Alzheimer's disease have a deficiency of cholinergic neurons in the CNS. This observation led to the development of anticholinesterases as possible remedies for the loss of cognitive function. *Tacrine* [TAK-reen] was the first to become available, but it has been replaced by the others because of its hepatotoxicity. Despite the ability of *donepezil* [doe-NEP-e-zil], *rivastigmine* [ri-va-STIG-meen], and

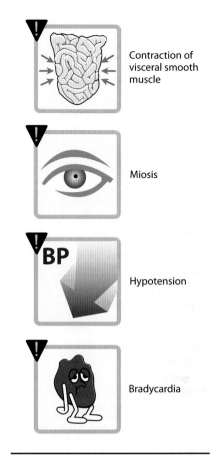

Contraction of visceral smooth muscle

Miosis

Hypotension

Bradycardia

Figure 4.9
Some actions of *physostigmine*.

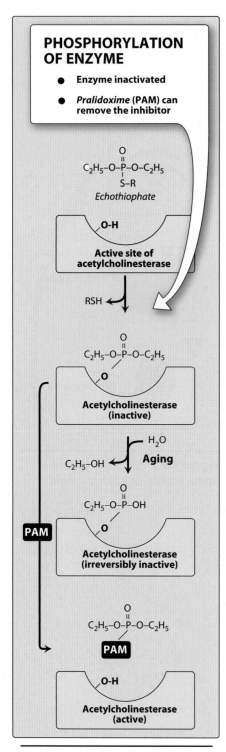

PHOSPHORYLATION OF ENZYME

- Enzyme inactivated
- *Pralidoxime* (PAM) can remove the inhibitor

Figure 4.10
Covalent modification of acetyl-cholinesterase by *echothiophate*; also shown is the reactivation of the enzyme with *pralidoxime*.
R = $(CH_3)_3N^+-CH_2-CH_2-$

galantamine [gaa-LAN-ta-meen] to delay the progression of the disease, none can stop its progression. Gastrointestinal distress is their primary adverse effect (see p. 102).

VI. INDIRECT-ACTING CHOLINERGIC AGONSISTS: ANTICHOLINESTERASES (IRREVERSIBLE)

A number of synthetic organophosphate compounds have the capacity to bind covalently to acetylcholinesterase. The result is a long-lasting increase in acetylcholine at all sites where it is released. Many of these drugs are extremely toxic and were developed by the military as nerve agents. Related compounds, such as *parathion*, are employed as insecticides.

A. Echothiophate

1. **Mechanism of action:** *Echothiophate* [ek-oe-THI-oh-fate] is an organophosphate that covalently binds via its phosphate group to the serine-OH group at the active site of acetylcholinesterase (Figure 4.10). Once this occurs, the enzyme is permanently inactivated, and restoration of acetylcholinesterase activity requires the synthesis of new enzyme molecules. Following covalent modification of acetyl-cholinesterase, the phosphorylated enzyme slowly releases one of its ethyl groups (see Figure 4.10). The loss of an alkyl group, which is called aging, makes it impossible for chemical reactivators, such as *pralidoxime* (see below), to break the bond between the remaining drug and the enzyme.

2. **Actions:** Actions include generalized cholinergic stimulation, paralysis of motor function (causing breathing difficulties), and convulsions. *Echothiophate* produces intense miosis and, thus, has found therapeutic use. *Atropine* in high dosage can reverse many of the muscarinic and some of the central effects of *echothiophate*.

3. **Therapeutic uses:** An ophthalmic solution of the drug is used directly in the eye for the chronic treatment of open-angle glaucoma. The effects may last for up to one week after a single administration. *Echothiophate* is not a first-line agent in the treatment of glaucoma. In addition to its other side effects, the potential risk for causing cataracts limits the use of *echothiophate*.

4. **Reactivation of acetylcholinesterase:** *Pralidoxime* can reactivate inhibited acetylcholinesterase. However, it is unable to penetrate into the CNS. The presence of a charged group allows it to approach an anionic site on the enzyme, where it essentially displaces the phosphate group of the organophosphate and regenerates the enzyme. If given before aging of the alkylated enzyme occurs, it can reverse the effects of *echothiophate*, except for those in the CNS. With the newer nerve agents, which produce aging of the enzyme complex within seconds, *pralidoxime* is less effective. *Pralidoxime* is a weak acetylcholinesterase inhibitor and, at higher doses, may cause side effects similar to other acetylcholinsterase inhibitors (Figures 4.6 and 4.9).

A summary of the actions of some of the cholinergic agonists is presented in Figure 4.11.

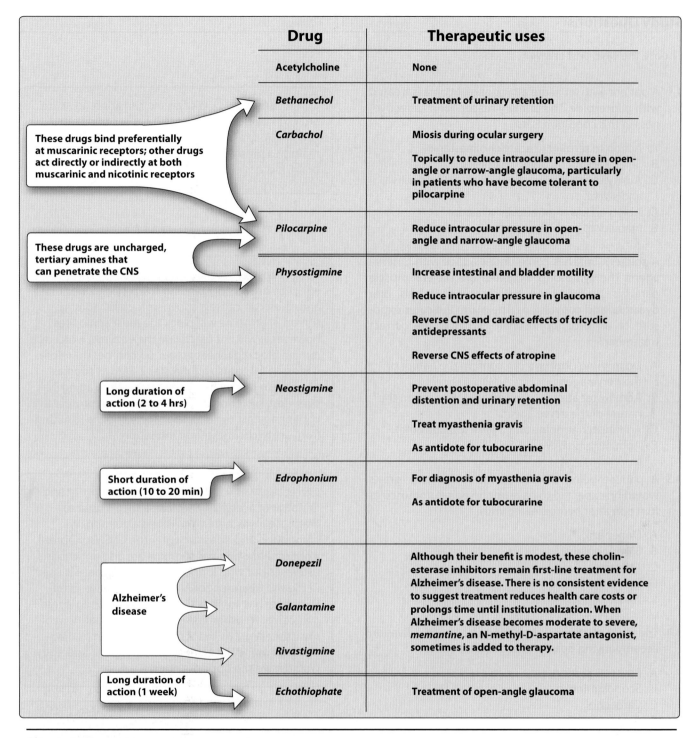

Figure 4.11
Summary of actions of some cholinergic agonists.

Study Questions

Choose the ONE best answer.

4.1 A patient with an acute attack of glaucoma is treated with pilocarpine. The primary reason for its effectiveness in this condition is its:

   A. Action to terminate acetylcholinesterase.
   B. Selectivity for nicotinic receptors.
   C. Ability to inhibit secretions, such as tears, saliva, and sweat.
   D. Ability to lower intraocular pressure.
   E. Inability to enter the brain.

Correct answer = D. Pilocarpine can abort an acute attack of glaucoma, because it causes pupillary constriction to lower intraocular pressure. It binds mainly to muscarinic receptors and can enter the brain. It is not effective in inhibiting secretions.

4.2 A soldier's unit has come under attack with a nerve agent. The symptoms exhibited are skeletal muscle paralysis, profuse bronchial secretions, miosis, bradycardia, and convulsions. The alarm indicates exposure to an organophosphate. What is the correct treatment?

   A. Do nothing until you can confirm the nature of the nerve agent.
   B. Administer atropine, and attempt to confirm the nature of the nerve agent.
   C. Administer atropine and 2-PAM (pralidoxime).
   D. Administer 2-PAM.

Correct answer = C. Organophosphates exert their effect by irreversibly binding to acetylcholinesterase and, thus, can cause a cholinergic crisis. Administration of atropine will block the muscarinic sites; however, it will not reactivate the enzyme, which will remain blocked for a long period of time. Therefore, it is essential to also administer 2-PAM as soon as possible to reactivate the enzyme before aging occurs. Administering 2-PAM alone will not protect the patient against the effects of acetylcholine resulting from acetylcholinesterase inhibition.

4.3 A patient being diagnosed for myasthenia gravis would be expected to have improved neuromuscular function after being treated with:

   A. Donepezil.
   B. Edrophonium.
   C. Atropine.
   D. Echothiophate.
   E. Neostigmine.

Correct answer = B. Edrophonium is a short-acting inhibitor of acetylcholinesterase that is used to diagnose myasthenia gravis. It is a quaternary compound and does not enter the CNS. Doneprezil, isoflurophate, and neostigmine are also anticholinesterases but with longer actions. Donepezil is used in the the treatment of Alzheimer's disease. Echothiophate has some activity in treating open-angle glaucoma. Neostigmine is used in the treatment of myasthenia gravis but is not employed in its diagnosis. Atropine is a cholinergic antagonist and, thus, would have the opposite effects.

4.4 The drug of choice for treating decreased salivation accompanying head and neck irradiation is:

   A. Physostigmine.
   B. Scopolamine.
   C. Carbachol.
   D. Acetylcholine.
   E. Pilocarpine.

Correct answer = E. Pilocarpine has proven to be beneficial in this situation. All the others except scopolamine are cholinergic agonists. However, their ability to stimulate salivation is less than that of pilocarpine, and their other effects are more troublesome.

Cholinergic Antagonists

5

I. OVERVIEW

The cholinergic antagonists (also called cholinergic blockers, parasympatholytics or anticholinergic drugs) bind to cholinoceptors, but they do not trigger the usual receptor-mediated intracellular effects. The most useful of these agents selectively block muscarinic synapses of the parasympathetic nerves. The effects of parasympathetic innervation are thus interrupted, and the actions of sympathetic stimulation are left unopposed. A second group of drugs, the ganglionic blockers, show a preference for the nicotinic receptors of the sympathetic and parasympathetic ganglia. Clinically, they are the least important of the anticholinergic drugs. A third family of compounds, the neuromuscular blocking agents, interfere with transmission of efferent impulses to skeletal muscles. These agent are used as adjuvants in anesthesia during surgery. Figure 5.1 summarizes the cholinergic antagonists discussed in this chapter.

II. ANTIMUSCARINIC AGENTS

Commonly known as antimuscarinics, these agents (for example, *atropine* and *scopolamine*) block muscarinic receptors (Figure 5.2), causing inhibition of all muscarinic functions. In addition, these drugs block the few exceptional sympathetic neurons that are cholinergic, such as those innervating salivary and sweat glands. In contrast to the cholinergic agonists, which have limited usefulness therapeutically, the cholinergic blockers are beneficial in a variety of clinical situations. Because they do not block nicotinic receptors, the antimuscarinic drugs have little or no action at skeletal neuromuscular junctions or autonomic ganglia. [Note: A number of antihistaminic and antidepressant drugs also have antimuscarinic activity.]

A. Atropine

Atropine [A-troe-peen], a tertiary amine belladonna alkaloid, has a high affinity for muscarinic receptors, where it binds competitively, preventing acetylcholine from binding to those sites (Figure 5.3). *Atropine* acts both centrally and peripherally. Its general actions last about 4 hours except when placed topically in the eye, where the action may last for days.

1. Actions:

a. **Eye:** *Atropine* blocks all cholinergic activity on the eye, resulting in persistent mydriasis (dilation of the pupil, see Figure 4.6, p. 46), unresponsiveness to light, and cycloplegia (inability to focus for near vision). In patients with narrow-angle glaucoma,

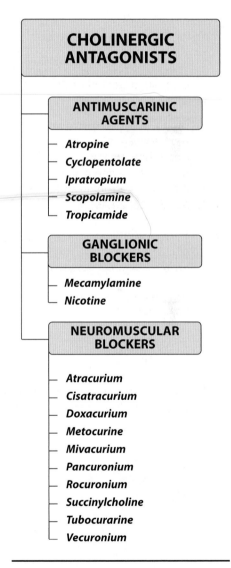

CHOLINERGIC ANTAGONISTS

ANTIMUSCARINIC AGENTS
- *Atropine*
- *Cyclopentolate*
- *Ipratropium*
- *Scopolamine*
- *Tropicamide*

GANGLIONIC BLOCKERS
- *Mecamylamine*
- *Nicotine*

NEUROMUSCULAR BLOCKERS
- *Atracurium*
- *Cisatracurium*
- *Doxacurium*
- *Metocurine*
- *Mivacurium*
- *Pancuronium*
- *Rocuronium*
- *Succinylcholine*
- *Tubocurarine*
- *Vecuronium*

Figure 5.1
Summary of cholinergic antagonists.

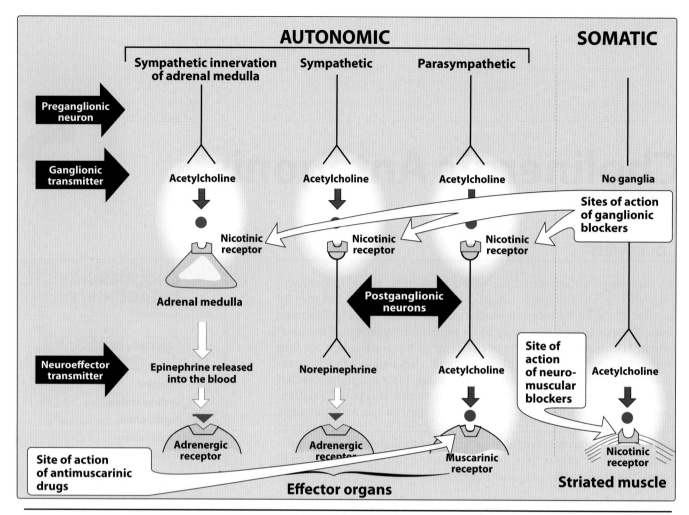

Figure 5.2
Sites of actions of cholinergic antagonists.

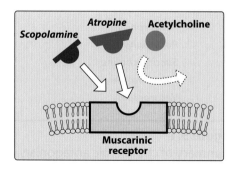

Figure 5.3
Competition of *atropine* and *scopolamine* with acetylcholine for the muscarinic receptor.

intraocular pressure may rise dangerously. Shorter-acting agents, such as the antimuscarinic *tropicamide*, or an α-adrenergic drug, like *phenylephrine*, are generally favored for producing mydriasis in ophthalmic examinations.

b. Gastrointestinal (GI): *Atropine* can be used as an antispasmodic to reduce activity of the GI tract. *Atropine* and *scopolamine* (which is discussed below) are probably the most potent drugs available that produce this effect. Although gastric motility is reduced, hydrochloric acid production is not significantly affected. Thus, the drug is not effective in promoting healing of peptic ulcer. [Note: *Pirenzepine* (see p. 47), an M_1-muscarinic antagonist, does reduce gastric acid secretion at doses that do not antagonize other systems.]

c. Urinary system: *Atropine* is also employed to reduce hypermotility states of the urinary bladder. It is still occasionally used in enuresis (involuntary voiding of urine) among children, but α-adrenergic agonists with fewer side effects may be more effective.

d. Cardiovascular: *Atropine* produces divergent effects on the cardiovascular system, depending on the dose (Figure 5.4). At low doses, the predominant effect is a decreased cardiac rate (bradycardia). Originally thought to be due to central activation of vagal efferent outflow, the effect is now known to result from blockade of the M_1 receptors on the inhibitory prejunctional (or presynaptic) neurons, thus permitting increased acetylcholine release. With higher doses of *atropine*, the M_2 receptors on the sinoatrial node are blocked, and the cardiac rate increases modestly. This generally requires at least 1 mg of *atropine*, which is a higher dose than ordinarily given. Arterial blood pressure is unaffected, but at toxic levels, *atropine* will dilate the cutaneous vasculature.

e. Secretions: *Atropine* blocks the salivary glands, producing a drying effect on the oral mucous membranes (xerostomia). The salivary glands are exquisitely sensitive to *atropine*. Sweat and lacrimal glands are also affected. [Note: Inhibition of secretions by sweat glands can cause elevated body temperature.]

2. Therapeutic uses:

a. Ophthalmic: In the eye, topical *atropine* exerts both mydriatic and cycloplegic effects, and it permits the measurement of refractive errors without interference by the accommodative capacity of the eye. [Note: *Phenylephrine* or similar α-adrenergic drugs are preferred for pupillary dilation if cycloplegia is not required. Also, individuals 40 years of age and older have decreased ability to accommodate, and drugs are not necessary for an accurate refraction.] Shorter-acting antimuscarinics (*cyclopentolante* and *tropicamide*) have largely replaced *atropine* due to prolonged mydriasis observed with *atropine* (7–14 days versus 6–24 hours with other agents). *Atropine* may induce an acute attack of eye pain due to sudden increases in eye pressure in individuals with narrow-angle glaucoma.

b. Antispasmodic: *Atropine* is used as an antispasmodic agent to relax the GI tract and bladder.

c. Antidote for cholinergic agonists: *Atropine* is used for the treatment of overdoses of cholinesterase inhibitor insecticides and some types of mushroom poisoning (certain mushrooms contain cholinergic substances that block cholinesterases). Massive doses of the antagonist may be required over a long period of time to counteract the poisons. The ability of *atropine* to enter the central nervous system (CNS) is of particular importance. The drug also blocks the effects of excess acetylcholine resulting from acetylcholinesterase inhibitors, such as *physostigmine*.

d. Antisecretory: The drug is sometimes used as an antisecretory agent to block secretions in the upper and lower respiratory tracts prior to surgery.

3. Pharmacokinetics: *Atropine* is readily absorbed, partially metabolized by the liver, and eliminated primarily in the urine. It has a half-life of about 4 hours.

4. Adverse effects: Depending on the dose, *atropine* may cause dry mouth, blurred vision, "sandy eyes," tachycardia, and constipation.

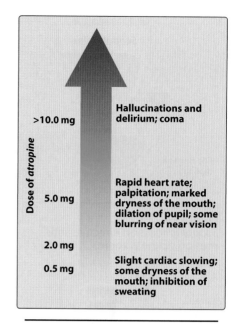

Figure 5.4
Dose-dependent effects of *atropine*.

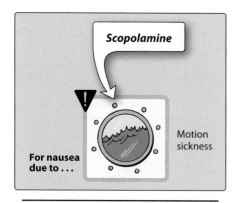

Figure 5.5
Scopolamine is an effective anti-motion sickness agent.

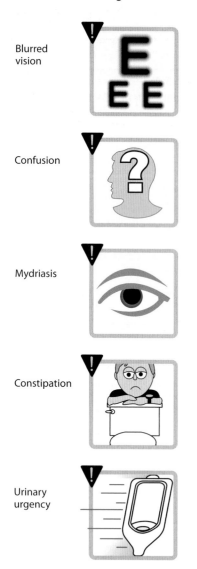

Blurred vision

Confusion

Mydriasis

Constipation

Urinary urgency

Figure 5.6
Adverse effects commonly observed with cholinergic antagonists.

Effects on the CNS include restlessness, confusion, hallucinations, and delirium, which may progress to depression, collapse of the circulatory and respiratory systems, and death. Low doses of cholinesterase inhibitors such as *physostigmine* may be used to overcome *atropine* toxicity. In older individuals, the use of *atropine* to induce mydriasis and cycloplegia is considered to be too risky, because it may exacerbate an attack of glaucoma in someone with a latent condition. In other older individuals, *atropine* may induce urinary retention that is troublesome. Children are sensitive to effects of *atropine*—in particular, the rapid increases in body temperature that it may elicit. This may be dangerous in children.

B. Scopolamine

Scopolamine [skoe-POL-a-meen], another tertiary amine belladonna alkaloid, produces peripheral effects similar to those of *atropine*. However, *scopolamine* has greater action on the CNS (unlike with *atropine*, CNS effects are observed at therapeutic doses) and a longer duration of action in comparison to those of *atropine*. It has some special actions as indicated below.

1. **Actions:** *Scopolamine* is one of the most effective anti–motion sickness drugs available (Figure 5.5). *Scopolamine* also has the unusual effect of blocking short-term memory. In contrast to *atropine*, *scopolamine* produces sedation, but at higher doses it can produce excitement instead. *Scopolamine* may produce euphoria and is subject to abuse.

2. **Therapeutic uses:** Although similar to *atropine*, therapeutic use of *scopolamine* is limited to prevention of motion sickness (for which it is particularly effective) and to blocking short-term memory. [Note: As with all such drugs used for motion sickness, it is much more effective prophylactically than for treating motion sickness once it occurs. The amnesic action of *scopolamine* makes it an important adjunct drug in anesthetic procedures.]

3. **Pharmacokinetics and adverse effects:** These aspects are similar to those of *atropine*.

C. Ipratropium

Inhaled *ipratropium* [i-pra-TROE-pee-um], a quaternary derivative of *atropine*, is useful in treating asthma in patients who are unable to take adrenergic agonists. *Ipratropium* is also beneficial in the management of chronic obstructive pulmonary disease. It is inhaled for these conditions. Because of its positive charge, it does not enter the systemic circulation or the CNS, isolating its effects to the pulmonary system. Important characteristics of the muscarinic antagonists are summarized in Figures 5.6 and 5.7.

D. Tropicamide and cyclopentolate

These agents are used as ophthalmic solutions for similar conditions as *atropine* (mydriasis and cyclopegia). Their duration of action is shorter than that of *atropine*; *tropicamide* produces mydriasis for 6 hours and *cyclopentolate* for 24 hours.

III. GANGLIONIC BLOCKERS

Ganglionic blockers specifically act on the nicotinic receptors of both parasympathetic and sympathetic autonomic ganglia. Some also block the ion channels of the autonomic ganglia. These drugs show no selectivity toward the parasympathetic or sympathetic ganglia and are not effective as neuromuscular antagonists. Thus, these drugs block the entire output of the autonomic nervous system at the nicotinic receptor. Except for nicotine, the other drugs mentioned in this category are nondepolarizing, competitive antagonists. The responses observed are complex and unpredictable, making it impossible to achieve selective actions. Therefore, ganglionic blockade is rarely used therapeutically. However, ganglionic blockers often serve as tools in experimental pharmacology.

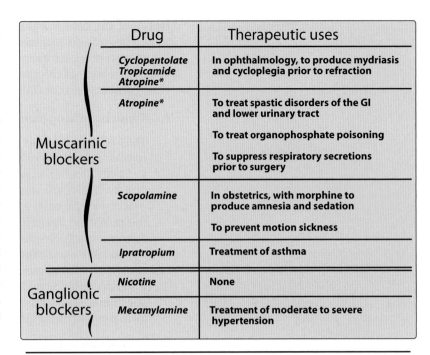

	Drug	Therapeutic uses
Muscarinic blockers	*Cyclopentolate Tropicamide Atropine**	In ophthalmology, to produce mydriasis and cycloplegia prior to refraction
	*Atropine**	To treat spastic disorders of the GI and lower urinary tract
		To treat organophosphate poisoning
		To suppress respiratory secretions prior to surgery
	Scopolamine	In obstetrics, with morphine to produce amnesia and sedation
		To prevent motion sickness
	Ipratropium	Treatment of asthma
Ganglionic blockers	*Nicotine*	None
	Mecamylamine	Treatment of moderate to severe hypertension

Figure 5.7
Summary of cholinergic antagonists. *Contraindicated in narrow-angle glaucoma. GI = gastrointestinal.

A. Nicotine

A component of cigarette smoke, nicotine [NIC-oh-teen] is a poison with many undesirable actions. It is without therapeutic benefit and is deleterious to health. [Note: Nicotine is available as patches, lozenges, gums, and other forms. Patches are available for application to the skin. The drug is absorbed and is effective in reducing the craving for nicotine in people who wish to stop smoking.] Depending on the dose, nicotine depolarizes autonomic ganglia, resulting first in stimulation and then in paralysis of all ganglia. The stimulatory effects are complex due to effects on both sympathetic and parasympathetic ganglia. The effects include increased blood pressure and cardiac rate (due to release of transmitter from adrenergic terminals and from the adrenal medulla) and increased peristalsis and secretions. At higher doses, the blood pressure falls because of ganglionic blockade, and activity both in the GI tract and bladder musculature ceases. (See p. 118 for a full discussion of nicotine.)

B. Mecamylamine

Mecamylamine [mek-a-MILL-a-meen] produces a competitive nicotinic blockade of the ganglia. The duration of action is about 10 hours after a single administration. The uptake of the drug via oral absorption is good, in contrast to that of *trimethaphan*. As with *trimethaphan*, it is primarily used to lower blood pressure in emergency situations.

IV. NEUROMUSCULAR BLOCKING DRUGS

These drugs block cholinergic transmission between motor nerve endings and the nicotinic receptors on the neuromuscular end plate of skeletal muscle (see Figure 5.2). These neuromuscular blockers are structural analogs of acetylcholine, and they act either as antagonists (nondepolarizing type) or agonists (depolarizing type) at the receptors on the end plate of the neuromuscular junction. Neuromuscular blockers are clinically useful during surgery for producing complete muscle relaxation, without having to employ higher anesthetic doses to achieve comparable muscular relaxation. Agents are also useful in facilitating intubation as well. A second group of muscle relaxants, the central muscle relaxants, are used to control spastic muscle tone. These drugs include *diazepam*, which binds at γ-aminobutyric acid (GABA) receptors; *dantrolene*, which acts directly on muscles by interfering with the release of calcium from the sarcoplasmic reticulum; and *baclofen*, which probably acts at GABA receptors in the CNS.

A. Nondepolarizing (competitive) blockers

The first drug that was found to be capable of blocking the skeletal neuromuscular junction was curare, which the native hunters of the Amazon in South America used to paralyze game. The drug *tubocurarine* [too-boe-kyoo-AR-een] was ultimately purified and introduced into clinical practice in the early 1940s. Although *tubocurarine* is considered to be the prototype agent in this class, it has been largely replaced by other agents due to side effects (see Figure 5.10). The neuromuscular blocking agents have significantly increased the safety of anesthesia, because less anesthetic is required to produce muscle relaxation, allowing patients to recover quickly and completely after surgery. Note: Higher doses of anesthesia may produce respiratory paralysis and cardiac depression, increasing recovery time after surgery.]

1. Mechanism of action:

a. At low doses: Nondepolarizing neuromuscular blocking drugs interact with the nicotinic receptors to prevent the binding of acetylcholine (Figure 5.8). These drugs thus prevent depolarization of the muscle cell membrane and inhibit muscular contraction. Because these agents compete with acetylcholine at the receptor without stimulating the receptor, they are called competitive blockers. Their action can be overcome by increasing the concentration of acetylcholine in the synaptic gap—for example, by administration of cholinesterase inhibitors, such as *neostigmine*, *pyridostigmine*, or *edrophonium*. Anesthesiologists often employ this strategy to shorten the duration of the neuromuscular blockade.

b. At high doses: Nondepolarizing blockers can block the ion channels of the end plate. This leads to further weakening of neuromuscular transmission, and it reduces the ability of acetylcholinesterase inhibitors to reverse the actions of nondepolarizing muscle relaxants.

2. Actions:
Not all muscles are equally sensitive to blockade by competitive blockers. Small, rapidly contracting muscles of the face and eye are most susceptible and are paralyzed first, followed by the fingers. Thereafter, the limbs, neck, and trunk muscles are paralyzed. Then the intercostal muscles are affected, and lastly, the diaphragm muscles are paralyzed. Those agents (for example, *tubocurarine*, *mivacurium*, and *atracurium*), which release histamine, can produce a fall in blood pressure, flushing, and bronchoconstriction.

3. Therapeutic uses:
These blockers are used therapeutically as adjuvant drugs in anesthesia during surgery to relax skeletal muscle. These agents are also used to facilitate intubation as well as during orthopedic surgery.

4. Pharmacokinetics:
All neuromuscular blocking agents are injected intravenously, because their uptake via oral absorption is mini-

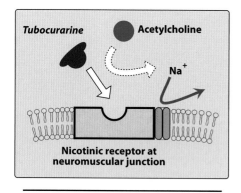

Figure 5.8
Mechanism of action of competitive neuromuscular blocking drugs.

mal. These agents possess two or more quaternary amines in their bulky ring structure, making them orally ineffective. They penetrate membranes very poorly and do not enter cells or cross the blood-brain barrier. Many of the drugs are not metabolized; their actions are terminated by redistribution (Figure 5.9). For example, *tubocurarine*, *pancuronium*, *mivacurium*, *metocurine*, and *doxacurium* are excreted in the urine unchanged. *Atracurium* is degraded spontaneously in the plasma and by ester hydrolysis. [Note: *Atracurium* has been replaced by its isomer, *cisatracurium*. *Atracurium* releases histamine and is metabolized to laudanosine, which can provoke seizures. *Cisatracurium*, which has the same pharmacokinetic properties as *atracurium*, is less likely to have these effects.] The aminosteroid drugs (*vecuronium* and *rocuronium*) are deacetylated in the liver, and their clearance may be prolonged in patients with hepatic disease. These drugs are also excreted unchanged in the bile. The choice of an agent will depend on how quickly muscle relaxation is needed and on the duration of the muscle relaxation. The onset and duration of action as well as other characteristics of the neuromuscular blocking drugs are shown in Figure 5.10.

5. **Adverse effects:** In general, agents are safe with minimal side effects. The adverse effects of the specific neuromuscular blocking drugs are shown in Figure 5.10.

6. **Drug interactions:**

   a. **Cholinesterase inhibitors:** Drugs such as *neostigmine*, *physostigmine*, *pyridostigmine*, and *edrophonium* can overcome the action of nondepolarizing neuromuscular blockers, but with increased dosage, cholinesterase inhibitors can cause a depolarizing block as a result of elevated acetylcholine concentrations at the end-plate membrane. If the neuromuscular blocker has entered the ion channel, cholinesterase inhibitors are not as effective in overcoming blockade.

   b. **Halogenated hydrocarbon anesthetics:** Drugs such as *halothane* act to enhance neuromuscular blockade by exerting a stabilizing action at the neuromuscular junction. These agents sensitize the neuromusclular junction to the effects of neuromuscular blockers.

   c. **Aminoglycoside antibiotics:** Drugs such as *gentamicin* or *tobramycin* inhibit acetylcholine release from cholinergic nerves by competing with calcium ions. They synergize with *tubocurarine* and other competitive blockers, enhancing the blockade.

   d. **Calcium-channel blockers:** These agents may increase the neuromuscular block of *tubocurarine* and other competitive blockers as well as depolarizing blockers.

B. Depolarizing agents

1. **Mechanism of action:** The depolarizing neuromuscular blocking drug *succinylcholine* [suk-sin-ill-KOE-leen] attaches to the nicotinic receptor and acts like acetylcholine to depolarize the junction (Figure 5.11). Unlike acetylcholine, which is instantly destroyed by acetylcholinesterase, the depolarizing agent persists at high concentrations in the synaptic cleft, remaining attached to the receptor for a relative-

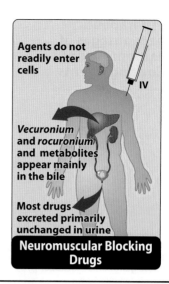

Figure 5.9
Pharmacokinetics of the neuromuscular blocking drugs. IV = intravenous.

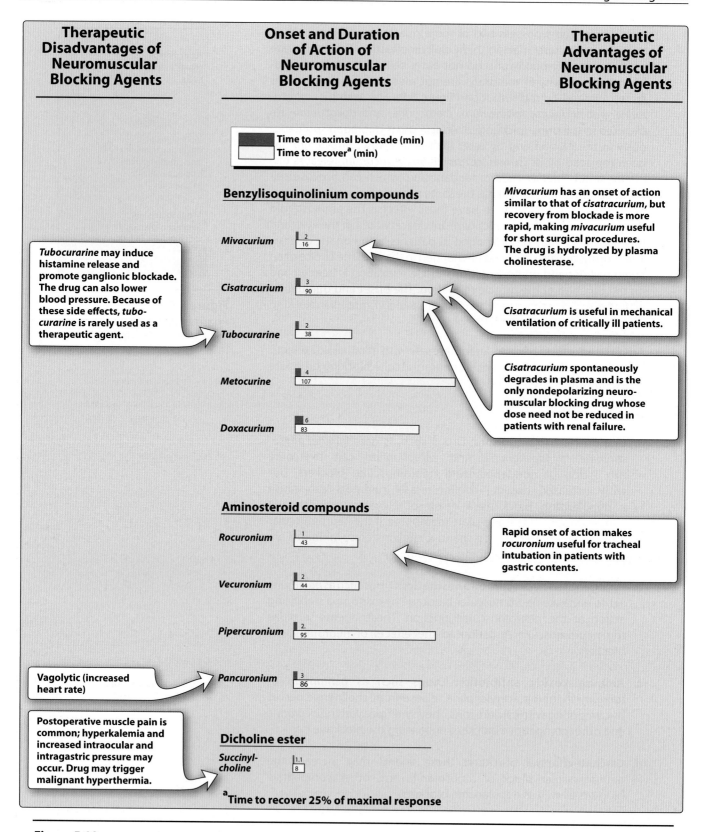

| Therapeutic Disadvantages of Neuromuscular Blocking Agents | Onset and Duration of Action of Neuromuscular Blocking Agents | Therapeutic Advantages of Neuromuscular Blocking Agents |

Time to maximal blockade (min)
Time to recover[a] (min)

Benzylisoquinolinium compounds

Mivacurium 2 / 16

Cisatracurium 3 / 90

Tubocurarine 2 / 38

Metocurine 4 / 107

Doxacurium 6 / 83

Aminosteroid compounds

Rocuronium 1 / 43

Vecuronium 2 / 44

Pipercuronium 2. / 95

Pancuronium 3 / 86

Dicholine ester

Succinyl-choline 1.1 / 8

[a] Time to recover 25% of maximal response

Tubocurarine may induce histamine release and promote ganglionic blockade. The drug can also lower blood pressure. Because of these side effects, *tubocurarine* is rarely used as a therapeutic agent.

Vagolytic (increased heart rate)

Postoperative muscle pain is common; hyperkalemia and increased intraocular and intragastric pressure may occur. Drug may trigger malignant hyperthermia.

Mivacurium has an onset of action similar to that of *cisatracurium*, but recovery from blockade is more rapid, making *mivacurium* useful for short surgical procedures. The drug is hydrolyzed by plasma cholinesterase.

Cisatracurium is useful in mechanical ventilation of critically ill patients.

Cisatracurium spontaneously degrades in plasma and is the only nondepolarizing neuromuscular blocking drug whose dose need not be reduced in patients with renal failure.

Rapid onset of action makes *rocuronium* useful for tracheal intubation in patients with gastric contents.

Figure 5.10
Onset and duration of action of neuromuscular blocking drugs (center column), with a summary of therapeutic considerations.

ly longer time and providing a constant stimulation of the receptor. [Note: The duration of action of *succinylcholine* is dependent on diffusion from the motor end plate and hydrolysis by plasma cholinesterase.] The depolarizing agent first causes the opening of the sodium channel associated with the nicotinic receptors, which results in depolarization of the receptor (Phase I). This leads to a transient twitching of the muscle (fasciculations). Continued binding of the depolarizing agent renders the receptor incapable of transmitting further impulses. With time, continuous depolarization gives way to gradual repolarization as the sodium channel closes or is blocked. This causes a resistance to depolarization (Phase II) and a flaccid paralysis.

2. **Actions:** The sequence of paralysis may be slightly different, but as with the competitive blockers, the respiratory muscles are paralyzed last. *Succinylcholine* initially produces short-lasting muscle fasciculations, followed within a few minutes by paralysis. The drug does not produce a ganglionic block except at high doses, but it does have weak histamine-releasing action. Normally, the duration of action of *succinylcholine* is extremely short, because this drug is rapidly broken down by plasma cholinesterase. However, *succinylcholine* that gets to the neuromuscular junction is not metabolized by acetylcholinesterase, allowing the agent to bind to nicotinic receptors, and redistribution to plasma is necessary for metabolism (therapeutic benefits last only for a few minutes). [Note: Genetic variants in which plasma cholinesterase levels are low or absent leads to prolonged neuromuscular paralysis.]

3. **Therapeutic uses:** Because of its rapid onset and short duration of action, *succinylcholine* is useful when rapid endotracheal intubation is required during the induction of anesthesia (a rapid action is essential if aspiration of gastric contents is to be avoided during intubation). It is also employed during electroconvulsive shock treatment.

4. **Pharmacokinetics:** *Succinylcholine* is injected intravenously. Its brief duration of action (several minutes) results from redistribution and rapid hydrolysis by plasma cholinesterase. It therefore is usually given by continuous infusion.

5. **Adverse effects:**

   a. **Hyperthermia:** When *halothane* (see p. 133) is used as an anesthetic, administration of *succinylcholine* has occasionally caused malignant hyperthermia (with muscular rigidity and hyperpyrexia) in genetically susceptible people (see Figure 5.10). This is treated by rapidly cooling the patient and by administration of *dantrolene*, which blocks release of Ca^{2+} from the sarcoplasmic reticulum of muscle cells, thus reducing heat production and relaxing muscle tone.

   b. **Apnea:** Administration of *succinylcholine* to a patient who is genetically deficient in plasma cholinesterase or has an atypical form of the enzyme can lead to prolonged apnea due to paralysis of the diaphragm.

   c. **Hyperkalemia:** *Succinylcholine* increases potassium release from intracellular stores. This may be particularly dangerous in burn patients or patients with massive tissue damage in which postassium is been rapidly lost from within cells.

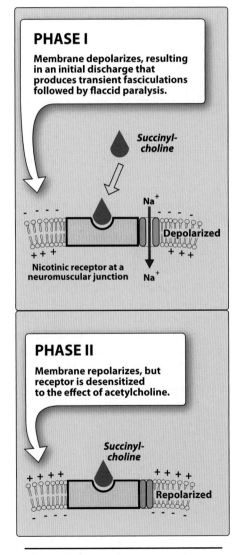

Figure 5.11
Mechanism of action of depolarizing neuromuscular blocking drugs.

Study Questions

Choose the ONE best answer.

5.1 A 75-year-old man who was a smoker is diagnosed with chronic obstructive pulmonary disease and suffers from occasional bronchospasm. Which of the following would be effective in treating him?

A. Ipratropium aerosol.
B. Scopolamine patches.
C. Mecamylamine.
D. Oxygen.

Correct answer = A. This is a drug of choice, especially in a patient who cannot tolerate an adrenergic agonist, which would dilate the bronchioles. Scopolamine's main effect is atropinic, and, is the most effective anti–motion sickness drug. Mecamylamine is a ganglionic blocker and completely inappropriate in this situation. Oxygen would improve aeration but would not dilate the bronchial musculature.

5.2 Which of the following may precipitate an attack of open-angle glaucoma if instilled into the eye?

A. Physostigmine.
B. Atropine.
C. Pilocarpine.
D. Echothiophate.

Correct answer = B. The mydriatic effect of atropine can result in the narrowing of the canal of Schlemm leading to an increase in intraocular pressure. The other agents would cause miosis.

5.3 The prolonged apnea sometimes seen in patients who have undergone an operation in which *succinylcholine* was employed as a muscle relaxant has been shown to be due to:

A. Urinary atony.
B. Depressed levels of plasma cholinesterase.
C. A mutation in acetylcholinesterase.
D. A mutation in the nicotinic receptor at the neuromuscular junction.

Correct answer = B. These patients have a genetic deficiency of the nonspecific plasma cholinesterase that is required for the termination of succinylcholine's action.

5.4 A 50-year-old male farm worker is brought to the emergency room. He was found confused in the orchard and since then has lost consciousness. His heart rate is 45, and his blood pressure is 80/40 mm Hg. He is sweating and salivating profusely. Which of the following treatments is indicated?

A. Physostigmine.
B. Norepinephrine.
C. Trimethaphan.
D. Atropine.
E. Edrophonium.

Correct answer = D. The patient is exhibiting signs of cholinergic stimulation. Because he is a farmer, insecticide poisoning is a likely diagnosis. Thus, either intravenous or intramuscular doses of atropine are indicated to antagonize the muscarinic symptoms. Physostigmine and edrophonium are cholinesterase inhibitors and would exacerbate the problem. Norepinephrine would not be effective in combatting the cholinergic stimulation. Trimethaphan, being a ganglionic blocker, would also worsen the condition.

Adrenergic Agonists

6

I. OVERVIEW

The adrenergic drugs affect receptors that are stimulated by norepinephrine or *epinephrine*. Some adrenergic drugs act directly on the adrenergic receptor (adrenoceptor) by activating it and are said to be sympathomimetic. Others, which will be dealt with in Chapter 7, block the action of the neurotransmitters at the receptors (sympatholytics), whereas still other drugs affect adrenergic function by interrupting the release of norepinephrine from adrenergic neurons. This chapter describes agents that either directly or indirectly stimulate adrenoceptors (Figure 6.1).

II. THE ADRENERGIC NEURON

Adrenergic neurons release norepinephrine as the primary neurotransmitter. These neurons are found in the central nervous system (CNS) and also in the sympathetic nervous system, where they serve as links between ganglia and the effector organs. The adrenergic neurons and receptors, located either presynaptically on the neuron or postsynaptically on the effector organ, are the sites of action of the adrenergic drugs (Figure 6.2).

A. Neurotransmission at adrenergic neurons

Neurotransmission in adrenergic neurons closely resembles that already described for the cholinergic neurons (see p. 43), except that norepinephrine is the neurotransmitter instead of acetylcholine. Neurotransmission takes place at numerous bead-like enlargements called varicosities. The process involves five steps: synthesis, storage, release, and receptor binding of norepinephrine, followed by removal of the neurotransmitter from the synaptic gap (Figure 6.3).

1. **Synthesis of norepinephrine:** Tyrosine is transported by a Na^+-linked carrier into the axoplasm of the adrenergic neuron, where it is hydroxylated to dihydroxyphenylalanine (DOPA) by tyrosine hydroxylase.[1] This is the rate-limiting step in the formation of norepinephrine. DOPA is then decarboxylated by the enzyme dopa decarboxylase (aromatic L-amino acid decarboxylase) to form *dopamine* in the cytoplasm of the presynaptic neuron.

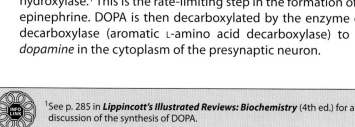

[1]See p. 285 in ***Lippincott's Illustrated Reviews: Biochemistry*** (4th ed.) for a discussion of the synthesis of DOPA.

ADRENERGIC AGONISTS

DIRECT-ACTING

- Albuterol
- Clonidine
- Dobutamine*
- Dopamine*
- Epinephrine*
- Formoterol
- Isoproterenol*
- Metaproterenol
- Methoxamine
- Norepinephrine*
- Phenylephrine
- Piruterol
- Salmeterol
- Terbutaline

INDIRECT-ACTING

- Amphetamine
- Cocaine
- Tyramine

DIRECT and INDIRECT ACTING (mixed action)

- Ephedrine
- Pseudoephrine

Figure 6.1
Summary of adrenergic agonists. Agents marked with an asterisk (*) are catecholamines.

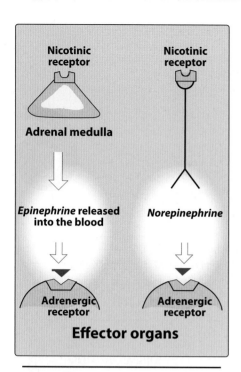

Figure 6.2
Sites of actions of adrenergic agonists.

2. **Storage of norepinephrine in vesicles:** *Dopamine* is then transported into synaptic vesicles by an amine transporter system that is also involved in the reuptake of preformed norepinephrine. This carrier system is blocked by *reserpine* (see p. 90). *Dopamine* is hydroxylated to form norepinephrine by the enzyme, dopamine β-hydroxylase. [Note: Synaptic vesicles contain *dopamine* or norepinephrine plus adenosine triphosphate (ATP), and β-hydroxylase, as well as other cotransmitters.] In the adrenal medulla, norepinephrine is methylated to yield *epinephrine*, both of which are stored in chromaffin cells. On stimulation, the adrenal medulla releases about 80 percent *epinephrine* and 20 percent norepinephrine directly into the circulation.

3. **Release of norepinephrine:** An action potential arriving at the nerve junction triggers an influx of calcium ions from the extracellular fluid into the cytoplasm of the neuron. The increase in calcium causes vesicles inside the neuron to fuse with the cell membrane and expel (exocytose) their contents into the synapse. This release is blocked by drugs such as *guanethidine* (see p. 91).

4. **Binding to α receptor:** Norepinephrine released from the synaptic vesicles diffuses across the synaptic space and binds to either postsynaptic receptors on the effector organ or to presynaptic receptors on the nerve ending. The recognition of norepinephrine by the membrane receptors triggers a cascade of events within the cell, resulting in the formation of intracellular second messengers that act as links (transducers) in the communication between the neurotransmitter and the action generated within the effector cell. Adrenergic receptors use both the cyclic adenosine monophosphate (cAMP) second-messenger system,[2] and the phosphatidylinositol cycle,[3] to transduce the signal into an effect.

5. **Removal of norepinephrine:** Norepinephrine may 1) diffuse out of the synaptic space and enter the general circulation, 2) be metabolized to O-methylated derivatives by postsynaptic cell membrane–associated catechol O-methyltransferase (COMT) in the synaptic space, or 3) be recaptured by an uptake system that pumps the norepinephrine back into the neuron. The uptake by the neuronal membrane involves a sodium/potassium-activated ATPase that can be inhibited by tricyclic antidepressants, such as *imipramine*, or by *cocaine* (see Figure 6.3). Uptake of norepinephrine into the presynaptic neuron is the primary mechanism for termination of norepinephrine's effects.

6. **Potential fates of recaptured norepinephrine:** Once norepinephrine reenters the cytoplasm of the adrenergic neuron, it may be taken up into adrenergic vesicles via the amine transporter system and be sequestered for release by another action potential, or it may persist in a protected pool. Alternatively, norepinephrine can be oxidized by monoamine oxidase (MAO) present in neuronal mitochondria. The inactive products of norepinephrine metabolism are excreted in the urine as vanillylmandelic acid, metanephrine, and normetanephrine.

[2]See p. 94 in *Lippincott's Illustrated Reviews: Biochemistry* (4th ed.) for a discussion of the cyclic AMP second messenger system.
[3]See p. 205 in *Lippincott's Illustrated Reviews: Biochemistry* (4th ed.) for a discussion of the phosphatidylinositol cycle.

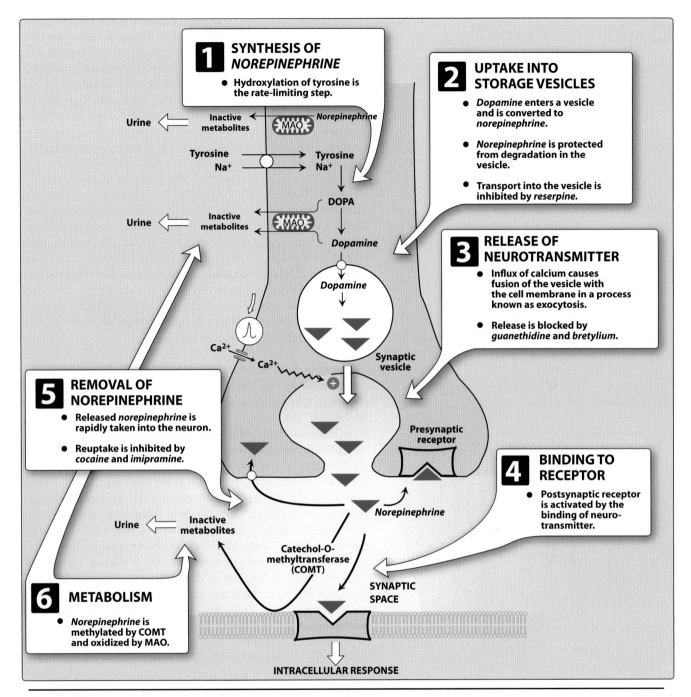

Figure 6.3
Synthesis and release of *norepinephrine* from the adrenergic neuron. (MAO = monoamine oxidase.)

B. Adrenergic receptors (adrenoceptors)

In the sympathetic nervous system, several classes of adrenoceptors can be distinguished pharmacologically. Two families of receptors, designated α and β, were initially identified on the basis of their responses to the adrenergic agonists *epinephrine*, norepinephrine, and *isoproterenol*. The use of specific blocking drugs and the cloning of genes have revealed the molecular identities of a number of receptor subtypes. These proteins belong to a multigene family. Alterations in the primary structure of the receptors influence their affinity for various agents.

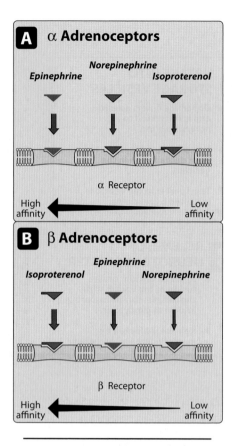

Figure 6.4
Types of adrenergic receptors.

1. α_1 and α_2 **Receptors:** The α-adrenoceptors show a weak response to the synthetic agonist *isoproterenol*, but they are responsive to the naturally occurring catecholamines *epinephrine* and norepinephrine (Figure 6.4). For α receptors, the rank order of potency is *epinephrine* $\geq$ norepinephrine $>>$ *isoproterenol*. The α-adrenoceptors are subdivided into two subgroups, α_1 and α_2, based on their affinities for α agonists and blocking drugs. For example, the α_1 receptors have a higher affinity for *phenylephrine* than do the α_2 receptors. Conversely, the drug *clonidine* selectively binds to α_2 receptors and has less effect on α_1 receptors.

a. α_1 **Receptors:** These receptors are present on the post-synaptic membrane of the effector organs and mediate many of the classic effects—originally designated as α-adrenergic—involving constriction of smooth muscle. Activation of α_1 receptors initiates a series of reactions through a G protein activation of phospholipase C, resulting in the generation of inositol-1,4,5-trisphosphate (IP_3) and diacylglycerol (DAG) from phosphatidylinositol. IP_3 initiates the release of Ca^{2+} from the endoplasmic reticulum into the cytosol, and DAG turns on other proteins within the cell (Figure 6.5).

b. α_2 **Receptors:** These receptors, located primarily on presynaptic nerve endings and on other cells, such as the β cell of the pancreas, and on certain vascular smooth muscle cells, control adrenergic neuromediator and insulin output, respectively. When a sympathetic adrenergic nerve is stimulated, the released norepinephrine traverses the synaptic cleft and interacts with the α_1 receptors. A portion of the released norepinephrine "circles back" and reacts with α_2 receptors on the neuronal membrane (see Figure 6.5). The stimulation of the α_2 receptor causes feedback inhibition of the ongoing release of norepinephrine from the stimulated adrenergic neuron. This inhibitory action decreases further output from the adrenergic neuron and serves as a local modulating mechanism for reducing sympathetic neuromediator output when there is high sympathetic activity. [Note: In this instance these receptors are acting as inhibitory autoreceptors.] α_2 Receptors are also found on presynpatic parasympathetic neurons. Norepinephrine released from a presynaptic sympathetic neuron can diffuse to and interact with these receptors, inhibiting acetylcholine release [Note: In these instances these receptors are behaving as inhibitory heteroreceptors.] This is another local modulating mechanism to control autonomic activity in a given area. In contrast to α_1 receptors, the effects of binding at α_2 receptors are mediated by inhibition of adenylyl cyclase and a fall in the levels of intracellular cAMP.

c. **Further subdivisions:** The α_1 and α_2 receptors are further divided into α_{1A}, α_{1B}, α_{1C}, and α_{1D} and into α_{2A}, α_{2B}, α_{2C}, and α_{2D}. This extended classification is necessary for understanding the selectivity of some drugs. For example, *tamsulosin* is a selective α_{1A} antagonist that is used to treat benign prostate hyperplasia. The drug is clinically useful because it targets α_{1A} receptors found primarily in the urinary tract and prostate gland.

2. **β Receptors:** β Receptors exhibit a set of responses different from those of the α receptors. These are characterized by a strong response to *isoproterenol*, with less sensitivity to *epinephrine* and norepinephrine (see Figure 6.4). For β receptors, the rank order of potency is *isoproterenol* > *epinephrine* > norepinephrine. The β-adrenoceptors can be subdivided into three major subgroups, β_1, β_2, and β_3, based on their affinities for adrenergic agonists and antagonists, although several others have been identified by gene cloning. [It is known that β_3 receptors are involved in lipolysis but their role in other specific reactions are not known] . β_1 Receptors have approximately equal affinities for *epinephrine* and norepinephrine, whereas β_2 receptors have a higher affinity for *epinephrine* than for norepinephrine. Thus, tissues with a predominance of β_2 receptors (such as the vasculature of skeletal muscle) are particularly responsive to the hormonal effects of circulating *epinephrine* released by the adrenal medulla. Binding of a neurotransmitter at any of the three β receptors results in activation of adenylyl cyclase and, therefore, increased concentrations of cAMP within the cell.

3. **Distribution of receptors:** Adrenergically innervated organs and tissues tend to have a predominance of one type of receptor. For example, tissues such as the vasculature to skeletal muscle have both α_1 and β_2 receptors, but the β_2 receptors predominate. Other tissues may have one type of receptor exclusively, with practically no significant numbers of other types of adrenergic receptors. For example, the heart contains predominantly β_1 receptors.

4. **Characteristic responses mediated by adrenoceptors:** It is useful to organize the physiologic responses to adrenergic stimulation according to receptor type, because many drugs preferentially stimulate or block one type of receptor. Figure 6.6 summarizes the most prominent effects mediated by the adrenoceptors. As a generalization, stimulation of α_1 receptors characteristically produces vasoconstriction (particularly in skin and abdominal viscera) and an increase in total peripheral resistance and blood pressure. Conversely, stimulation of β_1 receptors characteristically causes cardiac stimulation, whereas stimulation of β_2 receptors produces vasodilation (in skeletal vascular beds) and bronchiolar relaxation.

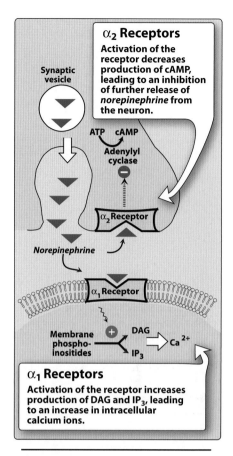

Figure 6.5
Second messengers mediate the effects of α receptors. DAG = diacylglycerol; IP_3 = inositol trisphosphate; ATP = adenosine triphosphate; cAMP = cyclic adenosine monophosphate.

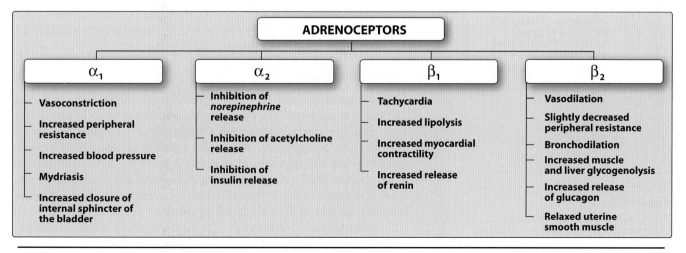

Figure 6.6
Major effects mediated by α and β adrenoceptors.

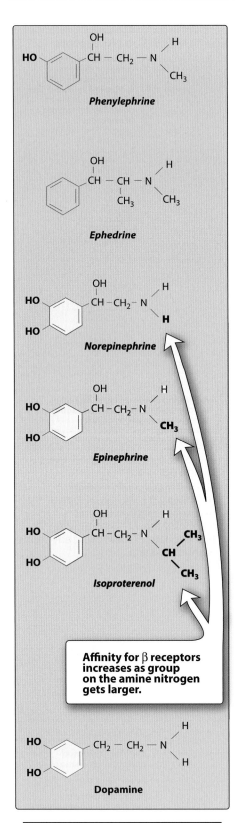

Figure 6.7
Structures of several important adrenergic agonists. Drugs containing the catechol ring are shown in yellow.

5. **Desensitization of receptors:** Prolonged exposure to the catecholamines reduces the responsiveness of these receptors, a phenomenon known as desensitization. Three mechanisms have been suggested to explain this phenomenon: 1) sequestration of the receptors so that they are unavailable for interaction with the ligand; 2) down-regulation, that is, a disappearance of the receptors either by destruction or decreased synthesis; and 3) an inability to couple to G protein, because the receptor has been phosphorylated on the cytoplasmic side by either protein kinase A or β-adrenergic receptor kinase.

III. CHARACTERISTICS OF ADRENERGIC AGONISTS

Most of the adrenergic drugs are derivatives of β-phenylethylamine (Figure 6.7). Substitutions on the benzene ring or on the ethylamine side chains produce a great variety of compounds with varying abilities to differentiate between α and β receptors and to penetrate the CNS. Two important structural features of these drugs are the number and location of OH substitutions on the benzene ring and the nature of the substituent on the amino nitrogen.

A. Catecholamines

Sympathomimetic amines that contain the 3,4-dihydroxybenzene group (such as *epinephrine*, norepinephrine, *isoproterenol*, and *dopamine*) are called catecholamines. These compounds share the following properties:

1. **High potency:** Drugs that are catechol derivatives (with –OH groups in the 3 and 4 positions on the benzene ring) show the highest potency in directly activating α or β receptors.

2. **Rapid inactivation:** Not only are the catecholamines metabolized by COMT postsynaptically and by MAO intraneuronally, they are also metabolized in other tissues. For example, COMT is in the gut wall, and MAO is in the liver and gut wall. Thus, catecholamines have only a brief period of action when given parenterally, and they are ineffective when administered orally because of inactivation.

3. **Poor penetration into the CNS:** Catecholamines are polar and, therefore, do not readily penetrate into the CNS. Nevertheless, most of these drugs have some clinical effects (anxiety, tremor, and headaches) that are attributable to action on the CNS.

B. Noncatecholamines

Compounds lacking the catechol hydroxyl groups have longer half-lives, because they are not inactivated by COMT. These include *phenylephrine*, *ephedrine*, and *amphetamine*. *Phenylephrine*, an analog of *epinephrine*, has only a single –OH at position 3 on the benzene ring, whereas *ephedrine* lacks hydroxyls on the ring but has a methyl substitution at the α-carbon. These are poor substrates for MAO and, thus, show a prolonged duration of action, because MAO is an important route of detoxification. Increased lipid solubility of many of the noncatecholamines (due to lack of polar hydroxyl groups) permits greater access to the CNS. [Note: *Ephedrine* and *amphetamine* may act indirectly by causing the release of stored catecholamines.]

C. Substitutions on the amine nitrogen

The nature and bulk of the substituent on the amine nitrogen is important in determining the β selectivity of the adrenergic agonist. For example, *epinephrine*, with a $-CH_3$ substituent on the amine nitrogen, is more potent at β receptors than norepinephrine, which has an unsubstituted amine. Similarly, *isoproterenol*, with an isopropyl substituent $-CH(CH_3)_2$ on the amine nitrogen (see Figure 6.7), is a strong β agonist with little α activity (see Figure 6.4).

D. Mechanism of action of the adrenergic agonists

1. **Direct-acting agonists:** These drugs act directly on α or β receptors, producing effects similar to those that occur following stimulation of sympathetic nerves or release of the hormone *epinephrine* from the adrenal medulla (Figure 6.8). Examples of direct-acting agonists include *epinephrine*, norepinephrine, *isoproterenol*, and *phenylephrine*.

2. **Indirect-acting agonists:** These agents, which include *amphetamine,* cocaine and tyramine, may block the uptake of norepinephrine (uptake blockers) or are taken up into the presynaptic neuron and cause the release of norepinephrine from the cytoplasmic pools or vesicles of the adrenergic neuron (see Figure 6.8). As with neuronal stimulation, the norepinephrine then traverses the synapse and binds to the α or β receptors. Examples of uptake blockers and agents that cause norepinephrine release include *cocaine* and amphetamines, respectively.

3. **Mixed-action agonists:** Some agonists, such as *ephedrine, pseudoephedrine* and *metaraminol*, have the capacity both to stimulate adrenoceptors directly and to release norepinephrine from the adrenergic neuron (see Figure 6.8).

IV. DIRECT-ACTING ADRENERGIC AGONISTS

Direct-acting agonists bind to adrenergic receptors without interacting with the presynaptic neuron. The activated receptor initiates synthesis of second messengers and subsequent intracellular signals. As a group, these agents are widely used clinically.

A. Epinephrine

Epinephrine [ep-i-NEF-rin] is one of four catecholamines—*epinephrine*, norepinephrine, *dopamine*, and *dobutamine*—commonly used in therapy. The first three catecholamines occur naturally in the body as neurotransmitters; the latter is a synthetic compound. *Epinephrine* is synthesized from tyrosine in the adrenal medulla and released, along with small quantities of norepinephrine, into the bloodstream. *Epinephrine* interacts with both α and β receptors. At low doses, β effects (vasodilation) on the vascular system predominate, whereas at high doses, α effects (vasoconstriction) are strongest.

1. **Actions:**

   a. **Cardiovascular:** The major actions of *epinephrine* are on the cardiovascular system. *Epinephrine* strengthens the contractility of the myocardium (positive inotropic: $β_1$ action) and increases its rate of contraction (positive chronotropic: $β_1$ action). Cardiac

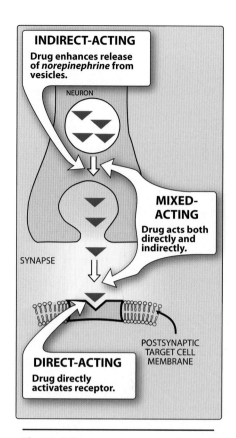

Figure 6.8
Sites of action of direct-, indirect-, and mixed-acting adrenergic agonists.

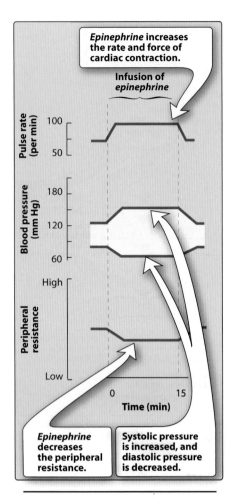

Figure 6.9
Cardiovascular effects of intravenous infusion of low doses of *epinephrine*.

output therefore increases. With these effects comes increased oxygen demands on the myocardium. *Epinephrine* constricts arterioles in the skin, mucous membranes, and viscera (α effects), and it dilates vessels going to the liver and skeletal muscle (β_2 effects). Renal blood flow is decreased. Therefore, the cumulative effect is an increase in systolic blood pressure, coupled with a slight decrease in diastolic pressure (Figure 6.9).

b. Respiratory: *Epinephrine* causes powerful bronchodilation by acting directly on bronchial smooth muscle (β_2 action). This action relieves all known allergic- or histamine-induced bronchoconstriction. In the case of anaphylactic shock, this can be lifesaving. In individuals suffering from an acute asthmatic attack, *epinephrine* rapidly relieves the dyspnea (labored breathing) and increases the tidal volume (volume of gases inspired and expired). *Epinephrine* also inhibits the release of allergy mediators such as histamines from mast cells.

c. Hyperglycemia: *Epinephrine* has a significant hyperglycemic effect because of increased glycogenolysis in the liver (β_2 effect), increased release of glucagon (β_2 effect), and a decreased release of insulin (α_2 effect). These effects are mediated via the cAMP mechanism.

d. Lipolysis: *Epinephrine* initiates lipolysis through its agonist activity on the β receptors of adipose tissue, which upon stimulation activate adenylyl cyclase to increase cAMP levels. Cyclic AMP stimulates a hormone-sensitive lipase, which hydrolyzes triacylglycerols to free fatty acids and glycerol.[4]

2. **Biotransformations:** *Epinephrine*, like the other catecholamines, is metabolized by two enzymatic pathways: MAO, and COMT, which has S-adenosylmethionine as a cofactor (see Figure 6.3). The final metabolites found in the urine are metanephrine and vanillylmandelic acid. [Note: Urine also contains normetanephrine, a product of norepinephrine metabolism.]

3. **Therapeutic uses**

   a. Bronchospasm: *Epinephrine* is the primary drug used in the emergency treatment of any condition of the respiratory tract when bronchoconstriction has resulted in diminished respiratory exchange. Thus, in treatment of acute asthma and anaphylactic shock, *epinephrine* is the drug of choice; within a few minutes after subcutaneous administration, greatly improved respiratory exchange is observed. Administration may be repeated after a few hours. However, selective β_2 agonists, such as *albuterol*, are presently favored in the chronic treatment of asthma because of a longer duration of action and minimal cardiac stimulatory effect.

---

 [4]See p. 190 in ***Lippincott's Illustrated Reviews: Biochemistry*** (4th ed.) for a discussion of hormone-sensitive lipase activity.

b. **Glaucoma:** In ophthalmology, a two-percent *epinephrine* solution may be used topically to reduce intraocular pressure in open-angle glaucoma. It reduces the production of aqueous humor by vasoconstriction of the ciliary body blood vessels.

c. **Anaphylactic shock:** *Epinephrine* is the drug of choice for the treatment of Type I hypersensitivity reactions in response to allergens.

d. **Cardiac arrest:** *Epinephrine* may be used to restore cardiac rhythm in patients with cardiac arrest regardless of the cause.

e. **Anesthetics:** Local anesthetic solutions usually contain 1:100,000 parts *epinephrine*. The effect of the drug is to greatly increase the duration of the local anesthesia. It does this by producing vasoconstriction at the site of injection, thereby allowing the local anesthetic to persist at the injection site before being absorbed into the circulation and metabolized. Very weak solutions of *epinephrine* (1:100,000) can also be used topically to vasoconstrict mucous membranes to control oozing of capillary blood.

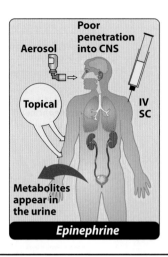

Figure 6.10
Pharmacokinetics of *epinephrine*.

4. **Pharmacokinetics:** *Epinephrine* has a rapid onset but a brief duration of action (due to rapid degradation). In emergency situations, *epinephrine* is given intravenously for the most rapid onset of action. It may also be given subcutaneously, by endotracheal tube, by inhalation, or topically to the eye (Figure 6.10). Oral administration is ineffective, because *epinephrine* and the other catecholamines are inactivated by intestinal enzymes. Only metabolites are excreted in the urine.

5. **Adverse effects:**

a. **CNS disturbances:** *Epinephrine* can produce adverse CNS effects that include anxiety, fear, tension, headache, and tremor.

b. **Hemorrhage:** The drug may induce cerebral hemorrhage as a result of a marked elevation of blood pressure.

c. **Cardiac arrhythmias:** *Epinephrine* can trigger cardiac arrhythmias, particularly if the patient is receiving digitalis.

d. **Pulmonary edema:** *Epinephrine* can induce pulmonary edema.

6. **Interactions:**

a. **Hyperthyroidism:** *Epinephrine* may have enhanced cardiovascular actions in patients with hyperthyroidism. If *epinephrine* is required in such an individual, the dose must be reduced. The mechanism appears to involve increased production of adrenergic receptors on the vasculature of the hyperthyroid individual, leading to a hypersensitive response.

b. **Cocaine:** In the presence of *cocaine*, *epinephrine* produces exaggerated cardiovascular actions. This is due to the ability of cocaine to prevent reuptake of catecholamines into the adrenergic neuron; thus, like norepinephrine, *epinephrine* remains at the receptor site for longer periods of time (see Figure 6.3).

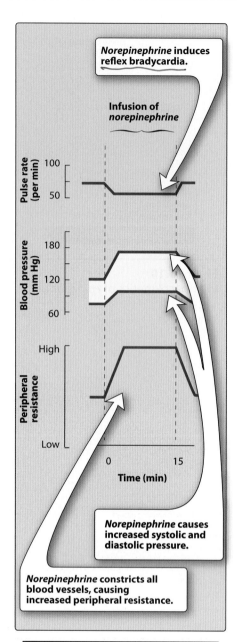

Figure 6.11
Cardiovascular effects of intravenous infusion of *norepinephrine*.

c. Diabetes: *Epinephrine* increases the release of endogenous stores of glucose. In the diabetic, dosages of insulin may have to be increased.

d. β-Blockers: These agents prevent *epinephrine*'s effects on β receptors, leaving α-receptor stimulation unopposed. This may lead to an increase in peripheral resistance and an increase in blood pressure.

e. Inhalation anesthetics: Inhalational anesthetics sensitize the heart to the effects of *epinephrine,* which may lead to tachycardia.

B. Norepinephrine

Because norepinephrine [nor-ep-i-NEF-rin] is the neuromediator of adrenergic nerves, it should theoretically stimulate all types of adrenergic receptors. In practice, when the drug is given in therapeutic doses to humans, the α-adrenergic receptor is most affected.

1. Cardiovascular actions:

a. Vasoconstriction: Norepinephrine causes a rise in peripheral resistance due to intense vasoconstriction of most vascular beds, including the kidney (α_1 effect). Both systolic and diastolic blood pressures increase (Figure 6.11). [Note: Norepinephrine causes greater vasoconstriction than does *epinephrine,* because it does not induce compensatory vasodilation via β_2 receptors on blood vessels supplying skeletal muscles, etc. The weak β_2 activity of norepinephrine also explains why it is not useful in the treatment of asthma.]

b. Baroreceptor reflex: In isolated cardiac tissue, norepinephrine stimulates cardiac contractility; however, in vivo, little if any cardiac stimulation is noted. This is due to the increased blood pressure that induces a reflex rise in vagal activity by stimulating the baroreceptors. This reflex bradycardia is sufficient to counteract the local actions of norepinephrine on the heart, although the reflex compensation does not affect the positive inotropic effects of the drug (see Figure 6.11).

c. Effect of atropine pretreatment: If *atropine,* which blocks the transmission of vagal effects, is given before norepinephrine, then norepinephrine stimulation of the heart is evident as tachycardia.

2. Therapeutic uses: Norepinephrine is used to treat shock, because it increases vascular resistance and, therefore, increases blood pressure. However, *metaraminol* is favored, because it does not reduce blood flow to the kidney, as does norepinephrine. Other actions of norepinephrine are not considered to be clinically significant. It is never used for asthma or in combination with local anesthetics. Norepinephrine is a potent vasoconstrictor and will cause extravasation (discharge of blood from vessel into tissues) along the injection site. [Note: When norepinephrine is used as a drug, it is sometimes called *levarterenol* [leev-are-TER-a-nole].]

3. Pharmacokinetics: Norepinephrine may be given IV for rapid onset of action. The duration of action is 1 to 2 minutes following the end of the infusion period. It is poorly absorbed after subcutaneous injection and is destroyed in the gut if administered orally. Metabolism is similar to that of *epinephrine*.

4. **Adverse effects:** These are similar to those of *epinephrine*. In addition, norepinephrine may cause blanching and sloughing of skin along injected vein (due to extreme vasoconstriction).

C. Isoproterenol

Isoproterenol [eye-soe-proe-TER-e-nole] is a direct-acting synthetic catecholamine that predominantly stimulates both β₁- and β₂-adrenergic receptors. Its nonselectivity is one of its drawbacks and the reason why it is rarely used therapeutically. Its action on α receptors is insignificant.

1. **Actions:**

    a. **Cardiovascular:** *Isoproterenol* produces intense stimulation of the heart to increase its rate and force of contraction, causing increased cardiac output (Figure 6.12). It is as active as *epinephrine* in this action and, therefore, is useful in the treatment of atrioventricular block or cardiac arrest. *Isoproterenol* also dilates the arterioles of skeletal muscle (β₂ effect), resulting in decreased peripheral resistance. Because of its cardiac stimulatory action, it may increase systolic blood pressure slightly, but it greatly reduces mean arterial and diastolic blood pressure (see Figure 6.12).

    b. **Pulmonary:** A profound and rapid bronchodilation is produced by the drug (β₂ action, Figure 6.13). *Isoproterenol* is as active as *epinephrine* and rapidly alleviates an acute attack of asthma when taken by inhalation (which is the recommended route). This action lasts about 1 hour and may be repeated by subsequent doses.

    c. **Other effects:** Other actions on β receptors, such as increased blood sugar and increased lipolysis, can be demonstrated but are not clinically significant.

2. **Therapeutic uses:** *Isoproterenol* is now rarely used as a bronchodilator in asthma. It can be employed to stimulate the heart in emergency situations.

3. **Pharmacokinetics:** *Isoproterenol* can be absorbed systemically by the sublingual mucosa but is more reliably absorbed when given parenterally or as an inhaled aerosol. It is a marginal substrate for COMT and is stable to MAO action.

4. **Adverse effects:** The adverse effects of *isoproterenol* are similar to those of *epinephrine*.

D. Dopamine

Dopamine [DOE-pa-meen], the immediate metabolic precursor of norepinephrine, occurs naturally in the CNS in the basal ganglia, where it functions as a neurotransmitter, as well as in the adrenal medulla. *Dopamine* can activate α- and β-adrenergic receptors. For example, at higher doses, it can cause vasoconstriction by activating α₁ receptors, whereas at lower doses, it stimulates β₁ cardiac receptors. In addition, D₁ and D₂ dopaminergic receptors, distinct from the α- and β-adrenergic receptors, occur in the peripheral mesenteric and renal vascular beds, where binding of *dopamine* produces vasodilation. D₂ receptors are

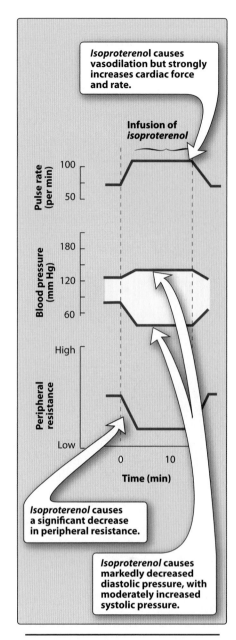

Figure 6.12
Cardiovascular effects of intravenous infusion of *isoproterenol*.

mimics   epinephrine

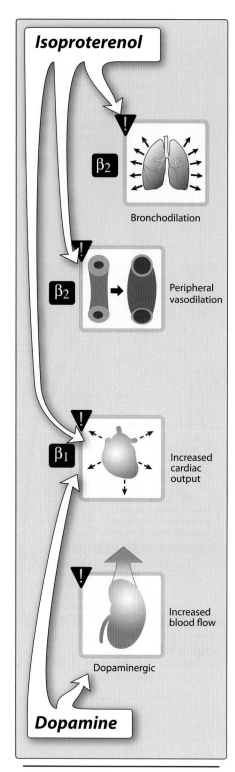

Figure 6.13
Clinically important actions of
isoproterenol and *dopamine*.

also found on presynaptic adrenergic neurons, where their activation interferes with norepinephrine release.

1. **Actions:**

   a. **Cardiovascular:** *Dopamine* exerts a stimulatory effect on the β_1 receptors of the heart, having both inotropic and chronotropic effects (see Figure 6.13). At very high doses, *dopamine* activates α_1 receptors on the vasculature, resulting in vasoconstriction.

   b. **Renal and visceral:** *Dopamine* dilates renal and splanchnic arterioles by activating dopaminergic receptors, thus increasing blood flow to the kidneys and other viscera (see Figure 6.13). These receptors are not affected by α- or β-blocking drugs. Therefore, *dopamine* is clinically useful in the treatment of shock, in which significant increases in sympathetic activity might compromise renal function. [Note: Similar *dopamine* receptors are found in the autonomic ganglia and in the CNS.]

2. **Therapeutic uses:** *Dopamine* is the drug of choice for shock and is given by continuous infusion. It raises the blood pressure by stimulating the β_1 receptors on the heart to increase cardiac output, and α_1 receptors on blood vessels to increase total peripheral resistance. In addition, it enhances perfusion to the kidney and splanchnic areas, as described above. An increased blood flow to the kidney enhances the glomerular filtration rate and causes sodium diuresis. In this regard, *dopamine* is far superior to norepinephrine, which diminishes the blood supply to the kidney and may cause renal shutdown.

3. **Adverse effects:** An overdose of *dopamine* produces the same effects as sympathetic stimulation. *Dopamine* is rapidly metabolized to homovanillic acid by MAO or COMT, and its adverse effects (nausea, hypertension, arrhythmias) are therefore short-lived.

E. **Dobutamine**

1. **Actions:** *Dobutamine* [doe-BYOO-ta-meen] is a synthetic, direct-acting catecholamine that is a β_1-receptor agonist. It is available as a racemic mixture. One of the stereoisomers has a stimulatory activity. It increases cardiac rate and output with few vascular effects.

2. **Therapeutic uses:** *Dobutamine* is used to increase cardiac output in congestive heart failure (see p. 194) as well as for inotropic support after cardiac surgery. The drug increases cardiac output with little change in heart rate, and it does not significantly elevate oxygen demands of the myocardium—a major advantage over other sympathomimetic drugs.

3. **Adverse effects:** *Dobutamine* should be used with caution in atrial fibrillation, because the drug increases atrioventricular conduction. Other adverse effects are the same as those for *epinephrine*. Tolerance may develop on prolonged use.

F. **Oxymetazoline**

Oxymetazoline [ok-see-met-AZ-of-leen] is a direct-acting synthetic adrenergic agonist that stimulates both α_1- and α_2-adrenergic receptors. It is primarily used locally in the eye or the nose as a vasoconstrictor. *Oxymetazoline* is found in many over-the-counter short-term nasal spray decongestant products as well as in ophthalmic drops for the relief of redness of the eyes associated with swimming, colds, or contact lens. The mechanism of action of *oxymetazoline* is direct stimulation of α receptors on blood vessels supplying the nasal mucosa and the conjunctiva to reduce blood flow and decrease congestion. *Oxymetazoline* is absorbed in the systemic circulation regardless of the route of administration and may produce nervousness, headaches, and trouble sleeping. When administered in the nose, burning of the nasal mucosa and sneezing may occur. Rebound congestion is observed with long-term use.

G. Phenylephrine

Phenylephrine [fen-ill-EF-rin] is a direct-acting, synthetic adrenergic drug that binds primarily to α receptors and favors α_1 receptors over α_2 receptors. It is not a catechol derivative and, therefore, not a substrate for COMT. *Phenylephrine* is a vasoconstrictor that raises both systolic and diastolic blood pressures. It has no effect on the heart itself but rather induces reflex bradycardia when given parenterally. It is often used topically on the nasal mucous membranes and in ophthalmic solutions for mydriasis. *Phenylephrine* acts as a nasal decongestant and produces prolonged vasoconstriction. The drug is used to raise blood pressure and to terminate episodes of supraventricular tachycardia (rapid heart action arising both from the atrioventricular junction and atria). Large doses can cause hypertensive headache and cardiac irregularities.

H. Methoxamine

Methoxamine [meth-OX-a-meen] is a direct-acting, synthetic adrenergic drug that binds primarily to α receptors, with α_1 receptors favored over α_2 receptors. *Methoxamine* raises blood pressure by stimulating α_1 receptors in the arterioles, causing vasoconstriction. This causes an increase in total peripheral resistance. Because of its effects on the vagus nerve, *methoxamine* is used clinically to relieve attacks of paroxysmal supraventricular tachycardia. It is also used to overcome hypotension during surgery involving *halothane* anesthetics. In contrast to most other adrenergic drugs, *methoxamine* does not tend to trigger cardiac arrhythmias in the heart, which is sensitized by these general anesthetics. Adverse effects include hypertensive headache and vomiting.

I. Clonidine

Clonidine [KLOE-ni-deen] is an α_2 agonist that is used in essential hypertension to lower blood pressure because of its action in the CNS (see p. 225). It can be used to minimize the symptoms that accompany withdrawal from opiates or benzodiazepines. *Clonidine* acts centrally to produce inhibition of sympathetic vasomotor centers, decreasing sympathetic outflow to the periphery.

J. Metaproterenol

Metaproterenol [met-a-proe-TER-a-nole], although chemically similar to *isoproterenol*, is not a catecholamine, and it is resistant to methylation by COMT. It can be administered orally or by inhalation. The drug acts primarily at β_2 receptors, producing little effect on the heart. *Metaproterenol* produces dilation of the bronchioles and improves airway function. The drug is useful as a bronchodilator in the treatment of asthma and to reverse bronchospasm (Figure 6.14).

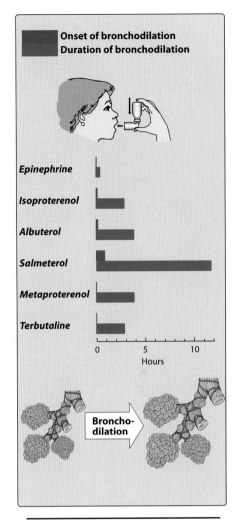

Figure 6.14
Onset and duration of bronchodilation effects of inhaled adrenergic agonists.

K. Albuterol, pirbuterol, and terbutaline

Albuterol [al-BYOO-ter-ole], *pirbuterol* [peer-BYOO-ter-ole], and *terbutaline* [ter-BYOO-te-leen] are short-acting β₂ agonists used primarily as bronchodilators and administered by a metered-dose inhaler (see Figure 6.14). Compared with the nonselective β-adrenergic agonists, such as *metaproterenol*, these drugs produce equivalent bronchodilation with less cardiac stimulation.

L. Salmeterol and formoterol

Salmeterol [sal-ME-ter-ole] and *formoterol* [for-MOH-ter-ole] are β₂-adrenergic selective, long-acting bronchodilators. A single dose by a metered-dose inhalation device, such as a dry powder inhaler, provides sustained bronchodilation over 12 hours, compared with less than 3 hours for *albuterol*. Unlike *formoterol*, however, *salmeterol* has a somewhat delayed onset of action (see Figure 6.14). These agents are not recommended as monotherapy and are highly efficacious when combined with a corticorsteroid. *Salmeterol* and *formoterol* are the agents of choice for treating nocturnal asthma in symptomatic patients taking other asthma medications.

V. INDIRECT-ACTING ADRENERGIC AGONISTS

Indirect-acting adrenergic agonists cause norepinephrine release from presynaptic terminals or inhibit the uptake of norepinephrine (see Figure 6.8). They potentiate the effects of norepinephrine produced endogenously, but these agents do not directly affect postsynaptic receptors.

A. Amphetamine

The marked central stimulatory action of *amphetamine* [am-FET-a-meen] is often mistaken by drug abusers as its only action. However, the drug can increase blood pressure significantly by α-agonist action on the vasculature as well as β-stimulatory effects on the heart. Its peripheral actions are mediated primarily through the blockade of norepinephrine uptake and cellular release of stored catecholamines; thus, *amphetamine* is an indirect-acting adrenergic drug. The actions and uses of amphetamines are discussed under stimulants of the CNS (see p. 121). The CNS stimulant effects of *amphetamine* and its derivatives have led to their use for treating hyperactivity in children, narcolepsy, and appetite control. Its use in pregnancy should be avoided because of adverse effects on development of the fetus.

B. Tyramine

Tyramine [TIE-ra-meen] is not a clinically useful drug, but it is important because it is found in fermented foods, such as ripe cheese and Chianti wine (see MAO inhibitors, p. 145). It is a normal byproduct of tyrosine metabolism. Normally, it is oxidized by MAO in the gastrointestinal tract, but if the patient is taking MAO inhibitors, it can precipitate serious vasopressor episodes. Like amphetamines, tyramine can enter the nerve terminal and displace stored norepinephrine. The released catecholamine then acts on adrenoceptors.

C. Cocaine

Cocaine [koe-KANE] is unique among local anesthetics in having the ability to block the Na⁺/K⁺-activated ATPase (required for cellular uptake of norepinephrine) on the cell membrane of the adrenergic neuron. Consequently, norepinephrine accumulates in the synaptic space, resulting in enhancement of sympathetic activity and potentiation of the actions of *epinephrine* and norepinephrine. Therefore, small doses of the catecholamines produce greatly magnified effects in an individual taking *cocaine* as compared to those in one who is not. In addition, the duration of action of *epinephrine* and norepinephrine is increased. Like amphetamines, it can increase blood pressure by α-agonist actions and β-stimulatory effects. [Note: *Cocaine* as a CNS stimulant and drug of abuse is discussed on p. 118.]

VI. MIXED-ACTION ADRENERGIC AGONISTS

Mixed-action drugs induce the release of norepinephrine from presynaptic terminals, and they activate adrenergic receptors on the postsynaptic membrane (see Figure 6.8).

A. Ephedrine and pseudoephedrine

Ephedrine [e-FED-rin], and *pseudoephedrine* [soo-doe-e-FED-rin] are plant alkaloids, that are now made synthetically. These drugs are mixed-action adrenergic agents. They not only release stored norepinephrine from nerve endings (see Figure 6.8) but also directly stimulate both α and β receptors. Thus, a wide variety of adrenergic actions ensue that are similar to those of *epinephrine*, although less potent. *Ephedrine* and *pseudoephedrine* are not catechols and are poor substrates for COMT and MAO; thus, these drugs have a long duration of action. *Ephedrine* and *pseudoephedrine* have excellent absorption orally and penetrate into the CNS; however, *pseudoephedrine* has fewer CNS effects. *Ephedrine* is eliminated largely unchanged in the urine, and *pseudoephedrine* undergoes incomplete hepatic metabolism before elimination in the urine. *Ephedrine* raises systolic and diastolic blood pressures by vasoconstriction and cardiac stimulation. *Ephedrine* produces bronchodilation, but it is less potent than *epinephrine* or *isoproterenol* in this regard and produces its action more slowly. It is therefore sometimes used prophylactically in chronic treatment of asthma to prevent attacks rather than to treat the acute attack. *Ephedrine* enhances contractility and improves motor function in myasthenia gravis, particularly when used in conjunction with anticholinesterases (see p. 50). *Ephedrine* produces a mild stimulation of the CNS. This increases alertness, decreases fatigue, and prevents sleep. It also improves athletic performance. *Ephedrine* has been used to treat asthma, as a nasal decongestant (due to its local vasoconstrictor action), and to raise blood pressure. *Pseudoephedrine* is primarily used to treat nasal and sinus congestion or congestion of the eustachian tubes. [Note: The clinical use of *ephedrine* is declining due to the availability of better, more potent agents that cause fewer adverse effects. *Ephedrine*-containing herbal supplements (mainly ephedra-containing products) were banned by the U.S. Food and Drug Administration in April 2004 because of life-threatening cardiovascular reactions. *Pseudoephedrine* has been illegally converted to *methamphetamine*. Thus, products containing *pseudoephedrine* have certain restrictions and must be kept behind the sales counter.]

Important characteristics of the adrenergic agonists are summarized in Figures 6.15, 6.16 and 6.17.

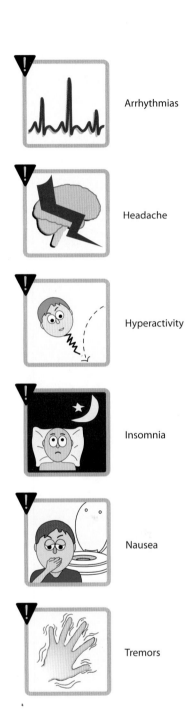

Figure 6.15
Some adverse effects observed with adrenergic agonists.

TISSUE	RECEPTOR TYPE	ACTION	OPPOSING ACTIONS
Heart			
• Sinus and AV	β₁	↑ Automaticity	Cholinergic receptors
• Conduction pathway	β₁	↑ Conduction velocity, automaticity	Cholinergic receptors
• Myofibrils	β₁	↑ Contractility, automaticity	
Vascular smooth muscle	β₂	Vasodilation	α-Adrenergic receptors
Bronchial smooth muscle	β₂	Bronchodilation	Cholinergic receptors
Kidneys	β₁	↑ Renin release	α₁-Adrenergic receptors
Liver	β₂	↑ Glucose metabolism, lipolysis	α₁-Adrenergic receptors
Adipose tissue	β₃	↑ Lipolysis	α₂-Adrenergic receptors
Skeletal muscle	β₂	↑ Potassium uptake, glycogenolysis Dilates arteries to skeletal muscle	—
Eye-ciliary muscle	β₂	Relaxation	Cholinergic receptors
GI tract	β₂	↓ Motility	Cholinergic receptors
Gall bladder	β₂	Relaxation	Cholinergic receptors
Urinary bladder detrusor muscle	β₂	Relaxation	Cholinergic receptors
Uterus	β₂	Relaxation	Oxytocin

Figure 6.16
Summary of β-adrenergic receptors

DRUG	RECEPTOR SPECIFICITY	THERAPEUTIC USES
Epinephrine	α_1, α_2 β_1, β_2	**Acute asthma** **Treatment of open-angle glaucoma** **Anaphylactic shock** **In local anesthetics to increase duration of action**
Norepinephrine	α_1, α_2 β_1	**Treatment of shock**
Isoproterenol	β_1, β_2	**As a cardiac stimulant**
Dopamine	Dopaminergic α_1, β_1	**Treatment of shock** **Treatment of congestive heart failure** **Raise blood pressure**
Dobutamine	β_1	**Treatment of congestive heart failure**
Oxymetazoline	α_1	**As a nasal decongestant**
Phenylephrine	α_1	**As a nasal decongestant** **Raise blood pressure** **Treatment of paroxysmal supraventricular tachycardia**
Methoxamine	α_1	**Treatment of supraventricular tachycardia**
Clonidine	α_2	**Treatment of hypertension**
Metaproterenol	$\beta_2 > \beta_1$	**Treatment of bronchospasm and asthma**
Albuterol *Pirbuterol* *Terbutaline*	β_2	**Treatment of bronchospasm (short acting)**
Salmeterol *Formoterol*	β_2	**Treatment of bronchospasm (long acting)**
Amphetamine	α, β, CNS	**As a CNS stimulant in treatment of children with attention deficit syndrome, narcolepsy, and appetite control**
Ephedrine *Pseudoephedrine*	α, β, CNS	**Treatment of asthma** **As a nasal decongestant** **Raise blood pressure**

CATECHOLAMINES
- Rapid onset of action
- Brief duration of action
- Not administered orally
- Do not penetrate the blood-brain barrier

NONCATECHOL-AMINES

Compared to catecholamines:
- Longer duration of action
- All can be administered orally

Figure 6.17
Summary of the therapeutic uses of adrenergic agonists.

Study Questions

Choose the ONE best answer.

6.1 A 68-year-old man presents to the emergency department with acute heart failure. You decide that this patient requires immediate drug therapy to improve his cardiac function. Which one of the following drugs would be most beneficial?

   A. Albuterol.
   B. Dobutamine.
   C. Epinephrine.
   D. Norepinephrine.
   E. Phenylephrine.

6.2 Remedies for nasal stuffiness often contain which one of the following drugs?

   A. Albuterol.
   B. Atropine.
   C. Epinephrine.
   D. Norepinephrine.
   E. Phenylephrine.

6.3 Which one of the following drugs, when administered intravenously, can decrease blood flow to the skin, increase blood flow to skeletal muscle, and increase the force and rate of cardiac contraction?

   A. Epinephrine.
   B. Isoproterenol.
   C. Norepinephrine.
   D. Phenylephrine.
   E. Terbutaline.

6.4 The following circles represent pupillary diameter in one eye prior to and following the topical application of Drug X:

Control   Drug X

Which of the following is most likely to be Drug X?

   A. Physostigmine.
   B. Acetylcholine.
   C. Terbutaline.
   D. Phenylephrine.
   E. Isoproterenol.

Correct answer = B. Dobutamine increases cardiac output without significantly increasing heart rate—a complicating condition in heart failure. Because epinephrine can significantly increase heart rate, it is not usually employed for acute heart failure. Both norepinephrine and phenylephrine have significant α_1-receptor–stimulating properties. The subsequent increase in blood pressure would worsen the heart failure. Albuterol, a β_2-selective–receptor agonist, would not improve contractility of the heart significantly.

Correct answer = E. Phenylephrine is an α agonist that constricts the nasal mucosa, thereby decreasing airway resistance. Norepinephrine and epinephrine also constrict the mucosa but have much too short a duration of action. Albuterol is a β_2 agonist and has no effect on mucosal volume. Atropine, a muscarinic antagonist, only dries the mucosa—it does not decrease its volume.

Correct answer = A. Exogenous epinephrine stimulates α and β receptors equally well, leading to the constriction of blood vessels in tissues such as skin and dilation of other blood vessels in tissues such as skeletal muscle. Epinephrine also has positive chronotropic and inotropic effects in the heart. Exogenous norepinephrine constricts blood vessels only and causes a reflex bradycardia because of its strong α-adrenergic–stimulating properties. Phenylephrine has similar effects. Isoproterenol stimulates β receptors and would not cause vasoconstriction of cutaneous vessels.

Correct answer = D. Phenylephrine is the only drug in the list that causes mydriasis, because it stimulates α receptors. Both physostigmine and acetylcholine cause pupillary constriction. The β-blockers, terbutaline and isoproterenol, do not influence pupillary diameter.

Adrenergic Antagonists

7

I. OVERVIEW

The adrenergic antagonists (also called blockers or sympatholytic agents) bind to adrenoceptors but do not trigger the usual receptor-mediated intracellular effects. These drugs act by either reversibly or irreversibly attaching to the receptor, thus preventing its activation by endogenous catecholamines. Like the agonists, the adrenergic antagonists are classified according to their relative affinities for α or β receptors in the peripheral nervous system. [Note: Antagonists that block dopamine receptors are most important in the central nervous system (CNS) and are therefore considered in that section (see p. 151).] The receptor-blocking drugs discussed in this chapter are summarized in Figure 7.1.

II. α-ADRENERGIC BLOCKING AGENTS

Drugs that block α-adrenoceptors profoundly affect blood pressure. Because normal sympathetic control of the vasculature occurs in large part through agonist actions on α-adrenergic receptors, blockade of these receptors reduces the sympathetic tone of the blood vessels, resulting in decreased peripheral vascular resistance. This induces a reflex tachycardia resulting from the lowered blood pressure. [Note: β receptors, including β_1-adrenoceptors on the heart, are not affected by α blockade.] The α-adrenergic blocking agents, *phenoxybenzamine* and *phentolamine*, have limited clinical applications.

A. Phenoxybenzamine

Phenoxybenzamine [fen-ox-ee-BEN-za-meen] is nonselective, linking covalently to both α_1-postsynaptic and α_2-presynaptic receptors (Figure 7.2). The block is irreversible and noncompetitive, and the only mechanism the body has for overcoming the block is to synthesize new adrenoceptors, which requires a day or more. Therefore, the actions of *phenoxybenzamine* last about 24 hours after a single administration. After the drug is injected, a delay of a few hours occurs before α blockade develops, because the molecule must undergo biotransformation to the active form.

1. Actions:

a. Cardiovascular effects: By blocking α receptors, *phenoxybenzamine* prevents vasoconstriction of peripheral blood vessels by endogenous catecholamines. The decreased peripheral resistance provokes a reflex tachycardia. Furthermore, the

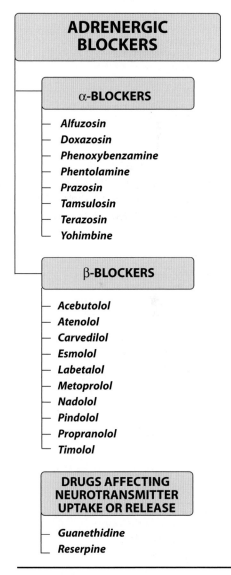

ADRENERGIC BLOCKERS

α-BLOCKERS

— *Alfuzosin*
— *Doxazosin*
— *Phenoxybenzamine*
— *Phentolamine*
— *Prazosin*
— *Tamsulosin*
— *Terazosin*
— *Yohimbine*

β-BLOCKERS

— *Acebutolol*
— *Atenolol*
— *Carvedilol*
— *Esmolol*
— *Labetalol*
— *Metoprolol*
— *Nadolol*
— *Pindolol*
— *Propranolol*
— *Timolol*

DRUGS AFFECTING NEUROTRANSMITTER UPTAKE OR RELEASE

— *Guanethidine*
— *Reserpine*

Figure 7.1
Summary of blocking agents and drugs affecting neurotransmitter uptake or release.

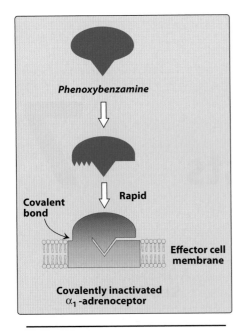

Figure 7.2
Covalent inactivation of α_1 adrenoceptor by *phenoxybenzamine*.

ability to block presynaptic inhibitory α_2 receptors in the heart can contribute to an increased cardiac output. [Note: These receptors when blocked will result in more norepinephrine release, which stimulates β receptors on the heart to increase cardiac output]. Thus, the drug has been unsuccessful in maintaining lowered blood pressure in hypertension and has been discontinued for this purpose.

  b. Epinephrine reversal: All α-adrenergic blockers reverse the α-agonist actions of *epinephrine*. For example, the vasoconstrictive action of *epinephrine* is interrupted, but vasodilation of other vascular beds caused by stimulation of β receptors is not blocked. Therefore, the systemic blood pressure decreases in response to *epinephrine* given in the presence of *phenoxybenzamine* (Figure 7.3). [Note: The actions of norepinephrine are not reversed but are diminished, because norepinephrine lacks significant β-agonist action on the vasculature.] *Phenoxybenzamine* has no effect on the actions of *isoproterenol*, which is a pure β agonist (see Figure 7.3).

2. **Therapeutic uses:** *Phenoxybenzamine* is used in the treatment of pheochromocytoma, a catecholamine-secreting tumor of cells derived from the adrenal medulla. Prior to surgical removal of the tumor, patients are treated with *phenoxybenzamine* to preclude the hypertensive crisis that can result from manipulation of the tissue. This drug is also useful in the chronic management of these tumors, particularly when the catecholamine-secreting cells are diffuse and, therefore, inoperable. *Phenoxybenzamine* or *phentolamine* are sometimes effective in treating Raynaud's disease. Autonomic hyperreflexia, which predisposes paraplegics to strokes, can be managed with *phenoxybenzamine*.

3. **Adverse effects:** *Phenoxybenzamine* can cause postural hypotension, nasal stuffiness, nausea, and vomiting. It can inhibit ejaculation. The drug also may induce reflex tachycardia, mediated by the baroreceptor reflex, and is contraindicated in patients with decreased coronary perfusion.

B. Phentolamine

In contrast to *phenoxybenzamine*, *phentolamine* [fen-TOLE-a-meen] produces a competitive block of α_1 and α_2 receptors. The drug's action lasts for approximately 4 hours after a single administration. Like *phenoxybenzamine*, it produces postural hypotension and causes *epinephrine* reversal. *Phentolamine*-induced reflex cardiac stimulation and tachycardia are mediated by the baroreceptor reflex and by blocking the α_2 receptors of the cardiac sympathetic nerves. The drug can also trigger arrhythmias and anginal pain, and it is contraindicated in patients with decreased coronary perfusion. *Phentolamine* is also used for the short-term management of pheochromocytoma. *Phentolamine* is now rarely used for the treatment of impotence (it can be injected intracavernosally to produce vasodilation of penile arteries).

C. Prazosin, terazosin, doxazosin, alfuzosin, and tamsulosin

Prazosin [PRAY-zoe-sin], *terazosin* [ter-AY-zoe-sin], *doxazosin* [dox-AY-zoe-sin], and *tamsulosin* [tam-SUE-loh-sin] are selective competitive blockers of the α_1 receptor. In contrast to *phenoxybenzamine* and *phen-*

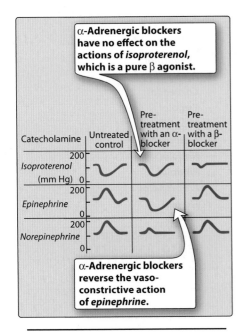

Figure 7.3
Summary of effects of adrenergic blockers on the changes in blood pressure induced by *isoproterenol*, *epinephrine*, and *norepinephrine*.

tolamine, the first three drugs are useful in the treatment of hypertension. *Tamsulosin* and *alfuzosin* [al-FYOO-zoe-sin] are indicated for the treatment of benign prostatic hypertrophy (also known as benign prostatic hyperplasia or BPH). Metabolism leads to inactive products that are excreted in the urine except for those of *doxazosin*, which appear in the feces. *Doxazosin* is the longest acting of these drugs.

1. **Cardiovascular effects:** All of these agents decrease peripheral vascular resistance and lower arterial blood pressure by causing the relaxation of both arterial and venous smooth muscle. *Tamsulosin* has the least effect on blood pressure. These drugs, unlike *phenoxybenzamine* and *phentolamine*, cause minimal changes in cardiac output, renal blood flow, and the glomerular filtration rate.

2. **Therapeutic uses:** Individuals with elevated blood pressure who have been treated with one of these drugs do not become tolerant to its action. However, the first dose of these drugs produces an exaggerated orthostatic hypotensive response that can result in syncope (fainting). This action, termed a "first-dose" effect, may be minimized by adjusting the first dose to one-third or one-fourth of the normal dose and by giving the drug at bedtime. An increase in the risk of congestive heart failure has been reported when α_1-receptor blockers have been used as monotherapy in hypertension. The α_1-receptor antagonists have been used as an alternative to surgery in patients with symptomatic BPH. Blockade of the α receptors decreases tone in the smooth muscle of the bladder neck and prostate and improves urine flow. *Tamsulosin* is a more potent inhibitor of the α_{1A} receptors found on the smooth muscle of the prostate. This selectivity accounts for *tamsulosin's* minimal effect on blood pressure. [Note: *Finasteride* and *dutasteride* inhibit 5α-reductase, preventing the conversion of testosterone to dihydrotestosterone. These drugs are approved for the treatment of BPH by reducing prostate volume in selected patients (see. p. 309)]

3. **Adverse effects:** α_1 Blockers may cause dizziness, a lack of energy, nasal congestion, headache, drowsiness, and orthostatic hypotension (although to a lesser degree than that observed with *phenoxybenzamine* and *phentolamine*). An additive antihypertensive effect occurs when *prazosin* is given with either a diuretic or a β-blocker, thereby necessitating a reduction in its dose. Due to a tendency to retain sodium and fluid, *prazosin* is frequently used along with a diuretic. Male sexual function is not as severely affected by these drugs as it is by *phenoxybenzamine* and *phentolamine*; however, by blocking α receptors in the ejaculatory ducts and impairing smooth muscle contraction, inhibition of ejaculation and retrograde ejaculation have been reported. Figure 7.4 summarizes some adverse effects observed with α-blockers.

D. Yohimbine

Yohimbine [yo-HIM-bean] is a selective competitive α_2 blocker. It is found as a component of the bark of the yohimbe tree and is sometimes used as a sexual stimulant. *Yohimbine* works at the level of the CNS to increase sympathetic outflow to the periphery. It directly blocks α_2 receptors and has been used to relieve vasoconstriction associated with Raynaud's disease. *Yohimbine* is contraindicated in CNS and cardiovascular conditions because it is a CNS and cardiovascular stimulant.

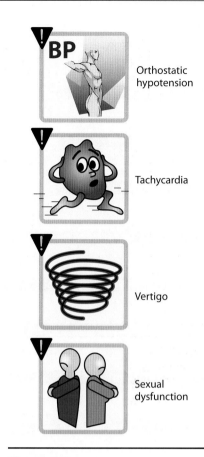

Orthostatic hypotension

Tachycardia

Vertigo

Sexual dysfunction

Figure 7.4
Some adverse effects commonly observed with nonselective α-adrenergic blocking agents.

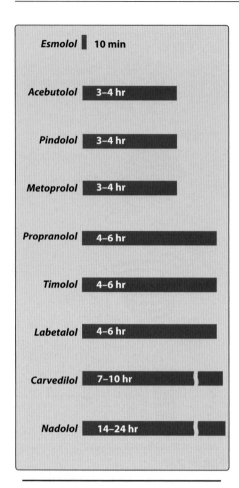

Figure 7.5
Elimination half-lives for some β-blockers.

III. β-ADRENERGIC BLOCKING AGENTS

All the clinically available β-blockers are competitive antagonists. Non-selective β-blockers act at both β₁ and β₂ receptors, whereas cardioselective β antagonists primarily block β₁ receptors [Note: There are no clinically useful β₂ antagonists]. These drugs also differ in intrinsic sympathomimetic activity, in CNS effects, and in pharmacokinetics (Figure 7.5). Although all β-blockers lower blood pressure in hypertension, they do not induce postural hypotension, because the α-adrenoceptors remain functional. Therefore, normal sympathetic control of the vasculature is maintained. β-Blockers are also effective in treating angina, cardiac arrhythmias, myocardial infarction, congestive heart failure, hyperthyroidism, and glaucoma, as well as serving in the prophylaxis of migraine headaches. [Note: The names of all β-blockers end in "-olol" except for *labetalol* and *carvedilol*.]

A. Propranolol: A nonselective β antagonist

Propranolol [proe-PRAN-oh-lole] is the prototype β-adrenergic antagonist and blocks both β₁ and β₂ receptors. Sustained-release preparations for once-a-day dosing are available.

1. Actions:

a. Cardiovascular: *Propranolol* diminishes cardiac output, having both negative inotropic and chronotropic effects (Figure 7.6). It directly depresses sinoatrial and atrioventricular activity. The resulting bradycardia usually limits the dose of the drug. Cardiac output, work, and oxygen consumption are decreased by blockade of β₁ receptors; these effects are useful in the treatment of angina (see p. 211). The β-blockers are effective in attenuating supraventricular cardiac arrhythmias but generally are not effective against ventricular arrhythmias (except those induced by exercise).

b. Peripheral vasoconstriction: Blockade of β receptors prevents β₂-mediated vasodilation (see Figure 7.6). The reduction in cardiac output leads to decreased blood pressure. This hypotension triggers a reflex peripheral vasoconstriction that is reflected in reduced blood flow to the periphery. On balance, there is a gradual reduction of both systolic and diastolic blood pressures in hypertensive patients. No postural hypotension occurs, because the α₁-adrenergic receptors that control vascular resistance are unaffected.

c. Bronchoconstriction: Blocking β₂ receptors in the lungs of susceptible patients causes contraction of the bronchiolar smooth muscle (see Figure 7.6). This can precipitate a respiratory crisis in patients with chronic obstructive pulmonary disease (COPD) or asthma. β-Blockers, and in particular nonselective ones, are thus contraindicated in patients with COPD or asthma.

d. Increased Na⁺ retention: Reduced blood pressure causes a decrease in renal perfusion, resulting in an increase in Na⁺ retention and plasma volume (see Figure 7.6). In some cases, this compensatory response tends to elevate the blood pressure. For these patients, β-blockers are often combined with a diuretic to prevent Na⁺ retention. By inhibiting β receptors, renin production is also prevented, contributing to Na⁺ retention.

e. **Disturbances in glucose metabolism:** β-blockade leads to decreased glycogenolysis and decreased glucagon secretion. Therefore, if a Type I (formerly insulin-dependent) diabetic is to be given *propranolol*, very careful monitoring of blood glucose is essential, because pronounced hypoglycemia may occur after insulin injection. β-Blockers also attenuate the normal physiologic response to hypoglycemia.

f. **Blocked action of isoproterenol:** All β-blockers, including *propranolol*, have the ability to block the actions of *isoproterenol* on the cardiovascular system. Thus, in the presence of a β-blocker, *isoproterenol* does not produce either the typical cardiac stimulation or reductions in mean arterial pressure and diastolic pressure (see Figure 7.3). [Note: In the presence of a β-blocker, *epinephrine* no longer lowers diastolic blood pressure or stimulates the heart, but its vasoconstrictive action (mediated by α receptors) remains unimpaired. The actions of norepinephrine on the cardiovascular system are mediated primarily by α receptors and are, therefore, unaffected.]

2. **Therapeutic effects:**

a. **Hypertension:** *Propranolol* lowers blood pressure in hypertension by several different mechanisms of action. Decreased cardiac output is the primary mechanism, but inhibition of renin release from the kidney and decreased sympathetic outflow from the CNS also contribute to *propranolol's* antihypertensive effects (see p. 220).

b. **Glaucoma:** β-Blockers, particularly topically applied *timolol*, are effective in diminishing intraocular pressure in glaucoma. This occurs by decreasing the secretion of aqueous humor by the ciliary body. Many patients with glaucoma have been maintained with these drugs for years. They neither affect the ability of the eye to focus for near vision nor change pupil size, as do the cholinergic drugs. However, in an acute attack of glaucoma, *pilocarpine* is still the drug of choice. The β-blockers are only used to treat this disease chronically.

c. **Migraine:** *Propranolol* is also effective in reducing migraine episodes when used prophylactically (see p. 526). β-Blockers are valuable in the treatment of chronic migraine, in which they decrease the incidence and severity of the attacks. The mechanism may depend on the blockade of catecholamine-induced vasodilation in the brain vasculature. [Note: During an attack, the usual therapy with *sumatriptan* or other drugs is used.]

d. **Hyperthyroidism:** *Propranolol* and other β-blockers are effective in blunting the widespread sympathetic stimulation that occurs in hyperthyroidism. In acute hyperthyroidism (thyroid storm), β-blockers may be lifesaving in protecting against serious cardiac arrhythmias.

e. **Angina pectoris:** *Propranolol* decreases the oxygen requirement of heart muscle and, therefore, is effective in reducing the chest pain on exertion that is common in angina. *Propranolol* is therefore

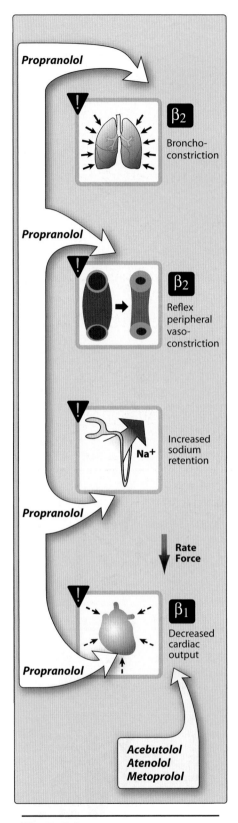

Figure 7.6
Actions of *propranolol* and other β-blockers.

useful in the chronic management of stable angina, but not for acute treatment. Tolerance to moderate exercise is increased, and this is measurable by improvement in the electrocardiogram. However, treatment with *propranolol* does not allow strenuous physical exercise, such as tennis.

f. Myocardial infarction: *Propranolol* and other β-blockers have a protective effect on the myocardium. Thus, patients who have had one myocardial infarction appear to be protected against a second heart attack by prophylactic use of β-blockers. In addition, administration of a β-blocker immediately following a myocardial infarction reduces infarct size and hastens recovery. The mechanism for these effects may be a blocking of the actions of circulating catecholamines, which would increase the oxygen demand in an already ischemic heart muscle. *Propranolol* also reduces the incidence of sudden arrhythmic death after myocardial infarction.

3. Adverse effects:

a. Bronchoconstriction: *Propranolol* has a serious and potentially lethal side effect when administered to an asthmatic (Figure 7.7). An immediate contraction of the bronchiolar smooth muscle prevents air from entering the lungs. Deaths by asphyxiation have been reported for asthmatics who were inadvertently administered the drug. Therefore, *propranolol* must never be used in treating any individual with COPD or asthma.

b. Arrhythmias: Treatment with β-blockers must never be stopped quickly because of the risk of precipitating cardiac arrhythmias, which may be severe. The β-blockers must be tapered off gradually for 1 week. Long-term treatment with a β antagonist leads to up-regulation of the β-receptor. On suspension of therapy, the increased receptors can worsen angina or hypertension.

c. Sexual impairment: Because sexual function in the male occurs through α-adrenergic activation, β-blockers do not affect normal ejaculation or the internal bladder sphincter function. On the other hand, some men do complain of impaired sexual activity. The reasons for this are not clear, and they may be independent of β-receptor blockade.

d. Disturbances in metabolism: β-Blockade leads to decreased glycogenolysis and decreased glucagon secretion. Fasting hypoglycemia may occur. [Note: Cardioselective β-blockers are preferred in treating asthmatic patients who use insulin (see β$_1$-selective antagonists).]

e. Drug interactions: Drugs that interfere with the metabolism of *propranolol*, such as *cimetidine, fluoxetine, paroxetine,* and *ritonavir*, may potentiate its antihypertensive effects. Conversely, those that stimulate its metabolism, such as barbiturates, *phenytoin,* and *rifampin,* can decrease its effects.

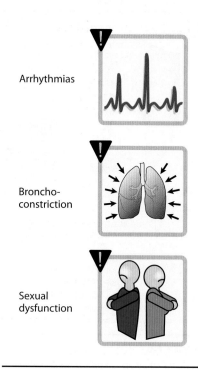

Arrhythmias

Broncho-
constriction

Sexual
dysfunction

Figure 7.7
Adverse effects commonly observed in individuals treated with *propranolol*.

B. Timolol and nadolol: Nonselective β antagonists

Timolol [TIM-o-lole] and *nadolol* [NAH-doh-lole] also block β$_1$- and β$_2$-adrenoceptors and are more potent than *propranolol*. *Nadolol* has a very long duration of action (see Figure 7.5). *Timolol* reduces the production of aqueous humor in the eye. It is used topically in the treatment of chronic open-angle glaucoma and, occasionally, for systemic treatment of hypertension.

C. Acebutolol, atenolol, metoprolol, and esmolol: Selective β₁ antagonists

Drugs that preferentially block the β₁ receptors have been developed to eliminate the unwanted bronchoconstrictor effect (β₂ effect) of *propranolol* seen among asthmatic patients. Cardioselective β-blockers, such as *acebutolol* [a-se-BYOO-toe-lole], *atenolol* [a-TEN-oh-lole], and *metoprolol* [me-TOE-proe-lole], antagonize β₁ receptors at doses 50- to 100-fold less than those required to block β₂ receptors. This cardioselectivity is thus most pronounced at low doses and is lost at high doses. [Note: *Acebutolol* has some intrinsic agonist activity.]

1. **Actions:** These drugs lower blood pressure in hypertension and increase exercise tolerance in angina (see Figure 7.6). *Esmolol* [EZ-moe-lole] has a very short lifetime (see Figure 7.5) due to metabolism of an ester linkage. It is only given intravenously if required during surgery or diagnostic procedures (for example, cystoscopy). In contrast to *propranolol*, the cardiospecific blockers have relatively little effect on pulmonary function, peripheral resistance, and carbohydrate metabolism. Nevertheless, asthmatics treated with these agents must be carefully monitored to make certain that respiratory activity is not compromised.

2. **Therapeutic use in hypertension:** The cardioselective β-blockers are useful in hypertensive patients with impaired pulmonary function. Because these drugs have less effect on peripheral vascular β₂ receptors, coldness of extremities, a common side effect of β-blocker therapy, is less frequent. Cardioselective β-blockers are useful in diabetic hypertensive patients who are receiving insulin or oral hypoglycemic agents.

D. Pindolol and acebutolol: Antagonists with partial agonist activity

1. **Actions:**

   a. **Cardiovascular:** *Acebutolol* and *pindolol* [PIN-doe-lole] are not pure antagonists; instead, they have the ability to weakly stimulate both β₁ and β₂ receptors (Figure 7.8) and are said to have intrinsic sympathomimetic activity (ISA). These partial agonists stimulate the β receptor to which they are bound, yet they inhibit stimulation by the more potent endogenous catecholamines, *epinephrine* and norepinephrine. The result of these opposing actions is a much diminished effect on cardiac rate and cardiac output compared to that of β-blockers without ISA.

   b. **Decreased metabolic effects:** Blockers with ISA minimize the disturbances of lipid and carbohydrate metabolism that are seen with other β-blockers.

2. **Therapeutic use in hypertension:** β-Blockers with ISA are effective in hypertensive patients with moderate bradycardia, because a further decrease in heart rate is less pronounced with these drugs. Carbohydrate metabolism is less affected with *acebutolol* and *pin-*

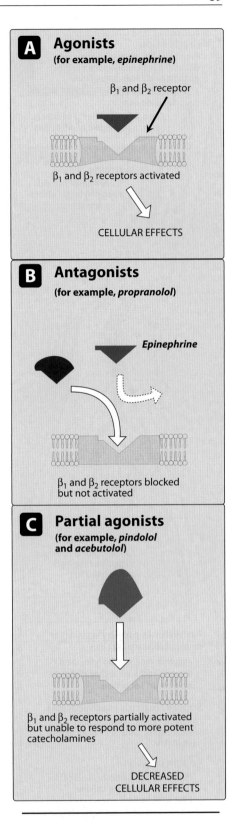

Figure 7.8
Comparison of agonists, antagonists, and partial agonists of β adrenoceptors.

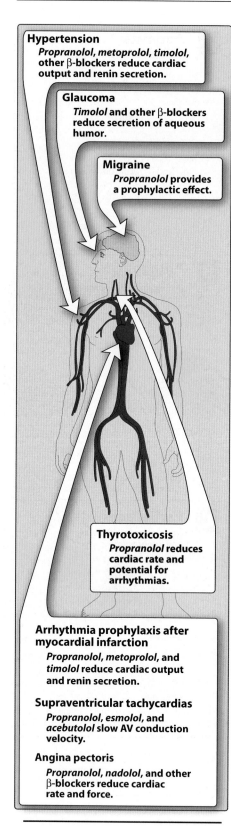

Hypertension
Propranolol, metoprolol, timolol, other β-blockers reduce cardiac output and renin secretion.

Glaucoma
Timolol and other β-blockers reduce secretion of aqueous humor.

Migraine
Propranolol provides a prophylactic effect.

Thyrotoxicosis
Propranolol reduces cardiac rate and potential for arrhythmias.

Arrhythmia prophylaxis after myocardial infarction
Propranolol, metoprolol, and *timolol* reduce cardiac output and renin secretion.

Supraventricular tachycardias
Propranolol, esmolol, and *acebutolol* slow AV conduction velocity.

Angina pectoris
Propranolol, nadolol, and other β-blockers reduce cardiac rate and force.

Figure 7.9
Some clinical applications of β-blockers. AV = atrioventricular.

dolol than it is with *propranolol*, making them valuable in the treatment of diabetics. [Note: The β blockers with ISA are not used as antiarrhythmic agents due to their partial agonist effect.] Figure 7.9 summarizes some of the indications for β-blockers.

E. Labetalol and carvedilol: Antagonists of both α- and β-adrenoceptors

1. **Actions:** *Labetalol* [lah-BET-a-lole] and *carvedilol* [CAR-ve-dil-ol] are reversible β-blockers with concurrent α_1-blocking actions that produce peripheral vasodilation, thereby reducing blood pressure. They contrast with the other β-blockers that produce peripheral vasoconstriction, and they are therefore useful in treating hypertensive patients for whom increased peripheral vascular resistance is undesirable. They do not alter serum lipid or blood glucose levels. *Carvedilol* also decreases lipid peroxidation and vascular wall thickening, effects that have benefit in heart failure.

2. **Therapeutic use in hypertension:** *Labetalol* is useful for treating the elderly or black hypertensive patient in whom increased peripheral vascular resistance is undesirable. [Note: In general, black hypertensive patients are not well controlled with β-blockers.] *Labetalol* may be employed as an alternative to *methyldopa* in the treatment of pregnancy-induced hypertension. Intravenous *labetalol* is also used to treat hypertensive emergencies, because it can rapidly lower blood pressure (see p. 227).

3. **Adverse effects:** Orthostatic hypotension and dizziness are associated with α_1 blockade. Figure 7.10 summarizes the receptor specificities and uses of the β-adrenergic antagonists.

IV. DRUGS AFFECTING NEUROTRANSMITTER RELEASE OR UPTAKE

As noted on p. 119, some agonists, such as *amphetamine* and *tyramine*, do not act directly on the adrenoceptor. Instead, they exert their effects indirectly on the adrenergic neuron by causing the release of neurotransmitter from storage vesicles. Similarly, some agents act on the adrenergic neuron, either to interfere with neurotransmitter release or to alter the uptake of the neurotransmitter into the adrenergic nerve. However, due to the advent of newer and more effective agents, with fewer side effects, these agents are rarely used therapeutically. These agents are included in this chapter due to their unique mechanisms of action and historical value.

A. Reserpine

Reserpine [re-SER-peen], a plant alkaloid, blocks the Mg^{2+}/adenosine triphosphate–dependent transport of biogenic amines, norepinephrine, *dopamine*, and *serotonin* from the cytoplasm into storage vesicles in the adrenergic nerves of all body tissues. This causes the ultimate depletion of biogenic amines. Sympathetic function, in general, is impaired because of decreased release of norepinephrine. The drug has a slow onset, a long duration of action, and effects that persist for many days after discontinuation.

B. Guanethidine

Guanethidine [gwahn-ETH-i-deen] blocks the release of stored norepinephrine as well as displaces norepinephrine from storage vesicles (thus producing a transient increase in blood pressure). This leads to gradual depletion of norepinephrine in nerve endings except for those in the CNS. *Guanethidine* commonly causes orthostatic hypotension and interferes with male sexual function. Supersensitivity to norepinephrine due to depletion of the amine can result in hypertensive crisis in patients with pheochromocytoma.

C. Cocaine

Although cocaine inhibits norepinephrine uptake, it is an adrenergic agonist. See page 78 for discussion.

DRUG	RECEPTOR SPECFICITY	THERAPEUTIC USES
Propranolol	β_1, β_2	Hypertension Glaucoma Migraine Hyperthyroidism Angina pectoris Myocardial infarction
Nadolol *Timolol*	β_1, β_2	Glaucoma Hypertension
Acebutolol[1] *Atenolol* *Esmolol* *Metoprolol*	β_1	Hypertension
Pindolol[1]	β_1, β_2	Hypertension
Carvedilol *Labetalol*	$\alpha_1, \beta_1, \beta_2$	Hypertension Congestive heart failure

Figure 7.10
Summary of β-adrenergic antagonists. [1]*Acebutolol* and *pindolol* are partial agonists.

Study Questions

Choose the ONE best answer.

7.1 The graphs below depict the changes in blood pressure caused by the intravenous administration of epinephrine before and after an unknown Drug X.

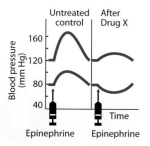

Which of the following drugs is most likely Drug X?

A. Atropine.
B. Phenylephrine.
C. Physostigmine.
D. Prazosin.
E. Propranolol.

Correct answer = D. The dose of epinephrine increased both systolic and diastolic pressures, but because epinephrine dilates some and constricts other vessel beds, the rise in diastolic pressure is not as much. There is a marked increase in the pulse pressure. An α-blocker, such as prazosin, prevents the peripheral vasoconstrictor effects of epinephrine, leaving the vasodilator (β₂-stimulation) unopposed. This results in a marked decrease in the diastolic pressure coupled with a slight increase in systolic pressure due to increased cardiac output. This phenomenon is known as "epinephrine reversal," and it is characteristic of the effect of α-blockers on the cardiovascular effects of epinephrine. None of the other drugs has α-blocking activity and, therefore, cannot produce this interaction.

7.2 A 38-year-old male has recently started monotherapy for mild hypertension. At his most recent office visit, he complains of tiredness and not being able to complete three sets of tennis. Which one of the following drugs is he most likely to be taking for hypertension?

A. Albuterol.
B. Atenolol.
C. Ephedrine.
D. Phentolamine.
E. Prazosin.

Correct answer = B. Atenolol is a β₁ antagonist and is effective in lowering blood pressure in patients with hypertension. Side effects of β-blockers include fatigue and exercise intolerance. Albuterol and ephedrine are not antihypertensive medications. Phentolamine and prazosin are antihypertensive drugs, but the side effects of α antagonists are not characterized by these symptoms.

7.3 A 60-year-old asthmatic man comes in for a checkup and complains that he is having some difficulty in "starting to urinate." Physical examination indicates that the man has a blood pressure of 160/100 mm Hg and a slightly enlarged prostate. Which of the following medications would be useful in treating both of these conditions?

A. Doxazosin.
B. Labetalol.
C. Phentolamine.
D. Propranolol.
E. Isoproterenol.

Correct answer = A. Doxazosin is an competitive blocker at the α₁ receptor and lowers blood pressure. In addition, it blocks the α receptors in the smooth muscle of the bladder neck and prostate to improve urine flow. Labetalol and propranolol, although effective for treating the hypertension, are contraindicated in an asthmatic. They would not improve urine flow. Phentolamine has too many adverse effects to be used as a hypertensive agent. Isoproterenol is a β agonist and is not employed as a hypertensive, nor would it affect urinary function.

Neurodegenerative Diseases

8

I. OVERVIEW

Most drugs that affect the central nervous system (CNS) act by altering some step in the neurotransmission process. Drugs affecting the CNS may act presynaptically by influencing the production, storage, release, or termination of action of neurotransmitters. Other agents may activate or block postsynaptic receptors. This chapter provides an overview of the CNS, with a focus on those neurotransmitters that are involved in the actions of the clinically useful CNS drugs. These concepts are useful in understanding the etiology and treatment strategies of Parkinson's and Alzheimer's diseases—the two neurodegenerative disorders that respond to drug therapy (Figure 8.1).

II. NEUROTRANSMISSION IN THE CNS

In many ways, the basic functioning of neurons in the CNS is similar to that of the autonomic nervous system described in Chapter 3. For example, transmission of information in the CNS and in the periphery both involve the release of neurotransmitters that diffuse across the synaptic space to bind to specific receptors on the postsynaptic neuron. In both systems, the recognition of the neurotransmitter by the membrane receptor of the postsynaptic neuron triggers intracellular changes. However, several major differences exist between neurons in the peripheral autonomic nervous system and those in the CNS. The circuitry of the CNS is much more complex than that of the autonomic nervous system, and the number of synapses in the CNS is far greater. The CNS, unlike the peripheral autonomic nervous system, contains powerful networks of inhibitory neurons that are constantly active in modulating the rate of neuronal transmission. In addition, the CNS communicates through the use of more than 10 (and perhaps as many as 50) different neurotransmitters. In contrast, the autonomic nervous system uses only two primary neurotransmitters, acetylcholine and norepinephrine. Figure 8.2 describes some of the more important neurotransmitters in the CNS.

ANTI-PARKINSON DRUGS

- *Amantadine*
- *Apomorphine*
- *Benztropine*
- *Biperiden*
- *Bromocriptine*
- *Carbidopa*
- *Entacapone*
- *Levodopa*
- *Pramipexole*
- *Procyclidine*
- *Rasagiline*
- *Ropinirole*
- *Rotigotine*
- *Selegiline (Deprenyl)*
- *Tolcapone*
- *Trihexyphenidyl*

ANTI-ALZHEIMER DRUGS

- *Donepezil*
- *Galantamine*
- *Memantine*
- *Rivastigmine*
- *Tacrine*

Figure 8.1
Summary of agents used in the treatment of Parkinson's and Alzheimer's diseases.

NEUROTRANSMITTER		POSTSYNAPTIC EFFECTS
BIOGENIC AMINES	**Acetylcholine**	**Excitatory:** Involved in arousal, short-term memory, learning and movement.
	Norepinephrine	**Excitatory:** Involved in arousal, wakefulness, mood, and cardiovascular regulation.
	Dopamine	**Excitatory:** Involved in emotion, reward systems and motor control.
	Serotonin	**Excitatory/Inhibitory:** Feeding behavior, control of body temperature, modulation of sensory pathways including nociception (stimulation of pain nerve sensors), regulation of mood and emotion, and sleep/wakefulness.
AMINO ACIDS	**GABA**	**Inhibitory:** Increases Cl⁻ flux into the postsynaptic neuron, resulting in hyperpolarization. Mediates the majority of inhibitory postsynaptic potentials.
	Glycine	**Inhibitory:** Increases Cl⁻ flux into the postsynaptic neuron, resulting in hyperpolarization.
	Glutamate	**Excitatory:** Mediates excitatory Na⁺ influx into the postsynaptic neuron.
NEURO-PEPTIDES	**Substance P**	**Excitatory:** Mediates nociception (pain) within the spinal cord.
	Met-enkephalin	**Generally inhibitory:** Mediates analgesia as well as other central nervous system effects.

Figure 8.2
Summary of some neurotransmitters of the central nervous system. GABA = γ-aminobutyric acid.

III. SYNAPTIC POTENTIALS

In the CNS, receptors at most synapses are coupled to ion channels; that is, binding of the neurotransmitter to the postsynaptic membrane receptors results in a rapid but transient opening of ion channels. Open channels allow specific ions inside and outside the cell membrane to flow down their concentration gradients. The resulting change in the ionic composition across the membrane of the neuron alters the postsynaptic potential, producing either depolarization or hyperpolarization of the postsynaptic membrane, depending on the specific ions that move and the direction of their movement.

A. Excitatory pathways

Neurotransmitters can be classified as either excitatory or inhibitory, depending on the nature of the action they elicit. Stimulation of excitatory neurons causes a movement of ions that results in a depolarization of the postsynaptic membrane. These excitatory postsynaptic potentials (EPSP) are generated by the following: 1) Stimulation of an excitatory neuron causes the release of neurotransmitter molecules, such as glutamate or acetylcholine, which bind to receptors on the postsynaptic cell membrane. This causes a transient increase in the permeability of sodium (Na⁺) ions. 2) The influx of Na⁺ causes a weak depolarization or EPSP that moves the postsynaptic potential toward its firing threshold. 3) If the number of stimulated excitatory neurons increases, more excitatory neurotransmitter is released. This ultimately causes the EPSP depolarization of the postsynaptic cell to pass a threshold, thereby generating an all-or-none action potential. [Note: The generation of a nerve impulse typically reflects the activation of synaptic receptors by thousands of excitatory neurotransmitter molecules released from many nerve fibers.] (See Figure 8.3 for an example of an excitatory pathway.)

B. Inhibitory pathways

Stimulation of inhibitory neurons causes movement of ions that results in a hyperpolarization of the postsynaptic membrane. These inhibitory postsynaptic potentials (IPSP) are generated by the following: 1)

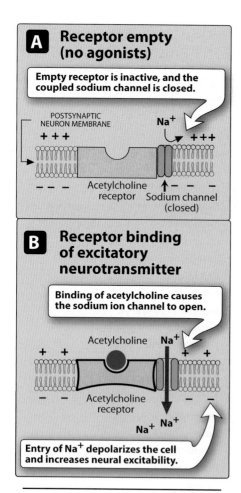

A **Receptor empty (no agonists)**

Empty receptor is inactive, and the coupled sodium channel is closed.

POSTSYNAPTIC NEURON MEMBRANE
+ + +   Na⁺   + + +

Acetylcholine receptor   Sodium channel (closed)

B **Receptor binding of excitatory neurotransmitter**

Binding of acetylcholine causes the sodium ion channel to open.

Acetylcholine   Na⁺

Acetylcholine receptor

Na⁺ Na⁺

Entry of Na⁺ depolarizes the cell and increases neural excitability.

Figure 8.3
Binding of the excitatory neurotransmitter, acetylcholine, causes depolarization of the neuron.

generally contraindicated in parkinsonian patients, because these potently block dopamine receptors and produce a parkinsonian syndrome themselves. However low doses of certain "atypical" antipsychotic agents are sometimes employed to treat levodopa-induced psychiatric symptoms.

B. Selegiline and rasagiline   *MAO - B inhibitors*

Selegiline [seh-LEDGE-ah-leen], also called *deprenyl* [DE-pre-nill], selectively inhibits MAO Type B (which metabolizes dopamine) at low to moderate doses but does not inhibit MAO Type A (which metabolizes norepinephrine and serotonin) unless given at above recommended doses, where it loses its selectivity. By thus decreasing the metabolism of dopamine, *selegiline* has been found to increase dopamine levels in the brain (Figure 8.10). Therefore, it enhances the actions of *levodopa* when these drugs are administered together. *Selegiline* substantially reduces the required dose of *levodopa*. Unlike nonselective MAO inhibitors, *selegiline* at recommended doses has little potential for causing hypertensive crises. However, if *selegiline* is administered at high doses, the selectivity of the drug is lost, and the patient is at risk for severe hypertension. [Note: Early reports of possible neuroprotective effects of *selegiline* have not been supported by long-term studies.] *Selegiline* is metabolized to methamphetamine and *amphetamine*, whose stimulating properties may produce insomnia if the drug is administered later than midafternoon. (See p. 148 for the use of *selegiline* in treating depression). *Rasagiline* [ra-SA-gi-leen], an irreversible and selective inhibitor of brain (MAO) Type B, has five times the potency of *selegiline*. Unlike *selegiline*, it is not metabolized to an amphetamine-like substance.

C. Catechol-O-methyltransferase inhibitors   *Capones*

Normally, the methylation of *levodopa* by catechol-O-methyltransferase (COMT) to 3-O-methyldopa is a minor pathway for *levodopa* metabolism. However, when peripheral dopamine decarboxylase activity is inhibited by *carbidopa*, a significant concentration of 3-O-methyldopa is formed that competes with *levodopa* for active transport into the CNS (Figure 8.11). Inhibition of COMT by *entacapone* [en-TA-ka-pone] or *tolcapone* [TOLE-ka-pone] leads to decreased plasma concentrations of 3-O-methyldopa, increased central uptake of *levodopa*, and greater concentrations of brain dopamine. Both of these agents have been demonstrated to reduce the symptoms of "wearing-off" phenomena seen in patients on *levodopa–carbidopa*. *Entacapone* and *tolcapone* are nitrocatechol derivatives that selectively and reversibly inhibit COMT. The two drugs differ primarily in their pharmacokinetics and in some adverse effects.

1. **Pharmacokinetics:** Oral absorption of both drugs occurs readily and is not influenced by food. They are extensively bound to plasma albumin (>98 percent), with limited volumes of distribution. *Tolcapone* differs from *entacapone* in that the former penetrates the blood-brain barrier and inhibits COMT in the CNS. However, the inhibition of COMT in the periphery appears to be the primary therapeutic action. *Tolcapone* has a relatively long duration of action (probably due to its affinity for the enzyme) compared to *entacapone*, which requires more frequent dosing. Both drugs are extensively metabolized and eliminated in the feces and urine. Dosage may need to be adjusted in patients with moderate or severe cirrhosis.

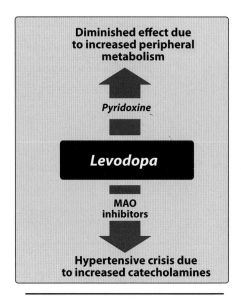

Figure 8.9
Some drug interactions observed with *levodopa*.

meth + amphetamine → selegiline

Capones → Reduce methylation of levadopa in levadopa / carbadopa pts to stop "wearing-off"

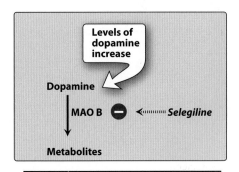

Figure 8.10
Action of *selegiline* (*deprenyl*) in dopamine metabolism. MAO = monoamine oxidase Type B.

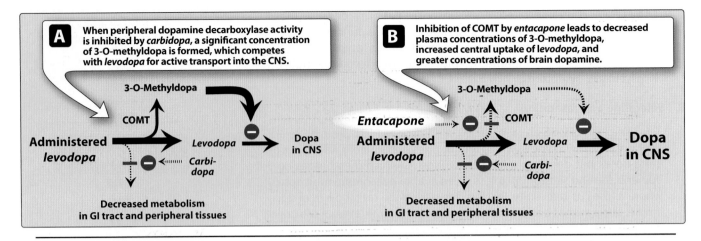

A When peripheral dopamine decarboxylase activity is inhibited by *carbidopa*, a significant concentration of 3-O-methyldopa is formed, which competes with *levodopa* for active transport into the CNS.

B Inhibition of COMT by *entacapone* leads to decreased plasma concentrations of 3-O-methyldopa, increased central uptake of *levodopa*, and greater concentrations of brain dopamine.

Figure 8.11
Effect of *entacapone* on dopa concentration in the central nervous system (CNS). COMT = catechol-O-methyltransferase.

2. **Adverse effects:** Both drugs exhibit adverse effects that are observed in patients taking *levodopa–carbidopa,* including diarrhea, postural hypotension, nausea, anorexia, dyskinesias, hallucinations, and sleep disorders. Most seriously, fulminating hepatic necrosis is associated with *tolcapone* use. Therefore, it should be used—along with appropriate hepatic function monitoring—only in patients in whom other modalities have failed. *Entacapone* does not exhibit this toxicity and has largely replaced *tolcapone.*

D. **Dopamine-receptor agonists**

This group of anti-Parkinson compounds includes *bromocriptine,* an ergot derivative, and two newer, nonergot drugs, *ropinirole, pramipexole* and *rotigotine*. These agents have durations of action longer than that of *levodopa* and, thus, have been effective in patients exhibiting fluctuations in their response to *levodopa*. Initial therapy with the newer drugs is associated particularly with less risk of developing dyskinesias and motor fluctuations when compared to patients started with *levodopa* therapy. *Bromocriptine, pramipexole,* and *ropinirole* are all effective in patients with advanced Parkinson's disease complicated by motor fluctuations and dyskinesias. However, these drugs are ineffective in patients who have shown no therapeutic response to *levodopa*. *Apomorphine* is also used in severe and advanced stages of the disease as an injectable dopamine agonist to supplement the oral medications commonly prescribed.

1. **Bromocriptine:** *Bromocriptine* [broe-moe-KRIP-teen], a derivative of the vasoconstrictive alkaloid, ergotamine, is a dopamine-receptor agonist. The dose is increased gradually during a period of 2 to 3 months. Side effects severely limit the utility of the dopamine agonists (Figure 8.12). The actions of *bromocriptine* are similar to those of *levodopa,* except that hallucinations, confusion, delirium, nausea, and orthostatic hypotension are more common, whereas dyskinesia is less prominent. In psychiatric illness, *bromocriptine* and *levodopa* may cause the mental condition to worsen. Serious cardiac problems may develop, particularly in patients with a history of myocardial infarction. In patients with peripheral vascular disease, a worsening of the vasospasm occurs, and in patients with peptic ulcer, there is a

worsening of the ulcer. Because *bromocriptine* is an ergot derivative, it has the potential to cause pulmonary and retroperitoneal fibrosis.

2. **Apomorphine, pramipexole, ropinirole, and rotigotine:** These are nonergot dopamine agonists that have been approved for the treatment of Parkinson's disease. *Pramipexole* [pra-mi-PEX-ole] and *ropinirole* [roe-PIN-i-role] are agonists at dopamine receptors. *Apomorphine* [A-po-mor-feen] and *rotigotine* [ro-TI-go-teen] are newer dopamine agonists available in injectable and transdermal delivery systems, respectively. *Apomorphine* is meant to be used for the acute management of the hypomobility "off" phenomenon. These agents alleviate the motor deficits in both *levodopa*-naïve patients (patients who have never been treated with *levodopa*) and patients with advanced Parkinson's disease who are taking *levodopa*. Dopamine agonists may delay the need to employ *levodopa* therapy in early Parkinson's disease and may decrease the dose of *levodopa* in advanced Parkinson's disease. Unlike the ergotamine derivatives, *pramipexole* and *ropinirole* do not exacerbate peripheral vasospasm, nor do they cause fibrosis. Nausea, hallucinations, insomnia, dizziness, constipation, and orthostatic hypotension are among the more distressing side effects of these drugs; dyskinesias are less frequent than with *levodopa*. The dependence of *pramipexole* on renal function for its elimination cannot be overly stressed. For example, *cimetidine*, which inhibits renal tubular secretion of organic bases, increases the half-life of *pramipexole* by 40 percent. The fluoroquinolone antibiotics (see p. 387) and other inhibitors of the CYP450-1A2 hepatic enzyme have been shown to inhibit the metabolism of *ropinirole* and to enhance the AUC (area under the concentration vs. time curve) by some 80 percent. *Rotigotine* is a dopamine agonist used in the treatment of the signs and symptoms of early stage Parkinson's disease. It is administered as a once-daily transdermal patch that provides even pharmacokinetics over 24 hours. Figures 8.13 summarizes some properties of these dopamine agonists.

E. Amantadine

It was accidentally discovered that the antiviral drug *amantadine* [a-MAN-ta-deen], which is effective in the treatment of influenza (see p. 437), has an antiparkinsonism action. *Amantadine* has several effects on a number of neurotransmitters implicated in causing parkinsonism, including increasing the release of dopamine, blockading cholinergic receptors, and inhibiting the N-methyl-D-aspartate (NMDA) type of glutamate receptors. Current evidence supports an action at NMDA receptors as the primary action at therapeutic concentrations. [Note: If

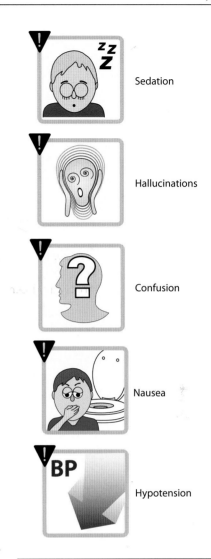

Figure 8.12
Some adverse effects of dopamine agonists.

Ropinirole → CYP 450
Pramipexole – Renal

	Pramipexole	Ropinirole	Rotigotine
Bioavailability	>90%	55%	45%
V_d	7 L/kg	7.5 L/kg	84 L/kg
Half-life	8 hours[1]	6 hours	7 hours[3]
Metabolism	Negligible	Extensive	Extensive
Elimination	Renal	Renal[2]	Renal[2]

Figure 8.13
Pharmacokinetic properties of dopamine agonists of *pramipexole*, *ropinirole* and *rotigotine*. V_d = volume of distribution. [1]Increases to 12 hours in patients older than 65 years; [2]Less than 10 percent excreted unchanged; [3]Administered as a once-daily transdermal patch.

dopamine release is already at a maximum, *amantadine* has no effect.] The drug may cause restlessness, agitation, confusion, and hallucinations, and at high doses, it may induce acute toxic psychosis. Orthostatic hypotension, urinary retention, peripheral edema, and dry mouth also may occur. *Amantadine* is less efficacious than *levodopa*, and tolerance develops more readily. However, *amantadine* has fewer side effects. The drug has little effect on tremor, but it is more effective than the anticholinergics against rigidity and bradykinesia.

F. Antimuscarinic agents

The antimuscarinic agents are much less efficacious than *levodopa* and play only an adjuvant role in antiparkinsonism therapy. The actions of *benztropine* [BENZ-tro-peen], *trihexyphenidyl* [tri-hex-ee FEN-i-dill], *procyclidine* [pro-CY-cli-deen], and *biperiden* [bi-PER-i den] are similar, although individual patients may respond more favorably to one drug. All of these drugs can induce mood changes and produce xerostomia (dryness of the mouth) and visual problems, as do all muscarinic blockers. They interfere with gastrointestinal peristalsis and are contraindicated in patients with glaucoma, prostatic hyperplasia, or pyloric stenosis. Blockage of cholinergic transmission produces effects similar to augmentation of dopaminergic transmission (again, because of the creation of an imbalance in the dopamine/acetylcholine ratio, see Figure 8.6). Adverse effects are similar to those caused by high doses of *atropine*—for example, pupillary dilation, confusion, hallucination, sinus tachycardia, urinary retention, constipation, and dry mouth.

VII. DRUGS USED IN ALZHEIMER'S DISEASE

Pharmacologic intervention for Alzheimer's disease is only palliative and provides modest short-term benefit. None of the currently available therapeutic agents have been shown to alter the underlying neurodegenerative process. Dementia of the Alzheimer's type (versus the other forms of dementia that will not be addressed in this discussion, such as multi-infarct dementia or Lewy body dementia) has three distinguishing features: 1) accumulation of senile plaques (β-amyloid accumulations), 2) formation of numerous neurofibrillary tangles, and 3) loss of cortical neurons—particularly cholinergic neurons. Current therapies are aimed at either improving cholinergic transmission within the CNS or preventing excitotoxic actions resulting from overstimulation of N-methyl-D-aspartic acid (NMDA)-glutamate receptors in selected brain areas.

A. Acetylcholinesterase inhibitors

Numerous studies have linked the progressive loss of cholinergic neurons and, presumably, cholinergic transmission within the cortex to the memory loss that is a hallmark symptom of Alzheimer's disease. It is postulated that inhibition of acetylcholinesterase (AChE) within the CNS will improve cholinergic transmission, at least at those neurons that are still functioning. Currently, four reversible AChE inhibitors are approved for the treatment of mild to moderate Alzheimer's disease. They are *donepezil* [dah-NE-peh-zeel], *galantamine* [ga-LAN-ta-meen], *rivastigmine* [ri-va-STIG-meen], and *tacrine* [TAK-reen]. Except for *galantamine*, which is competitive, all are uncompetitive inhibitors of AChE and appear to have some selectivity for AChE in the CNS as compared to the periphery. *Galantamine* may also be acting as an allosteric modulator of the nicotinic receptor in the CNS and, therefore, secondarily increase cholinergic neurotransmission through a separate mechanism. At best, these compounds provide a modest reduction in the rate of loss of cognitive functioning in Alzheimer's patients. *Rivastigmine* is hydrolyzed by AChE to a carbamylate metabolite and has no interactions with drugs that alter the activity of P450-dependent enzymes. The other agents are substrates for P450 and have a potential for such interactions. Common adverse effects include nausea, diarrhea, vomiting, anorexia, tremors, bradycardia, and muscle cramps—all of which are predicted by the actions of the drugs to enhance cholinergic neurotransmission (Figure 8.14). Unlike the others, *tacrine* is associated with hepatotoxicity.

B. NMDA-receptor antagonist

Stimulation of glutamate receptors in the CNS appears to be critical for the formation of certain memories; however, *overstimulation* of glutamate receptors, particularly of the NMDA type, has been shown to result in excitotoxic effects on neurons and is suggested as a mechanism for neurodegenerative or apoptotic (programmed cell death) processes. Binding of glutamate to the NMDA receptor assists in the opening of an associated ion channel that allows Na^+ and, particularly, Ca^{2+} to enter the neuron. Unfortunately, *excess* intracellular Ca^{2+} can activate a number of processes that ultimately damage neurons and lead to apoptosis. Antagonists of the NMDA-glutamate receptor are often neuroprotective, preventing the loss of neurons following ischemic and other injuries. *Memantine* [MEM-an-teen] is a dimethyl adamantane derivative. *Memantine* acts by physically blocking the NMDA receptor–associated ion channel, but at therapeutic doses, only a fraction of these channels are actually blocked. This partial blockade may allow *memantine* to limit Ca^{2+} influx into the neuron such that toxic intracellular levels are not achieved during NMDA receptor overstimulation, while still permitting sufficient Ca^{2+} flow through unblocked channels to preserve other vital processes that depend on Ca^{2+} (or Na^+) influx through these channels. This is in contrast to psychotoxic agents such as *phencyclidine,* which occupy and block nearly all of these channels. In short term studies, *memantine* has been shown to slow the rate of memory loss in both vascular-associated and Alzheimer's dementia in patients with moderate to severe cognitive losses. However, there is no evidence that *memantine* prevents or slows the neurodegeneration in patients with Alzheimer's disease or is more effective than the AChE inhibitors. *Memantine* is well tolerated, with few dose-dependent adverse events. Expected side effects, such as confusion, agitation, and restlessness, are indistinguishable from the symptoms of Alzheimer's disease. Given it's different mechanism of action and possible neuroprotective effects, *memantine* is often given in combination with an AChE inhibitor. Long-term data showing a significant effect of this combination is not available.

VIII. DRUGS USED IN AMYOTROPHIC LATERAL SCLEROSIS

Though not indicated for the treatment of Alzheimer's disease, another NMDA-receptor antagonist is indicated for the management of amyotrophic lateral sclerosis (ALS). *Riluzole* [RI-lu-zole] blocks glutamate, sodium channels and calcium channels. It may improve the survival time and delay the need for ventilator support in patients suffering from ALS.

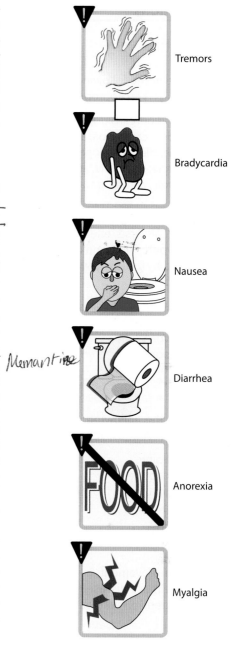

Figure 8.14
Adverse effects of acetylcholinesterase inhibitors.

Study Questions

Choose the ONE best answer.

8.1 Which one of the following combinations of antiparkinson drugs is an appropriate therapy?

 A. Amantadine, carbidopa, and entacapone.
 B. Levodopa, carbidopa, and entacapone.
 C. Pramipexole, carbidopa, and entacapone.
 D. Ropinirole, selegiline, and entacapone.
 E. Ropinirole, carbidopa, and selegiline.

Correct answer = B. To reduce the dose of levodopa and its peripheral side effects, the peripheral decarboxylase inhibitor, carbidopa, is coadministered. As a result of this combination, more levodopa is available for metabolism by COMT to 3-methyldopa, which competes with dopa for the active transport processes into the CNS. By administering entacapone (inhibitor of COMT), the competing product is not formed, and more dopa enters the brain. The other choices are not appropriate, because neither peripheral decarboxylase nor COMT nor MAO metabolizes amantadine or the direct-acting dopamine agonists, ropinirole and pramipexole.

8.2 Peripheral adverse effects of levodopa, including nausea, hypotension, and cardiac arrhythmias, can be diminished by including which of the following drugs in the therapy?

 A. Amantadine.
 B. Bromocriptine.
 C. Carbidopa.
 D. Entacapone.
 E. Ropinirole.

Correct answer = C. Carbidopa inhibits the peripheral decarboxylation of levodopa to dopamine, thereby diminishing the gastrointestinal and cardiovascular side effects of levodopa.

8.3 Which of the following antiparkinson drugs may cause peripheral vasospasm?

 A. Amantadine.
 B. Bromocriptine.
 C. Carbidopa.
 D. Entacapone.
 E. Ropinirole.

Correct answer = B. Bromocriptine is a dopamine-receptor agonist that may cause vasospasm; it is contraindicated in patients with peripheral vascular disease. Ropinirole directly stimulates dopamine receptors, but it does not cause vasospasm. The other drugs do not act directly on dopamine receptors.

8.4 Modest improvement in the memory of patients with Alzheimer's disease may occur with drugs that increase transmission at which of the following receptors?

 A. Adrenergic.
 B. Cholinergic.
 C. Dopaminergic.
 D. GABAergic.
 E. Serotonergic.

Correct answer = B. Acetylcholinesterase inhibitors, such as rivastigmine, increase cholinergic transmission in the CNS and may cause a modest delay in the progression of Alzheimer's disease.

Anxiolytic and Hypnotic Drugs

9

I. OVERVIEW

Anxiety is an unpleasant state of tension, apprehension, or uneasiness—a fear that seems to arise from a sometimes unknown source. Disorders involving anxiety are the most common mental disturbances. The physical symptoms of severe anxiety are similar to those of fear (such as tachycardia, sweating, trembling, and palpitations) and involve sympathetic activation. Episodes of mild anxiety are common life experiences and do not warrant treatment. However, the symptoms of severe, chronic, debilitating anxiety may be treated with antianxiety drugs (sometimes called anxiolytic or minor tranquilizers) and/or some form of behavioral or psychotherapy. Because many of the antianxiety drugs also cause some sedation, the same drugs often function clinically as both anxiolytic and hypnotic (sleep-inducing) agents. In addition, some have anticonvulsant activity. Figure 9.1 summarizes the anxiolytic and hypnotic agents. Though also indicated for certain anxiety disorders, the selective serotonin reuptake inhibitors (SSRIs) will be presented in the chapter discussing antidepressants.

II. BENZODIAZEPINES

Benzodiazepines are the most widely used anxiolytic drugs. They have largely replaced barbiturates and *meprobamate* in the treatment of anxiety, because the benzodiazepines are safer and more effective (Figure 9.2).

A. Mechanism of action

The targets for benzodiazepine actions are the γ-aminobutyric acid (GABA$_A$) receptors. [Note: GABA is the major inhibitory neurotransmitter in the central nervous system (CNS).] These receptors are primarily composed of α, β and γ subunit families of which a combination of five or more span the postsynaptic membrane (Figure 9.3). Depending on the types, number of subunits, and brain region localization, the activation of the receptors results in different pharmacologic effects. Benzodiazepines modulate the GABA effects by binding to a specific, high-affinity site located at the interface of the α subunit and the γ$_2$ subunit (see Figure 9.3). [Note: These binding sites are sometimes labeled benzodiazepine receptors. Two benzodiazepine receptor subtypes commonly found in the CNS have been designated as BZ$_1$ and BZ$_2$ receptor depending on whether their composition includes the α$_1$ subunit or the α$_2$ subunit, respectively. The benzodiazepine receptor locations in the CNS parallel those of the GABA neu-

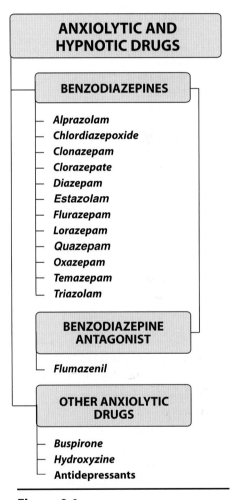

ANXIOLYTIC AND HYPNOTIC DRUGS

BENZODIAZEPINES

— *Alprazolam*
— *Chlordiazepoxide*
— *Clonazepam*
— *Clorazepate*
— *Diazepam*
— *Estazolam*
— *Flurazepam*
— *Lorazepam*
— *Quazepam*
— *Oxazepam*
— *Temazepam*
— *Triazolam*

BENZODIAZEPINE ANTAGONIST

— *Flumazenil*

OTHER ANXIOLYTIC DRUGS

— *Buspirone*
— *Hydroxyzine*
— *Antidepressants*

Figure 9.1
Summary of anxiolytic and hypnotic drugs.
(Figure continues on next page.)

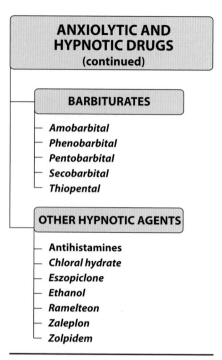

Figure 9.1 (continued)
Summary of anxiolytic and hypnotic drugs.

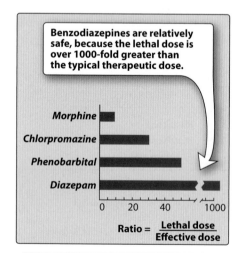

Figure 9.2
Ratio of lethal dose to effective dose for *morphine* (an opioid, see Chapter 14), *chlorpromazine* (a neuroleptic, see Chapter 13), and the anxiolytic, hypnotic drugs, *phenobarbital* and *diazepam*.

rons. Binding of GABA to its receptor triggers an opening of a chloride channel, which leads to an increase in chloride conductance (see Figure 9.3). Benzodiazepines increase the frequency of channel openings produced by GABA. The influx of chloride ions causes a small hyperpolarization that moves the postsynaptic potential away from its firing threshold and, thus, inhibits the formation of action potentials. [Note: Binding of a benzodiazepine to its receptor site will increase the affinity of GABA for the GABA-binding site (and vice versa) without actually changing the total number of sites.] The clinical effects of the various benzodiazepines correlate well with each drug's binding affinity for the GABA receptor–chloride ion channel complex.

B. Actions

The benzodiazepines have neither antipsychotic activity nor analgesic action, and they do not affect the autonomic nervous system. All benzodiazepines exhibit the following actions to a greater or lesser extent:

1. **Reduction of anxiety:** At low doses, the benzodiazepines are anxiolytic. They are thought to reduce anxiety by selectively enhancing GABAergic transmission in neurons having the α_2 subunit in their $GABA_A$ receptors, thereby inhibiting neuronal circuits in the limbic system of the brain.

2. **Sedative and hypnotic actions:** All of the benzodiazepines used to treat anxiety have some sedative properties, and some can produce hypnosis (artificially produced sleep) at higher doses. Their effects have been shown to be mediated by the α_1-$GABA_A$ receptors.

3. **Anterograde amnesia:** The temporary impairment of memory with use of the benzodiazepines is also mediated by the α_1-$GABA_A$ receptors. This also impairs a person's ability to learn and form new memories.

4. **Anticonvulsant:** Several of the benzodiazepines have anticonvulsant activity and some are used to treat epilepsy (status epilepticus) and other seizure disorders. This effect is partially, although not completely, mediated by α_1-$GABA_A$ receptors.

5. **Muscle relaxant:** At high doses, the benzodiazepines relax the spasticity of skeletal muscle, probably by increasing presynaptic inhibition in the spinal cord, where the α_2-$GABA_A$ receptors are largely located. *Baclofen* is a muscle relaxant that is believed to affect $GABA_b$ receptors at the level of the spinal cord.

C. Therapeutic uses

The individual benzodiazepines show small differences in their relative anxiolytic, anticonvulsant, and sedative properties. However, the duration of action varies widely among this group, and pharmacokinetic considerations are often important in choosing one benzodiazepine over another.

1. **Anxiety disorders:** Benzodiazepines are effective for the treatment of the anxiety symptoms secondary to panic disorder, generalized anxiety disorder, social anxiety disorder, performance anxiety, posttraumatic stress disorder, obsessive-compulsive disorder, and the extreme anxiety sometimes encountered with specific phobias, such as fear of flying. The benzodiazepines are also useful in treat-

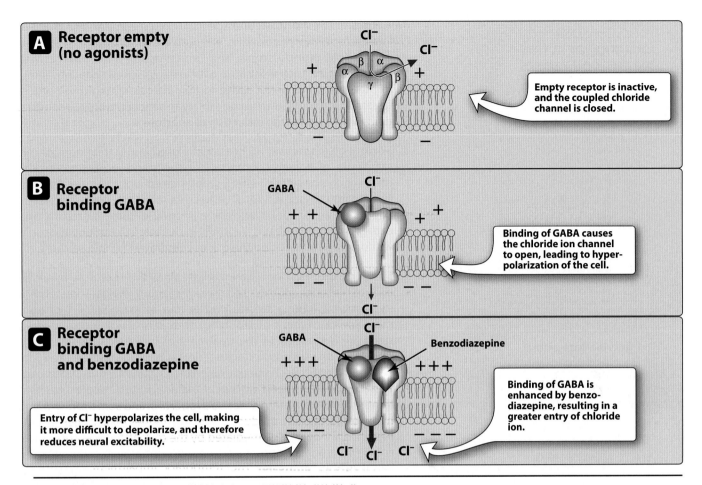

Figure 9.3
Schematic diagram of benzodiazepine–GABA–chloride ion channel complex. GABA = γ–aminobutyric acid.

ing the anxiety that accompanies some forms of depression and schizophrenia. These drugs should not be used to alleviate the normal stress of everyday life. They should be reserved for continued severe anxiety, and then should only be used for short periods of time because of their addiction potential. The longer-acting agents, such as *clonazepam* [kloe-NAZ-e-pam], *lorazepam* [lor-AZ-e-pam], and *diazepam* [dye-AZ-e-pam], are often preferred in those patients with anxiety that may require treatment for prolonged periods of time. The antianxiety effects of the benzodiazepines are less subject to tolerance than the sedative and hypnotic effects. [Note: Tolerance—that is, decreased responsiveness to repeated doses of the drug—occurs when used for more than one to two weeks. Cross-tolerance exists among this group of agents with ethanol. It has been shown that tolerance is associated with a decrease in GABA receptor density.] For panic disorders, *alprazolam* [al-PRAY-zoe-lam] is effective for short- and long-term treatment, although it may cause withdrawal reactions in about 30 percent of sufferers.

2. **Muscular disorders:** *Diazepam* is useful in the treatment of skeletal muscle spasms, such as occur in muscle strain, and in treating spasticity from degenerative disorders, such as multiple sclerosis and cerebral palsy.

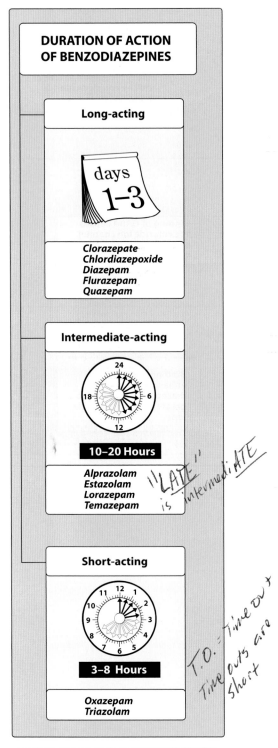

DURATION OF ACTION OF BENZODIAZEPINES

Long-acting

days 1-3

Clorazepate
Chlordiazepoxide
Diazepam
Flurazepam
Quazepam

Intermediate-acting

10–20 Hours

Alprazolam
Estazolam
Lorazepam
Temazepam

"LATE" is intermediATE

Short-acting

3–8 Hours

Oxazepam
Triazolam

T.O. = Time Out | Time outs are short

Figure 9.4
Comparison of the durations of action of the benzodiazepines.

3. **Amnesia:** The shorter-acting agents are often employed as premedication for anxiety-provoking and unpleasant procedures, such as endoscopic, bronchoscopic, and certain dental procedures as well as angioplasty. They also cause a form of conscious sedation, allowing the person to be receptive to instructions during these procedures. *Midazolam* [mi-DAY-zoe-lam] is an injectable-only benzodiazepine also used for the induction of anesthesia.

4. **Seizures:** *Clonazepam* is occasionally used in the treatment of certain types of epilepsy, whereas *diazepam* and *lorazepam* are the drugs of choice in terminating grand mal epileptic seizures and status epilepticus (see p. 174). Due to cross-tolerance, *chlordiazepoxide* [klor-di-az-e-POX-ide], *clorazepate* [klor-AZ-e-pate], *diazepam*, and *oxazepam* [ox-AZ-e-pam] are useful in the acute treatment of alcohol withdrawal and reducing the risk of withdrawal-related seizures.

5. **Sleep disorders:** Not all benzodiazepines are useful as hypnotic agents, although all have sedative or calming effects. They tend to decrease the latency to sleep onset and increase Stage II of non-rapid eye movement (REM) sleep. Both REM sleep and slow-wave sleep are decreased. In the treatment of insomnia, it is important to balance the sedative effect needed at bedtime with the residual sedation ("hangover") upon awakening. Commonly prescribed benzodiazepines for sleep disorders include long-acting *flurazepam* [flure-AZ-e-pam], intermediate-acting *temazepam* [te-MAZ-e-pam], and short-acting *triazolam* [trye-AY-zoe-lam]. Unlike the benzodiazepines, at usual hypnotic doses, the nonbenzodiazepine drugs, *zolpidem*, *zaleplon*, and *eszopiclone*, do not significantly alter the various sleep stages and, hence, are often the preferred hypnotics (see p. 113). This may be due to their relative selectivity for the BZ_1 receptor.

a. **Flurazepam:** This long-acting benzodiazepine significantly reduces both sleep-induction time and the number of awakenings, and it increases the duration of sleep. *Flurazepam* has a long-acting effect (Figure 9.4) and causes little rebound insomnia. With continued use, the drug has been shown to maintain its effectiveness for up to 4 weeks. *Flurazepam* and its active metabolites have a half-life of approximately 85 hours, which may result in daytime sedation and accumulation of the drug.

b. **Temazepam:** This drug is useful in patients who experience frequent wakening. However, the peak sedative effect occurs 1 to 3 hours after an oral dose; therefore, it should be given 1 to 2 hours before the desired bedtime.

c. **Triazolam:** This benzodiazepine has a relatively short duration of action and, therefore, is used to induce sleep in patients with recurring insomnia. Whereas *temazepam* is useful for insomnia caused by the inability to stay asleep, *triazolam* is effective in treating individuals who have difficulty in going to sleep. Tolerance frequently develops within a few days, and withdrawal of the drug often results in rebound insomnia, leading the patient to demand another prescription or higher dose. Therefore, this drug is best used intermittently rather than daily. In general, hypnotics should be given for only a limited time, usually less than 2 to 4 weeks.

D. Pharmacokinetics

1. **Absorption and distribution:** The benzodiazepines are lipophilic, and they are rapidly and completely absorbed after oral administration and distribute throughout the body.

2. **Duration of actions:** The half-lives of the benzodiazepines are very important clinically, because the duration of action may determine the therapeutic usefulness. The benzodiazepines can be roughly divided into short-, intermediate-, and long-acting groups (see Figure 9.4). The longer-acting agents form active metabolites with long half-lives. However, with some benzodiazepines, the clinical durations of action do not always correlate with actual half-lives (otherwise we would, conceivably, give a dose of *diazepam* every other day or even less often given its active metabolites). This may be due to receptor dissociation rates in the CNS and subsequent redistribution elsewhere.

3. **Fate:** Most benzodiazepines, including *chlordiazepoxide* and *diazepam*, are metabolized by the hepatic microsomal system to compounds that are also active. For these benzodiazepines, the apparent half-life of the drug represents the combined actions of the parent drug and its metabolites. The drugs' effects are terminated not only by excretion but also by redistribution. The benzodiazepines are excreted in the urine as glucuronides or oxidized metabolites. All the benzodiazepines cross the placental barrier and may depress the CNS of the newborn if given before birth. Nursing infants may also become exposed to the drugs in breast milk.

E. Dependence

Psychological and physical dependence on benzodiazepines can develop if high doses of the drugs are given over a prolonged period. Abrupt discontinuation of the benzodiazepines results in withdrawal symptoms, including confusion, anxiety, agitation, restlessness, insomnia, tension, and rarely, seizures. Because of the long half-lives of some benzodiazepines, withdrawal symptoms may occur slowly and last a number of days after discontinuation of therapy. Benzodiazepines with a short elimination half-life, such as *triazolam*, induce more abrupt and severe withdrawal reactions than those seen with drugs that are slowly eliminated, such as *flurazepam* (Figure 9.5).

F. Adverse effects

1. **Drowsiness and confusion:** These effects are the two most common side effects of the benzodiazepines. Ataxia occurs at high doses and precludes activities that require fine motor coordination, such as driving an automobile. Cognitive impairment (decreased long-term recall and acquisition of new knowledge) can occur with use of benzodiazepines. *Triazolam*, one of the most potent oral benzodiazepines with the most rapid elimination, often shows a rapid development of tolerance, early morning insomnia, and daytime anxiety, along with amnesia and confusion.

2. **Precautions:** Benzodiazepines should be used cautiously in treating patients with liver disease. They should be avoided in patients with acute narrow-angle glaucoma. Alcohol and other CNS depressants enhance the sedative-hypnotic effects of the benzodiazepines. Benzodiazepines are, however, considerably less dangerous than the

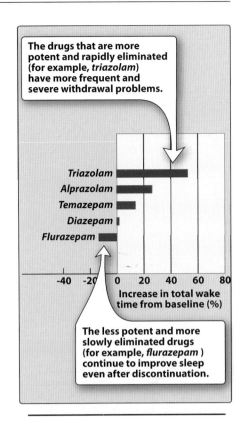

The drugs that are more potent and rapidly eliminated (for example, *triazolam*) have more frequent and severe withdrawal problems.

The less potent and more slowly eliminated drugs (for example, *flurazepam*) continue to improve sleep even after discontinuation.

Figure 9.5
Frequency of rebound insomnia resulting from discontinuation of benzodiazepine therapy.

older anxiolytic and hypnotic drugs. As a result, a drug overdose is seldom lethal unless other central depressants, such as alcohol, are taken concurrently.

III. BENZODIAZEPINE ANTAGONIST

Flumazenil [floo-MAZ-eh-nill] is a GABA-receptor antagonist that can rapidly reverse the effects of benzodiazepines. The drug is available for intravenous administration only. Onset is rapid but duration is short, with a half-life of about 1 hour. Frequent administration may be necessary to maintain reversal of a long-acting benzodiazepine. Administration of *flumazenil* may precipitate withdrawal in dependent patients or cause seizures if a benzodiazepine is used to control seizure activity. Seizures may also result if the patient ingests tricyclic antidepressants. Dizziness, nausea, vomiting, and agitation are the most common side effects.

IV. OTHER ANXIOLYTIC AGENTS

A. Buspirone

Buspirone [byoo-SPYE-rone] is useful in the treatment of generalized anxiety disorder and has an efficacy comparable to that of the benzodiazepines. The actions of *buspirone* appear to be mediated by serotonin (5-HT$_{1A}$) receptors, although other receptors could be involved, because *buspirone* displays some affinity for DA$_2$ dopamine receptors and 5-HT$_{2A}$ serotonin receptors. Thus, its mode of action differs from that of the benzodiazepines. [Note: "5-HT" and not "S" is the accepted abbreviation for serotonin (5-hydroxytryptamine) receptors.] In addition, *buspirone* lacks the anticonvulsant and muscle-relaxant properties of the benzodiazepines and causes only minimal sedation. However, it causes hypothermia and can increase prolactin and growth hormone. *Buspirone* undergoes metabolism by CYP3A4; thus, its half-life is shortened if taken with *rifampin* and lengthened if taken with *erythromycin*—an inducer and an inhibitor of the enzyme, respectively. The frequency of adverse effects is low, with the most common effects being headaches, dizziness, nervousness, and light-headedness. Sedation and psychomotor and cognitive dysfunction are minimal, and dependence is unlikely. *Buspirone* has the disadvantage of a slow onset of action. Figure 9.6 compares some of the common adverse effects of *buspirone* and the benzodiazepine *alprazolam*.

B. Hydroxyzine

Hydroxyzine [hye-DROX-i-zeen] is an antihistamine with antiemetic activity. It has a low tendency for habituation and, thus, is useful for patients with anxiety who have a history of drug abuse. It is also often used for sedation prior to dental procedures or surgery. Drowsiness is a possible adverse effect (see p. 552).

C. Antidepressants

Many antidepressants have proven efficacy in managing the long-term symptoms of chronic anxiety disorders and should be seriously considered as first-line agents, especially in patients with concerns for addiction or dependence or a history of addiction or dependence to other substances. The SSRIs, TCAs, *venlafaxine*, *duloxetine* and MAOIs all have potential usefulness in treating anxiety. Please refer to Chapter 12 for a discussion of the antidepressant agents.

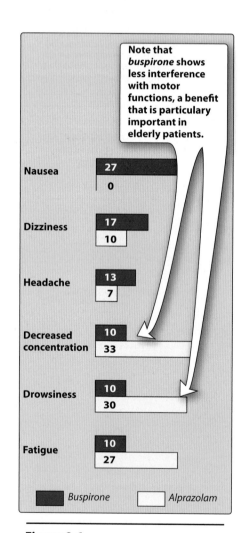

Figure 9.6
Comparison of common adverse effects of *buspirone* and *alprazolam*. Results are expressed as the percentage of patients showing each symptom.

V. BARBITURATES

The barbiturates were formerly the mainstay of treatment to sedate the patient or to induce and maintain sleep. Today, they have been largely replaced by the benzodiazepines, primarily because barbiturates induce tolerance, drug-metabolizing enzymes, physical dependence, and are associated with very severe withdrawal symptoms. Foremost is their ability to cause coma in toxic doses. Certain barbiturates, such as the very short-acting *thiopental*, are still used to induce anesthesia (see p. 135).

A. Mechanism of action

The sedative-hypnotic action of the barbiturates is due to their interaction with $GABA_A$ receptors, which enhances GABAergic transmission. The binding site is distinct from that of the benzodiazepines. Barbiturates potentiate GABA action on chloride entry into the neuron by prolonging the duration of the chloride channel openings. In addition, barbiturates can block excitatory glutamate receptors. Anesthetic concentrations of *pentobarbital* also block high-frequency sodium channels. All of these molecular actions lead to decreased neuronal activity.

B. Actions

Barbiturates are classified according to their duration of action (Figure 9.7). For example, *thiopental* [thye-oh-PEN-tal], which acts within seconds and has a duration of action of about 30 minutes, is used in the intravenous induction of anesthesia. By contrast, *phenobarbital* [fee-noe-BAR-bi-tal], which has a duration of action greater than a day, is useful in the treatment of seizures (see p. 178). *Pentobarbital* [pen-toe-BAR-bi-tal], *secobarbital* [see-koe-BAR-bi-tal], and *amobarbital* [am-oh-BAR-bi-tal] are short-acting barbiturates, which are effective as sedative and hypnotic (but not antianxiety) agents.

1. **Depression of CNS:** At low doses, the barbiturates produce sedation (calming effect, reducing excitement). At higher doses, the drugs cause hypnosis, followed by anesthesia (loss of feeling or sensation), and finally, coma and death. Thus, any degree of depression of the CNS is possible, depending on the dose. Barbiturates do not raise the pain threshold and have no analgesic properties. They may even exacerbate pain. Chronic use leads to tolerance.

2. **Respiratory depression:** Barbiturates suppress the hypoxic and chemoreceptor response to CO_2, and overdosage is followed by respiratory depression and death.

3. **Enzyme induction:** Barbiturates induce P450 microsomal enzymes in the liver. Therefore, chronic barbiturate administration diminishes the action of many drugs that are dependent on P450 metabolism to reduce their concentration.

C. Therapeutic uses

1. **Anesthesia:** Selection of a barbiturate is strongly influenced by the desired duration of action. The ultrashort-acting barbiturates, such as *thiopental*, are used intravenously to induce anesthesia.

2. **Anticonvulsant:** *Phenobarbital* is used in long-term management of tonic-clonic seizures, status epilepticus, and eclampsia. *Phenobarbital* has been regarded as the drug of choice for treatment of young chil-

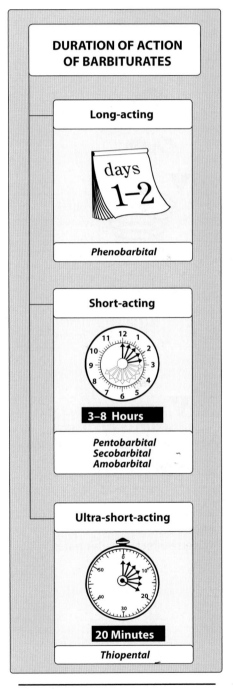

Figure 9.7
Barbiturates classified according to their durations of action.

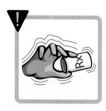

Potential
for Addiction

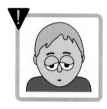

Drowsiness

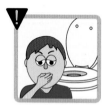

Nausea

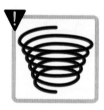

Vertigo

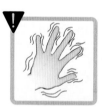

Tremors

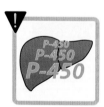

Enzyme
Induction

Figure 9.8
Adverse effect of barbiturates.

dren with recurrent febrile seizures. However, *phenobarbital* can depress cognitive performance in children, and the drug should be used cautiously. *Phenobarbital* has specific anticonvulsant activity that is distinguished from the nonspecific CNS depression.

3. **Anxiety:** Barbiturates have been used as mild sedatives to relieve anxiety, nervous tension, and insomnia. When used as hypnotics, they suppress REM sleep more than other stages. However, most have been replaced by the benzodiazepines.

D. Pharmacokinetics

Barbiturates are absorbed orally and distributed widely throughout the body. All barbiturates redistribute in the body from the brain to the splanchnic areas, to skeletal muscle, and finally, to adipose tissue. This movement is important in causing the short duration of action of *thiopental* and similar short-acting derivatives. They readily cross the placenta and can depress the fetus. Barbiturates are metabolized in the liver, and inactive metabolites are excreted in the urine.

E. Adverse effects

1. **CNS:** Barbiturates cause drowsiness, impaired concentration, and mental and physical sluggishness (Figure 9.8). The CNS depressant effects of barbiturates synergize with those of *ethanol*.

2. **Drug hangover:** Hypnotic doses of barbiturates produce a feeling of tiredness well after the patient wakes. This drug hangover may lead to impaired ability to function normally for many hours after waking. Occasionally, nausea and dizziness occur.

3. **Precautions:** As noted previously, barbiturates induce the P450 system and, therefore, may decrease the duration of action of drugs that are metabolized by these hepatic enzymes. Barbiturates increase porphyrin synthesis, and are contraindicated in patients with acute intermittent porphyria.

4. **Physical dependence:** Abrupt withdrawal from barbiturates may cause tremors, anxiety, weakness, restlessness, nausea and vomiting, seizures, delirium, and cardiac arrest. Withdrawal is much more severe than that associated with opiates and can result in death.

5. **Poisoning:** Barbiturate poisoning has been a leading cause of death resulting from drug overdoses for many decades. Severe depression of respiration is coupled with central cardiovascular depression, and results in a shock-like condition with shallow, infrequent breathing. Treatment includes artificial respiration and purging the stomach of its contents if the drug has been recently taken. [Note: No specific barbiturate antagonist is available.] Hemodialysis may be necessary if large quantities have been taken. Alkalinization of the urine often aids in the elimination of *phenobarbital* .

VI. OTHER HYPNOTIC AGENTS

A. Zolpidem

The hypnotic *zolpidem* [ZOL-pi-dem] is not a benzodiazepine in structure, but it acts on a subset of the benzodiazepine receptor family, BZ₁. *Zolpidem* has no anticonvulsant or muscle-relaxing properties. It shows few withdrawal effects, and exhibits minimal rebound insomnia, and little or no tolerance occurs with prolonged use. *Zolpidem* is rapidly absorbed from the gastrointestinal tract, and it has a rapid onset of action and short elimination half-life (about 2 to 3 hours). [Note: An extended-release formulation is now available.] *Zolpidem* undergoes hepatic oxidation by the cytochrome P450 system to inactive products. Thus, drugs such as *rifampin*, which induce this enzyme system, shorten the half-life of *zolpidem,* and drugs that inhibit the CYP3A4 isoenzyme may increase the half-life this drug. Adverse effects of *zolpidem* include nightmares, agitation, headache, gastrointestinal upset, dizziness, and daytime drowsiness.

B. Zaleplon

Zaleplon (ZAL-e-plon) is very similar to *zolpidem* in its hypnotic actions, but it causes fewer residual effects on psychomotor and cognitive functions compared to *zolpidem* or the benzodiazepines. This may be due to its rapid elimination, with a half-life that approximately 1 hour. The drug is metabolized by CYP3A4 (see p. 15).

C. Eszopiclone

Eszopiclone [es-ZOE-pi-clone] is an oral nonbenzodiazepine hypnotic (also utilizing the BZ_1 receptor similar to *zolpidem* and *zaleplon*) and is also used for treating insomnia. *Eszopiclone* been shown to be effective for up to 6 months compared to a placebo. *Eszopiclone* is rapidly absorbed (time to peak, 1 hour), extensively metabolized by oxidation and demethylation via the cytochrome enzyme system and mainly excreted in the urine. Elimination half-life is approximately 6 hours. Adverse events reported with *eszopiclone* include anxiety, dry mouth, headache, peripheral edema, somnolence, and unpleasant taste.

D. Ramelteon

Ramelteon [ram-EL-tee-on] is a selective agonist at the MT_1 and MT_2 subtypes of melatonin receptors. Normally, light stimulating the retina transmits a signal to the suprachiasmatic nucleus (SCN) of the hypothalamus, that in turn relays a signal via a lengthy nerve pathway to the pineal gland that inhibits the release of melatonin from the gland. As darkness falls and light ceases to strike the retina, melatonin release from the pineal gland is no longer inhibited, and the gland begins to secrete melatonin. Stimulation of MT_1 and MT_2 receptors by melatonin in the SCN is able to induce and promote sleep and is thought to maintain the circadian rhythm underlying the normal sleep-wake cycle. *Ramelteon* is indicated for the treatment of insomnia in which falling asleep (increased sleep latency) is the primary complaint. The potential for abuse of *ramelteon* is believed to be minimal, and no evidence of dependence or withdrawal effects has been observed. Therefore, *ramelteon* can be administered long-term. Common adverse effects of *ramelteon* include dizziness, fatigue, and somnolence. *Ramelteon* may also increase prolactin levels.

E. Chloral hydrate

Chloral hydrate [KLOR-al-HYE-drate] is a trichlorinated derivative of acetaldehyde that is converted to the active metabolite, trichloroethanol, in the body. The drug is an effective sedative and hypnotic that induces sleep in about 30 minutes and the duration of sleep is about 6 hours. *Chloral hydrate* is irritating to the gastrointestinal tract and causes epigastric distress. It also produces an unusual, unpleasant taste sensation. It synergizes with *ethanol*.

F. Antihistamines

Nonprescription antihistamines with sedating properties, such as *diphenhydramine* and *doxylamine*, are effective in treating mild types of insomnia. However, these drugs are usually ineffective for all but the milder forms of situational insomnia. Furthermore, they have numerous undesirable side effects (such as anticholinergic effects) that make them less useful than the benzodiazepines. These sedative antihistamines are marketed in numerous over-the-counter products.

G. Ethanol

Ethanol (*ethyl alcohol*) has anxiolytic and sedative effects, but its toxic potential outweighs its benefits. Alcoholism is a serious medical and social problem. *Ethanol* [ETH-an-ol] is a CNS depressant, producing sedation and, ultimately, hypnosis with increasing dosage. *Ethanol* has a shallow dose–response curve; therefore, sedation occurs over a wide dosage range. It is readily absorbed orally and has a volume of distribution close to that of total body water. *Ethanol* is metabolized primarily in the liver, first to acetaldehyde by alcohol dehydrogenase and then to acetate by aldehyde dehydrogenase (Figure 9.9). Elimination is mostly through the kidney, but a fraction is excreted through the lungs. *Ethanol* synergizes with many other sedative agents and can produce severe CNS depression with benzodiazepines, antihistamines, or barbiturates. Chronic consumption can lead to severe liver disease, gastritis, and nutritional deficiencies. Cardiomyopathy is also a consequence of heavy drinking. The treatment of choice for alcohol withdrawal are the benzodiazepines. *Carbamazepine* is effective in treating convulsive episodes during withdrawal.

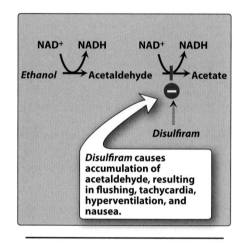

Figure 9.9
Metabolism of *ethanol*, and the effect of *disulfiram*. NAD$^+$ = oxidized form of nicotinamide-adenine dinucleotide; NADH = reduced form of nicotinamide-adenine dinucleotide.

1. **Disulfiram:** *Disulfiram* [dye-SUL-fi-ram] blocks the oxidation of acetaldehyde to acetic acid by inhibiting aldehyde dehydrogenase (see Figure 9.9). This results in the accumulation of acetaldehyde in the blood, causing flushing, tachycardia, hyperventilation, and nausea. *Disulfiram* has found some use in the patient seriously desiring to stop alcohol ingestion. A conditioned avoidance response is induced so that the patient abstains from alcohol to prevent the unpleasant effects of *disulfiram*-induced acetaldehyde accumulation.

2. **Naltrexone:** *Naltrexone* [nal-TREX-own] is a long-acting opiate antagonist (available orally or as a long-acting injectable) that is U.S. Food and Drug Administration–approved for the treatment of alcohol dependence and should be utilized in conjunction with supportive psychotherapy. It is better tolerated than *disulfiram* and does not produce the aversive reaction that *disulfiram* does.

3. **Acamprosate:** An agent utilized in alcohol dependence treatment programs with an as yet poorly understood mechanism of action that should also be utilized in conjunction with supportive psychotherapy.

Figure 9.10 summarizes the therapeutic disadvantages and advantages of some of the anxiolytic and hypnotic drugs.

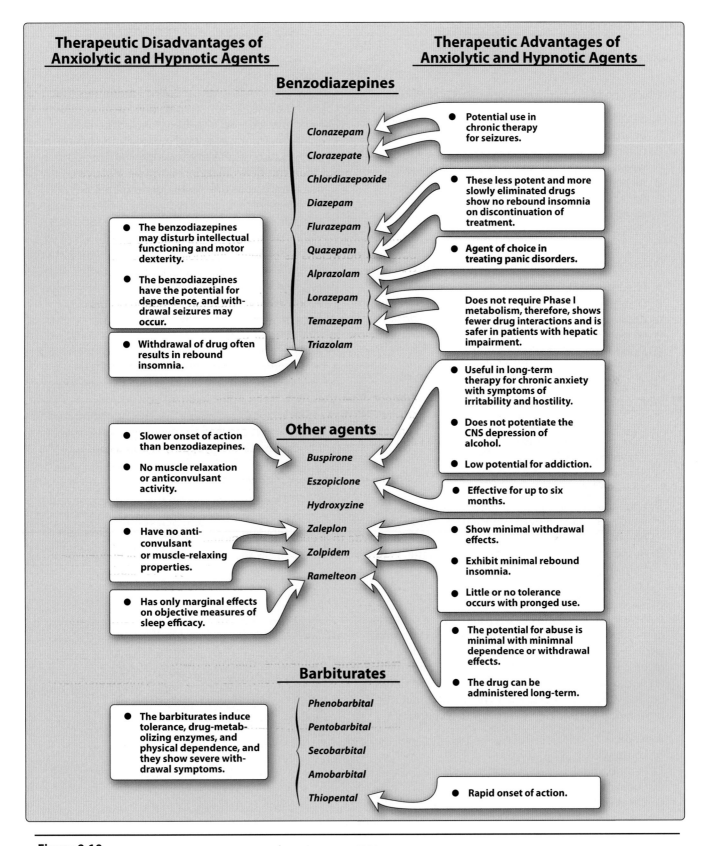

Figure 9.10
Therapeutic disadvantages and advantages of some anxiolytic and hypnotic agents. CNS = central nervous system.

Study Questions

Choose the ONE best answer.

9.1 Which one of the following statements is correct?

A. Benzodiazepines directly open chloride channels.
B. Benzodiazepines show analgesic actions.
C. Clinical improvement of anxiety requires 2 to 4 weeks of treatment with benzodiazepines.
D. All benzodiazepines have some sedative effects.
E. Benzodiazepines, like other CNS depressants, readily produce general anesthesia.

Correct answer = D. Although all benzodiazepines can cause sedation, the drugs labeled "benzodiazepines" in Figure 9.1 are promoted for the treatment of sleep disorder. Benzodiazepines enhance the binding of GABA to its receptor, which increases the permeability of chloride. The benzodiazepines do not relieve pain but may reduce the anxiety associated with pain. Unlike the tricyclic antidepressants and the monoamine oxidase inhibitors, the benzodiazepines are effective within hours of administration. Benzodiazepines do not produce general anesthesia and, therefore, are relatively safe drugs with a high therapeutic index.

9.2 Which one of the following is a short-acting hypnotic?

A. Phenobarbital.
B. Diazepam.
C. Chlordiazepoxide.
D. Triazolam.
E. Flurazepam.

Correct answer = D. Triazolam is an ultrashort-acting drug used as an adjuvant to dental anesthesia.

9.3 Which one of the following statements is correct?

A. Phenobarbital shows analgesic properties.
B. Diazepam and phenobarbital induce the P450 enzyme system.
C. Phenobarbital is useful in the treatment of acute intermittent porphyria.
D. Phenobarbital induces respiratory depression, which is enhanced by the consumption of ethanol.
E. Buspirone has actions similar to those of the benzodiazepines.

Correct answer = D. Barbiturates and ethanol are a potentially lethal combination. Phenobarbital is unable to alter the pain threshold. Only phenobarbital strongly induces the synthesis of the hepatic cytochrome P450 drug-metabolizing system. Phenobarbital is contraindicated in the treatment of acute intermittent porphyria. Buspirone lacks the anticonvulsant and muscle-relaxant properties of the benzodiazepines and causes only minimal sedation.

9.4 A 45-year-old man who has been injured in a car accident is brought into the emergency room. His blood alcohol level on admission is 275 mg/dL. Hospital records show a prior hospitalization for alcohol-related seizures. His wife confirms that he has been drinking heavily for 3 weeks. What treatment should be provided to the patient if he goes into withdrawal?

A. None.
B. Lorazepam.
C. Pentobarbital.
D. Phenytoin.
E. Buspirone

Correct answer = B. It is important to treat the seizures associated with alcohol withdrawal. Benzodiazepines, such as chlordiazepoxide, diazepam, or the shorter-acting lorazepam, are effective in controlling this problem. They are less sedating than pentobarbital or phenytoin.

CNS Stimulants

10

I. OVERVIEW

This chapter describes two groups of drugs that act primarily to stimulate the central nervous system (CNS). The first group, the psychomotor stimulants, cause excitement and euphoria, decrease feelings of fatigue, and increase motor activity. The second group, the hallucinogens, or psychotomimetic drugs, produce profound changes in thought patterns and mood, with little effect on the brainstem and spinal cord. Figure 10.1 summarizes the CNS stimulants. As a group, the CNS stimulants have diverse clinical uses and are important as drugs of abuse, as are the CNS depressants described in Chapter 9 and the narcotics described in Chapter 14 (Figure 10.2).

II. PSYCHOMOTOR STIMULANTS

A. Methylxanthines

The methylxanthines include *theophylline* [thee-OFF-i-lin] which is found in tea; *theobromine* [thee-o-BRO-min], found in cocoa; and *caffeine* [kaf-EEN]. *Caffeine*, the most widely consumed stimulant in the world, is found in highest concentration in coffee, but it is also present in tea, cola drinks, chocolate candy, and cocoa.

1. **Mechanism of action:** Several mechanisms have been proposed for the actions of methylxanthines, including translocation of extracellular calcium, increase in cyclic adenosine monophosphate and cyclic guanosine monophosphate caused by inhibition of phosphodiesterase, and blockade of adenosine receptors. The latter most likely accounts for the actions achieved by the usual consumption of *caffeine*-containing beverages.

2. **Actions:**

   a. **CNS:** The *caffeine* contained in one to two cups of coffee (100–200 mg) causes a decrease in fatigue and increased mental alertness as a result of stimulating the cortex and other areas of the brain. Consumption of 1.5 g of *caffeine* (12 to 15 cups of coffee) produces anxiety and tremors. The spinal cord is stimulated only by very high doses (2–5 g) of *caffeine*. Tolerance can rapidly develop to the stimulating properties of *caffeine*; withdrawal consists of feelings of fatigue and sedation.

   b. **Cardiovascular system:** A high dose of *caffeine* has positive inotropic and chronotropic effects on the heart. [Note:

CNS STIMULANTS

PSYCHOMOTOR STIMULANTS

— *Amphetamine*
— *Armodafinil*
— *Atomoxetine*
— *Caffeine*
— *Cocaine*
— *Dextroamphetamine*
— *Lisdexamfetamine*
— *Methylphenidate*
— *Modafinil*
— *Nicotine*
— *Theobromine*
— *Theophylline*
— *Varenicline*

HALLUCINOGENS

— *Lysergic acid diethylamide (LSD)*
— *Phencyclidine (PCP)*
— *Tetrahydrocannabinol (THC)*

Figure 10.1
Summary of central nervous system (CNS) stimulants.

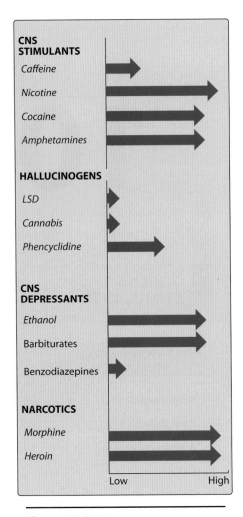

Figure 10.2
Relative potential for physical dependence on commonly abused substances.

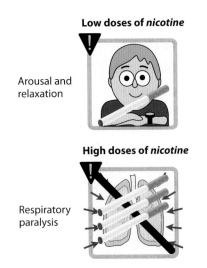

Figure 10.3
Actions of *nicotine* on the central nervous system.

Increased contractility can be harmful to patients with angina pectoris. In others, an accelerated heart rate can trigger premature ventricular contractions.]

   c. Diuretic action: *Caffeine* has a mild diuretic action that increases urinary output of sodium, chloride, and potassium.

   d. Gastric mucosa: Because all methylxanthines stimulate secretion of hydrochloric acid from the gastric mucosa, individuals with peptic ulcers should avoid beverages containing methylxanthines.

3. Therapeutic uses: *Caffeine* and its derivatives relax the smooth muscles of the bronchioles. [Note: Previously the mainstay of asthma therapy, *theophylline* has been largely replaced by other agents, such as β_2 agonists and corticosteroids.]

4. Pharmacokinetics: The methylxanthines are well absorbed orally. *Caffeine* distributes throughout the body, including the brain. The drugs cross the placenta to the fetus and is secreted into the mother's milk. All the methylxanthines are metabolized in the liver, generally by the CYP1A2 pathway, and the metabolites are then excreted in the urine.

5. Adverse effects: Moderate doses of *caffeine* cause insomnia, anxiety, and agitation. A high dosage is required for toxicity, which is manifested by emesis and convulsions. The lethal dose is about 10 g of *caffeine* (about 100 cups of coffee), which induces cardiac arrhythmias; death from *caffeine* is thus highly unlikely. Lethargy, irritability, and headache occur in users who have routinely consumed more than 600 mg of *caffeine* per day (roughly six cups of coffee per day) and then suddenly stop.

B. Nicotine

Nicotine [NIC-o-teen] is the active ingredient in tobacco. Although this drug is not currently used therapeutically (except in smoking cessation therapy, see p. 118), *nicotine* remains important, because it is second only to *caffeine* as the most widely used CNS stimulant and second only to alcohol as the most abused drug. In combination with the tars and carbon monoxide found in cigarette smoke, *nicotine* represents a serious risk factor for lung and cardiovascular disease, various cancers, as well as other illnesses. Dependency on the drug is not easily overcome.

1. Mechanism of action: In low doses, *nicotine* causes ganglionic stimulation by depolarization. At high doses, *nicotine* causes ganglionic blockade. *Nicotine* receptors exist at a number of sites in the CNS, which participate in the stimulant attributes of the drug.

2. Actions:

   a. CNS: *Nicotine* is highly lipid soluble and readily crosses the blood-brain barrier. Cigarette smoking or administration of low doses of *nicotine* produces some degree of euphoria and arousal as well as relaxation. It improves attention, learning, problem solving, and reaction time. High doses of *nicotine* result in central respiratory paralysis and severe hypotension caused by medullary paralysis (Figure 10.3). Nicotine is an appetite suppressant.

b. Peripheral effects: The peripheral effects of *nicotine* are complex. Stimulation of sympathetic ganglia as well as the adrenal medulla increases blood pressure and heart rate. Thus, use of tobacco is particularly harmful in hypertensive patients. Many patients with peripheral vascular disease experience an exacerbation of symptoms with smoking. For example, *nicotine*-induced vasoconstriction can decrease coronary blood flow, adversely affecting a patient with angina. Stimulation of parasympathetic ganglia also increases motor activity of the bowel. At higher doses, blood pressure falls, and activity ceases in both the gastrointestinal tract and bladder musculature as a result of a *nicotine*-induced block of parasympathetic ganglia.

3. **Pharmacokinetics:** Because *nicotine* is highly lipid soluble, absorption readily occurs via the oral mucosa, lungs, gastrointestinal mucosa, and skin. *Nicotine* crosses the placental membrane and is secreted in the milk of lactating women. By inhaling tobacco smoke, the average smoker takes in 1 to 2 mg of nicotine per cigarette (most cigarettes contain 6 to 8 mg of *nicotine*). The acute lethal dose is 60 mg. More than 90 percent of the *nicotine* inhaled in smoke is absorbed. Clearance of *nicotine* involves metabolism in the lung and the liver and urinary excretion. Tolerance to the toxic effects of *nicotine* develops rapidly, often within days after beginning usage.

4. **Adverse effects:** The CNS effects of *nicotine* include irritability and tremors. *Nicotine* may also cause intestinal cramps, diarrhea, and increased heart rate and blood pressure. In addition, cigarette smoking increases the rate of metabolism for a number of drugs.

5. **Withdrawal syndrome:** As with the other drugs in this class, *nicotine* is an addictive substance, and physical dependence on *nicotine* develops rapidly and can be severe (Figure 10.4). Withdrawal is characterized by irritability, anxiety, restlessness, difficulty concentrating, headaches, and insomnia. Appetite is affected, and gastrointestinal pain often occurs. [Note: Smoking cessation programs that combine pharmacologic and behavioral therapy are the most successful in helping individuals to stop smoking.] The transdermal patch and chewing gum containing *nicotine* have been shown to reduce *nicotine* withdrawal symptoms and to help smokers stop smoking. For example, the blood concentration of *nicotine* obtained from nicotine chewing gum is typically about one-half the peak level observed with smoking (Figure 10.5). *Bupropion*, an antidepressant (see p. 145), can reduce the craving for cigarettes.

C. Varenicline

Varenicline [ver-EN-e-kleen] is a partial agonist at $\alpha_4\beta_2$ neuronal nicotinic acetylcholine receptors in the CNS. Because it is only a partial agonist at these receptors, it produces less euphoric effects than those produced by *nicotine* itself (nicotine is a full agonist at these receptors). Thus, it is useful as an adjunct in the management of smoking cessation in patients with *nicotine* withdrawal symptoms. Additionally, *varenicline* tends to attenuate the rewarding effects of nicotine if a person relapses and uses tobacco. Patients should be monitored for suicidal thoughts, vivid nightmares and mood changes.

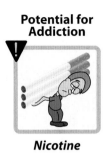

Potential for Addiction

Nicotine

Figure 10.4
Nicotine has potential for addiction.

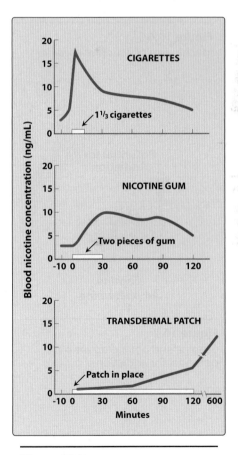

Figure 10.5
Blood concentrations of *nicotine* in individuals who smoked cigarettes, chewed nicotine gum, or received nicotine by transdermal patch.

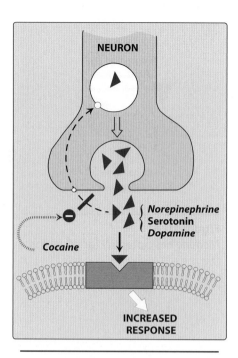

Figure 10.6
Mechanism of action of *cocaine*.

**Potential for
Addiction**

*Cocaine
Amphetamine*

Figure 10.7
Cocaine and *amphetamine* have
potential for addiction.

D. Cocaine

Cocaine [KOE-kane] is a widely available and highly addictive drug that is currently abused daily by more than 3 million people in the United States. Because of its abuse potential, *cocaine* is classified as a Schedule II drug by the U.S. Drug Enforcement Agency (see p. 541).

1. **Mechanism of action:** The primary mechanism of action underlying the central and peripheral effects of *cocaine* is blockade of reuptake of the monoamines (*norepinephrine*, serotonin, and *dopamine*) into the presynaptic terminals from which these neurotransmitters are released (Figure 10.6). This blockade is caused by *cocaine* binding to the monoaminergic reuptake transporters and, thus, potentiates and prolongs the CNS and peripheral actions of these monoamines. In particular, the prolongation of dopaminergic effects in the brain's pleasure system (limbic system) produces the intense euphoria that *cocaine* initially causes. Chronic intake of *cocaine* depletes *dopamine*. This depletion triggers the vicious cycle of craving for *cocaine* that temporarily relieves severe depression (Figure 10.7).

2. **Actions:**

   a. **CNS:** The behavioral effects of *cocaine* result from powerful stimulation of the cortex and brainstem. *Cocaine* acutely increases mental awareness and produces a feeling of well-being and euphoria similar to that caused by *amphetamine*. Like *amphetamine*, *cocaine* can produce hallucinations and delusions of paranoia or grandiosity. *Cocaine* increases motor activity, and at high doses, it causes tremors and convulsions, followed by respiratory and vasomotor depression.

   b. **Sympathetic nervous system:** Peripherally, *cocaine* potentiates the action of *norepinephrine*, and it produces the "fight or flight" syndrome characteristic of adrenergic stimulation. This is associated with tachycardia, hypertension, pupillary dilation, and peripheral vasoconstriction. Recent evidence suggests that the ability of baroreceptor reflexes to buffer the hypertensive effect may be impaired.

   c. **Hyperthermia:** *Cocaine* is unique among illicit drugs in that death can result not only as a function of dose but also from the drug's propensity to cause hyperthermia. [Note: Mortality rates for *cocaine* overdose rise in hot weather.] Even a small dose of intranasal *cocaine* impairs sweating and cutaneous vasodilatation. Perception of thermal discomfort is also decreased.

3. **Therapeutic uses:** *Cocaine* has a local anesthetic action that represents the only current rationale for the therapeutic use of *cocaine*. For example, *cocaine* is applied topically as a local anesthetic during eye, ear, nose, and throat surgery. Whereas the local anesthetic action of *cocaine* is due to a block of voltage-activated sodium channels, an interaction with potassium channels may contribute to the ability of *cocaine* to cause cardiac arrhythmias. [Note: *Cocaine* is the only local anesthetic that causes vasoconstriction. This effect is responsible for the necrosis and perforation of the nasal septum seen in association with chronic inhalation of *cocaine* powder.]

4. **Pharmacokinetics:** *Cocaine* is often self-administered by chewing, intranasal snorting, smoking, or intravenous (IV) injection. The peak effect occurs at 15 to 20 minutes after intranasal intake of *cocaine* powder, and the "high" disappears in 1 to 1.5 hours. Rapid but short-lived effects are achieved following IV injection of *cocaine* or by smoking the freebase form of the drug ("crack"). Because the onset of action is most rapid, the potential for overdosage and dependence is greatest with IV injection and crack smoking. *Cocaine* is rapidly de-esterified and demethylated to benzoylecgonine, which is excreted in the urine. Detection of this substance in the urine identifies a user.

5. **Adverse effects:**

   a. **Anxiety:** The toxic response to acute *cocaine* ingestion can precipitate an anxiety reaction that includes hypertension, tachycardia, sweating, and paranoia. Because of the irritability, many users take *cocaine* with alcohol. A product of *cocaine* metabolites and *ethanol* is cocaethylene, which is also psychoactive and believed to contribute to cardiotoxicity.

   b. **Depression:** Like all stimulant drugs, *cocaine* stimulation of the CNS is followed by a period of mental depression. Addicts withdrawing from *cocaine* exhibit physical and emotional depression as well as agitation. The latter symptom can be treated with benzodiazepines or phenothiazines.

   c. **Toxic effects:** *Cocaine* can induce seizures as well as fatal cardiac arrhythmias (Figure 10.8). Use of IV *diazepam* and *propranolol* may be required to control *cocaine*-induced seizures and cardiac arrhythmias, respectively. The incidence of myocardial infarction in *cocaine* users is unrelated to dose, to duration of use, or to route of administration. There is no marker to identify those individuals who may have life-threatening cardiac effects after taking *cocaine*.

E. **Amphetamine**

Amphetamine [am-FE-ta-meen] is a noncatecholaminergic sympathetic amine that shows neurologic and clinical effects quite similar to those of *cocaine*. *Dextroamphetamine* [dex-troe-am-FE-ta-meen] is the major member of this class of compounds. *Methamphetamine* [meth-am-FET-ah-mine] (also known as "speed") is a derivative of *amphetamine* that can be smoked, and it is preferred by many abusers.

1. **Mechanism of action:** As with *cocaine*, the effects of *amphetamine* on the CNS and peripheral nervous system are indirect; that is, both depend upon an elevation of the level of catecholamine neurotransmitters in synaptic spaces. *Amphetamine*, however, achieves this effect by releasing intracellular stores of catecholamines (Figure 10.9). Because *amphetamine* also inhibits monoamine oxidase (MAO), high levels of catecholamines are readily released into synaptic spaces. Despite different mechanisms of action, the behavioral effects of *amphetamine* and its derivatives are similar to those of *cocaine*.

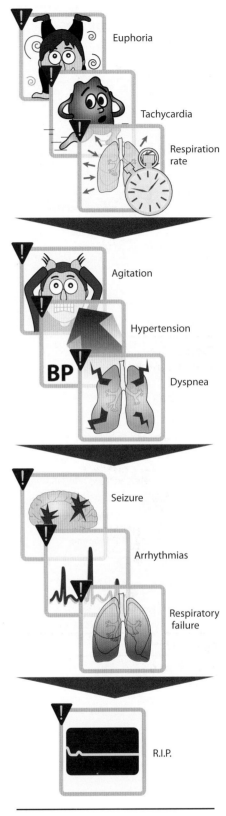

Figure 10.8
Major effects of *cocaine* use.

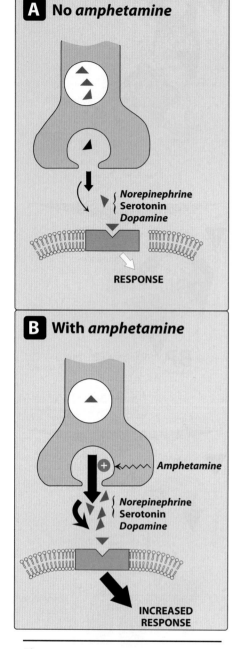

Figure 10.9
Mechanism of action of *amphetamine*.

2. **Actions:**

a. **CNS:** The major behavioral effects of *amphetamine* result from a combination of its *dopamine* and *norepinephrine* release-enhancing properties. *Amphetamine* stimulates the entire cerebrospinal axis, cortex, brainstem, and medulla. This leads to increased alertness, decreased fatigue, depressed appetite, and insomnia. These CNS stimulant effects of *amphetamine* and its derivatives have led to their use in therapy for hyperactivity in children, narcolepsy, and for appetite control. At high doses, psychosis and convulsions can ensue.

b. **Sympathetic nervous system:** In addition to its marked action on the CNS, *amphetamine* acts on the adrenergic system, indirectly stimulating the receptors through *norepinephrine* release.

3. **Therapeutic uses:** Factors that limit the therapeutic usefulness of *amphetamine* include psychological and physiological dependence similar to those with *cocaine* and the development of tolerance to the euphoric and anorectic effects with chronic use. [Note: Less tolerance to the toxic CNS effects (for example, convulsions) develops.]

a. **Attention deficit hyperactivity disorder (ADHD):** Some young children are hyperkinetic and lack the ability to be involved in any one activity for longer than a few minutes. *Dextroamphetamine* and the *amphetamine* derivative *methylphenidate* [meth-ill-FEN-i-date] are able to improve attention and to alleviate many of the behavioral problems associated with this syndrome, and to reduce the hyperkinesia that such children demonstrate. *Lisdexamfetamine* [lis-dex-am-FE-ta-meen] is a prodrug that is converted to the active component *dextroamphetamine* after gastrointestinal absorption and metabolism. The drug prolongs the patient's span of attention allowing better function in a school atmosphere. *Atomoxetine* [AT-oh-mox-e-teen] is a nonstimulant drug approved for ADHD in children and adults. [Note: It should not be taken by individuals on MAO inhibitors, and it is not recommended for patients with narrow-angle glaucoma.] Unlike *methylphenidate* which blocks *dopamine* reuptake, *atomoxetine* is a *norepinephrine* reuptake inhibitor. It is not habit forming and is not a controlled substance.

b. **Narcolepsy:** Narcolepsy is a relatively rare sleep disorder that is characterized by uncontrollable bouts of sleepiness during the day. It is sometimes accompanied by catalepsy, a loss in muscle control, or even paralysis brought on by strong emotions, such as laughter. However, it is the sleepiness for which the patient is usually treated with drugs such as *amphetamine* or *methylphenidate*. Recently, a newer drug, *modafinil* (moe-DA-fi-nil), and its R-enantiomer derivative, *armodafinil*, have become available to treat narcolepsy. *Modafinil* produces fewer psychoactive and euphoric effects as well as, alterations in mood, perception, thinking, and feelings typical of other CNS stimulants. It does promote wakefulness. The mechanism of action remains unclear but may involve the adrenergic and dopaminergic systems, although it has been shown to differ from that of *amphetamine*. *Modafinil* is effective orally. It is well distributed throughout the body and undergoes extensive hepatic metabolism. The metabolites are excreted in the urine. Headaches, nausea, and rhinitis are the primary adverse effects. There is some evidence to indicate the potential for abuse and physical dependence with *modafinil*.

4. **Pharmacokinetics:** *Amphetamine* is completely absorbed from the gastrointestinal tract, metabolized by the liver, and excreted in the urine. [Note: Administration of urinary alkalinizing agents will increase the non-ionized species of the drug and decrease its excretion.] *Amphetamine* abusers often administer the drugs by IV injection and by smoking. The euphoria caused by *amphetamine* lasts 4 to 6 hours, or four- to eight-fold longer than the effects of *cocaine*.

5. **Adverse effects:** The *amphetamines* may cause addiction, leading to dependence, tolerance, and drug-seeking behavior. In addition, they have the following undesirable effects.

   a. **Central effects:** Undesirable side effects of *amphetamine* usage include insomnia, irritability, weakness, dizziness, tremor, and hyperactive reflexes (Figure 10.10). *Amphetamine* can also cause confusion, delirium, panic states, and suicidal tendencies, especially in mentally ill patients. Chronic *amphetamine* use produces a state of "*amphetamine* psychosis" that resembles the psychotic episodes associated with schizophrenia. Whereas long-term *amphetamine* use is associated with psychic and physical dependence, tolerance to its effects may occur within a few weeks. Overdoses of *amphetamine* are treated with *chlorpromazine* or *haloperidol*, which relieve the CNS symptoms as well as the hypertension because of their α-blocking effects. The anorectic effect of *amphetamine* is due to its action in the lateral hypothalamic feeding center. 3,4-Methylenedioxymethamphetamine (also known as MDMA, or Ecstasy) is a synthetic derivative of *methamphetamine* with both stimulant and hallucinogenic properties (see p. 537).

   b. **Cardiovascular effects:** In addition to its CNS effects, *amphetamine* causes palpitations, cardiac arrhythmias, hypertension, anginal pain, and circulatory collapse. Headache, chills, and excessive sweating may also occur. Because of its cardiovascular effects, *amphetamine* should not be given to patients with cardiovascular disease or those receiving MAO inhibitors.

   c. **Gastrointestinal system effects:** *Amphetamine* acts on the gastrointestinal system, causing anorexia, nausea, vomiting, abdominal cramps, and diarrhea. Administration of *sodium bicarbonate* will increase the reabsorption of *dextroamphetamine* from the renal tubules into the bloodstream.

   d. **Contraindications:** Patients with hypertension, cardiovascular disease, hyperthyroidism, or glaucoma should not be treated with this drug, nor should patients with a history of drug abuse.

F. **Methylphenidate**

Methylphenidate has CNS stimulant properties similar to those of *amphetamine* and may also lead to abuse, although its addictive poten-

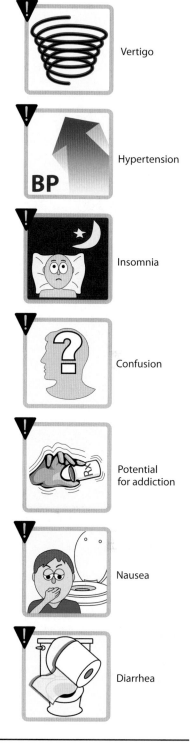

Vertigo

Hypertension

Insomnia

Confusion

Potential for addiction

Nausea

Diarrhea

Figure 10.10
Adverse effects of amphetamines.

tial is controversial. It is a Schedule II drug (see p. 541). It is presently one of the most prescribed medications in children. It is estimated that *methylphenidate* is taken daily by 4 to 6 million children in the United States for ADHD. The pharmacologically active isomer, *dexmethylphenidate*, has been approved in the United States for the treatment of ADHD.

1. **Mechanism of action:** Children with ADHD may produce weak *dopamine* signals, which suggests that usually interesting activities provide fewer rewards to these children. At present, the basis for the stimulant effect of *methylphenidate* is not understood. However, a recent study using positron-emission tomography has opened up some interesting possibilities. It showed that *methylphenidate* is a more potent *dopamine* transport inhibitor than *cocaine*, thus making more *dopamine* available. [Note: *Methylphenidate* may have less potential for abuse than *cocaine*, because it enters the brain much more slowly than *cocaine* and, thus, does not increase *dopamine* levels as rapidly.]

2. **Therapeutic uses:** *Methylphenidate* has been used for several decades in the treatment of ADHD in children aged 6 to 16. It is also effective in the treatment of narcolepsy. Unlike *methylphenidate*, *dexmethylphenidate* is not indicated in the treatment of narcolepsy.

3. **Pharmacokinetics:** Both *methylphenidate* and *dexmethylphenidate* are readily absorbed on oral administration. Concentrations in the brain exceed those in the plasma. The de-esterified product, ritalinic acid, is excreted in the urine.

4. **Adverse reactions:** Gastrointestinal effects are the most common. These include abdominal pain and nausea. Other reactions include anorexia, insomnia, nervousness, and fever. In seizure patients, *methylphenidate* seems to increase the seizure frequency, especially if the patient is taking antidepressants. *Methylphenidate* is contraindicated in patients with glaucoma.

5. **Drug interactions:** Studies have shown that *methylphenidate* can interfere in the metabolism of *warfarin*, *diphenylhydantoin*, *phenobarbital*, *primidone*, and the tricyclic antidepressants.

III. HALLUCINOGENS

A few drugs have, as their primary action, the ability to induce altered perceptual states reminiscent of dreams. Many of these altered states are accompanied by bright, colorful changes in the environment and by a plasticity of constantly changing shapes and color. The individual under the influence of these drugs is incapable of normal decision making, because the drug interferes with rational thought. These compounds are known as hallucinogens or psychotomimetic drugs.

A. Lysergic acid diethylamide

Multiple sites in the CNS are affected by *lysergic acid diethylamide (LSD)*. The drug shows serotonin (5-HT) agonist activity at presynaptic 5-HT$_1$ receptors in the midbrain, and also stimulates 5-HT$_2$ receptors. Activation of the sympathetic nervous system occurs, which causes pupillary dilation, increased blood pressure, piloerection, and increased body temperature. Taken orally, low doses of *LSD* can induce hallucinations with brilliant colors. Mood alteration also occurs. Tolerance

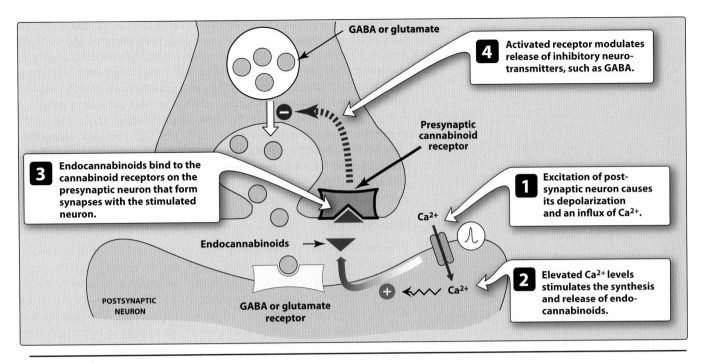

Figure 10.11
Cannabinoid receptor. GABA = γ-aminobutyric aid.

and physical dependence have occurred, but true dependence is rare. Adverse effects include hyperreflexia, nausea, and muscular weakness. High doses may produce long-lasting psychotic changes in susceptible individuals. *Haloperidol* and other neuroleptics can block the hallucinatory action of *LSD* and quickly abort the syndrome.

B. Tetrahydrocannabinol

The main psychoactive alkaloid contained in marijuana is Δ^9-*tetrahydrocannabinol* [tet-ra-hi-dro-can-NAB-i-nol] (*THC*), which is available as *dronabinol* [droe-NAB-i-nol]. Depending on the social situation, *THC* can produce euphoria, followed by drowsiness and relaxation. In addition to affecting short-term memory and mental activity, *THC* decreases muscle strength and impairs highly skilled motor activity, such as that required to drive a car. Its wide range of effects include appetite stimulation, xerostomia, visual hallucinations, delusions, and enhancement of sensory activity. *THC* receptors, designated CB1 receptors, have been found on inhibitory presynaptic nerve terminals that interact synaptically with pyramidal neurons. CB1 is coupled to a G protein. Interestingly, like the endogenous ligands of the opioid system, endocannabinoids have been identified in the CNS. These compounds, which bind to the CB1 receptors, are membrane-derived and are synthesized on demand, and they may act as local neuromodulators (Figure 10.11). The action of *THC* is believed to be mediated through the CB1 receptors but is still under investigation. The effects of THC appear immediately after the drug is smoked, but maximum effects take about 20 minutes. By 3 hours, the effects largely disappear. *Dronabinol* is administered orally and has a peak effect in 2 to 4 hours. Its psychoactive effects can last up to 6 hours, but its appetite-stimulant effects may persist for 24 hours. It is highly lipid soluble and has a large volume of distribution. *THC* itself is extensively metabolized by the mixed-function oxidases. Elimination

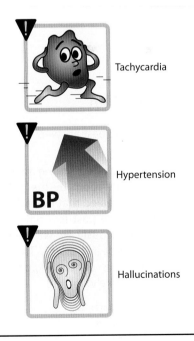

Tachycardia

Hypertension

Hallucinations

Figure 10.12
Adverse effects of *tetrahydrocannabinol*.

is largely through the biliary route. Adverse effects include increased heart rate, decreased blood pressure, and reddening of the conjunctiva. At high doses, a toxic psychosis develops (Figure 10.12). Tolerance and mild physical dependence occur with continued, frequent use of the drug. *Dronabinol* is indicated as an appetite stimulant for patients with acquired immunodeficiency syndrome who are losing weight. It is also sometimes given for the severe emesis caused by some cancer chemotherapeutic agents (see p. 337). The CB1-receptor antagonist, *rimonabant* [ri-MOH-nah-bant], is effective in the treatment of obesity and has been found to decrease appetite and body weight in humans. *Rimonabant* has also been found to induce psychiatric disturbances, such as anxiety and depression, during clinical trials.

C. Phencyclidine

Phencyclidine [fen-SYE-kli-deen] (also known as PCP, or "angel dust") inhibits the reuptake of *dopamine*, 5-HT, and *norepinephrine*. The major action of *phencyclidine* is to block the ion channel regulated by the NMDA subtype of glutamate receptor. This action prevents the passage of critical ions (particularly Ca^{2+}) through the channel. *Phencyclidine* also has anticholinergic activity but, surprisingly, produces hypersalivation. *Phencyclidine*, an analog of ketamine, causes dissociative anesthesia (insensitivity to pain, without loss of consciousness) and analgesia. In this state, it produces numbness of extremities, staggered gait, slurred speech, and muscular rigidity. Sometimes, hostile and bizarre behavior occurs. At increased dosages, anesthesia, stupor, or coma result, but strangely, the eyes may remain open. Increased sensitivity to external stimuli exists, and the CNS actions may persist for a week. Tolerance often develops with continued use.

Study Question

Choose the ONE best answer.

10.1 A very agitated young male was brought to the emergency room by the police. Psychiatric examination revealed that he had snorted cocaine several times in the past few days, the last time being 10 hours previously. He was given a drug that sedated him, and he fell asleep. The drug that was used to counter this patient's apparent cocaine wihdrawal was very likely:

A. Phenobarbital.
B. Lorazepam.
C. Cocaine.
D. Hydroxyzine.
E. Fluoxetine.

Correct answer = B. The anxiolytic properties of benzodiazepines, such as lorazepam, make them the drugs of choice in treating the anxiety and agitation of cocaine withdrawal. Lorazepam also has hypnotic properties. Phenobarbital has hypnotic properties, but its anxiolytic properties are inferior to those of the benzodiazepines. Cocaine itself could counteract the agitation of withdrawal, but its use would not be proper therapy. Hydroxyzine, an antihistamine, is effective as a hypnotic, and it is sometimes used to deal with anxiety, especially if emesis is a problem. Fluoxetine is an antidepressant with no immediate effects on anxiety.

Anesthetics

11

I. OVERVIEW

General anesthesia is essential to surgical practice, because it renders patients analgesic, amnesic, and unconscious, and provides muscle relaxation and suppression of undesirable reflexes. No single drug is capable of achieving these effects both rapidly and safely. Rather, several different categories of drugs are utilized to produce optimal anesthesia (Figure 11.1). Preanesthetic medication serves to calm the patient, relieve pain, and protect against undesirable effects of the subsequently administered anesthetic or the surgical procedure. Skeletal muscle relaxants facilitate intubation and suppress muscle tone to the degree required for surgery. Potent general anesthetics are delivered via inhalation or intravenous injection. With the exception of *nitrous oxide*, modern inhaled anesthetics are all volatile, halogenated hydrocarbons that derive from early research and clinical experience with *diethyl ether* and *chloroform*. On the other hand, intravenous general anesthetics consist of a number of chemically unrelated drug types that are commonly used for the rapid induction of anesthesia.

II. PATIENT FACTORS IN SELECTION OF ANESTHESIA

During the preoperative phase, the anesthesiologist selects drugs that provide a safe and efficient anesthetic regimen based on the nature of the surgical or diagnostic procedure as well as on the patient's physiologic, pathologic, and pharmacologic state.

A. Status of organ systems

1. **Liver and kidney:** Because the liver and kidney not only influence the long-term distribution and clearance of anesthetic agents but can also be the target organs for toxic effects, the physiologic status of these organs must be considered. Of particular concern is that the release of fluoride, bromide, and other metabolic products of the halogenated hydrocarbons can affect these organs, especially if the metabolites accumulate with repeated anesthetic administration over a short period of time.

2. **Respiratory system:** The condition of the respiratory system must be considered if inhalation anesthetics are indicated. For example, asthma and ventilation or perfusion abnormalities complicate control of an inhalation anesthetic. All inhaled anesthetics depress the respiratory system. Additionally, they also are bronchodilators.

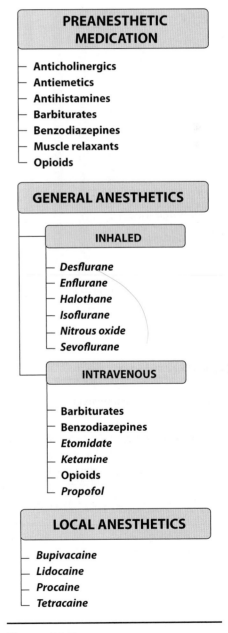

PREANESTHETIC MEDICATION
- Anticholinergics
- Antiemetics
- Antihistamines
- Barbiturates
- Benzodiazepines
- Muscle relaxants
- Opioids

GENERAL ANESTHETICS

INHALED
- *Desflurane*
- *Enflurane*
- *Halothane*
- *Isoflurane*
- *Nitrous oxide*
- *Sevoflurane*

INTRAVENOUS
- Barbiturates
- Benzodiazepines
- *Etomidate*
- *Ketamine*
- Opioids
- *Propofol*

LOCAL ANESTHETICS
- *Bupivacaine*
- *Lidocaine*
- *Procaine*
- *Tetracaine*

Figure 11.1
Summary of anesthetics.

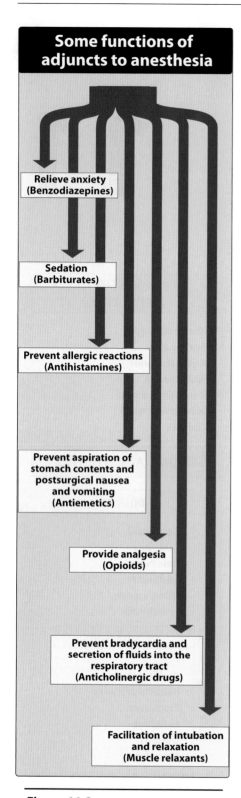

Figure 11.2
Components of balanced anesthesia.

3. **Cardiovascular system:** Whereas the hypotensive effect of most anesthetics is sometimes desirable, ischemic injury of tissues could follow reduced perfusion pressure. If a hypotensive episode during a surgical procedure necessitates treatment, a vasoactive substance is administered. This is done after consideration of the possibility that some anesthetics, such as *halothane*, may sensitize the heart to the arrhythmogenic effects of sympathomimetic agents.

4. **Nervous system:** The existence of neurologic disorders (for example, epilepsy or myasthenia gravis) influences the selection of an anesthetic. So, too, would a patient history suggestive of a genetically determined sensitivity to halogenated hydrocarbon–induced malignant hyperthermia.

5. **Pregnancy:** Some precautions should be kept in mind when anesthetics and adjunct drugs are administered to a pregnant woman. There has been at least one report that transient use of *nitrous oxide* can cause aplastic anemia in the unborn child. Oral clefts have occurred in the fetuses of women who have received benzodiazepines. *Diazepam* should not be used routinely during labor, because it results in temporary hypotonia and altered thermoregulation in the newborn.

B. **Concomitant use of drugs**

1. **Multiple adjunct agents:** Commonly, surgical patients receive one or more of the following preanesthetic medications: benzodiazepines, such as *midazolam* or *diazepam*, to allay anxiety and facilitate amnesia; barbiturates, such as *pentobarbital*, for sedation; antihistamines, such as *diphenhydramine*, for prevention of allergic reactions, or *ranitidine*, to reduce gastric acidity; antiemetics, such as *ondansetron*, to prevent the possible aspiration of stomach contents; opioids, such as *fentanyl*, for analgesia; and/or anticholinergics, such as *scopolamine*, for their amnesic effect and to prevent bradycardia and secretion of fluids into the respiratory tract (Figure 11.2). These agents facilitate smooth induction of anesthesia, and when administered continuously, they also lower the dose of anesthetic required to maintain the desired level of surgical (Stage III) anesthesia. However, such coadministration can also enhance undesirable anesthetic effects (for example, hypoventilation), and it may produce negative effects that are not observed when each drug is given individually.

2. **Concomitant use of additional nonanesthetic drugs:** Surgical patients may be chronically exposed to agents for the treatment of the underlying disease as well as to drugs of abuse that alter the response to anesthetics. For example, alcoholics have elevated levels of hepatic microsomal enzymes involved in the metabolism of barbiturates, and drug abusers may be overly tolerant of opioids.

III. INDUCTION, MAINTENANCE, AND RECOVERY FROM ANESTHESIA

Anesthesia can be divided into three stages: induction, maintenance, and recovery. Induction is defined as the period of time from the onset of administration of the anesthetic to the development of effective surgical anesthesia in the patient. Maintenance provides a sustained surgical anesthesia.

Recovery is the time from discontinuation of administration of the anesthesia until consciousness and protective physiologic reflexes are regained. Induction of anesthesia depends on how fast effective concentrations of the anesthetic drug reach the brain; recovery is the reverse of induction and depends on how fast the anesthetic drug diffuses from the brain.

A. Induction

During induction, it is essential to avoid the dangerous excitatory phase (Stage II delirium) that was observed with the slow onset of action of some earlier anesthetics (see below). Thus, general anesthesia is normally induced with an intravenous anesthetic like *thiopental*, which produces unconsciousness within 25 seconds after injection. At that time, additional inhalation or intravenous drugs comprising the selected anesthetic combination may be given to produce the desired depth of surgical (Stage III) anesthesia. [Note: This often includes coadministration of an intravenous skeletal muscle relaxant to facilitate intubation and relaxation. Currently used muscle relaxants include *pancuronium, doxacurium, rocuronium, vecuronium, cisatricurium, atracurium, mevacurium* and *succinylcholine.*] For children, without intravenous access, nonpungent agents, such as *halothane* or *sevoflurane*, are used to induce general anesthesia. This is termed inhalation induction.

B. Maintenance of anesthesia

Maintenance is the period during which the patient is surgically anesthetized. After administering the selected anesthetic mixture, the anesthesiologist monitors the patient's vital signs and response to various stimuli throughout the surgical procedure to carefully balance the amount of drug inhaled and/or infused with the depth of anesthesia. Anesthesia is usually maintained by the administration of volatile anesthetics, because these agents offer good minute-to-minute control over the depth of anesthesia. Opioids, such as *fentanyl*, are often used for pain along with inhalation agents, because the latter are not good analgesics.

C. Recovery

Postoperatively, the anesthesiologist withdraws the anesthetic mixture and monitors the return of the patient to consciousness. For most anesthetic agents, recovery is the reverse of induction; that is, redistribution from the site of action (rather than metabolism of the anesthetic) underlies recovery. The anesthesiologist continues to monitor the patient to be sure that he or she is fully recovered with normal physiologic functions (for example, is able to breathe on his/her own). Patients are observed for delayed toxic reactions, such as hepatotoxicity caused by halogenated hydrocarbons.

D. Depth of anesthesia

The depth of anesthesia has been divided into four sequential stages. Each stage is characterized by increased central nervous system (CNS) depression, which is caused by accumulation of the anesthetic drug in the brain (Figure 11.3). These stages were discerned and defined with *ether*, which produces a slow onset of anesthesia. However, with *halothane* and other commonly used anesthetics, the stages are difficult to characterize clearly because of the rapid onset of anesthesia.

1. **Stage I—Analgesia:** Loss of pain sensation results from interference with sensory transmission in the spinothalamic tract. The patient is

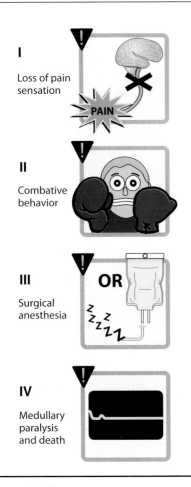

I

Loss of pain
sensation

PAIN

II

Combative
behavior

III   OR

Surgical
anesthesia

IV

Medullary
paralysis
and death

Figure 11.3
Stages of anesthesia. OR = operating

conscious and conversational. Amnesia and a reduced awareness of pain occur as Stage II is approached.

2. **Stage II—Excitement:** The patient experiences delirium and possibly violent, combative behavior. There is a rise and irregularity in blood pressure. The respiratory rate may increase. To avoid this stage of anesthesia, a short-acting barbiturate, such as *thiopental*, is given intravenously before inhalation anesthesia is administered.

3. **Stage III—Surgical anesthesia:** Regular respiration and relaxation of the skeletal muscles occur in this stage. Eye reflexes decrease progressively, until the eye movements cease and the pupil is fixed. Surgery may proceed during this stage.

4. **Stage IV—Medullary paralysis:** Severe depression of the respiratory and vasomotor centers occur during this stage. Death can rapidly ensue unless measures are taken to maintain circulation and respiration.

IV. INHALATION ANESTHETICS

Inhaled gases are the mainstay of anesthesia and are used primarily for the maintenance of anesthesia after administration of an intravenous agent. No one anesthetic is superior to another under all circumstances. Inhalation anesthetics have a benefit that is not available with intravenous agents, because the depth of anesthesia can be rapidly altered by changing the concentration of the drug. Inhalation anesthetics are also reversible, because most are rapidly eliminated from the body by exhalation.

A. Common features of inhalation anesthetics

Modern inhalation anesthetics are nonflammable, nonexplosive agents that include the gas *nitrous oxide* as well as a number of volatile, halogenated hydrocarbons. As a group, these agents decrease cerebrovascular resistance, resulting in increased perfusion of the brain. They also cause bronchodilation and decrease both minute ventilation (volume of air per unit time moved into or out of the lungs) and hypoxic pulmonary vasoconstriction (increased pulmonary vascular resistance in poorly aerated regions of the lungs, which allows redirection of pulmonary blood flow to regions that are richer in oxygen content). The movement of these agents from the lungs to the different body compartments depends upon their solubility in blood and tissues as well as on blood flow. These factors play a role not only in induction but also in recovery.

B. Potency

The potency of inhaled anesthetics is defined quantitatively as the median alveolar concentration (MAC). This is the end-tidal concentration of anesthetic gas needed to eliminate movement among 50 percent of patients challenged by a standardized skin incision. [Note: MAC is the median effective dose (ED_{50}) of the anesthetic.] MAC is usually expressed as the percentage of gas in a mixture required to achieve the effect. Numerically, MAC is small for potent anesthetics, such as *halothane*, and large for less potent agents, such as *nitrous oxide*. Therefore, the inverse of MAC is an index of the potency of the anesthetic. MAC values are useful in comparing pharmacologic effects of different anesthetics (Figure 11.4). The more lipid soluble an anesthetic, the lower the concentration of anesthetic needed to produce anesthesia and, thus, the higher the potency of the anesthetic.

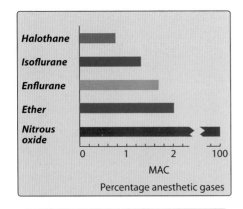

Halothane
Isoflurane
Enflurane
Ether
Nitrous oxide

0   1   2   100

MAC

Percentage anesthetic gases

Figure 11.4
Minimal alveolar concentrations (MAC) for anesthetic gases.

C. Uptake and distribution of inhalation anesthetics

The partial pressure of an anesthetic gas at the origin of the respiratory pathway is the driving force that moves the anesthetic into the alveolar space and, thence, into the blood, which delivers the drug to the brain and various other body compartments. Because gases move from one compartment to another within the body according to partial pressure gradients, a steady state is achieved when the partial pressure in each of these compartments is equivalent to that in the inspired mixture. The time course for attaining this steady state is determined by the following factors:

1. **Alveolar wash-in:** This term refers to the replacement of the normal lung gases with the inspired anesthetic mixture. The time required for this process is directly proportional to the functional residual capacity of the lung and inversely proportional to the ventilatory rate; it is independent of the physical properties of the gas. As the partial pressure builds within the lung, anesthetic transfer from the lung begins.

2. **Anesthetic uptake:** Anesthetic uptake is the product of gas solubility in the blood, cardiac output, and the anesthetic gradient between alveolar and venous partial pressure gradients.

   a. **Solubility in the blood:** This is determined by a physical property of the anesthetic molecule called the blood/gas partition coefficient, which is the ratio of the total amount of gas in the blood relative to the gas equilibrium phase (Figure 11.5). Drugs with low versus high solubility in blood differ in their speed of induction of anesthesia. For example, when an anesthetic gas with low blood solubility, such as *nitrous oxide*, diffuses from the alveoli into the circulation, little of the anesthetic dissolves in the blood. Therefore, the equilibrium between the inhaled anesthetic and arterial blood occurs rapidly, and relatively few additional molecules of anesthetic are required to raise arterial anesthetic partial pressure—that is, steady state is rapidly achieved. In contrast, an anesthetic gas with high blood solubility, such as *halothane*, dissolves more completely in the blood, and greater amounts of the anesthetic and longer periods of time are required to raise arterial partial pressure. This results in increased times of induction as well as recovery and slower changes in the depth of anesthesia in response to alterations in the concentration of the inhaled drug. Figure 11.6 illustrates the uptake curves for some inhalation anesthetics. The solubility in blood is ranked in the following order: *halothane > enflurane > isoflurane > sevoflurane > desflurane > nitrous oxide.*

   b. **Cardiac output:** It is obvious that cardiac output affects the delivery of anesthetic to tissues. Low cardiac output will result in slow delivery of the anesthetic.

   c. **Alveolar to venous partial pressure gradient of the anesthetic:** This is the driving force of anesthetic delivery. For all practical purposes, the pulmonary end-capillary anesthetic partial pressure may be considered as the anesthetic alveolar partial pressure if the patient does not have severe lung diffusion disease. The arterial circulation distributes the anesthetic to various tissues, and the pressure gradient drives free anesthetic

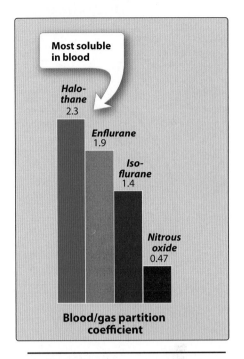

Figure 11.5
Blood/gas partition coefficients for some inhalation anesthetics.

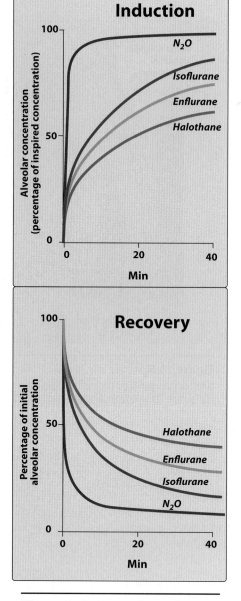

Figure 11.6
Changes in the alveolar blood concentrations of some inhalation anesthetics over time. N₂0 = nitrous oxide.

gas into tissues. As the venous circulation returns blood depleted of anesthetic to the lung, more gas moves into the blood from the lung according to the partial pressure difference. Over time, the partial pressure in the venous blood closely approximates the partial pressure in the inspired mixture; that is, no further net anesthetic uptake from the lung occurs.

3. **Effect of different tissue types on anesthetic uptake:** The time required for a particular tissue to achieve a steady state with the partial pressure of an anesthetic gas in the inspired mixture is inversely proportional to the blood flow to that tissue; that is, faster flow results in a more rapidly achieved steady state. It is also directly proportional to the capacity of that tissue to store anesthetic; that is, a larger capacity results in a longer time required to achieve steady state. Capacity, in turn, is directly proportional to the tissue's volume and the tissue/blood solubility coefficient of the anesthetic molecules. Four major tissue compartments determine the time course of anesthetic uptake.

   a. **Brain, heart, liver, kidney, and endocrine glands:** These highly perfused tissues rapidly attain a steady state with the partial pressure of anesthetic in the blood.

   b. **Skeletal muscles:** These are poorly perfused during anesthesia. This, and the fact that they have a large volume, prolong the time required to achieve steady state.

   c. **Fat:** This tissue is also poorly perfused. However, potent general anesthetics are very lipid soluble. Therefore, fat has a large capacity to store anesthetic. This combination of slow delivery to a high-capacity compartment prolongs the time required to achieve steady state.

   d. **Bone, ligaments, and cartilage:** These are poorly perfused and have a relatively low capacity to store anesthetic. Therefore, these tissues have only a slight impact on the time course of anesthetic distribution in the body.

4. **Washout:** When the administration of an inhalation anesthetic is discontinued, the body becomes the "source" that drives the anesthetic into the alveolar space. The same factors that influence attainment of steady state with an inspired anesthetic determine the time course of clearance of the drug from the body. Thus, *nitrous oxide* exits the body faster than *halothane* (see Figure 11.6).

D. Mechanism of action

No specific receptor has been identified as the locus of general anesthetic action. Indeed, the fact that chemically unrelated compounds produce the anesthetic state argues against the existence of such a receptor. The focus is now on interactions of the inhaled anesthetics with proteins comprising ion channels. For example, the general anesthetics increase the sensitivity of the γ-aminobutyric acid (GABA_A) receptors to the neurotransmitter, GABA, at clinically effective concentrations of the drug. This causes a prolongation of the inhibitory chloride ion current after a pulse of GABA release. Postsynaptic neuronal excitability is thus diminished (Figure 11.7). Other receptors are also affected by volatile anesthetics; for example, the activity of the inhibitory glycine receptors in the spinal motor neurons is increased. In addition, the inhalation anesthetics block the excitatory postsynaptic current of the nicotinic receptors. The mechanism by which the anesthetics perform these modulatory roles is not understood.

E. Halothane

This agent is the prototype to which newer inhalation anesthetics have been compared. When *halothane* (HAL-oh-thane) was introduced, its ability to induce the anesthetic state rapidly and to allow quick recovery—and the fact that it was nonexplosive—made it an anesthetic of choice. However, with the recognition of the adverse effects discussed below and the availability of other anesthetics that cause fewer complications, *halothane* is largely being replaced in the United States.

1. **Therapeutic uses:** Whereas *halothane* is a potent anesthetic, it is a relatively weak analgesic. Thus, *halothane* is usually coadministered with *nitrous oxide*, opioids, or local anesthetics. *Halothane* relaxes both skeletal and uterine muscle, and it can be used in obstetrics when uterine relaxation is indicated. *Halothane* is not hepatotoxic in pediatric patients (unlike its potential effect on adults, see below), and combined with its pleasant odor, this makes it suitable in children for inhalation induction.

2. **Pharmacokinetics:** *Halothane* is oxidatively metabolized in the body to tissue-toxic hydrocarbons (for example, trifluoroethanol) and bromide ion. These substances may be responsible for the toxic reaction that some patients (especially females) develop after *halothane* anesthesia. This reaction begins as a fever, followed by anorexia, nausea, and vomiting, and patients may exhibit signs of hepatitis. [Note: Although the incidence of this reaction is low—approximately 1 in 10,000 individuals—50 percent of affected patients will die of hepatic necrosis. To avoid this condition, *halothane* anesthesia is not repeated at intervals of less than 2 to 3 weeks.]

3. **Adverse effects:**

   a. **Cardiac effects:** Like other halogenated hydrocarbons, *halothane* is vagomimetic and causes *atropine*-sensitive bradycardia. In addition, *halothane* has the undesirable property of causing cardiac arrhythmias. [Note: These are especially serious if hypercapnia (increased arterial carbon dioxide partial pressure) develops due to reduced alveolar ventilation or an increase in the plasma concentration of catecholamines.] *Halothane*, like the other halogenated anesthetics, produces concentration-dependent hypotension. Should it become necessary to counter excessive hypotension during *halothane* anesthesia, it is recommended that a direct-acting vasoconstrictor, such as *phenylephrine*, be given.

   b. **Malignant hyperthermia:** In a very small percentage of patients, all of the halogenated hydrocarbon anesthetics—as well as the muscle relaxant *succinylcholine*—have the potential to induce malignant hyperthermia. Whereas the etiology of this condition is poorly understood, recent investigations have identified a dramatic increase in the myoplasmic calcium ion concentration. Strong evidence indicates that malignant hyperthermia is due

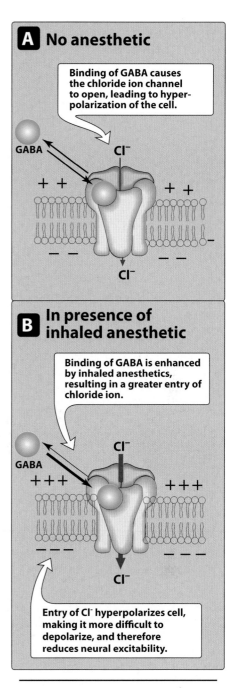

Figure 11.7
An example of modulation of a ligand-gated membrane channel modulated by inhaled anesthetics. GABA = γ-aminobutyric acid.

to an excitation–contraction coupling defect. Burn victims and individuals with Duchenne dystrophy, myotonia, osteogenesis imperfecta, and central-core disease are susceptible to malignant hyperthermia. Should a patient exhibit the characteristic symptoms of malignant hyperthermia, *dantrolene* is given as the anesthetic mixture is withdrawn. Therefore, *dantrolene* should be available for emergency use when needed. The patient must be carefully monitored and supported for respiratory, circulatory, and renal problems.

F. Enflurane

This gas is less potent than *halothane*, but it produces rapid induction and recovery. About 2 percent of the anesthetic is metabolized to fluoride ion, which is excreted by the kidney. Therefore, *enflurane* [EN-floo-rane] is contraindicated in patients with kidney failure. *Enflurane* anesthesia exhibits the following differences from *halothane* anesthesia: fewer arrhythmias, less sensitization of the heart to catecholamines, and greater potentiation of muscle relaxants due to a more potent "*curare*-like" effect. A disadvantage of *enflurane* is that it causes CNS excitation at twice the MAC and also at lower doses if hyperventilation reduces the partial pressure of carbon dioxide. For this reason, it is not used in patients with seizure disorders.

G. Isoflurane

This halogenated anesthetic is widely used in the United States. It is a very stable molecule that undergoes little metabolism; as a result, little fluoride is produced. *Isoflurane* [eye-soe-FLURE-ane] is not tissue toxic. Unlike the other halogenated anesthetic gases, *isoflurane* does not induce cardiac arrhythmias and does not sensitize the heart to the action of catecholamines. However, it produces concentration-dependent hypotension due to peripheral vasodilation. It also dilates the coronary vasculature, increasing coronary blood flow and oxygen consumption by the myocardium. This property may make it beneficial in patients with ischemic heart disease. [Note: All halogenated inhalation anesthetics have been reported to cause hepatitis, but at a much lower incidence than with *halothane*. For example, *isoflurane* does so in 1 in 500,000 individuals.]

H. Desflurane

The rapidity with which *desflurane* causes anesthesia and emergence has made it a popular anesthetic for outpatient surgery. However, *desflurane* [DES-flure-ane] has a low volatility and, thus, must be delivered using a special vaporizer. Like *isoflurane*, it decreases vascular resistance and perfuses all major tissues very well. Because it is irritating to the airway and can cause laryngospasm, coughing, and excessive secretions, *desflurane* is not used to induce extended anesthesia. Its degradation is minimal; thus, tissue toxicity is rare.

I. Sevoflurane

Sevoflurane [see-voe-FLOO-rane] has low pungency, allowing rapid uptake without irritating the airway during induction, thus making it suitable for induction in children. It is replacing *halothane* for this purpose. The drug has low solubility in blood and is rapidly taken up and excreted. Recovery is faster than with other anesthetics. It is metabolized by the liver, releasing fluoride ions; thus, like *enflurane*, it may prove to be nephrotoxic.

J. Nitrous oxide

Nitrous oxide [NYE-truss-OX-ide] ("laughing gas") is a potent analgesic but a weak general anesthetic. For example, *nitrous oxide* is frequently employed at concentrations of 30 percent in combination with oxygen for analgesia, particularly in dental surgery. However, *nitrous oxide* at 80 percent (without adjunct agents) cannot produce surgical anesthesia. It is therefore frequently combined with other, more potent agents to attain pain-free anesthesia. *Nitrous oxide* is poorly soluble in blood and other tissues, allowing it to move very rapidly in and out of the body. [Note: *Nitrous oxide* can concentrate the halogenated anesthetics in the alveoli when they are concomitantly administered because of its fast uptake from the alveolar gas. This phenomenon is known as the "second gas effect."] Within closed body compartments, *nitrous oxide* can increase the volume (for example, causing a pneumothorax) or increase the pressure (for example, in the sinuses), because it replaces nitrogen in the various air spaces faster than the nitrogen leaves. Furthermore, its speed of movement allows *nitrous oxide* to retard oxygen uptake during recovery, thus causing diffusion hypoxia. This anesthetic does not depress respiration, nor does it produce muscle relaxation. Under the usual circumstances of coadministration with other anesthetics, it also has moderate to no effect on the cardiovascular system or on increasing cerebral blood flow, and it is the least hepatotoxic of the inhalation anesthetics. It is therefore probably the safest of these anesthetics, provided that at least 20 percent oxygen is always administered simultaneously.

Some characteristics of the inhalation anesthetics are summarized in Figure 11.8

V. INTRAVENOUS ANESTHETICS

Intravenous anesthetics are often used for the rapid induction of anesthesia, which is then maintained with an appropriate inhalation agent. They rapidly induce anesthesia and must therefore be injected slowly. Recovery from intravenous anesthetics is due to redistribution from sites in the CNS.

A. Barbiturates

Thiopental is a potent anesthetic but a weak analgesic. It is an ultrashort-acting barbiturate and has a high lipid solubility. When agents such as *thiopental* and *methohexital* [meth-oh-HEX-i-tal] are administered intravenously, they quickly enter the CNS and depress function, often in less than 1 minute. However, diffusion out of the brain can occur very rapidly as well because of redistribution of the drug to other body tissues, including skeletal muscle and, ultimately, adipose tissue (Figure 11.9). [Note: This latter site serves as a reservoir of drugs from which the agent slowly leaks out and is metabolized and excreted.] The short duration of anesthetic action is due to the decrease of its concentration in the brain to a level below that necessary to produce anesthesia. These drugs may remain in the body for relatively long periods of time after their administration, because only about 15 percent of the dose of barbiturates entering the circulation is metabolized by the liver per hour. Thus, metabolism of *thiopental* is much slower than its tissue redistribution. The barbiturates are not significantly analgesic and, therefore, require some type of supplementary analgesic administration during anesthesia to avoid objectionable changes in blood pressure and autonomic function. *Thiopental* has minor effects on the cardiovascular system, but

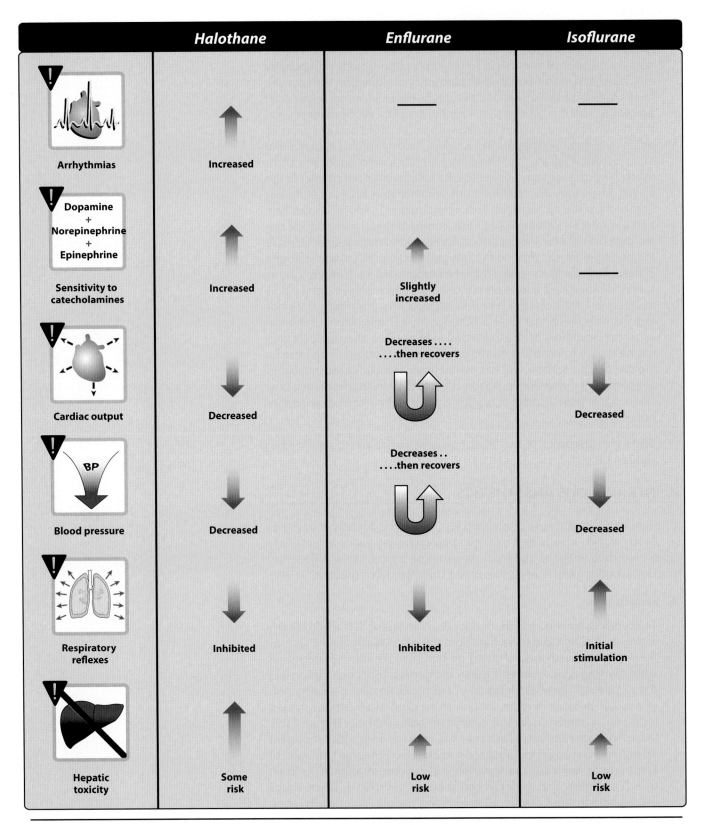

Figure 11.8
Characteristics of some inhalation anesthetics.

it may contribute to severe hypotension in patients with hypovolemia or shock. All barbiturates can cause apnea, coughing, chest wall spasm, laryngospasm, and bronchospasm. [Note: The latter is of particular concern for asthmatic patients.] Barbiturates are contraindicated in patients with acute intermittent or variegate porphyria.

B. Benzodiazepines

The benzodiazepines are used in conjunction with anesthetics to sedate the patient. The most commonly employed is *midazolam*, which is available in many formulations, including oral. *Diazepam* and *lorazepam* are alternatives. All three facilitate amnesia while causing sedation.

C. Opioids

Because of their analgesic property, opioids are frequently used together with anesthetics; for example, the combination of *morphine* and *nitrous oxide* provides good anesthesia for cardiac surgery. The choice of opioid used perioperatively is based primarily on the duration of action needed. The most frequently employed opioids are *fentanyl* and its congeners, *sufentanil* or *remifentanil*, because they induce analgesia more rapidly than *morphine* does. They are administered either intravenously, epidurally, or intrathecally. Opioids are not good amnesics, and they can all cause hypotension, respiratory depression, and muscle rigidity as well as postanesthetic nausea and vomiting. Opioid effects can be antagonized by *naloxone* (see p. 168).

D. Etomidate

Etomidate (eh-TOE-mid-ate) is used to induce anesthesia. It is a hypnotic agent but lacks analgesic activity. Its water solubility is poor, so *etomidate* is formulated in a propylene glycol solution. Induction is rapid, and the drug is short-acting. It is only used for patients with coronary artery disease or cardiovascular dysfunction, such as shock. *Etomidate* is hydrolyzed in the liver. Among its benefits are little to no effect on the heart and circulation. Its adverse effects include a decrease in plasma cortisol and aldosterone levels, which can persist for up to 8 hours. This is apparently due to inhibition of 11-β-hydroxylase.[1] [Note: *Etomidate* should not be infused for an extended time, because prolonged suppression of these hormones can be hazardous.] Venous pain can occur, and skeletal muscle movements are not uncommon. The latter are managed by administration of benzodiazepines and opioids.

E. Ketamine

Ketamine [KET-a-meen], a short-acting, nonbarbiturate anesthetic, induces a dissociated state in which the patient is unconscious but appears to be awake and does not feel pain. This dissociative anesthesia provides sedation, amnesia, and immobility. *Ketamine* interacts with the N-methyl-D-aspartate receptor. It also stimulates the central sympathetic outflow, which, in turn, causes stimulation of the heart and increased blood pressure and cardiac output. This property is especially beneficial in patients with either hypovolemic or cardiogenic shock as well as in patients with asthma. *Ketamine* is therefore used when circulatory depression is undesirable. On the other hand, these effects miti-

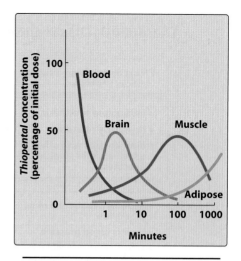

Figure 11.9
Redistribution of *thiopental* from brain to muscle and adipose tissue.

[1]See p. 237 in ***Lippincott's Illustrated Reviews: Biochemistry*** (4th ed.) for a discussion of steroid biosynthesis.

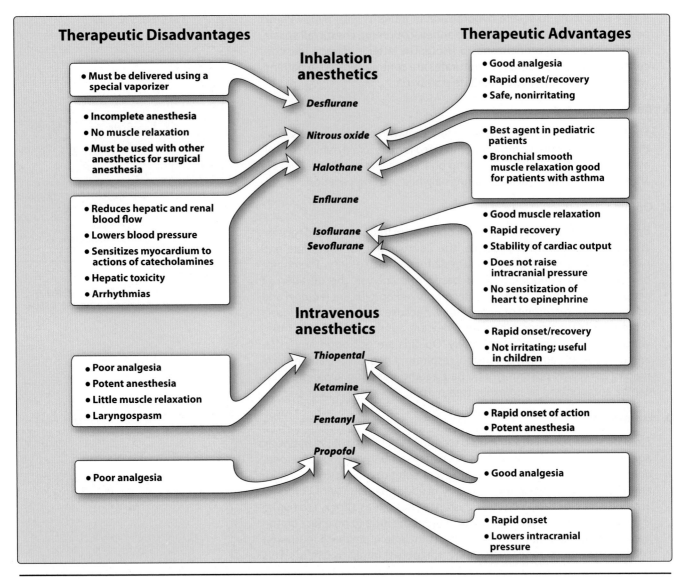

Figure 11.10
Therapeutic disadvantages and advantages of some anesthetic agents.

gate against the use of *ketamine* in hypertensive or stroke patients. The drug is lipophilic and enters the brain circulation very quickly, but like the barbiturates, it redistributes to other organs and tissues. It is metabolized in the liver, but small amounts can be excreted unchanged. *Ketamine* is employed mainly in children and young adults for short procedures. However, it is not widely used, because it increases cerebral blood flow and induces postoperative hallucinations ("nightmares"), particularly in adults.

F. Propofol

Propofol [pro-POF-ol] is an intravenous sedative/hypnotic used in the induction or maintenance of anesthesia. Onset is smooth and occurs within about 40 seconds of administration. Supplementation with narcotics for analgesia is required. Whereas *propofol* facilitates depression in the CNS, it is occasionally accompanied by excitatory phenomena, such as muscle twitching, spontaneous movement, or hiccups. *Propofol* decreases blood pressure without depressing the myocardium. It also reduces intracranial pressure. *Propofol* is widely used and has replaced *thiopental* as the first choice for anesthesia induction and sedation, because it produces a euphoric feeling in the patient and does not cause postanesthetic nausea and vomiting. It has much less of a depressant effect than the volatile anesthetics on CNS-evoked potentials, such as somatosensory evoked potentials. This makes *propofol* very useful for such surgeries as resection of spinal tumors, in which somatosensory evoked potentials are monitored to assess spinal cord functions.

Some therapeutic advantages and disadvantages of the anesthetic agents are summarized in Figure 11.10.

VI. LOCAL ANESTHETICS

Local anesthetics are generally applied locally and block nerve conduction of sensory impulses from the periphery to the CNS. [Note: Some of these agents do have additional uses—for example, the antiarrhythmic effect of *lidocaine*—and they are then administered by other routes.] Local anesthetics abolish sensation (and, in higher concentrations, motor activity) in a limited area of the body without producing unconsciousness (for example, during spinal anesthesia). The small, unmyelinated nerve fibers that conduct impulses for pain, temperature, and autonomic activity are most sensitive to actions of local anesthetics. The most widely used of these compounds are *bupivacaine* [byoo-PIV-ah-kane], *lidocaine* [LYE-doe-kane], *mepivacaine* [me-PIV-a-kane], *procaine* [PRO-kane], *ropivacaine* [roe-PIV-a-kane], and *tetracaine* [TET-ra-kane]. Of these, *lidocaine* is the most frequently employed. At physiologic pH, these compounds are charged; it is this ionized form that interacts with the protein receptor of the Na^+ channel to inhibit its function and, thereby, achieve local anesthesia. [Note: The natural product, *cocaine*, was recognized years ago as a local anesthetic. However, its toxicity and abuse have limited its use to topical application in anesthesia of the upper respiratory tract.] The local anesthetics differ pharmacokinetically as to onset and duration of action (Figure 11.11). By adding the vasoconstrictor *epinephrine* to the local anesthetic, the rate of anesthetic absorption is decreased. This both minimizes systemic toxicity and increases the duration of action. Adverse effects result from systemic absorption of toxic amounts of the locally applied anesthetic. Seizures and cardiovascular collapse are the most significant of these systemic effects. *Bupivacaine* is noted for its cardiotoxicity. *Mepivacaine* should not be used in obstetric anesthesia due to its increased toxicity to the neonate. Allergic reactions may be encountered with *procaine*, which is metabolized to *p*-aminobenzoic acid.

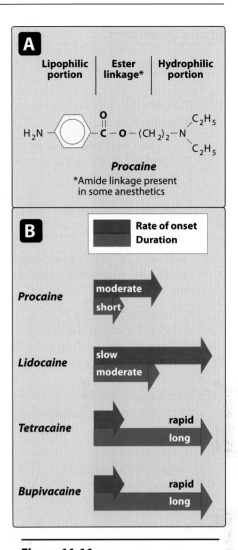

Figure 11.11
A. Structural formula of *procaine*.
B. Pharmacokinetic properties of local anesthetics.

Study Questions

Choose the ONE best answer.

11.1 Halogenated anesthetics may produce malignant hyperthermia in:

    A. Patients with poor renal function.
    B. Patients allergic to the anesthetic.
    C. Pregnant women.
    D. Alcoholics.
    E. Patients with a genetic defect in muscle calcium regulation.

> Correct answer = E. All patients undergoing anesthesia must be carefully assessed and monitored for possible adverse reactions. Malignant hyperthermia occurs in a small population who have a genetic defect and also receive succinylcholine. The other conditions are not known to dispose to malignant hperthermia.

11.2 Children with asthma undergoing a surgical procedure are frequently anesthetized with sevoflurane, because it:

    A. Is rapidly taken up.
    B. Does not irritate the airway.
    C. Has a low nephrotoxic potential.
    D. Does not undergo metabolism.

> Correct answer = B. Sevoflurane is an inhalation anesthetic with low pungency. It is nonirritative and, therefore, less likely to cause laryngospasm. Choice A is true; induction and recovery are rapid. However, Choices C and D are false.

11.3 Which one of the following is most likely to require administration of a muscle relaxant?

    A. Ethyl ether.
    B. Halothane.
    C. Methoxyflurane.
    D. Benzodiazepines.
    E. Nitrous oxide.

> Correct answer = E. Nitrous oxide has virtually no muscle-relaxing properties. Ethylether, methoxyflurane, and benzodiazepine produce good muscle relaxation; halothane produces moderate muscle relaxation.

11.4 Which one of the following is a potent intravenous anesthetic but a weak analgesic?

    A. Thiopental.
    B. Benzodiazepines.
    C. Ketamine.
    D. Etomidate.
    E. Isoflurane.

> Correct answer = A. Thiopental is a potent anesthetic but a weak analgesic. It is the most widely used intravenously administered general anesthetic. It is an ultrashort-acting barbiturate and has a high lipid solubility.

11.5 Which one of the following is a potent analgesic but a weak anesthetic?

    A. Methoxyflurane.
    B. Succinylcholine.
    C. Diazepam.
    D. Halothane.
    E. Nitrous oxide.

> Correct answer = E. Nitrous oxide is a potent analgesic but a weak general anesthetic. It is frequently employed at concentrations of 30 percent in combination with oxygen for analgesia, particularly in dental surgery.

Antidepressants

12

I. OVERVIEW

Depression is a serious disorder that afflicts approximately 14 million adults in the United States each year. The lifetime prevalence rate of depression in the United States has been estimated to include 16 percent of adults (21 percent of women, 13 percent of men), or more than 32 million people. The symptoms of depression are intense feelings of sadness, hopelessness, and despair, as well as the inability to experience pleasure in usual activities, changes in sleep patterns and appetite, loss of energy, and suicidal thoughts. Mania is characterized by the opposite behavior—that is, enthusiasm, rapid thought and speech patterns, extreme self-confidence, and impaired judgment. [Note: Depression and mania are different from schizophrenia (see p. 151), which produces disturbances in thought.]

II. MECHANISM OF ANTIDEPRESSANT DRUGS

Most clinically useful antidepressant drugs potentiate, either directly or indirectly, the actions of norepinephrine and/or serotonin in the brain. (See Figure 12.1 for a summary of the antidepressant agents.) This, along with other evidence, led to the biogenic amine theory, which proposes that depression is due to a deficiency of monoamines, such as norepinephrine and serotonin, at certain key sites in the brain. Conversely, the theory envisions that mania is caused by an overproduction of these neurotransmitters. However, the amine theory of depression and mania is overly simplistic. It fails to explain why the pharmacologic effects of any of the antidepressant and antimania drugs on neurotransmission occur immediately, whereas the time course for a therapeutic response occurs over several weeks. Furthermore, the potency of the antidepressant drugs in blocking neurotransmitter uptake often does not correlate with clinically observed antidepressant effects. This suggests that decreased uptake of neurotransmitter is only an initial effect of the drugs, which may not be directly responsible for the antidepressant effects. It has been proposed that presynaptic inhibitory receptor densities in the brain decrease over a 2- to 4-week period with antidepressant drug use. This down-regulation of inhibitory receptors permits greater synthesis and release of neurotransmitters into the synaptic cleft and enhanced signaling in the postsynaptic neurons, presumably leading to a therapeutic response (Figure 12.2).

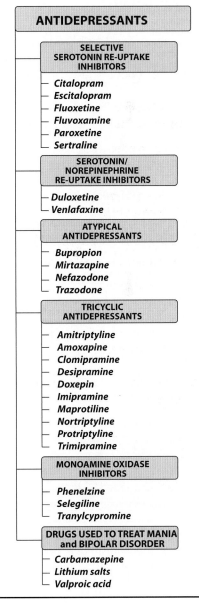

ANTIDEPRESSANTS

SELECTIVE SEROTONIN RE-UPTAKE INHIBITORS
- Citalopram
- Escitalopram
- Fluoxetine
- Fluvoxamine
- Paroxetine
- Sertraline

SEROTONIN/ NOREPINEPHRINE RE-UPTAKE INHIBITORS
- Duloxetine
- Venlafaxine

ATYPICAL ANTIDEPRESSANTS
- Bupropion
- Mirtazapine
- Nefazodone
- Trazodone

TRICYCLIC ANTIDEPRESSANTS
- Amitriptyline
- Amoxapine
- Clomipramine
- Desipramine
- Doxepin
- Imipramine
- Maprotiline
- Nortriptyline
- Protriptyline
- Trimipramine

MONOAMINE OXIDASE INHIBITORS
- Phenelzine
- Selegiline
- Tranylcypromine

DRUGS USED TO TREAT MANIA and BIPOLAR DISORDER
- Carbamazepine
- Lithium salts
- Valproic acid

Figure 12.1
Summary of antidepressants.

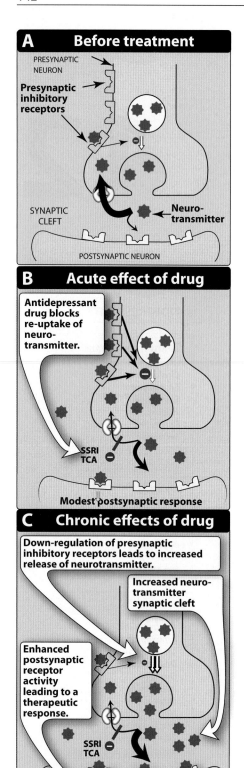

Figure 12.2
Proposed mechanism of action of selective serotonin re-uptake inhibitors (SSRI) and tricyclic antidepressant (TCA) drugs.

III. SELECTIVE SEROTONIN REUPTAKE INHIBITORS

The selective serotonin reuptake inhibitors (SSRIs) are a group of chemically diverse antidepressant drugs that specifically inhibit serotonin reuptake, having 300- to 3000-fold greater selectivity for the serotonin transporter as compared to the norepinephrine transporter. This contrasts with the tricyclic antidepressants (see p. 145) that nonselectively inhibit the uptake of norepinephrine and serotonin (Figure 12.3). Both of these antidepressant drug classes exhibit little ability to block the dopamine transporter. Moreover, the SSRIs have little blocking activity at muscarinic, α-adrenergic, and histaminic H₁ receptors. Therefore, common side effects associated with tricyclic antidepressants, such as orthostatic hypotension, sedation, dry mouth, and blurred vision, are not commonly seen with the SSRIs. Because they have fewer adverse effects and are relatively safe even in overdose, the SSRIs have largely replaced tricyclic antidepressants and monoamine oxidase inhibitors as the drugs of choice in treating depression. SSRIs include *fluoxetine* [floo-OX-e-teen] (the prototypic drug), *citalopram* [sye-TAL-oh-pram], *escitalopram* [es-sye-TAL-oh-pram], *fluvoxamine* [floo-VOX-e-meen], *paroxetine* [pa-ROX-e-teen], and *sertraline* [SER-tra-leen]. Both *citalopram* and *fluoxetine* are racemic mixtures, of which the respective S-enantiomers are the more potent inhibitors of the serotonin reuptake pump. *Escitalopram* is the pure S-enatiomer of *citalopram*.

A. Actions

The SSRIs block the reuptake of serotonin, leading to increased concentrations of the neurotransmitter in the synaptic cleft and, ultimately, to greater postsynaptic neuronal activity. Antidepressants, including SSRIs, typically take at least 2 weeks to produce significant improvement in mood, and maximum benefit may require up to 12 weeks or more (Figure 12.4). However, none of the antidepressants are uniformly effective. Approximately 40 percent of depressed patients treated with adequate doses for 4 to 8 weeks do not respond to the antidepressant agent. Patients that do not respond to one antidepressant may respond to another, and approximately 80 percent or more will respond to at least one antidepressant drug. [Note: These drugs do not usually produce central nervous system (CNS) stimulation or mood elevation in normal individuals.]

B. Therapeutic uses

The primary indication for SSRIs is depression, for which they are as effective as the tricyclic antidepressants. A number of other psychiatric disorders also respond favorably to SSRIs, including obsessive-compulsive disorder (the only approved indication for *fluvoxamine*), panic disorder, generalized anxiety disorder, posttraumatic stress disorder, social anxiety disorder, premenstrual dysphoric disorder, and bulimia nervosa (only *fluoxetine* is approved for this last indication).

C. Pharmacokinetics

All of the SSRIs are well absorbed after oral administration. Peak levels are seen in approximately 2 to 8 hours on average. Food has little effect on absorption (except with *sertraline*, for which food increases its absorption). Only *sertraline* undergoes significant first-pass metabolism. All of these agents are well distributed, having volumes of distribution far in excess of body weight (15–30 L/kg). The majority of SSRIs have plasma half-lives that range between 16 and 36 hours. Metabolism by P450-dependent enzymes and glucuronide or sulfate conjugation occur extensively. [Note: These metabolites do not generally contribute to the pharmacologic activity.] *Fluoxetine* differs from the other members of the class in two respects. First, it has a much longer half-life (50 hours) and is available as a sustained-release preparation allowing once-weekly dosing. Second, the metabolite of the S-enantiomer, S-norfluoxetine, is as potent as the parent compound. The half-life of the metabolite is quite long, averaging 10 days. *Fluoxetine* and *paroxetine* are potent inhibitors of a hepatic cytochrome P450 isoenzyme (CYP2D6) responsible for the elimination of tricyclic antidepressant drugs, neuroleptic drugs, and some antiarrhythmic and β-adrenergic–antagonist drugs. [Note: About seven percent of the Caucasian population lack this P450 enzyme and, therefore, metabolize *fluoxetine*, and other substrates of this enzyme, very slowly. These individuals may be referred to in the literature as poor metabolizers.] Other cytochrome enzymes (CYP2C9/19, CYP3A4, CYP1A2) are involved with SSRI metabolism and may also be inhibited to various degrees by the SSRIs and, thus, may affect the metabolism of multiple medications. Excretion of the SSRIs is primarily through the kidneys, except for *paroxetine* and *sertraline*, which also undergo fecal excretion (35 and 50 percent, respectively). Dosages of all of these drugs should be adjusted downward in patients with hepatic impairment.

D. Adverse effects

Although the SSRIs are considered to have fewer and less severe adverse effects than the tricyclic antidepressants and monoamine oxidase inhibitors, the SSRIs are not without troublesome adverse effects, such as, headache, sweating, anxiety and agitation, gastrointestinal effects (nausea, vomiting, diarrhea), weakness and fatigue, sexual dysfunction, changes in weight, sleep disturbances (insomnia and somnolence), and the above-mentioned potential for drug-drug interactions (Figure 12.5).

1. **Sleep disturbances:** *Paroxetine* and *fluvoxamine* are generally more sedating than activating, and they may be useful in patients who have difficulty sleeping. Conversely, patients who are fatigued or complaining of excessive somnolence may benefit from one of the more activating antidepressants, such as *fluoxetine or sertraline*.

2. **Sexual dysfunction:** Loss of libido, delayed ejaculation, and anorgasmia are underreported side effects often noted by clinicians but not prominently featured in the list of standard side effects. One option for managing SSRI-induced sexual dysfunction is to replace the offending antidepressant with an antidepressant having fewer sexual side effects, such as *bupropion* or *mirtazapine*. Alternatively, the dose of the drug may be reduced. In men with erectile dysfunction and depression, treatment with *sildenafil*, *vardenafil*, or *tadalafil* (see p. 341) may improve sexual function.

3. **Use in children and teenagers:** Antidepressants should be used cautiously in children and teenagers, because about 1 out of 50 children becomes more suicidal as a result of SSRI treatment. Pediatric patients should be observed for worsening depression and suicidal thinking whenever any antidepressant is started or its dose is increased or decreased.

4. **Overdoses:** Large intakes of SSRIs do not usually cause cardiac arrhythmias (compared to the arrhythmia risk for the tricyclic antidepressants), but seizures are a possibility because all antidepressants

DRUG	UPTAKE INHIBITION	
	Nor-epinephrine	Serotonin
Selective serotonin re-uptake inhibitor		
Fluoxetine	0	++++
Selective serotonin/ norepinephrine re-uptake inhibitors		
Venlafaxine	++*	++++
Duloxetine	++++	++++
Tricyclic antidepressant	++++	+++
Imipramine		

Figure 12.3
Relative receptor specificity of some antidepressant drugs. *Venlafaxine* inhibits norepinephrine re-uptake only at high doses. ++++ = very strong affinity; +++ = strong affinity; ++ = moderate affinity; + = weak affinity; 0 = little or no affinity.

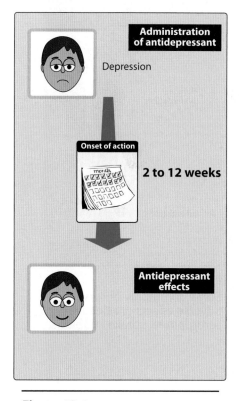

Figure 12.4
Onset of therapeutic effects of the major antidepressant drugs (tricyclic antidepressants, selective serotonin re-uptake inhibitors, and monoamine oxidase inhibitors) requires several weeks.

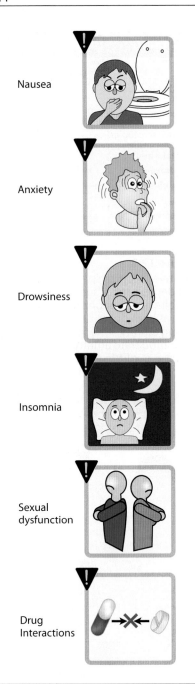

Nausea

Anxiety

Drowsiness

Insomnia

Sexual
dysfunction

Drug
Interactions

Figure 12.5
Some commonly observed
adverse effects of selective
serotonin re-uptake inhibitors.

may lower the seizure threshold. All SSRIs have the potential to cause a serotonin syndrome that may include the symptoms of hyperthermia, muscle rigidity, sweating, myoclonus (clonic muscle twitching), and changes in mental status and vital signs when used in the presence of a monoamine oxidase inhibitor or another highly serotonergic drug. Therefore, extended periods of washout for each drug class should occur prior to the administration of the other class of drugs.

5. **Discontinuation syndrome:** Whereas all of the SSRIs have the potential for causing a discontinuation syndrome after their abrupt withdrawal, the agents with the shorter half-lives and having inactive metabolites have a higher risk for such an adverse reaction. *Fluoxetine* has the lowest risk of causing an SSRI discontinuation syndrome. Possible signs and symptoms of such a serotonin-related discontinuation syndrome include headache, malaise and flu-like symptoms, agitation and irritability, nervousness, and changes in sleep pattern.

IV. SEROTONIN-NOREPINEPHRINE REUPTAKE INHIBITORS

Venlafaxine [VEN-la-fax-een] and *duloxetine* (doo-LOX-e-teen) selectively inhibit the re-uptake of both serotonin and norepinephrine (Figure 12.6). These agents, termed selective serotonin-norepinephrine reuptake inhibitors (SNRIs), may be effective in treating depression in patients in whom SSRIs are ineffective. Furthermore, depression is often accompanied by chronic painful symptoms, such as backache and muscle aches, against which SSRIs are also relatively ineffective. This pain is, in part, modulated by serotonin and norepinephrine pathways in the CNS. Both SNRIs and tricyclic antidepressants, with their dual actions of inhibiting both serotonin and norepinephrine reuptake are sometimes effective in relieving physical symptoms of neuropathic pain, such as diabetic peripheral neuropathy. However, the SNRIs, unlike the tricyclic antidepressants, have little activity at adrenergic, muscarinic, or histamine receptors and, thus, have fewer of these receptor-mediated adverse effects than the tricyclic antidepressants (see Figure 12.3). Both *venlafaxine* and *duloxetine* may precipitate a discontinuation syndrome if treatment is abruptly stopped.

A. Venlafaxine

Venlafaxine is a potent inhibitor of serotonin reuptake and, at medium to higher doses, is an inhibitor of norepinephrine re-uptake. It is also a mild inhibitor of dopamine reuptake at high doses. *Venlafaxine* has minimal inhibition of the cytochrome P450 isoenzymes and is a substrate of the CYP2D6 isoenzyme. The half-life of the parent compound plus its active metabolite is approximately 11 hours. *Venlafaxine* is only 27 percent bound to plasma protein and is not expected to be involved in protein displacement interactions. The most common side effects of *venlafaxine* are nausea, headache, sexual dysfunction, dizziness, insomnia, sedation, and constipation. At high doses, there may be an increase in blood pressure and heart rate.

B. Duloxetine

Duloxetine inhibits serotonin and norepinephrine reuptake at all doses. It is extensively metabolized in the liver to numerous metabolites. *Duloxetine* should not be administered to patients with hepatic insufficiency. Metabolites are excreted in the urine, and the use of *duloxetine* is not recommended in patients with end-stage renal disease.

Food delays the absorption of the drug. The half-life is approximately 12 hours. *Duloxetine* is highly bound to plasma protein. Gastrointestinal side effects are common with *duloxetine*, including nausea, dry mouth, and constipation. Diarrhea and vomiting are seen less often. Insomnia, dizziness, somnolence, and sweating are also seen. Sexual dysfunction also occurs along with the possible risk for an increase in either blood pressure or heart rate.

V. ATYPICAL ANTIDEPRESSANTS

The atypical antidepressants are a mixed group of agents that have actions at several different sites. This group includes *bupropion* [byoo-PROE-pee-on], *mirtazapine* [mir-TAZ-a-peen], *nefazodone* [nef-AY-zoe-done], and *trazodone* [TRAZ-oh-done]. They are not any more efficacious than the tricyclic antidepressants or SSRIs, but their side effect profiles are different.

A. Bupropion

This drug acts as a weak dopamine and norepinephrine reuptake inhibitor to alleviate the symptoms of depression. Its short half-life may require more than once-a-day dosing or the administration of an extended-release formulation. *Bupropion* is unique in that it assists in decreasing the craving and attenuating the withdrawal symptoms for *nicotine* in tobacco users trying to quit smoking. Side effects may include dry mouth, sweating, nervousness, tremor, a very low incidence of sexual dysfunction, and an increased risk for seizures at high doses. *Bupropion* is metabolized by the CYP2D6 pathway and is considered to have a relatively low risk for drug-drug interactions.

B. Mirtazapine

This drug enhances serotonin and norepinephrine neurotransmission via mechanisms related to its ability to block presynaptic α_2 receptors. Additionally, it may owe at least some of its antidepressant activity to its ability to block 5-HT$_2$ receptors. It is a sedative because of its potent antihistaminic activity, but it does not cause the antimuscarinic side effects of the tricyclic antidepressants, or interfere with sexual functioning, as do the SSRIs. Increased appetite and weight gain frequently occur. *Mirtazapine* is markedly sedating, which may be used to advantage in depressed patients having difficulty sleeping.

C. Nefazodone and trazodone

These drugs are weak inhibitors of serotonin reuptake. Their therapeutic benefit appears to be related to their ability to block postsynaptic 5-HT$_{2A}$ receptors. With chronic use, these agents may desensitize 5-HT$_{1A}$ presynaptic autoreceptors and, thereby, increase serotonin release. Both agents are sedating, probably because of their potent H$_1$-blocking activity. *Trazodone* has been associated with causing priapism, and *nefazodone* has been associated with the risk for hepatotoxicity.

VI. TRICYCLIC ANTIDEPRESSANTS

The tricyclic antidepressants (TCAs) block norepinephrine and serotonin reuptake into the neuron and, thus, if discovered today, may be referred to as SNRIs except for their differences in adverse effects relative to this newer class of antidepressants. The TCAs include the tertiary amines *imipramine* [ee-MIP-ra-meen] (the prototype drug), *amitriptyline* [aye-mee-TRIP-ti-leen], *clomipramine* [kloe-MIP-ra-meen], *doxepin* [DOX-e-pin] and *trimipramine*

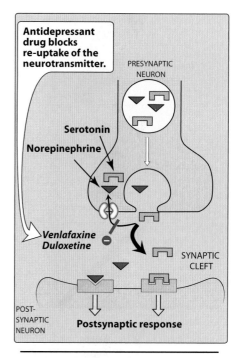

Figure 12.6
Proposed mechanism of action of selective serotonin/norepinephrine re-uptake inhibitor antidepressant drugs.

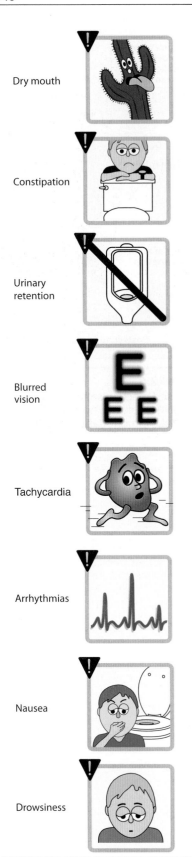

Dry mouth

Constipation

Urinary retention

Blurred vision

Tachycardia

Arrhythmias

Nausea

Drowsiness

Figure 12.7
Some commonly observed adverse effects of tricyclic antidepressants.

[trye-MIP-ra-meen]. The TCAs also include the secondary amines *desipramine* [dess-IP-ra-meen] and *nortriptyline* [nor-TRIP-ti-leen] (the respective N-demethylated metabolites of *imipramine* and *amitriptyline*) and *protriptyline* [proe-TRIP-ti-leen]. *Maprotiline* [ma-PROE-ti-leen] and *amoxapine* [a-MOX-a-peen] are related "tetracyclic" antidepressant agents and are commonly included in the general class of TCAs. All have similar therapeutic efficacy, and the choice of drug may depend on such issues as patient tolerance to side effects, prior response, preexisting medical conditions, and duration of action. Patients who do not respond to one TCA may benefit from a different drug in this group. These drugs are a valuable alternative for patients who do not respond to SSRIs.

A. Mechanism of action

1. **Inhibition of neurotransmitter reuptake:** TCAs and *amoxapine* are potent inhibitors of the neuronal reuptake of norepinephrine and serotonin into presynaptic nerve terminals (see Figure 12.2). At therapeutic concentrations, they do not block dopamine transporters. By blocking the major route of neurotransmitter removal, the TCAs cause increased concentrations of monoamines in the synaptic cleft, ultimately resulting in antidepressant effects. *Maprotiline* and *desipramine* are selective inhibitors of norepinephrine reuptake.

2. **Blocking of receptors:** TCAs also block serotonergic, α-adrenergic, histaminic, and muscarinic receptors (see Figure 12.3). It is not known if any of these actions produce their therapeutic benefit. However, actions at these receptors are probably responsible for many of the untoward effects of the TCAs. *Amoxapine* also blocks the D_2 receptor.

B. Actions

The TCAs elevate mood, improve mental alertness, increase physical activity, and reduce morbid preoccupation in 50 to 70 percent of individuals with major depression. The onset of the mood elevation is slow, requiring 2 weeks or longer (see Figure 12.4). These drugs do not commonly produce CNS stimulation or mood elevation in normal individuals. Physical and psychological dependence has been rarely reported, however, this necessitates slow withdrawal to minimize discontinuation syndromes and cholinergic rebound effects. These drugs, like all of the antidepressants, can be used for prolonged treatment of depression.

C. Therapeutic uses

The TCAs are effective in treating moderate to severe major depression. Some patients with panic disorder also respond to TCAs. *Imipramine* has been used to control bed-wetting in children (older than 6 years) by causing contraction of the internal sphincter of the bladder. At present, it is used cautiously because of the inducement of cardiac arrhythmias and other serious cardiovascular problems. The TCAs, particularly *amitriptyline*, have been used to treat migraine headache and chronic pain syndromes (for example, "neuropathic" pain) in a number of conditions for which the cause of the pain is unclear.

D. Pharmacokinetics

Tricyclic antidepressants are well absorbed upon oral administration. Because of their lipophilic nature, they are widely distributed and readily penetrate into the CNS. This lipid solubility also causes these drugs to have variable half-lives—for example, 4 to 17 hours for *imipramine*.

As a result of their variable first-pass metabolism in the liver, TCAs have low and inconsistent bioavailability. Therefore, the patient's response and plasma levels can be used to adjust dosage. The initial treatment period is typically 4 to 8 weeks. The dosage can be gradually reduced to improve tolerability unless relapse occurs. These drugs are metabolized by the hepatic microsomal system (and, thus, may be sensitive to agents that induce or inhibit the CYP450 isoenzymes) and conjugated with glucuronic acid. Ultimately, the TCAs are excreted as inactive metabolites via the kidney.

E. Adverse effects

Blockade of muscarinic receptors leads to blurred vision, xerostomia (dry mouth), urinary retention, constipation, and aggravation of narrow-angle glaucoma (Figure 12.7). These agents slow cardiac conduction similarly to *quinidine*, which may precipitate life-threatening arrhythmias should an overdose of one of these drugs be taken. The TCAs also block α-adrenergic receptors, causing orthostatic hypotension, dizziness, and reflex tachycardia. In clinical practice, this is the most serious problem in the elderly. *Imipramine* is the most likely and *nortriptyline* the least likely to cause orthostatic hypotension. Sedation may be prominent, especially during the first several weeks of treatment, and is related to the ability of these drugs to block histamine H_1 receptors. Weight gain is a common adverse effect of the TCAs. Sexual dysfunction, as evidenced by erectile dysfunction in men and anorgasmia in women, occurs in a significant minority of patients, but the incidence is still considered to be lower than the incidence of sexual dysfunction associated with the SSRIs.

1. **Precautions:** TCAs (like all antidepressants) should be used with caution in known manic-depressive patients, even during their depressed state, because antidepressants may cause a switch to manic behavior. The TCAs have a narrow therapeutic index; for example, five- to six-fold the maximal daily dose of *imipramine* can be lethal. Depressed patients who are suicidal should be given only limited quantities of these drugs and be monitored closely. Drug interactions with the TCAs are shown in Figure 12.8. The TCAs may exacerbate certain medical conditions, such as unstable angina, benign prostatic hyperplasia, epilepsy, and patients with preexisting arrhythmias. Caution should be exercised with their use in very young or very old patients as well.

VII. MONOAMINE OXIDASE INHIBITORS

Monoamine oxidase (MAO) is a mitochondrial enzyme found in nerve and other tissues, such as the gut and liver. In the neuron, MAO functions as a "safety valve" to oxidatively deaminate and inactivate any excess neurotransmitter molecules (norepinephrine, dopamine, and serotonin) that may leak out of synaptic vesicles when the neuron is at rest. The MAO inhibitors may irreversibly or reversibly inactivate the enzyme, permitting neurotransmitter molecules to escape degradation and, therefore, to both accumulate within the presynaptic neuron and leak into the synaptic space. This is believed to cause activation of norepinephrine and serotonin receptors, and it may be responsible for the indirect antidepressant action of these drugs. Three MAO inhibitors are currently available for treatment of depression: *phenelzine* [FEN-el-zeen], *tranylcypromine* [tran-il-SIP-roe-meen] and the agent that was prior-approved for Parkinson's disease, but is now also

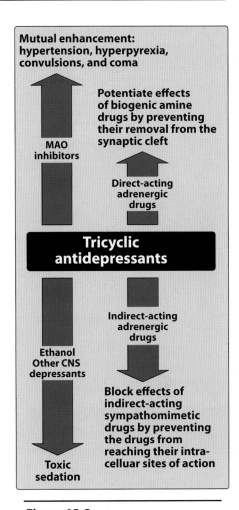

Mutual enhancement: hypertension, hyperpyrexia, convulsions, and coma

MAO inhibitors

Potentiate effects of biogenic amine drugs by preventing their removal from the synaptic cleft

Direct-acting adrenergic drugs

Tricyclic antidepressants

Indirect-acting adrenergic drugs

Ethanol Other CNS depressants

Block effects of indirect-acting sympathomimetic drugs by preventing the drugs from reaching their intracelluar sites of action

Toxic sedation

Figure 12.8
Drugs interacting with tricyclic antidepressants. CNS = central nervous system; MAO = monoamine oxidase.

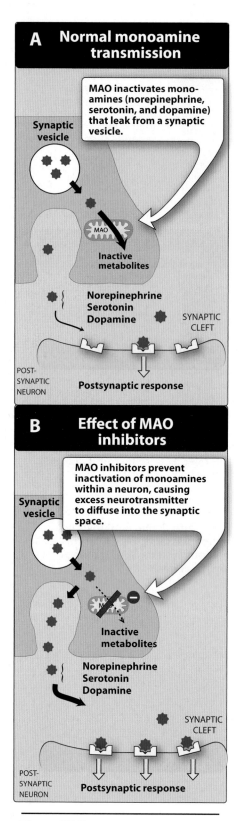

Figure 12.9
Mechanism of action of mono-amine oxidase (MAO) inhibitors.

approved for depression, *selegiline*, which is the first antidepressant available in a transdermal delivery system. Use of MAO inhibitors is now limited due to the complicated dietary restrictions required of patients taking MAO inhibitors.

A. Mechanism of action

Most MAO inhibitors, such as *phenelzine*, form stable complexes with the enzyme, causing irreversible inactivation. This results in increased stores of norepinephrine, serotonin, and dopamine within the neuron and subsequent diffusion of excess neurotransmitter into the synaptic space (Figure 12.9). These drugs inhibit not only MAO in the brain but also MAO in the liver and gut that catalyze oxidative deamination of drugs and potentially toxic substances, such as tyramine, which is found in certain foods. The MAO inhibitors therefore show a high incidence of drug-drug and drug-food interactions. *Selegiline* administered as the transdermal "patch" may produce less inhibition of hepatic MAO at low doses, because it avoids first-pass metabolism.

B. Actions

Although MAO is fully inhibited after several days of treatment, the antidepressant action of the MAO inhibitors, like that of the SSRIs and TCAs, is delayed several weeks. *Selegiline* and *tranylcypromine* have an amphetamine-like stimulant effect that may produce agitation or insomnia.

C. Therapeutic uses

The MAO inhibitors are indicated for depressed patients who are unresponsive or allergic to TCAs or who experience strong anxiety. Patients with low psychomotor activity may benefit from the stimulant properties of the MAO inhibitors. These drugs are also useful in the treatment of phobic states. A special subcategory of depression, called atypical depression, may respond to MAO inhibitors. Atypical depression is characterized by labile mood, rejection sensitivity, and appetite disorders. Despite their efficacy in treating depression, because of their risk for drug-drug and drug-food interactions, the MAO inhibitors are considered to be last-line agents in many treatment venues.

D. Pharmacokinetics

These drugs are well absorbed after oral administration, but antidepressant effects require at least 2 to 4 weeks of treatment. Enzyme regeneration, when irreversibly inactivated, varies, but it usually occurs several weeks after termination of the drug. Thus, when switching antidepressant agents, a minimum of 2 weeks of delay must be allowed after termination of MAO inhibitor therapy and the initiation of another antidepressant from any other class. MAO inhibitors are metabolized and excreted rapidly in the urine.

E. Adverse effects

Severe and often unpredictable side effects due to drug-food and drug-drug interactions limit the widespread use of MAO inhibitors. For example, tyramine, which is contained in certain foods, such as aged cheeses and meats, chicken liver, pickled or smoked fish such as anchovies or herring, and red wines, is normally inactivated by MAO in the gut. Individuals receiving an MAO inhibitor are unable to degrade tyramine obtained from the diet. Tyramine causes the release of large amounts of stored catecholamines from nerve terminals, resulting in occipital headache, stiff neck, tachycardia, nausea, hypertension, cardiac arrhythmias, seizures, and possibly, stroke. Patients must therefore be educated to avoid tyramine-containing foods. *Phentolamine* or *prazosin* are helpful in the management of tyramine-induced hypertension. [Note: Treatment with MAO inhibitors may be dangerous in severely depressed patients with suicidal tendencies. Purposeful consumption of tyramine-containing foods is a possibility.] Other possible side effects of treatment with MAO inhibitors include drowsiness, orthostatic hypotension, blurred vision, dry mouth, dysuria, and constipation. The MAO inhibitors and SSRIs should not be coadministered due to the risk of the life-threatening "serotonin syndrome." Both types of drugs require washout periods of at least 2 weeks before the other type is administered, with the exception of *fluoxetine,* which should be discontinued at least 6 weeks before a MAO inhibitor is initiated. Combination of MAO inhibitors and *bupropion* can produce seizures. Figure 12.10 summarizes the side effects of the antidepressant drugs.

VIII. TREATMENT OF MANIA AND BIPOLAR DISORDER

The treatment of bipolar disorder has increased in recent years, partly due to the increased recognition of the disorder and also due to the increase in the number of medications U.S. Food and Drug Administration (FDA)–approved for the treatment of mania. *Lithium salts* are used prophylactically for treating manic-depressive patients and in the treatment of manic episodes and, thus, is considered a "mood stabilizer." *Lithium* is effective in treating 60 to 80 percent of patients exhibiting mania and hypomania. Although many cellular processes are altered by treatment with *lithium salts*, the mode of action is unknown. [Note: *Lithium* is believed to attenuate signaling via receptors coupled to the phosphatidylinositol bisphosphate (PIP$_2$) second-messenger system. *Lithium* interferes with the resynthesis (recycling) of PIP$_2$, leading to its relative depletion in neuronal membranes of the CNS. PIP$_2$ levels in peripheral membranes are unaffected by *lithium*.] *Lithium* is given orally, and the ion is excreted by the kidney. *Lithium* salts can be toxic. Their safety factor and therapeutic index are extremely low— comparable to those of *digitalis*. Common adverse effects may include headache, dry mouth, polydipsia, polyuria, polyphagia, gastrointestinal distress (give *lithium* with food), fine hand tremor, dizziness, fatigue, dermatologic reactions, and sedation. Adverse effects due to higher plasma levels may include ataxia, slurred speech, coarse tremors, confusion, and convulsions. [Note: The diabetes insipidus that results from taking *lithium* can be treated with *amiloride*.] Thyroid function may be decreased and should be monitored. *Lithium* causes no noticeable effect on normal individuals. It is not a sedative, euphoriant, or depressant.

Several antiepileptic drugs, including most notably *carbamazepine, valproic acid, and lamotrigine,* have been identified and FDA-approved as "mood stabilizers" and have been successfully utilized in the treatment of bipolar disorder. Other agents that may improve manic symptoms include the older and newer antipsychotics. The atypical antipsychotics (*risperidone*, *olanzapine*, *ziprasidone*, *aripiprazole*, and *quetiapine*) have also received FDA approval for the management of mania. Benzodiazepines are also frequently used as adjunctive treatments for the acute stabilization of patients with mania. (See the respective chapters on these psychotropics for a more detailed description).

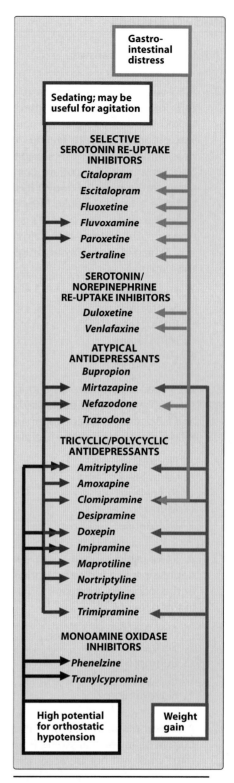

Figure 12.10
Side effects of some drugs used to treat depression.

Study Questions

Choose the ONE best answer.

12.1 A 55-year-old teacher began to experience changes in mood. He was losing interest in his work and lacked the desire to play his daily tennis match. He was preoccupied with feelings of guilt, worthlessness, and hopelessness. In addition to the psychiatric symptoms, the patient complained of muscle aches throughout his body. Physical and laboratory tests were unremarkable. After 6 weeks of therapy with fluoxetine, the patient's symptoms resolved. However, the patient complains of sexual dysfunction. Which of the following drugs might be useful in this patient?

A. Fluvoxamine.
B. Sertraline.
C. Citalopram.
D. Mirtazapine.
E. Lithium.

Correct answer = D. Sexual dysfunction commonly occurs with TCAs, SSRIs, and SNRIs. Mirtazapine is largely free from sexual side effects.

12.2 A 25-year-old woman has a long history of depressive symptoms accompanied by body aches. Physical and laboratory tests are unremarkable. Which of the following drugs might be useful in this patient?

A. Fluoxetine.
B. Sertraline.
C. Phenelzine.
D. Mirtazapine.
E. Duloxetine.

Correct answer = E. Duloxetine is an SNRI that can be used for depression accompanied by neuropathic pain. MAOs and SSRIs have little activity against neuropathic pain.

12.3 A 51-year-old woman with symptoms of major depression also has narrow-angle glaucoma. Which of the following antidepressants should be avoided in this patient?

A. Amitriptyline.
B. Sertraline.
C. Bupropion.
D. Mirtazepine.
E. Fluvoxamine.

Correct answer = A. Because of its potent antimuscarinic activity, amitriptyline should not be given to patients with glaucoma because of the risk of acute increases in ocular pressure. The other antidepressants all lack antagonist activity at the muscarinic receptor.

12.4 A 36-year-old man presents with symptoms of compulsive behavior. If anything is out of order, he feels that "work will not be accomplished effectively or efficiently." He realizes that his behavior is interfering with his ability to accomplish his daily tasks but cannot seem to stop himself. Which of the following drugs would be most helpful to this patient?

A. Imipramine.
B. Fluvoxamine.
C. Amitriptyline.
D. Tranylcypromine.
E. Lithium.

Correct answer = B. Selective serotonin reuptake inhibitors are particularly effective in treating obsessive-compulsive disorder; fluvoxamine is approved for this condition. The other drugs are ineffective in the treatment of obsessive-compulsive disorder.

Neuroleptics

13

I. OVERVIEW

The neuroleptic drugs (also called antipsychotic drugs, or major tranquilizers) are used primarily to treat schizophrenia, but they are also effective in other psychotic states, such as manic states with psychotic symptoms such as grandiosity or paranoia and hallucinations, and delirium. All currently available antipsychotic drugs that alleviate symptoms of schizophrenia decrease dopaminergic and/or serotonergic neurotransmission. The traditional or "typical" neuroleptic drugs (also called conventional or first-generation antipsychotics) are competitive inhibitors at a variety of receptors, but their antipsychotic effects reflect competitive blocking of dopamine receptors. These drugs vary in potency. For example, *chlorpromazine* is a low-potency drug, and *fluphenazine* is a high-potency agent (Figure 13.1). No one drug is clinically more effective than another. In contrast, the newer antipsychotic drugs are referred to as "atypical" (or second-generation antipsychotics), because they have fewer extrapyramidal adverse effects than the older, traditional agents. These drugs appear to owe their unique activity to blockade of both serotonin and dopamine (and, perhaps, other) receptors. Current antipsychotic therapy commonly employs the use of the atypical agents to minimize the risk of debilitating movement disorders associated with the typical drugs that act primarily at the D_2 dopamine receptor. All of the atypical antipsychotics exhibit an efficacy that is equivalent to, or occasionally exceeds, that of the typical neuroleptic agents. However, consistent differences in therapeutic efficacy among the individual atypical neuroleptics have not been established, and individual patient response and comorbid conditions must often be used as a guide in drug selection. Neuroleptic drugs are not curative and do not eliminate the fundamental and chronic thought disorder, but they often decrease the intensity of hallucinations and delusions and permit the person with schizophrenia to function in a supportive environment.

II. SCHIZOPHRENIA

Schizophrenia is a particular type of psychosis—that is, a mental disorder caused by some inherent dysfunction of the brain. It is characterized by delusions, hallucinations (often in the form of voices), and thinking or speech disturbances. This mental disorder is a common affliction, occurring among about one percent of the population. The illness often initially affects people during late adolescence or early adulthood and is a chronic and disabling disorder. Schizophrenia has a strong genetic component and probably reflects some fundamental biochemical abnormality, possibly a dysfunction of the mesolimbic or mesocortical dopaminergic neurons.

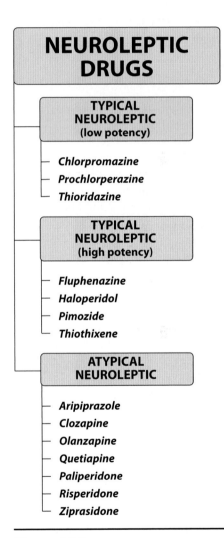

NEUROLEPTIC DRUGS

TYPICAL NEUROLEPTIC (low potency)
- *Chlorpromazine*
- *Prochlorperazine*
- *Thioridazine*

TYPICAL NEUROLEPTIC (high potency)
- *Fluphenazine*
- *Haloperidol*
- *Pimozide*
- *Thiothixene*

ATYPICAL NEUROLEPTIC
- *Aripiprazole*
- *Clozapine*
- *Olanzapine*
- *Quetiapine*
- *Paliperidone*
- *Risperidone*
- *Ziprasidone*

Figure 13.1
Summary of neuroleptic agents.

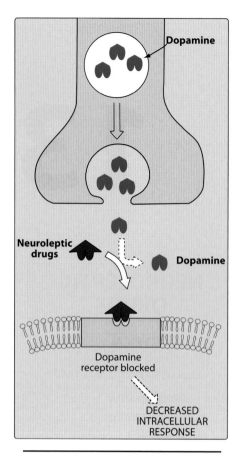

Figure 13.2
Dopamine-blocking actions
of neuroleptic drugs.

III. NEUROLEPTIC DRUGS

The neuroleptic drugs represent several diverse, heterocyclic structures with markedly different potencies. The tricyclic phenothiazine derivative, *chlorpromazine* [klor-PROE-ma-zeen], was the first neuroleptic drug used to treat schizophrenia. Antipsychotic drugs developed subsequently, such as *haloperidol* [hal-oh-PER-i-dole], are more than 100-fold as potent as *chlorpromazine* but have an increased ability to induce parkinson-like and other extrapyramidal effects. Furthermore, these more potent traditional drugs are no more effective than *chlorpromazine*.

A. Mechanism of action

1. **Dopamine receptor–blocking activity in the brain:** All of the older and most of the newer neuroleptic drugs block dopamine receptors in the brain and the periphery (Figure 13.2). Five types of dopamine receptors have been identified. D_1 and D_5 receptors activate adenylyl cyclase, often exciting neurons, whereas D_2, D_3 and D_4 receptors inhibit adenylyl cyclase, or mediate membrane K^+ channel opening leading to neuronal hyperpolarization. The neuroleptic drugs bind to these receptors to varying degrees. However, the clinical efficacy of the typical neuroleptic drugs correlates closely with their relative ability to block D_2 receptors in the mesolimbic system of the brain. On the other hand, the atypical drug *clozapine* [KLOE-za-peen] has higher affinity for the D_4 receptor and lower affinity for the D_2 receptor, which may partially explain its minimal ability to cause extrapyramidal side effects (EPS). (Figure 13.3 summarizes the receptor-binding properties of *clozapine*, *chlorpromazine*, and *haloperidol*.) The actions of the neuroleptic drugs are antagonized by agents that raise synaptic dopamine concentrations—for example, *levodopa* and amphetamines—or mimic dopamine at post-synaptic binding sites—for example, *bromocriptine*.

2. **Serotonin receptor–blocking activity in the brain:** Most of the newer atypical agents appear to exert part of their unique action through inhibition of serotonin receptors (5-HT), particularly 5-HT$_{2A}$ receptors. Thus, *clozapine* has high affinity for D_1, D_4, 5-HT$_2$, muscarinic, and α-adrenergic receptors, but it is also a dopamine D_2-receptor antagonist. *Risperidone* [ris-PEER-i-dohn] blocks 5-HT$_{2A}$ receptors to a greater extent than it does D_2 receptors, as does *olanzapine*. The atypical neuroleptic *aripiprazole* [a-rih-PIP-ra-zole] is a partial agonist at D_2 and 5-HT$_{1A}$ receptors as well as a blocker of 5-HT$_{2A}$ receptors. *Quetiapine* blocks D_2 receptors more potently than 5HT$_{2A}$ receptors but is relatively weak at blocking either receptor, and its low risk for EPS may also be related to the relatively short period of time it binds to the D_2 receptor.

B. Actions

The antipsychotic actions of neuroleptic drugs appear to reflect a blockade at dopamine and/or serotonin receptors. However, many of these agents also block cholinergic, adrenergic, and histaminergic receptors (Figure 13.4). It is unknown what role, if any, these actions have in alleviating the symptoms of psychosis. The undesirable side effects of these agents, however, are often a result of actions at these other receptors.

1. **Antipsychotic actions:** All of the neuroleptic drugs can reduce the hallucinations and delusions associated with schizophrenia (the so-

called "positive" symptoms) by blocking dopamine receptors in the mesolimbic system of the brain. The "negative" symptoms, such as blunted affect, anhedonia (not getting pleasure from normally pleasurable stimuli), apathy, and impaired attention, as well as cognitive impairment are not as responsive to therapy, particularly with the typical neuroleptics. Many atypical agents, such as *clozapine*, ameliorate the negative symptoms to some extent. All of the drugs also have a calming effect and reduce spontaneous physical movement. In contrast to the central nervous system (CNS) depressants, such as barbiturates, the neuroleptics do not depress the intellectual functioning of the patient as much, and motor incoordination is minimal. The antipsychotic effects usually take several days to weeks to occur, suggesting that the therapeutic effects are related to secondary changes in the corticostriatal pathways.

2. **Extrapyramidal effects:** Dystonias (sustained contraction of muscles leading to twisting distorted postures), parkinson-like symptoms, akathisia (motor restlessness), and tardive dyskinesia (involuntary movements of the tongue, lips, neck, trunk, and limbs) occur with chronic treatment. Blocking of dopamine receptors in the nigrostriatal pathway probably causes these unwanted movement symptoms. The atypical neuroleptics exhibit a lower incidence of these symptoms.

3. **Antiemetic effects:** With the exceptions of *aripiprazole* and *thioridazine* [thye-oh-RID-a-zeen], most of the neuroleptic drugs have antiemetic effects that are mediated by blocking D_2-dopaminergic receptors of the chemoreceptor trigger zone of the medulla. (See p. 335 for a discussion of emesis.) Figure 13.5 summarizes the antiemetic uses of neuroleptic agents, along with the therapeutic applications of other drugs that combat nausea. [Note: The atypical antipsychotic drugs are not used as antiemetics.]

4. **Antimuscarinic effects:** Some of the neuroleptics, particularly *thioridazine*, *chlorpromazine*, *clozapine*, and *olanzapine* [oh-LAN-za-peen], produce anticholinergic effects, including blurred vision, dry

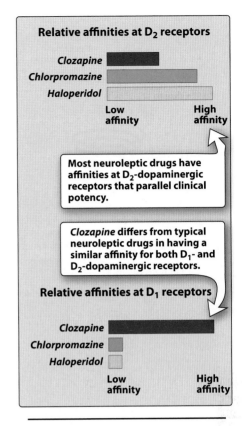

Relative affinities at D_2 receptors

Clozapine / Chlorpromazine / Haloperidol

Low affinity — High affinity

Most neuroleptic drugs have affinities at D_2-dopaminergic receptors that parallel clinical potency.

Clozapine differs from typical neuroleptic drugs in having a similar affinity for both D_1- and D_2-dopaminergic receptors.

Relative affinities at D_1 receptors

Clozapine / Chlorpromazine / Haloperidol

Low affinity — High affinity

Figure 13.3
Relative affinity of *clozapine, chlorpromazine,* and *haloperidol* at D_1- and D_2-dopaminergic receptors.

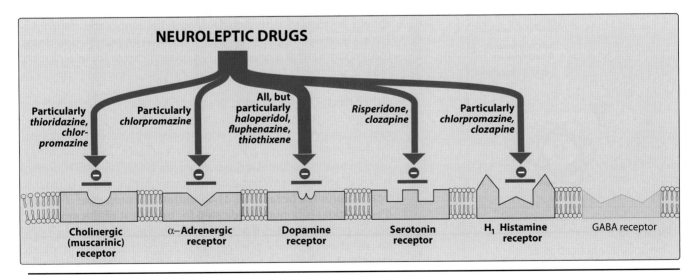

NEUROLEPTIC DRUGS

Particularly *thioridazine, chlorpromazine* → Cholinergic (muscarinic) receptor

Particularly *chlorpromazine* → α–Adrenergic receptor

All, but particularly *haloperidol, fluphenazine, thiothixene* → Dopamine receptor

Risperidone, clozapine → Serotonin receptor

Particularly *chlorpromazine, clozapine* → H_1 Histamine receptor

GABA receptor

Figure 13.4
Neuroleptic drugs block at dopaminergic and serotonergic receptors as well as at adrenergic, cholinergic, and histamine-binding receptors. GABA = γ-aminobutyric acid.

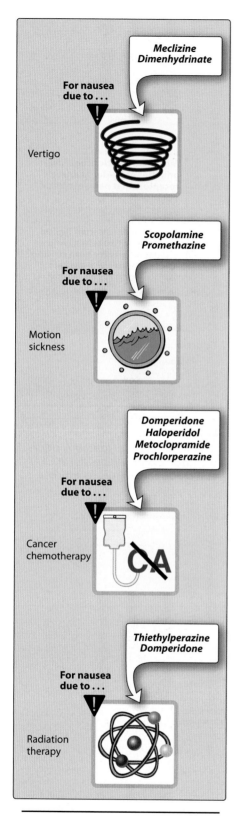

Figure 13.5
Therapeutic application of antiemetic agents.

mouth (exception: *clozapine* increase salivation), confusion, and inhibition of gastrointestinal and urinary tract smooth muscle, leading to constipation and urinary retention. This anticholinergic property may actually assist in reducing the risk of EPS with these agents.

5. **Other effects:** Blockade of α-adrenergic receptors causes orthostatic hypotension and light-headedness. The neuroleptics also alter temperature-regulating mechanisms and can produce poikilothermia (body temperature varies with the environment). In the pituitary, neuroleptics block D_2 receptors, leading to an increase in prolactin release. Atypical neuroleptics are less likely to produce prolactin elevations. Sedation occurs with those drugs that are potent antagonists of the H_1-histamine receptor, including *chlorpromazine, olanzapine, quetiapine,* and *clozapine.* Sexual dysfunction may also occur with the antipsychotics due to various receptor-binding characteristics.

C. **Therapeutic uses**

1. **Treatment of schizophrenia:** The neuroleptics are considered to be the only efficacious treatment for schizophrenia. Not all patients respond, and complete normalization of behavior is seldom achieved. The traditional neuroleptics are most effective in treating positive symptoms of schizophrenia (delusions, hallucinations, thought processing, and agitation). The newer agents with 5-HT_{2A} receptor–blocking activity may be effective in many patients who are resistant to the traditional agents, especially in treating the negative symptoms of schizophrenia (social withdrawal, blunted emotions, ambivalence, and reduced ability to relate to people). However, even the atypical antipsychotics do not consistently improve the negative symptoms of schizophrenia more than the older agents. [Note: *Clozapine* is reserved for the treatment of individuals who are unresponsive to other neuroleptics, because its use is associated with blood dyscrasias and other severe adverse effects].

2. **Prevention of severe nausea and vomiting:** The older neuroleptics (most commonly *prochlorperazine*) are useful in the treatment of drug-induced nausea (see p. 336). Nausea arising from motion should be treated with sedatives, antihistamines, and anticholinergics, however, rather than with the powerful neuroleptic drugs. [Note: Transdermal *scopolamine* is a drug of choice for treatment of motion sickness.]

3. **Other uses:** The neuroleptic drugs can be used as tranquilizers to manage agitated and disruptive behavior secondary to other disorders. Neuroleptics are used in combination with narcotic analgesics for treatment of chronic pain with severe anxiety. *Chlorpromazine* is used to treat intractable hiccups. *Promethazine* [proe-METH-a-zeen] is not a good antipsychotic drug; however, this agent is used in treating pruritus because of its antihistaminic properties. *Pimozide* [PI-moe-zide] is primarily indicated for treatment of the motor and phonic tics of Tourette's disorder. However, *risperidone* and *haloperidol* are also commonly prescribed for this tic disorder. Also, *risperidone* is now approved for the management of disruptive behavior and irritability secondary to autism.

D. Absorption and metabolism

After oral administration, the neuroleptics show variable absorption that is unaffected by food (except for *ziprasidone* and *paliperidone*, the absorption of which is increased with food). These agents readily pass into the brain, have a large volume of distribution, bind well to plasma proteins, and are metabolized to many different substances, usually by the cytochrome P450 system in the liver, particularly the CYP2D6, CYP1A2, and CYP3A4 isoenzymes. Some metabolites are active. *Fluphenazine decanoate*, *haloperidol decanoate*, and *risperidone* microspheres are slow-release (up to 2 to 4 weeks) injectable formulations of neuroleptics that are administered via deep gluteal intramuscular injection. These drugs are often used to treat outpatients and individuals who are noncompliant with oral medications. However, patients may still develop extrapyramidal symptoms (EPS), but the risk of EPS is lower with these long-acting, injectable formulations compared to their respective oral formulations. The neuroleptic drugs produce some tolerance but little physical dependence.

E. Adverse effects

Adverse effects of the neuroleptic drugs can occur in practically all patients and are significant in about 80 percent (Figure 13.6). Although antipsychotic drugs have an array of adverse effects, their therapeutic index is high.

1. **Extrapyramidal side effects:** The inhibitory effects of dopaminergic neurons are normally balanced by the excitatory actions of cholinergic neurons in the striatum. Blocking dopamine receptors alters this balance, causing a relative excess of cholinergic influence, which results in extrapyramidal motor effects. The maximal risk of appearance of the movement disorders is time and dose dependent, with dystonias occurring within a few hours to days of treatment, followed by akathisias (the inability to remain seated due to motor restlessness) occurring within days to weeks. Parkinson-like symptoms of bradykinesia, rigidity, and tremor usually occur within weeks to months of initiating treatment. Tardive dyskinesia, which can be irreversible, may occur after months or years of treatment.

   a. **Effect of anticholinergic drugs:** If cholinergic activity is also blocked, a new, more nearly normal balance is restored, and extrapyramidal effects are minimized. This can be achieved by administration of an anticholinergic drug, such as *benztropine*. The therapeutic trade-off will be fewer extrapyramidal effects in exchange for the side effects of muscarinic receptor blockade. [Note: Sometimes, the parkinson-like actions persist despite the anticholinergic drugs.] Those drugs that exhibit strong anticholinergic activity, such as *thioridazine*, show fewer extrapyramidal disturbances, because the cholinergic activity is strongly dampened. This contrasts with *haloperidol* and *fluphenazine*, which have low anticholinergic activity and produce extrapyramidal effects more frequently because of the preferential blocking of dopaminergic transmission without the blocking of cholinergic activity.

   b. **Atypical antipsychotics (clozapine and risperidone):** These drugs exhibit a lower potential for causing extrapyramidal symptoms and lower risk of tardive dyskinesia, which has been

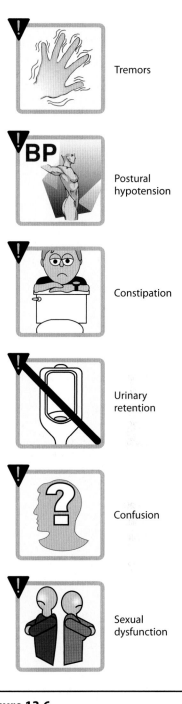

Tremors

Postural hypotension

Constipation

Urinary retention

Confusion

Sexual dysfunction

Figure 13.6
Adverse effects commonly observed in individuals treated with neuroleptic drugs.

attributed to their blockade of 5-HT$_{2A}$ receptors. These two drugs appear to be superior to *haloperidol* and *chlorpromazine* in treating some of the symptoms of schizophrenia, especially the negative symptoms. *Risperidone* should be included among the first-line antipsychotic drugs, whereas *clozapine* should be reserved for severely schizophrenic patients who are refractory to traditional therapy. *Clozapine* can produce bone marrow suppression, seizures, and cardiovascular side effects. The risk of severe agranulocytosis necessitates frequent monitoring of white-blood-cell counts. Paliperidone, the major active metabolite of *risperidone*, exhibits neuroleptic activity similar to that of the parent drug. The other atypical antipsychotics (*olanzapine, quetiapine, ziprasidone,* and *aripiprazole*) have proven efficacy in treating psychotic symptoms, but their efficacy is not considered to be consistently superior to that of the older neurolepitcs. However, their lower incidence of EPS commonly places these newer agents ahead of the older neuroleptics when treating patients with schizophrenia.

2. **Tardive dyskinesia:** Long-term treatment with neuroleptics can cause this motor disorder. Patients display involuntary movements, including lateral jaw movements and "fly-catching" motions of the tongue. A prolonged holiday from neuroleptics may cause the symptoms to diminish or disappear within a few months. However, in many individuals, tardive dyskinesia is irreversible and persists after discontinuation of therapy. Tardive dyskinesia is postulated to result from an increased number of dopamine receptors that are synthesized as a compensatory response to long-term dopamine-receptor blockade. This makes the neuron supersensitive to the actions of dopamine, and it allows the dopaminergic input to this structure to overpower the cholinergic input, causing excess movement in the patient.

3. **Neuroleptic malignant syndrome:** This potentially fatal reaction to neuroleptic drugs is characterized by muscle rigidity, fever, altered mental status and stupor, unstable blood pressure, and myoglobinemia. Treatment necessitates discontinuation of the neuroleptic and supportive therapy. Administration of *dantrolene* or *bromocriptine* may be helpful.

4. **Other effects:** Drowsiness occurs due to CNS depression and antihistaminic effects, usually during the first few weeks of treatment. Confusion is sometimes encountered. Those neuroleptics with potent antimuscarinic activity often produce dry mouth, urinary retention, constipation, and loss of accommodation. Others may block α-adrenergic receptors, resulting in lowered blood pressure and orthostatic hypotension. The neuroleptics depress the hypothalamus, affecting thermoregulation, and causing amenorrhea, galactorrhea, gynecomastia, infertility, and impotence. Significant weight gain is often a reason for noncompliance. It is also recommended that glucose and lipid profiles be monitored in patients taking antipsychotics due to the potential for the atypical agents to increase these laboratory parameters and the possible exacerbation of preexisting diabetes mellitus or hyperlipidemia.

5. **Cautions and contraindications:** Acute agitation accompanying withdrawal from alcohol or other drugs may be aggravated by the

neuroleptics. Stabilization with a simple sedative, such as a *benzodi-azepine*, is the preferred treatment. All antipsychotics may lower the seizure threshold, and *chlorpromazine* and *clozapine* are contraindicated in patients with seizure disorders. Therefore, the neuroleptics can also aggravate preexisting epilepsy, and they should be used with caution in patients with epilepsy. The high incidence of agranulocytosis with *clozapine* may limit its use to patients who are resistant to other drugs. All of the atypical antipsychotics also carry the warning of increased risk for mortality when used in elderly patients with dementia-related behavioral disturbances and psychosis.

F. Maintenance treatment

Patients who have had two or more psychotic episodes secondary to schizophrenia should receive maintenance therapy for at least 5 years, and some experts prefer indefinite therapy. There has been a greater emphasis in research and practice on identifying and aggressively managing first-episode psychosis to determine the benefits of antipsychotic agents in this population. Low doses of antipsychotic drugs are not as effective as higher-dose maintenance therapy in preventing relapse (Figure 13.7).

Figure 13.8 summarizes the therapeutic uses of some of the neuroleptic drugs.

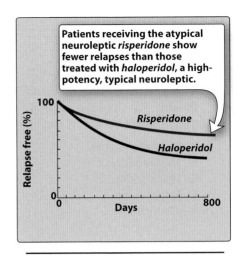

Figure 13.7
Rates of relapse among patients with schizophrenia after maintenance therapy with either *risperidone* or *haloperidol*.

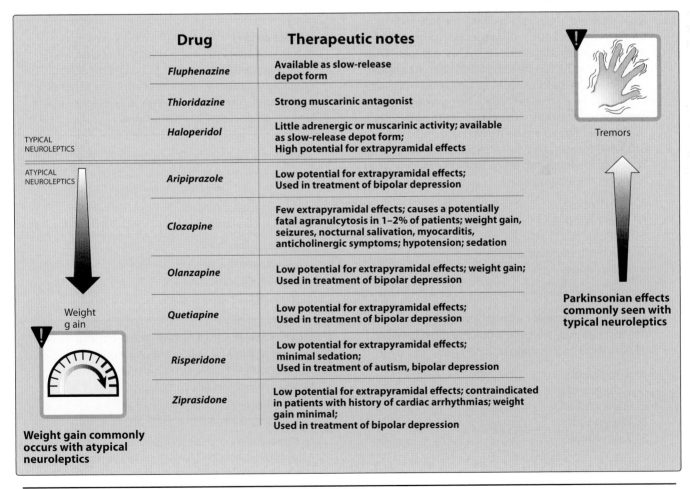

Figure 13.8
Summary of neuroleptic agents.

Study Questions

Choose the ONE best answer.

13.1 An adolescent male is newly diagnosed with schizophrenia. Which of the following neuroleptic agents
may improve his apathy and blunted affect?

A. Chlorpromazine.
B. Fluphenazine.
C. Haloperidol.
D. Risperidone.
E. Thioridazine.

Correct answer = D. Risperidone is the only neuroleptic on the list that has some benefit in improving
the negative symptoms of schizophrenia. All the
agents have the potential to diminish the hallucinations and delusional thought processes.

13.2 Which one of the following neuroleptics has been
shown to be a partial agonist at the D_2 receptor?

A. Aripiprazole.
B. Clozapine.
C. Haloperidol.
D. Risperidone.
E. Thioridazine.

Correct answer = A. Aripiprazole is the agent that
acts as a partial agonist at D_2 receptors. Theoretically,
the drug would enhance action at these receptors
when there is a low concentration of dopamine and
would block the actions of high concentrations of
dopamine. All the other drugs are only antagonistic
at D_2 receptors, with haloperidol being particularly
potent.

13.3 A 21-year-old male has recently begun pimozide
therapy for Tourette's disorder. He is brought to
the emergency department by his parents. They
describe that he has been having "different-appear-
ing tics" than before, such as prolonged contraction of the facial muscles. While being examined, he
experiences opisthotonus (spasm of the body where
the head and heels are bent backward and the body
is bowed forward. A type of extrapyramidal effect).
Which of the following drugs would be beneficial in
reducing these symptoms?

A. Benztropine.
B. Bromocriptine.
C. Lithium.
D. Prochlorperazine.
E. Risperidone.

Correct answer = A. The patient is experiencing
extrapyramidal symptoms due to pimozide, and a
muscarinic antagonist such as benztropine would be
effective in reducing the symptoms. The other drugs
would have no effect or, in the case of prochlorperazine, might increase the symptoms.

13.4 A 28-year-old woman with schizoid affective disorder and difficulty sleeping would be most benefited
by which of the following drugs?

A. Aripiprazole.
B. Chlorpromazine.
C. Haloperidol.
D. Risperidone.
E. Ziprasidone.

Correct answer = B. Chlorpromazine has significant
sedative activity as well as antipsychotic properties.
Of the choices, it is the drug most likely to alleviate this patient's major complaints, including her
insomnia.

Opioids

14

I. OVERVIEW

Management of pain is one of clinical medicine's greatest challenges. Pain is defined as an unpleasant sensation that can be either acute or chronic and that is a consequence of complex neurochemical processes in the peripheral and central nervous system (CNS). It is subjective, and the physician must rely on the patient's perception and description of his or her pain. Alleviation of pain depends on its type. In many cases—for example, with headaches or mild to moderate arthritic pain—nonsteroidal anti-inflammatory agents (NSAIDs, see Chapter 42) are effective. Neurogenic pain responds best to anticonvulsants (for example pregabalin, see p. 179), tricyclic antidepressants (for example, *amitriptyline,* see p. 145), or serotonin/norepinephrine reuptake inhibitors (for example, *duloxetine,* see p. 144) rather than NSAIDs or opioids. However, for severe or chronic malignant pain, opioids are usually the drugs of choice. Opioids are natural or synthetic compounds that produce *morphine*-like effects. [Note: The term "opiate" is reserved for drugs, such as *morphine* and *codeine,* obtained from the juice of the opium poppy.] All drugs in this category act by binding to specific opioid receptors in the CNS to produce effects that mimic the action of endogenous peptide neurotransmitters (for example, endorphins, enkephalins, and dynorphins). Although the opioids have a broad range of effects, their primary use is to relieve intense pain and the anxiety that accompanies it, whether that pain is from surgery or a result of injury or disease, such as cancer. However, their widespread availability has led to abuse of those opioids with euphoric properties. [Note: Dependence is seldom a problem in patients being treated for severe pain with these agents, as in cancer or acute pain in terminally ill patients.] Antagonists that can reverse the actions of opioids are also very important clinically for use in cases of overdose. Figure 14.1 lists the opioid agonists and antagonists discussed in this chapter.

II. OPIOID RECEPTORS

Opioids interact stereospecifically with protein receptors on the membranes of certain cells in the CNS, on nerve terminals in the periphery, and on cells of the gastrointestinal tract and other anatomic regions. The major effects of the opioids are mediated by three major receptor families. These are designated by the Greek letters μ (mu), κ (kappa), and δ (delta). Each receptor family exhibits a different specificity for the drug(s) it binds. The analgesic properties of the opioids are primarily mediated by the μ receptors; however, the κ receptors in the dorsal horn also contribute. For example, *butorphanol* and *nalbuphine* primarily owe their analgesic effect

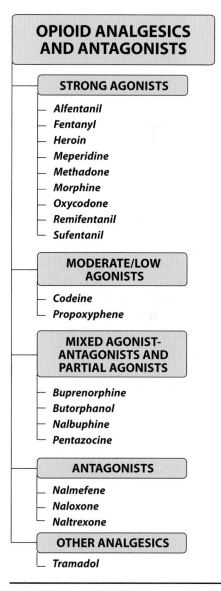

OPIOID ANALGESICS AND ANTAGONISTS

STRONG AGONISTS
- *Alfentanil*
- *Fentanyl*
- *Heroin*
- *Meperidine*
- *Methadone*
- *Morphine*
- *Oxycodone*
- *Remifentanil*
- *Sufentanil*

MODERATE/LOW AGONISTS
- *Codeine*
- *Propoxyphene*

MIXED AGONIST-ANTAGONISTS AND PARTIAL AGONISTS
- *Buprenorphine*
- *Butorphanol*
- *Nalbuphine*
- *Pentazocine*

ANTAGONISTS
- *Nalmefene*
- *Naloxone*
- *Naltrexone*

OTHER ANALGESICS
- *Tramadol*

Figure 14.1
Summary of opioid analgesics and antagonists.

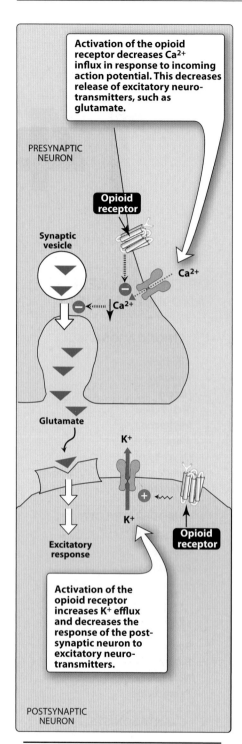

Activation of the opioid receptor decreases Ca²⁺ influx in response to incoming action potential. This decreases release of excitatory neurotransmitters, such as glutamate.

PRESYNAPTIC NEURON

Opioid receptor

Synaptic vesicle

Ca²⁺

Ca²⁺

Glutamate

K⁺

K⁺

Excitatory response

Opioid receptor

Activation of the opioid receptor increases K⁺ efflux and decreases the response of the postsynaptic neuron to excitatory neurotransmitters.

POSTSYNAPTIC NEURON

Figure 14.2
Mechanism of action of μ-opioid receptor agonists in the spinal cord.

to κ-receptor activation. The enkephalins interact more selectively with the δ receptors in the periphery. All three opioid receptors are members of the G protein–coupled receptor family and inhibit adenylyl cyclase.[1] They are also associated with ion channels, increasing postsynaptic K⁺ efflux (hyperpolarization) or reducing presynaptic Ca²⁺ influx, thus impeding neuronal firing and transmitter release (Figure 14.2).

A. Distribution of receptors

High densities of opioid receptors known to be involved in integrating information about pain are present in five general areas of the CNS. They have also been identified on the peripheral sensory nerve fibers and their terminals and on immune cells. [Note: There is considerable overlap of receptor types in these various areas.]

1. **Brainstem:** Opioid receptors influence respiration, cough, nausea and vomiting, blood pressure, pupillary diameter, and control of stomach secretions.

2. **Medial thalamus:** This area mediates deep pain that is poorly localized and emotionally influenced.

3. **Spinal cord:** Receptors in the substantia gelatinosa are involved with the receipt and integration of incoming sensory information, leading to the attenuation of painful afferent stimuli.

4. **Hypothalamus:** Receptors here affect neuroendocrine secretion.

5. **Limbic system:** The greatest concentration of opiate receptors in the limbic system is located in the amygdala. These receptors probably do not exert analgesic action, but they may influence emotional behavior.

6. **Periphery:** Opioids also bind to peripheral sensory nerve fibers and their terminals. As in the CNS, they inhibit Ca²⁺-dependent release of excitatory, proinflammatory substances (for example, substance P) from these nerve endings.

7. **Immune cells:** Opioid-binding sites have also been found on immune cells. The role of these receptors in nociception (response or sensitivity to painful stimuli) has not been determined.

III. STRONG AGONISTS

Morphine [MOR-feen] is the major analgesic drug contained in crude opium and is the prototype strong agonist. *Codeine* is present in crude opium in lower concentrations and is inherently less potent. These drugs show a high affinity for μ receptors and varying affinities for δ and κ receptors.

A. Morphine

1. **Mechanism of action:** Opioids exert their major effects by interacting with opioid receptors in the CNS and in other anatomic structures, such as the gastrointestinal tract and the urinary bladder. Opioids cause hyperpolarization of nerve cells, inhibition of nerve

[1]See p. 94 in *Lippincott's Illustrated Reviews: Biochemistry* (4th ed.) for a discussion of adenylyl cyclase.

firing, and presynaptic inhibition of transmitter release. *Morphine* acts at κ receptors in Lamina I and II of the dorsal horn of the spinal cord, and it decreases the release of substance P, which modulates pain perception in the spinal cord. *Morphine* also appears to inhibit the release of many excitatory transmitters from nerve terminals carrying nociceptive (painful) stimuli.

2. **Actions:**

   a. **Analgesia:** *Morphine* causes analgesia (relief of pain without the loss of consciousness). Opioids relieve pain both by raising the pain threshold at the spinal cord level and, more importantly, by altering the brain's perception of pain. Patients treated with *morphine* are still aware of the presence of pain, but the sensation is not unpleasant. However, when given to an individual free of pain, its effects may be unpleasant and may cause nausea and vomiting. The maximum analgesic efficacy and the addiction potential for representative agonists are shown in Figure 14.3.

   b. **Euphoria:** *Morphine* produces a powerful sense of contentment and well-being. Euphoria may be caused by disinhibition of the ventral tegmentum.

   c. **Respiration:** *Morphine* causes respiratory depression by reduction of the sensitivity of respiratory center neurons to carbon dioxide. This occurs with ordinary doses of *morphine* and is accentuated as the dose increases until, ultimately, respiration ceases. Respiratory depression is the most common cause of death in acute opioid overdose.

   d. **Depression of cough reflex:** Both *morphine* and *codeine* have antitussive properties. In general, cough suppression does not correlate closely with analgesic and respiratory depressant properties of opioid drugs. The receptors involved in the antitussive action appear to be different from those involved in analgesia.

   e. **Miosis:** The pinpoint pupil, characteristic of *morphine* use, results from stimulation of μ and κ receptors. *Morphine* excites the Edinger-Westphal nucleus of the oculomotor nerve, which causes enhanced parasympathetic stimulation to the eye (Figure 14.4). There is little tolerance to the effect, and all *morphine* abusers demonstrate pinpoint pupils. [Note: This is important diagnostically, because many other causes of coma and respiratory depression produce dilation of the pupil.]

   f. **Emesis:** *Morphine* directly stimulates the chemoreceptor trigger zone in the area postrema that causes vomiting.

   g. **Gastrointestinal tract:** *Morphine* relieves diarrhea and dysentery by decreasing the motility and increasing the tone of the intestinal circular smooth muscle. *Morphine* also increases the tone of the anal sphincter. Overall, *morphine* produces constipation, with little tolerance developing. It can also increase biliary tract pressure due to contraction of the gallbladder and constriction of the biliary sphincter.

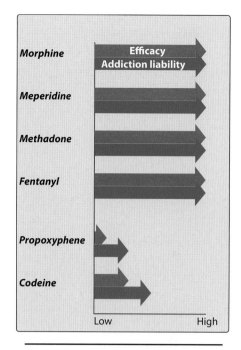

Figure 14.3
A comparison of the maximum efficacy and addiction/abuse liability of commonly used narcotic analgesics.

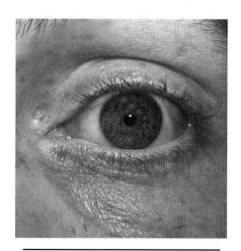

Figure 14.4
Morphine causes enhanced parasympathetic stimulation to the eye, resulting in pinpoint pupils.

h. Cardiovascular: *Morphine* has no major effects on the blood pressure or heart rate except at large doses, when hypotension and bradycardia may occur. Because of respiratory depression and carbon dioxide retention, cerebral vessels dilate and increase the cerebrospinal fluid (CSF) pressure. Therefore, *morphine* is usually contraindicated in individuals with severe brain injury.

i. Histamine release: *Morphine* releases histamine from mast cells, causing urticaria, sweating, and vasodilation. Because it can cause bronchoconstriction, asthmatics should not receive the drug.

j. Hormonal actions: *Morphine* inhibits release of gonadotropin-releasing hormone and corticotropin-releasing hormone, and it decreases the concentration of luteinizing hormone, follicle-stimulating hormone, adrenocorticotropic hormone, and β-endorphin. Testosterone and cortisol levels decrease. *Morphine* increases growth hormone release and enhances prolactin secretion. It increases antidiuretic hormone and, thus, leads to urinary retention. [Note: It also can inhibit the urinary bladder voiding reflex; thus, catheterization may be required.]

k. Labor: *Morphine* may prolong the second stage of labor by transiently decreasing the strength, duration, and frequency of uterine contractions.

3. Therapeutic uses:

a. Analgesia: Despite intensive research, few other drugs have been developed that are as effective as *morphine* in the relief of pain. Opioids induce sleep, and in clinical situations when pain is present and sleep is necessary, opiates may be used to supplement the sleep-inducing properties of benzodiazepines, such as *temazepam*. [Note: The sedative-hypnotic drugs are not usually analgesic, and they may have diminished sedative effect in the presence of pain.]

b. Treatment of diarrhea: *Morphine* decreases the motility and increases the tone of intestinal circular smooth muscle. [Note: This can cause constipation.]

c. Relief of cough: *Morphine* suppresses the cough reflex; however, *codeine* or *dextromethorphan* are more widely used for this purpose. *Codeine* has greater antitussive action than *morphine*.

d. Treatment of acute pulmonary edema: Intravenous (IV) *morphine* dramatically relieves dyspnea caused by pulmonary edema associated with left ventricular failure—possibly by its vasodilatory effect.

4. Pharmacokinetics:

a. Administration: Absorption of *morphine* from the gastrointestinal tract is slow and erratic. *Codeine*, by contrast, is well absorbed when given by mouth. Significant first-pass metabolism of *morphine* occurs in the liver; therefore, intramuscular, subcutaneous, or IV injections produce the most reliable responses. When used orally, *morphine* is commonly administered in an extended-release form to provide more consistent plasma levels. [Note: In cases of chronic pain associated with neoplastic disease, it has become common practice to use either the extended-release tablets orally or pumps that allow the patient to control the pain through self-administration, as show in Figure 14.5.] Opiates have been taken for nonmedical purposes by inhaling powders or smoke from burning crude opium, which provide a rapid onset of drug action.

b. **Distribution:** *Morphine* rapidly enters all body tissues, including the fetuses of pregnant women, and should not be used for analgesia during labor. Infants born of addicted mothers show physical dependence on opiates and exhibit withdrawal symptoms if opioids are not administered. Only a small percentage of *morphine* crosses the blood-brain barrier, because *morphine* is the least lipophilic of the common opioids. This contrasts with the more fat-soluble opioids, such as *fentanyl*, *methadone*, and *heroin*, which readily penetrate into the brain.

c. **Fate:** *Morphine* is conjugated in the liver to glucuronic acid. Morphine-6-glucuronide is a very potent analgesic, whereas the conjugate at position 3 is much less active. The conjugates are excreted primarily in the urine, with small quantities appearing in the bile. The duration of action of *morphine* is 4 to 6 hours when administered systemically to morphine-naïve individuals but considerably longer when injected epidurally, because its low lipophilicity prevents redistribution from the epidural space. [Note: A patient's age can influence the response to *morphine*. Elderly patients are more sensitive to the analgesic effects of the drug, possibly due to decreased metabolism or other factors, such as decreased lean body mass, renal function, etc. They should be treated with lower doses. Neonates should not receive *morphine* because of their low conjugating capacity.]

5. **Adverse effects:** Severe respiratory depression occurs and can result in death from acute opioid poisoning. A serious effect of the drug is stoppage of respiratory exchange in patients with emphysema or cor pulmonale. [Note: If employed in such individuals, respiration must be carefully monitored.] Other effects include vomiting, dysphoria, and allergy-enhanced hypotensive effects (Figure 14.6). The elevation of intracranial pressure, particularly in head injury, can be serious. *Morphine* enhances cerebral and spinal ischemia. In benign prostatic hyperplasia, *morphine* may cause acute urinary retention. Patients with adrenal insufficiency or myxedema may experience extended and increased effects from the opioids. *Morphine* should be used with cautiously in patients with bronchial asthma or liver failure.

6. **Tolerance and physical dependence:** Repeated use produces tolerance to the respiratory depressant, analgesic, euphoric, and sedative effects of *morphine*. However, tolerance usually does not develop to the pupil-constricting and constipating effects of the drug. Physical and psychological dependence readily occur with *morphine* and with some of the other agonists to be described (see Figure 14.3). Withdrawal produces a series of autonomic, motor, and psychological responses that incapacitate the individual and cause serious—almost unbearable—symptoms. However, it is very rare that the

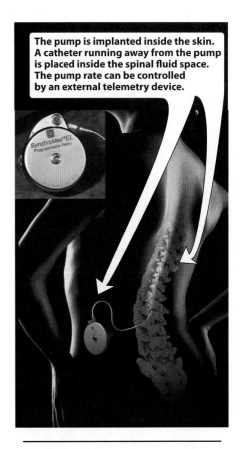

The pump is implanted inside the skin. A catheter running away from the pump is placed inside the spinal fluid space. The pump rate can be controlled by an external telemetry device.

SynchroMed®EL Programmable Pump

Figure 14.5
Implanted pump for delivery of morphine.

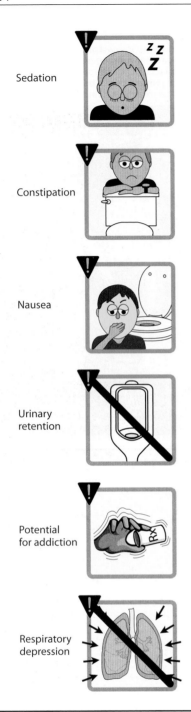

Sedation

Constipation

Nausea

Urinary retention

Potential for addiction

Respiratory depression

Figure 14.6
Adverse effects commonly observed in individuals treated with opioids.

effects are so profound as to cause death. [Note: Detoxification of *heroin-* or *morphine-*dependent individuals is usually accomplished through the oral administration of *methadone, buprenorphine* (see below), or *clonidine.*]

7. **Drug interactions:** The depressant actions of *morphine* are enhanced by phenothiazines, monoamine oxidase inhibitors, and tricyclic antidepressants (Figure 14.7). Low doses of *amphetamine* inexplicably enhance analgesia, as does *hydroxyzine.*

B. Meperidine

Meperidine [me-PER-i-deen] is a synthetic opioid structurally unrelated to *morphine.* It is used for acute pain.

1. **Mechanism of action:** *Meperidine* binds to opioid receptors, particularly μ receptors. However, it also binds well to κ receptors.

2. **Actions:** *Meperidine* causes a depression of respiration similar to that of *morphine,* but it has no significant cardiovascular action when given orally. On IV administration, *meperidine* produces a decrease in peripheral resistance and an increase in peripheral blood flow, and it may cause an increase in cardiac rate. As with *morphine, meperidine* dilates cerebral vessels, increases CSF pressure, and contracts smooth muscle (the latter to a lesser extent than does *morphine*). *Meperidine* does not cause pinpoint pupils but, rather, causes the pupils to dilate because of an *atropine*-like action.

3. **Therapeutic uses:** *Meperidine* provides analgesia for any type of severe pain. Unlike *morphine, meperidine* is not clinically useful in the treatment of diarrhea or cough. *Meperidine* produces less of an increase in urinary retention than does *morphine.* It has significantly less effects on uterine smooth muscle than morphine and is the opioid commonly employed in obstetrics (see below).

4. **Pharmacokinetics:** *Meperidine* is well absorbed from the gastrointestinal tract, and is useful when an orally administered, potent analgesic is needed. However, *meperidine* is most often administered parenterally. The drug has a duration of action of 2 to 4 hours, which is shorter than that of *morphine* (Figure 14.8). *Meperidine* is N-demethylated to normeperidine in the liver and is excreted in the urine. [Note: Because of its shorter action and different route of metabolism, *meperidine* is preferred over *morphine* for analgesia during labor.]

5. **Adverse effects:** Large or repetitive doses of *meperidine* can cause anxiety, tremors, muscle twitches, and rarely, convulsions due to the accumulation of a toxic metabolite, normeperidine. The drug differs from opioids in that when given in large doses, it dilates the pupil and causes hyperactive reflexes. Severe hypotension can occur when the drug is administered postoperatively. Due to its antimuscarinic action, patients may experience dry mouth and blurred vision. When used with major neuroleptics, depression is greatly enhanced. Administration to patients taking monoamine oxidase inhibitors can provoke severe reactions, such as convulsions and hyperthermia. *Meperidine* can cause dependence, and can substitute for *morphine* or *heroin* in opiate-dependent persons. Partial cross-tolerance with the other opioids occurs.

C. Methadone

Methadone [METH-a-done] is a synthetic, orally effective opioid that is approximately equal in potency to *morphine* but induces less euphoria and has a somewhat longer duration of action.

1. **Mechanism of action:** The actions of *methadone* are mediated by the μ receptors.

2. **Actions:** The analgesic activity of *methadone* is equivalent to that of *morphine* (see Figure 14.3). *Methadone* is well-absorbed when administered orally, in contrast to *morphine*, which is only partially absorbed from the gastrointestinal tract. The miotic and respiratory-depressant actions of *methadone* have average half-lives of 24 hours. Like *morphine*, *methadone* increases biliary pressure and is also constipating.

3. **Therapeutic uses:** *Methadone* is used as an analgesic as well as in the controlled withdrawal of dependent abusers from *heroin* and *morphine*. Orally administered, *methadone* is substituted for the injected opioid. The patient is then slowly weaned from *methadone*. *Methadone* causes a withdrawal syndrome that is milder but more protracted (days to weeks) than that of other opioids.

4. **Pharmacokinetics:** *Methadone* is readily absorbed following oral administration. It accumulates in tissues, where it remains bound to protein, from which it is slowly released. The drug is biotransformed in the liver and is excreted in the urine, mainly as inactive metabolites.

5. **Adverse effects:** *Methadone* can produce physical dependence like that of *morphine*.

D. Fentanyl

Fentanyl [FEN-ta-nil], which is chemically related to *meperidine*, has 100-fold the analgesic potency of *morphine* and is used in anesthesia. The drug is highly lipophilic and has a rapid onset and short duration of action (15 to 30 minutes). It is usually injected IV, epidurally, or intrathecally. Epidural *fentanyl* is used for analgesia postoperatively and during labor. An oral transmucosal preparation and a transdermal patch are also available. The transmucosal preparation is used in the treatment of cancer patients with breakthrough pain who are tolerant to opioids. The transdermal patch must be used with caution, because death resulting from hypoventilation has been known to occur. [Note: The transdermal patch creates a reservoir of the drug in the skin. Hence, the onset is delayed 12 hours, and the offset is prolonged.] *Fentanyl* is often used during cardiac surgery because of its negligible effects on myocardial contractility. Muscular rigidity, primarily of the abdomen and chest wall, is often observed with *fentanyl* use in anesthesia. *Fentanyl* is metabolized to inactive metabolites by the cytochrome P4503A4 system, and drugs that inhibit this isozyme can potentiate the effect of *fentanyl*. Most of the drug and metabolites are eliminated through the urine. Adverse effects of *fentanyl* are similar to those of other μ-receptor agonists. Because of life-threatening hypoventilation, the *fentanyl* patch is contraindicated in the management of acute and postoperative pain or pain that can be ameliorated with other analgesics. Unlike *meperidine*, it causes pupillary constriction.

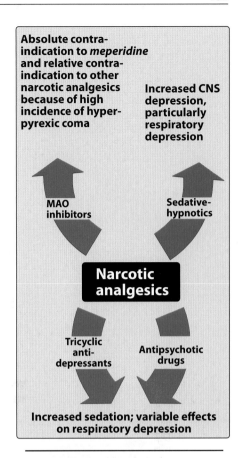

Figure 14.7
Drugs interacting with narcotic analgesics. CNS = central nervous system; MAO = monoamine oxidase.

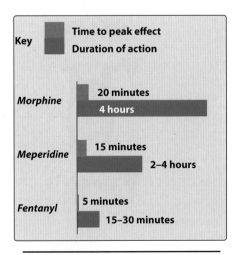

Figure 14.8
Time to peak effect and duration of action of several opioids administered intravenously.

E. Sufentanil, alfentanil, and remifentanil

Three drugs related to *fentanyl*—*sufentanil* [soo-FEN-ta-nil], *alfentanil* [al-FEN-ta-nil], and *remifentanil* [rem-i FEN-ta-nil]—differ in their potency and metabolic disposition. *Sufentanil* is even more potent than *fentanyl*, whereas the other two are less potent but much shorter-acting.

F. Heroin

Heroin [HAIR-o-in] does not occur naturally. It is produced by diacetylation of *morphine*, which leads to a three-fold increase in its potency. Its greater lipid solubility allows it to cross the blood-brain barrier more rapidly than *morphine*, causing a more exaggerated euphoria when the drug is taken by injection. *Heroin* is converted to *morphine* in the body, but its effects last about half as long. It has no accepted medical use in the United States.

G. Oxycodone

Oxycodone [ok-see-KOE-done] is a semisynthetic derivative of *morphine*. It is orally active and is sometimes formulated with *aspirin* or *acetaminophen*. It is used to treat moderate to severe pain and has many properties in common with *morphine*. *Oxycodone* is metabolized to products with lower analgesic activity. Excretion is via the kidney. Abuse of the sustained-release preparation (ingestion of crushed tablets) has been implicated in many deaths. It is important that the higher-dosage forms of the latter preparation be used only by patients who are tolerant to opioids.

IV. MODERATE AGONISTS

A. Codeine

The analgesic actions of *codeine* [KOE-deen] are due to its conversion to morphine, whereas the drug's antitussive effects are due to *codeine* itself. Thus, *codeine* is a much less potent analgesic than *morphine*, but it has a higher oral effectiveness. *Codeine* shows good antitussive activity at doses that do not cause analgesia. At commonly used doses, the drug has a lower potential for abuse than *morphine*, and it rarely produces dependence. *Codeine* produces less euphoria than *morphine*. *Codeine* is often used in combination with *aspirin* or *acetaminophen*. [Note: In most nonprescription cough preparations, *codeine* has been replaced by drugs such as *dextromethorphan*—a synthetic cough depressant that has relatively no analgesic action and a relatively low potential for abuse in usual antitussive doses.] Figure 14.9 shows some of the actions of *codeine*.

B. Propoxyphene

Propoxyphene [proe-POX-i-feen] is a derivative of *methadone*. The dextro isomer is used as an analgesic to relieve mild to moderate pain. The levo isomer is not analgesic, but it has antitussive action. *Propoxyphene* is a weaker analgesic than *codeine*, requiring approximately twice the dose to achieve an effect equivalent to that of *codeine*. *Propoxyphene* is often used in combination with *acetaminophen* for an analgesia greater than that obtained with either drug alone. It is well absorbed orally, with peak plasma levels occurring in 1 hour, and it is metabolized in the liver. *Propoxyphene* can produce nausea, anorexia, and constipation. In toxic doses, it can cause respiratory depression, convulsions, hallucinations, and confusion. When toxic doses are taken, a very serious prob-

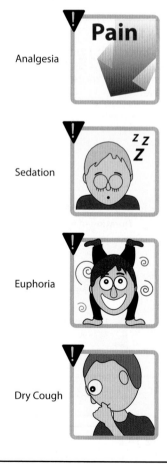

Figure 14.9
Some actions of *codeine*.

lem can arise in some individuals, with resultant cardiotoxicity and pulmonary edema. [Note: When used with alcohol and sedatives, severe CNS depression is produced, and death by respiratory depression and cardiotoxicity can result. Respiratory depression and sedation can be antagonized by *naloxone*, but the cardiotoxicity cannot.]

V. MIXED AGONIST-ANTAGONISTS AND PARTIAL AGONISTS

Drugs that stimulate one receptor but block another are termed mixed agonist-antagonists. The effects of these drugs depend on previous exposure to opioids. In individuals who have not recently received opioids (naïve patients), mixed agonist-antagonists show agonist activity and are used to relieve pain. In the patient with opioid dependence, the agonist-antagonist drugs may show primarily blocking effects—that is, produce withdrawal symptoms.

A. Pentazocine

Pentazocine [pen-TAZ-oh-seen] acts as an agonist on κ receptors and is a weak antagonist at μ and δ receptors. *Pentazocine* promotes analgesia by activating receptors in the spinal cord, and it is used to relieve moderate pain. It may be administered either orally or parenterally. *Pentazocine* produces less euphoria compared to *morphine*. In higher doses, the drug causes respiratory depression and decreases the activity of the gastrointestinal tract. High doses increase blood pressure and can cause hallucinations, nightmares, dysphoria, tachycardia, and dizziness. The latter properties have led to its decreased use. In angina, *pentazocine* increases the mean aortic pressure and pulmonary arterial pressure and, thus, increases the work of the heart. The drug decreases renal plasma flow. Despite its antagonist action, *pentazocine* does not antagonize the respiratory depression of *morphine*, but it can precipitate a withdrawal syndrome in a *morphine* abuser. Tolerance and dependence develop on repeated use.

B. Buprenorphine

Buprenorphine [byoo-pre-NOR-feen] is classified as a partial agonist, acting at the μ receptor. It acts like *morphine* in naïve patients, but it can also precipitate withdrawal in *morphine* users. A major use is in opiate detoxification, because it has a less severe and shorter duration of withdrawal symptoms compared to *methadone* (Figure 14.10). It causes little sedation, respiratory depression, and hypotension, even at high doses. In contrast to *methadone,* which is available only at specialized clinics, *buprenorphine* is approved for office-based detoxification or maintenance. *Buprenorphine* is administered sublingually or parenterally and has a long duration of action because of its tight binding to the μ receptor. The tablets are indicated for the treatment of opioid dependence. The injectable form is indicated for the relief of moderate to severe pain. It is metabolized by the liver and excreted in the bile and urine. Adverse effects include respiratory depression that cannot easily be reversed by *naloxone*, decreased (or, rarely, increased) blood pressure, nausea, and dizziness.

C. Nalbuphine and butorphanol

Nalbuphine [NAL byoo feen] and *butorphanol* [byoo-TOR-fa-nole], like *pentazocine*, play a limited role in the treatment of chronic pain. Neither is available for oral use. Their propensity to cause psychotomi-

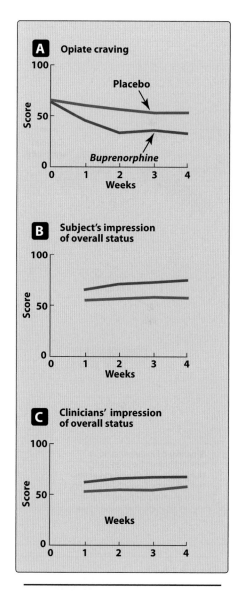

Figure 14.10
Scores for opiate craving and overall status in opioid-addicted patients assigned to office-based treatment with *buprenorphine* or placebo.

metic (actions mimics the symptoms of psychosis) effects is less than that of *pentazocine*. *Nalbuphine* does not affect the heart or increase blood pressure, in contrast to *pentazocine* and *butorphanol*. A benefit of all three medications is that they exhibit a ceiling effect for respiratory depression.

VI. OTHER ANALGESICS

A. Tramadol

Tramadol (TRA-ma-dole) is a centrally acting analgesic that binds to the µ-opioid receptor. In addition, it weakly inhibits reuptake of norepinephrine and serotonin. It is used to manage moderate to moderately severe pain. Its respiratory-depressant activity is less than that of *morphine*. *Naloxone* (see below) can only partially reverse the analgesia produced by *tramadol* or its active metabolite. The drug undergoes extensive metabolism, and one metabolite is active. Concurrent use with *carbamazepine* results in increased metabolism, presumably by induction of the cytochrome P450 2D6 system. [Note: *Quinidine*, which inhibits this isozyme, increases levels of *tramadol* when taken concurrently.] Anaphylactoid reactions have been reported. Of concern are the seizures that can occur, especially in patients taking selective serotonin reuptake inhibitors, tricyclic antidepressants, or in overdose. *Tramadol* should also be avoided in patients taking monoamine oxidase inhibitors.

VII. ANTAGONISTS

The opioid antagonists bind with high affinity to opioid receptors but fail to activate the receptor-mediated response. Administration of opioid antagonists produces no profound effects in normal individuals. However, in patients dependent on opioids, antagonists rapidly reverse the effect of agonists, such as *heroin*, and precipitate the symptoms of opiate withdrawal.

A. Naloxone

Naloxone [nal-OX-own] is used to reverse the coma and respiratory depression of opioid overdose. It rapidly displaces all receptor-bound opioid molecules and, therefore, is able to reverse the effect of a *heroin* overdose (Figure 14.11). Within 30 seconds of IV injection of *naloxone*, the respiratory depression and coma characteristic of high doses of *heroin* are reversed, causing the patient to be revived and alert. *Naloxone* has a half-life of 60 to 100 minutes. [Note: Because of its relatively short duration of action, a depressed patient who has been treated and recovered may lapse back into respiratory depression.] *Naloxone* is a competitive antagonist at µ, κ, and δ, receptors, with a 10-fold higher affinity for µ than for κ receptors. This may explain why *naloxone* readily reverses respiratory depression with only minimal reversal of the analgesia that results from agonist stimulation of κ receptors in the spinal cord. *Naloxone* produces no pharmacologic effects in normal individuals, but it precipitates withdrawal symptoms in opioid abusers. Figure 14.12 summarizes some of the signs and symptoms of opiate withdrawal.

B. Naltrexone

Naltrexone [nal-TREX-own] has actions similar to those of *naloxone*. It has a longer duration of action than *naloxone*, and a single oral dose of *naltrexone* blocks the effect of injected *heroin* for up to 48 hours. *Naltrexone* in combination with *clonidine*—and, sometimes, with *buprenorphine*—

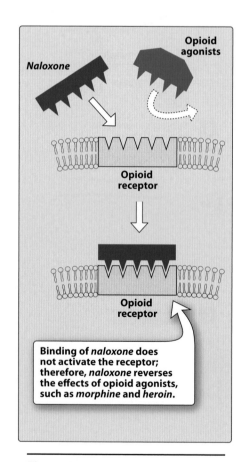

Figure 14.11
Competition of *naloxone* with opioid agonists.

Binding of *naloxone* does not activate the receptor; therefore, *naloxone* reverses the effects of opioid agonists, such as *morphine* and *heroin*.

is employed for rapid opioid detoxification. It may also be beneficial in treating chronic alcoholism by an unknown mechanism; however, benzodiazepines and *clonidine* are preferred. *Naltrexone* is hepatotoxic.

C. Nalmefene

Nalmefene [NAL-meh-freen] is a parenteral opioid antagonist with actions similar to that of *naloxone* and *naltrexone*. It can be administered IV, intramuscularly, or subcutaneously. Its half-life of 8 to 10 hours is significantly longer than that of *naloxone* and several opioid agonists.

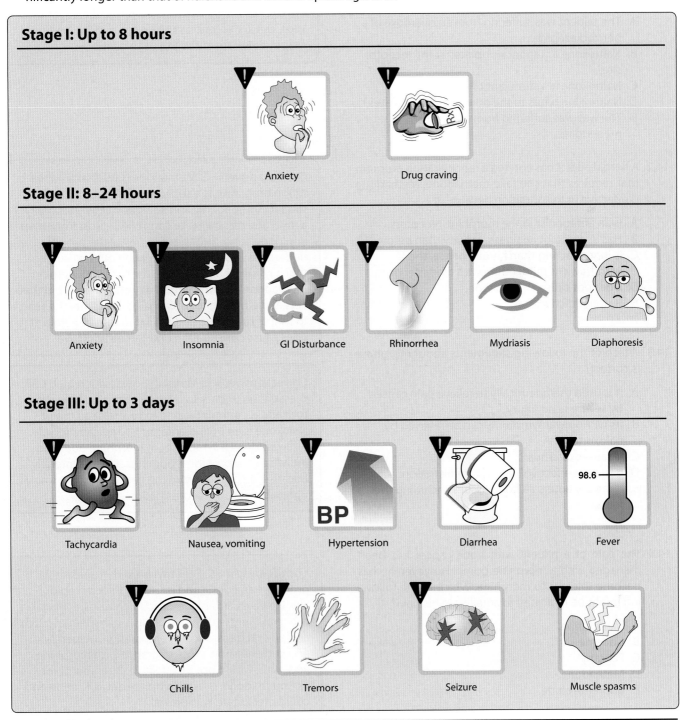

Figure 14.12
Opiate withdrawal syndrome.

Study Questions

Choose the ONE best answer.

14.1 A young man is brought into the emergency room. He is unconscious, and he has pupillary constriction and depressed respiration. You note needle marks on his legs. You administer naltrexone, and he awakens. This agent was effective because:

    A. The patient was suffering from an overdose of a benzodiazepine.
    B. Naltrexone antagonizes opiates at the receptor site.
    C. Naltrexone is a stimulant of the CNS.
    D. Naltrexone binds to the opioid and inactivates it.
    E. The was was suffering from an overdose of meperidine.

> Correct answer = B. The indications are that the patient is suffering from an overdose of an opioid, such as heroin. Naltrexone antagonizes the opioid by displacing it from the receptor. It is used in preference to naloxone, because it is longer acting and, thus, can act as long as the opiate is in the body. Meperidine causes the pupils to dilate.

14.2 A heroin addict has entered a rehabilitation program that requires that she take methadone. Methadone is effective in this situation because it:

    A. Is an antagonist at the morphine receptors.
    B. Has less potent analgesic activity than heroin.
    C. Is longer acting than heroin; hence, the withdrawal is milder than with the latter drug.
    D. Does not cause constipation.
    E. Is nonaddictive.

> Correct answer = C. Methadone is used in rehabilitation programs as a substitute for heroin. It has similar euphorigenic and analgesic activity, is orally active, and can be easily controlled. Most important, it is long acting, and the withdrawal the patient undergoes as she is being weaned off the drug is much milder than would be the case with heroin. Methadone is a synthetic, orally effective opioid that acts at the μ receptors. Its analgesic activity is equal to that of morphine and similar to that of heroin. It does cause constipation and can be addictive.

14.3 Which of the following statements about morphine is correct?

    A. It is used therapeutically to relieve pain caused by severe head injury.
    B. Its withdrawal symptoms can be relieved by naloxone.
    C. It causes diarrhea.
    D. It is most effective by oral administration.
    E. It rapidly enters all body tissues, including the fetus.

> Correct answer = E. Morphine causes increased CSF pressure secondary to dilation of cerebral vasculature and is contraindicated in severe head injury. Naloxone is an opioid antagonist and can precipitate withdrawal symptoms in morphine-addicted individuals. Morphine is administered parenterally, because absorption from the gastrointestinal tract is unreliable. It causes constipation.

14.4 The pain of a patient with bone cancer has been managed with a morphine pump. However, he has become tolerant to morphine. Which of the following might be indicated to ameliorate his pain?

    A. Meperidine.
    B. Codeine.
    C. Fentanyl.
    D. Methadone.
    E. Buprenorphine.

> Correct answer= C. Fentanyl is used in anesthesia. It produces analgesia and is usually injected epidurally. However, its analgesic action is also beneficial in cancer patients. It is available as a transdermal patch and an oral transmucosal preparation. Meperidine and codeine show cross-tolerance with morphine and, thus, would not be effective. Buprenorphine, like methadone, is used in opiate detoxification and could precipitate withdrawal.

Epilepsy

15

I. OVERVIEW

Epilepsy affects approximately 3 percent of individuals by the time they are 80 years old. About 10 percent of the population will have at least one seizure in their lifetime. Globally epilepsy is the third most common neurologic disorder after cerebrovascular and Alzheimer's disease. Epilepsy is not a single entity but, instead, an assortment of different seizure types and syndromes originating from several mechanisms that have in common the sudden, excessive, and synchronous discharge of cerebral neurons. This abnormal electrical activity may result in a variety of events, including loss of consciousness, abnormal movements, atypical or odd behavior, or distorted perceptions that are of limited duration but recur if untreated. The site of origin of the abnormal neuronal firing determines the symptoms that are produced. For example, if the motor cortex is involved, the patient may experience abnormal movements or a generalized convulsion. Seizures originating in the parietal or occipital lobe may include visual, auditory, or olfactory hallucinations. Drug or vagal nerve stimulator therapy is the most widely effective mode for the treatment of patients with epilepsy. It is expected that seizures can be controlled completely in approximately 70 to 80 percent of patients with one medication. It is estimated that approximately 10 to 15 percent of patients will require more than one drug and perhaps 10 percent may not achieve complete seizure control. A summary of antiseizure drugs is shown in Figure 15.1.

II. IDIOPATHIC AND SYMPTOMATIC SEIZURES

In most cases, epilepsy has no identifiable cause. Focal areas that are functionally abnormal may be triggered into activity by changes in any of a variety of environmental factors, including alteration in blood gases, pH, electrolytes, blood glucose level, sleep deprivation, alcohol intake, and stress. The neuronal discharge in epilepsy results from the firing of a small population of neurons in some specific area of the brain that is referred to as the primary focus. Anatomically, this focal area may appear to be normal. However, advances in technology have improved ability to detect abnormalities, and in some patients, neuroimaging techniques, such as magnetic resonance imaging (MRI), positron-emission tomography (PET) scans and single-photon-emission coherence tomography (SPECT) can identify areas of concern (Figure 15.2). Epilepsy can be labeled idiopathic or symptomatic depending if the etiology is unknown, or is secondary to an identifiable condition. There are also multiple specific epilepsy syndromes that have been classified and include symptoms other than seizures.

ANTIEPILEPTIC DRUGS

- Barbiturates
- Benzodiazepines
- *Carbamazepine*
- *Divalproex*
- *Ethosuximide*
- *Felbamate*
- *Gabapentin*
- *Lamotrigine*
- *Levetiracetam*
- *Oxcarbazepine*
- *Phenytoin*
- *Pregabalin*
- *Primidone*
- *Tiagabine*
- *Topiramate*
- *Zonisamide*

Figure 15.1
Summary of agents used in the treatment of epilepsy.

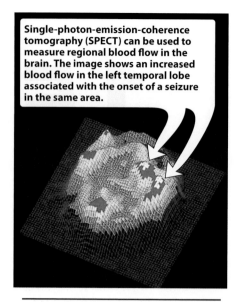

Single-photon-emission-coherence tomography (SPECT) can be used to measure regional blood flow in the brain. The image shows an increased blood flow in the left temporal lobe associated with the onset of a seizure in the same area.

Figure 15.2
Region of the brain in an epileptic individual showing increased blood flow during a seizure.

A. Idiopathic epilepsy

When no specific anatomic cause for the seizure, such as trauma or neoplasm, is evident, a patient may be diagnosed with idiopathic or cryptogenic (primary) epilepsy. These seizures may result from an inherited abnormality in the central nervous system (CNS). Patients are treated chronically with antiseizure drugs or vagal nerve stimulation. Most cases of epilepsy are idiopathic.

B. Symptomatic epilepsy

A number of causes, such as illicit drug use, tumors, head injury, hypoglycemia, meningeal infection, or rapid withdrawal of alcohol from an alcoholic, can precipitate seizures. When two or more seizures occur, then the patient may be diagnosed with symptomatic (secondary) epilepsy. Chronic treatment with antiseizure medications, vagal nerve stimulation and surgery are all appropriate treatments and may be used alone or in combination. In some cases when the cause of a single seizure can be determined and corrected, therapy may not be necessary. For example, a seizure that is caused by transient hypotension or is due to a drug reaction does not require chronic prophylactic therapy. In other situations, antiseizure drugs may be given until the primary cause of the seizures can be corrected.

III. CLASSIFICATION OF SEIZURES

It is important to correctly classify seizures to determine appropriate treatment. Seizures have been categorized by site of origin, etiology, electrophysiologic correlation, and clinical presentation. The International League Against Epilepsy developed a nomenclature for describing seizures, and it is considered to be the standard way to document seizures and epilepsy syndromes (Figure 15.3). Seizures have been classified into two broad groups: partial (or focal), and generalized. A diagnosis may classify the seizure as partial or primary generalized epilepsy depending on the onset.

A. Partial

Partial seizures involve only a portion of the brain, typically part of one lobe of one hemisphere. The symptoms of each seizure type depend on the site of neuronal discharge and on the extent to which the electrical activity spreads to other neurons in the brain. Consciousness is usually preserved. Partial seizures may progress, becoming generalized tonic-clonic seizures.

1. **Simple partial:** These seizures are caused by a group of hyperactive neurons exhibiting abnormal electrical activity, which are confined to a single locus in the brain. The electrical discharge does not spread, and the patient does not lose consciousness. The patient often exhibits abnormal activity of a single limb or muscle group that is controlled by the region of the brain experiencing the disturbance. The patient may also show sensory distortions. This activity may spread. Simple partial seizures may occur at any age.

2. **Complex partial:** These seizures exhibit complex sensory hallucinations, mental distortion, and loss of consciousness. Motor dysfunction may involve chewing movements, diarrhea, and/or urination. Consciousness is altered. Simple partial seizure activity may spread and become complex and then spread to a secondarily generalized convulsion. Partial seizures may occur at any age.

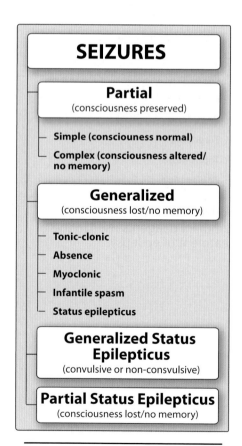

SEIZURES

Partial
(consciousness preserved)

- Simple (consciouness normal)
- Complex (consciousness altered/no memory)

Generalized
(consciousness lost/no memory)

- Tonic-clonic
- Absence
- Myoclonic
- Infantile spasm
- Status epilepticus

Generalized Status Epilepticus
(convulsive or non-consvulsive)

Partial Status Epilepticus
(consciousness lost/no memory)

Figure 15.3
Classification of epilepsy.

B. Generalized

Generalized seizures may begin locally, producing abnormal electrical discharges throughout both hemispheres of the brain. Primary generalized seizures may be convulsive or nonconvulsive, and the patient usually has an immediate loss of consciousness

1. **Tonic-clonic:** Seizures result in loss of consciousness, followed by tonic (continuous contraction) and clonic (rapid contraction and relaxation) phases. The seizure may be followed by a period of confusion and exhaustion due to the depletion of glucose and energy stores.

2. **Absence:** These seizures involve a brief, abrupt, and self-limiting loss of consciousness. The onset generally occurs in patients at 3 to 5 years of age and lasts until puberty or beyond. The patient stares and exhibits rapid eye-blinking, which lasts for 3 to 5 seconds. This seizure has a very distinct three-per-second spike and wave discharge seen on electroencephalogram.

3. **Myoclonic:** These seizures consist of short episodes of muscle contractions that may reoccur for several minutes. They generally occur after wakening and exhibit as brief jerks of the limbs. Myoclonic seizures occur at any age but usually begin around puberty or early adulthood.

4. **Febrile seizures:** Young children may develop seizures with illness accompanied by high fever. This may occur in siblings. The febrile seizures consist of generalized tonic-clonic convulsions of short duration and do not necessarily lead to a diagnosis of epilepsy.

5. **Status epilepticus:** In status epilepticus, two or more seizures recur without recovery of full consciousness between them. These may be partial or primary generalized, convulsive or nonconvulsive. Status epilepticus is life-threatening and requires emergency treatment.

C. Mechanism of action of antiepileptic drugs

Drugs that are effective in seizure reduction accomplish this by a variety of mechanisms, including blockade of voltage-gated channels (Na^+ or Ca^{2+}), enhancement of inhibitory GABAergic impulses, or interference with excitatory glutamate transmission. Some antiepileptic drugs appear to have multiple targets within the CNS, whereas the mechanism of action for some agents is poorly defined. The antiepilepsy drugs suppress seizures but do not "cure" or "prevent" epilepsy.

IV. DRUG CHOICE

Choice of drug treatment is based on the classification of the seizures being treated, patient specific variables (for example, age, comorbid medical conditions, lifestyle, and other preferences), and characteristics of the drug, including cost and interactions with other medications. For example, partial onset tonic-clonic seizures are treated differently than primary generalized seizures. Several drugs may be equally effective, and the toxicities of the agent and characteristics of the patient are major considerations in drug selection. In newly diagnosed patients, monotherapy is instituted with a single agent until seizures are controlled or toxicity occurs (Figure 15.4). Compared to those receiving combination therapy, patients receiving

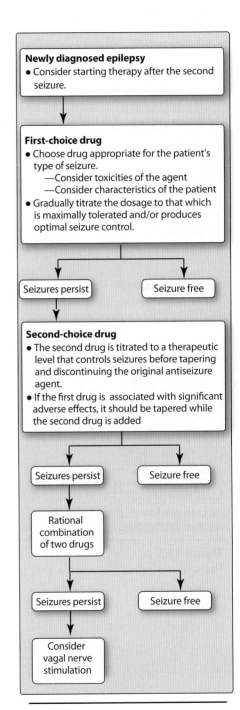

Figure 15.4
Therapeutic strategies for managing newly diagnosed epilepsy.

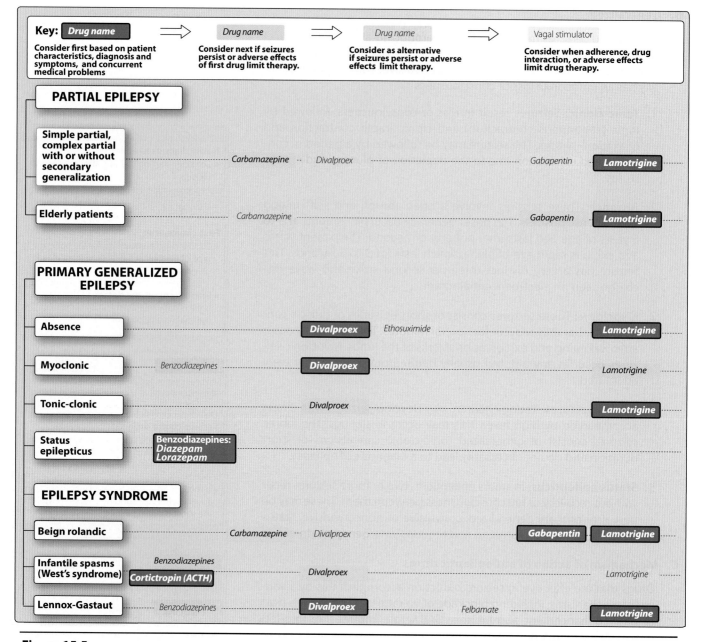

Key:

Drug name	⇒	Drug name	⇒	Drug name	⇒	Vagal stimulator
Consider first based on patient characteristics, diagnosis and symptoms, and concurrent medical problems		Consider next if seizures persist or adverse effects of first drug limit therapy.		Consider as alternative if seizures persist or adverse effects limit therapy.		Consider when adherence, drug interaction, or adverse effects limit drug therapy.

PARTIAL EPILEPSY

- **Simple partial, complex partial with or without secondary generalization** — Carbamazepine ·· Divalproex ········· Gabapentin — Lamotrigine
- **Elderly patients** ········· Carbamazepine ········· Gabapentin — Lamotrigine

PRIMARY GENERALIZED EPILEPSY

- **Absence** ········· Divalproex Ethosuximide ········· Lamotrigine
- **Myoclonic** ··· Benzodiazepines ··· Divalproex ········· Lamotrigine
- **Tonic-clonic** ········· Divalproex ········· Lamotrigine
- **Status epilepticus** — Benzodiazepines: Diazepam Lorazepam

EPILEPSY SYNDROME

- **Beign rolandic** ········· Carbamazepine ·· Divalproex ········· Gabapentin Lamotrigine
- **Infantile spasms (West's syndrome)** — Benzodiazepines Corticotropin (ACTH) ········· Divalproex ········· Lamotrigine
- **Lennox-Gastaut** ··· Benzodiazepines ··· Divalproex ········· Felbamate ········· Lamotrigine

Figure 15.5
Therapeutic indications for the anticonvulsant agents.

monotherapy exhibit better adherence and fewer side effects. If seizures are not controlled with the first drug, monotherapy with an alternate antiepileptic drug(s), or vagal nerve stimulation should be considered (see Figure 15.5). An awareness of the antiepileptic drugs available, including their mechanisms of action, pharmacokinetics, potential for drug-drug interactions, and adverse effects, is essential for successful therapy.

V. PRIMARY ANTIEPILEPTIC DRUGS

During the past 15 years, new antiepileptic drugs have been introduced, some of which have potential advantages in terms of pharmacokinetics, tolerability, and lesser risk for drug-drug interactions when compared with the

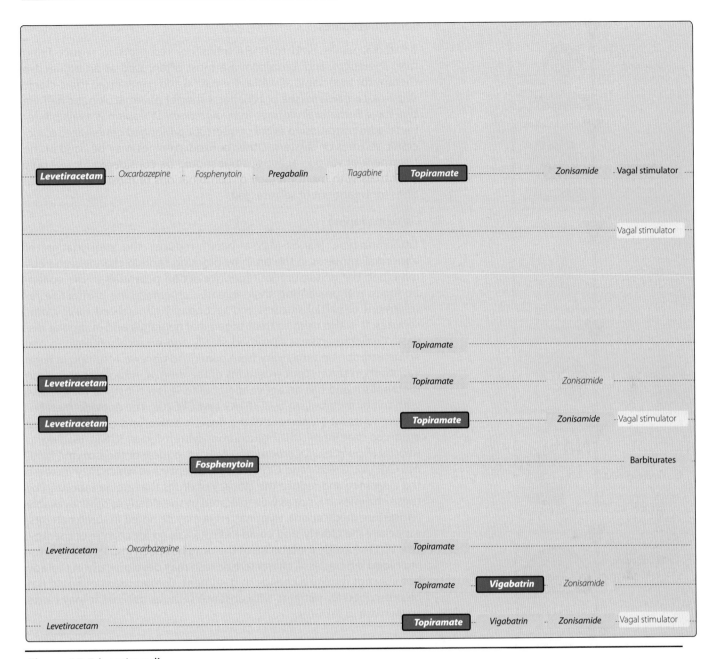

Figure 15.5 (continued)
Therapeutic indications for the anticonvulsant agents.

older agents used to treat epilepsy. These new drugs, which include *gabapentin, lamotrigine, topiramate, levetiracetam, oxcarbazepine, zonisamide*, are labeled "second generation" when compared with older antiepileptics, such as *phenobarbital, phenytoin, carbamazepine, ethosuximide, divalproex* and *valproic acid*. However, clinical studies have not shown that the second-generation drugs as a group are significantly better with respect to efficacy and in some cases, adverse effects than the older agents. For that reason, the authors have chosen to present the antiepileptic drugs in alphabetic order, rather than attempting to rank them by efficacy. Figure 15.6 shows the commonly encountered adverse effect of the antiepileptic drugs. In addition, an increased risk of suicidal behavior and suicidal ideation has been observed with many of the antiepileptic drugs.

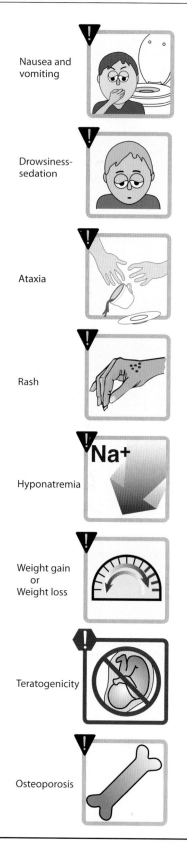

Nausea and vomiting

Drowsiness-sedation

Ataxia

Rash

Na⁺

Hyponatremia

Weight gain or Weight loss

Teratogenicity

Osteoporosis

Figure 15.6
Notable adverse effects of anti-seizure medications.

A. Benzodiazepines

Benzodiazepines bind to GABA inhibitory receptors to reduce firing rate. *Diazepam*, and *lorazepam* are most often used as an adjunctive therapy for myoclonic as well as for partial and generalized tonic-clonic seizures. *Lorazepam* (see p. 108) has a shorter pharmacokinetic half-life but stays in the brain longer than *diazepam*. *Diazepam* is available for rectal administration to avoid or interrupt prolonged generalized tonic-clonic seizures or clusters. Other benzodiazepines may be used in the treatment of various epilepsies but should be considered for use only after trials with monotherapy or combinations of most other medications for treatment of seizures fail.

B. Carbamazepine

Carbamazepine [kar-ba-MAZ-a peen] reduces the propagation of abnormal impulses in the brain by blocking sodium channels, thereby inhibiting the generation of repetitive action potentials in the epileptic focus and preventing their spread. *Carbamazepine* is effective for treatment of partial seizures and secondarily generalized tonic-clonic seizures. It is also used to treat trigeminal neuralgia and in bipolar disease. *Carbamazepine* is absorbed slowly and erratically following oral administration and may vary from generic to generic, resulting in large variations in serum concentrations of the drug. It induces its own drug metabolism and has an active metabolite. It is a substrate for CYP3A4 with minor metabolism by CYP1A2 and CYC2C8. The epoxide metabolite accounts for 25 percent of the dose, is active, and can be inhibited by drugs that inhibit UDP glucouronosyltransferase (UGT), leading to toxicity (Figure 15.7). *Carbamazepine* is an inducer of the isozyme families CYP1A2, CYP2C, and CYP3A and UGT enzymes which may increase the clearance and reduce the efficacy of drugs that are metabolized by these enzymes. It is not as well tolerated by the elderly as other available antiseizure medications. Hyponatremia may be noted in some patients, especially the elderly, and could indicate a need for change of therapy. The 10,11-epoxide metabolite of the drug has been implicated in causing blood dyscrasias. A characteristic rash may develop early in therapy but may not require a change in treatment. *Carbamazepine* should not be prescribed for patients with absence seizures because it may cause an increase in seizures.

C. Divalproex

Divalproex sodium is a combination of *sodium valproate* and *valproic acid* and is reduced to *valproate* when it reaches the gastrointestinal tract. It was developed to improve gastrointestinal tolerance of *valproic acid*. All of the available salt forms are equivalent in efficacy (*valproic acid* and *valproate sodium*). Commercial products are available in multiple-salt, dosage forms and extended-release formulations. Therefore the risk for medication errors is high, and it is essential to be familiar with all preparations. Proposed mechanisms of action include sodium channel blockade, blockade of GABA transaminase, and action at the T-type calcium channels. These many mechanisms provide a broad spectrum of activity against seizures. It is effective for the treatment of partial and primary generalized epilepsies. *Valproate* inhibits metabolism of the CYP2C9, UGT and epoxide hydrolase systems. *Valproate* is bound to albumin (greater than 90 percent), which can cause significant interactions with other highly protein bound drugs. Rare hepatic toxicity may cause a rise in hepatic enzymes in plasma, which should be monitored frequently. Teratogenicity is of great concern. Therefore all women of child-bearing age should be placed on other therapies and counseled about the potential for birth defects, including neural tube defects.

D. Ethosuximide

Ethosuximide [eth-oh-SUX-i-mide] reduces propagation of abnormal electrical activity in the brain, most likely by inhibiting T-type calcium channels. It is effective in treating only primary generalized absence seizures (see Figure 15.5). Use of *ethosuximide* is limited because of this very narrow spectrum.

E. Felbamate

Felbamate [FEL-ba-mate] has a broad spectrum of anticonvulsant action. The drug has multiple proposed mechanisms including 1) blocking voltage-dependent sodium channels, 2) competing with the glycine-coagonist binding site on the N-methyl-D-aspartate (NMDA) glutamate receptor, 3) blocking calcium channels, and 5) potentiation of GABA actions. It is an inhibitor of drugs metabolized by CYP2C19 and β-oxidation. It induces drugs metabolized by CYP3A4. It is reserved for use in refractory epilepsies (particularly Lennox-Gastaut syndrome) because of the risk of aplastic anemia (about 1:4000) and hepatic failure.

F. Gabapentin

Gabapentin [GA-ba-pen-tin] is an analog of GABA. However, it does not act at GABA receptors nor enhance GABA actions, nor is it converted to GABA. Its precise mechanism of action is not known. It is approved as adjunct therapy for partial seizures and for treatment of postherpetic neuralgia. *Gabapentin* exhibits nonlinear pharmacokinetics due to its uptake by a saturable transport system from the gut. *Gabapentin* does not bind to plasma proteins and is excreted unchanged through the kidneys. Reduced dosing is required in renal disease. *Gabapentin* has been shown to be well tolerated by the elderly population with partial seizures due to the relatively mild adverse effects and a good choice due to limited or no reported pharmacokinetic drug interactions.

G. Lamotrigine

Lamotrigine [la-MOE-tri-jeen] blocks sodium channels as well as high voltage–dependent calcium channels. *Lamotrigine* is effective in a wide variety of seizure disorders, including partial seizures, generalized seizures, typical absence seizures, and the Lennox-Gastaut syndrome. It is approved for use in bipolar disorder as well. *Lamotrigine* is metabolized primarily to the N-2 glucuronide through the UGT pathway. The half-life of *lamotrigine* (24–35 hours) is decreased by enzyme-inducing drugs (for example, *carbamazepine* and *phenytoin*) and increased by greater than 50 percent with addition of *valproate*. *Lamotrigine* dosages should be reduced when adding *valproate* to therapy unless the *valproate* is being added in a small dose to provide a boost to the *lamotrigine* serum concentration. Rapid titration to high serum concentrations of *lamotrigine* have been reported to cause a rash, which in some patients may progress to a serious, life-threatening reaction. *Lamotrigine* has also been shown to be well tolerated by the elderly population with partial seizures due to the relatively minor adverse effects when titrated slowly.

CYP1A2
> *Carbamazepine*

CYP2C8
> *Carbamazepine*

CYP2C9
> *Carbamazepine*
> *Divalproex*
> *Phenobarbital*
> *Phenytoin*

CYP2C19
> *Divalproex*
> *Felbamate*
> *Phenobarbital*
> *Phenytoin*
> *Zonisamide*

CYP3A4
> *Carbamazepine*
> *Ethosuximide*
> *Tiagabine*
> *Zonisamide*

UDP-glucuronsyltransferases
> *Divalproex*
> *Lamotrigine*
> *Lorazepam*

Figure 15.7
Metabolism of the antiepileptic drugs.

H. Levetiracetam

Levetiracetam [lee-ve-tye-RA-se-tam] is approved for adjunct therapy of partial onset seizures, myoclonic seizures, and primary generalized tonic-clonic seizures in adults and children. The exact mechanism of anticonvulsant action is unknown. It demonstrates high affinity for a synaptic vesicle protein (SV2A). In mice, this was associated with potent antiseizure action. The drug is well absorbed orally, and excretion is urinary, with most of the drug (66 percent) being unchanged. The drug does not interact with CYP or UGT metabolism systems. Side effects most often reported include dizziness, sleep disturbances, headache, and weakness.

I. Oxcarbazepine

Oxcarbazepine [ox-kar-BAY-zeh-peen] is a prodrug that is rapidly reduced to the 10-monohydroxy (MHD) metabolite which is responsible for its anticonvulsant activity. MHD blocks sodium channels preventing the spread of the abnormal discharge. Modulation of calcium channels is also a hypothesis. It is approved for use in adults and children with partial onset seizures. *Oxcarbazepine* is a less potent inducer of CYP3A4 and UGT than *carbamazepine*. The adverse effects profile is similar to that of other antiepileptic drugs with respect to nausea, vomiting, headache, and visual disturbance.

J. Phenobarbital

Phenobarbital [fee-noe-BAR-bih-tal] was synthesized in 1902 and brought to the market in 1912 by Bayer. The primary mechanism of action is the enhancement of inhibitory effects of GABA-mediated neurons (see p. 111). The primary use for *phenobarbital* in epilepsy is in treatment of status epilepticus. Due to interaction with the cytochrome P450 enzymes as an inducer, and adverse effects of sedation, cognitive impairment, and potential for osteoporosis, this drug should only be considered for chronic therapy once a patient is found to be refractory to many other drugs, and the benefits of therapy outweigh the multiple risks.

K. Phenytoin and fosphenytoin

Phenytoin [FEN-i-toin] blocks voltage-gated sodium channels by selectively binding to the channel in the inactive state and slowing its rate of recovery. At very high concentrations, *phenytoin* can block voltage-dependent calcium channels and interfere with the release of monoaminergic neurotransmitters. *Phenytoin* is effective for treatment of partial seizures and generalized tonic-clonic seizures and in the treatment of status epilepticus (see Figure 15.5). The drug is 90 percent bound to plasma albumin. *Phenytoin* is an inducer of drugs metabolized by the CYP2C, and CYP3A families and the UGT enzyme system. *Phenytoin* exhibits saturable enzyme metabolism at a low serum concentration; thus knowledge of zero- order pharmacokinetics and population parameters is important for dosing adjustment. Small increases in a daily dose can produce large increases in the plasma concentration, resulting in drug-induced toxicity (Figure 15.8). Depression of the CNS occurs particularly in the cerebellum and vestibular system, causing nystagmus and ataxia. The elderly are highly susceptible to this effect. Gingival hyperplasia may cause the gums to grow over the teeth. Long-term use may lead to development of peripheral neuropathies and osteoporosis.

Fosphenytoin [FOS-phen-i-toin] is a prodrug and is rapidly converted to *phenytoin* in the blood, providing high levels of *phenytoin* within minutes. *Fosphenytoin* may also be administered intramuscularly (IM). *Phenytoin sodium* should never be given IM because it can cause tissue damage and necrosis. *Fosphenytoin* is the drug of choice and standard of care for IV and IM administration. Due to sound-alike and look-alike names, there is a risk for medication error to occur. The trade name of *fosphenytoin* is Cerebyx®, which is easily confused with Celebrex®, the cyclooxygenase-2 inhibitor, and Celexa®, the antidepressant.

L. Pregabalin

Pregabalin [pree-GABA-lin] binds to the α_2-δ site, an auxiliary subunit of voltage-gated calcium channels in the CNS, inhibiting excitatory neurotransmitter release. The exact role this plays in treatment is not known, but the drug has proven effects on partial onset seizures, neuropathic pain associated with diabetic peripheral neuropathy, postherpetic neuralgia, and fibromyalgia. *Pregabalin* is greater than 90 percent eliminated renally, with no indication of CYP involvement. Drowsiness, blurred vision, weight gain, and peripheral edema have been reported.

M. Primidone

Primidone [PRIM-i-done] has two active metabolites, *phenobarbital* and phenylethylmalonamide, which have longer half-lives than the parent drug. Due to the nature of the long term adverse effects associated with *phenobarbital*, this drug should be considered for use only in those patients with refractory epilepsy.

N. Tiagabine

Tiagabine [ty-AG-a-been] blocks GABA uptake into presynaptic neurons, permitting more GABA to be available for receptor binding, thus, there is thought to be enhanced inhibitory activity. *Tiagabine* is effective in decreasing the number of seizures in patients with partial onset epilepsy. Binding to albumin and α_1-acid glycoprotein is greater than 95 percent, and metabolism is mainly completed by the CYP3A family of enzymes. Adverse effects include tiredness, dizziness, and gastrointestinal upset. There is some indication in postmarketing surveillance that seizures have occurred in patients who did not have epilepsy when the drug was used. *Tiagabine* has not been approved for use for any other indication.

O. Topiramate

Topiramate [toe-PEER-a-mate] possesses several actions that are believed to contribute to its broad spectrum of antiseizure activity. *Topiramate* blocks voltage-dependent sodium channels; it has been shown to increase the frequency of chloride channel opening by binding to the GABA$_A$ receptor. High-voltage calcium currents (L type) are reduced by *topiramate*. It is a carbonic anhydrase inhibitor and may act at glutamate (NMDA) sites. *Topiramate* is effective and approved for use in partial and primary generalized epilepsies. It is also approved for treatment of migraine. *Topiramate* is renally eliminated to a high degree, but it also has inactive metabolites. It inhibits CYP2C19 and is induced by *phenytoin*, and *carbamazepine*. *Lamotrigine* is reported to cause an increase in *topiramate* concentration. Coadministration of *topiramate* reduces *ethinyl estradiol*. Adverse effects include somnolence, weight loss, and paresthesias; renal stones are reported to occur at a higher

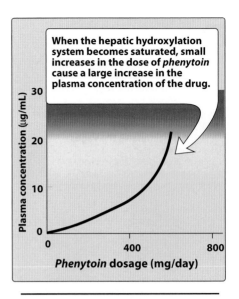

When the hepatic hydroxylation system becomes saturated, small increases in the dose of *phenytoin* cause a large increase in the plasma concentration of the drug.

Figure 15.8
Nonlinear effect of *phenytoin* dosage on the plasma concentration of the drug.

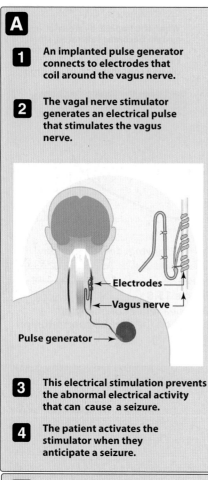

A

1 An implanted pulse generator connects to electrodes that coil around the vagus nerve.

2 The vagal nerve stimulator generates an electrical pulse that stimulates the vagus nerve.

Electrodes

Vagus nerve

Pulse generator

3 This electrical stimulation prevents the abnormal electrical activity that can cause a seizure.

4 The patient activates the stimulator when they anticipate a seizure.

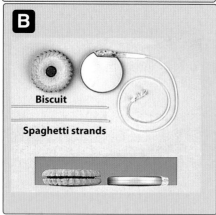

B

Biscuit

Spaghetti strands

Figure 15.9
Vagal nerve stimulation. A. Location of implanted stimulator. B. Size of device.

incidence than in a nontreated population. Glaucoma, oligohidrosis, and hyperthermia have also been reported. The latter are specifically related to the carbonic anhydrase activity.

P. Zonisamide

Zonisamide [zoe-NIS-a-mide] is a sulfonamide derivative that has a broad spectrum of action. The compound has multiple effects on neuronal systems thought to be involved in seizure generation. These include blockade of both voltage-gated sodium channels and T-type calcium currents. It has a limited amount of carbonic anhydrase activity. Cross reactivity with other sulfonamides should be reviewed and its use monitored in patients with reported allergies. *Zonisamide* is approved for use in patients with partial epilepsy. It is metabolized by the CYP3A4 isozyme and may, to a lesser extent, be affected by CYP3A5 and CYP2C19. In addition to the typical CNS adverse effects, *zonisamide* may cause kidney stones. Oligohidrosis has been reported, and patients should be monitored for increased body temperature and decreased sweating.

VI. VAGAL NERVE STIMULATION

Vagal nerve stimulation requires surgical implant of a small pulse generator with a battery and a lead wire for stimulus (Figure 15.9). The device is implanted and lead wires wrapped around the patient's vagal nerve. This device and treatment were approved in 1997. The device is also approved for treatment of depression. The mechanism of action is unknown. Because it has diffuse involvement with the neuronal circuits, there are a variety of mechanisms by which it may exert its affect on seizure control. Vagal nerve stimulation has been effective in treatment of partial onset seizures and has enabled reduction of drug therapy in some cases. It is an alternative for patients who have been refractory to multiple drugs, who are sensitive to the many adverse effects of antiseizure drugs, and who have difficulty adhering to medication schedules. Vagal nerve stimulation requires invasive procedure and is expensive.

VII. EPILEPSY IN PREGNANCY

Women with epilepsy are often very concerned about pregnancy and what the medications will do to the development of the baby. Planning is the most important component. All women should be on high doses of folic acid prior to conception. *Divalproex* and barbiturates should be avoided. Switching women to other drugs before pregnancy should be accomplished when possible. When seizures are controlled, maintenance medication should be reduced, if possible, to the lowest dose that provides control. If seizures are not controlled, medications and dosages should be adjusted. The frequency and severity of seizures may change during pregnancy. Women should be monitored regularly by the obstetrician as well as the neurologist. All women with epilepsy should register with the AED (Antiepileptic drug) Pregnancy Registry.

Figure 15.10 summarizes the antiepileptic drugs,

DRUG	MECHANISM OF ACTION	ADVERSE EFFECTS AND COMMENTS
Carbamazepine	Blocks Na⁺ channels	Hyponatremia, drowsiness, fatigue, dizziness, and blurred vision. Drug use has as been associated with Stevens-Johnson Syndrome. Blood dyscrasias: neutropenia, leukopenia, thrombocytopenia, pancytopenia, and anemias.
Divalproex	Multiple mechanisms of action	Weight gain, easy bruising, nausea, tremor, hair loss, weight gain, GI upset, liver damage, alopecia, and sedation. Hepatic failure, pancreatitis, and teratogenic effects such have been observed. Broad spectrum of antiseizure activity.
Ethosuximide	Blocks Ca²⁺ channels	Drowsiness, hyperactivity, nausea, sedation, GI upset, weight gain, lethargy, SLE, and rash. Blood dyscrasias can occur; periodic CBCs should be done. Abrupt discontinuance of drug may causes seizures.
Felbamate	Multiple mechanisms of action	Insomnia, dizziness, headache, ataxia, weight gain, and irritability. Aplastic anemia; hepatic failure. Broad spectrum of antiseizure activity. Requires patient to sign informed consent at dispensing.
Gabapentin	Unknown	Mild drowsiness, dizziness, ataxia, weight gain, and diarrhea. Few drug interactions. One-hundred percent renal elimination.
Lamotrigine	Multiple mechanisms of action	Nausea, drowsiness, dizziness, headache, and diplopia. Rash (Stevens-Johnson syndrome—potentially life-threatening). Broad spectrum of antiseizure activity.
Levetiracetam	Multiple mechanisms of action	Sedation, dizziness, headache, anorexia, fatigue, infections, and behavioral symptoms. Few drug interactions. Broad spectrum of antiseizure activity.
Oxcarbazepine	Blocks Na⁺ channels	Nausea, rash, hyponatremia, headache, sedation, dizziness, vertigo, ataxia, and diplopia.
Fosphenytoin	Blocks Na⁺ channels	Gingival hyperplasia, confusion, slurred speech, double vision, ataxia, sedation, dizziness, and hirsutism. Stevens-Johnson syndrome—potentially life-threatening. Not recommended for chronic use. Primary treatment for status epilepticus.
Pregabalin	Multiple mechanisms of action	Weight gain, somnolence, dizziness, headache, weight gain, diplopia, and ataxia. One hundred percent renal elimination.
Primidone	GABA receptor	Sedation, lethargy, behavioral changes, ataxia, hyperactivity, and nausea. Not recommended for chronic use.
Tiagabine	GABA receptor	Sedation, weight gain, fatigue, headache, tremor, dizziness, and anorexia. Multiple drug interactions.
Topiramate	Multiple mechanisms of action	Paresthesia, weight loss, nervousness, depression, anorexia, anxiety, tremor, cognitive complaints, headache, and oligohidrosis. Few drug interactions. Broad spectrum of antiseizure activity.
Zonisamide	Multiple mechanisms of action	Nausea, anorexia, ataxia, confusion, difficulty concentrating, sedation, paresthesia and oligohidrosis. Broad spectrum of antiseizure activity.

Figure 15.10
Summary of antiepileptic drugs. CBC = complete blood count; GABA = γ-aminobutyric acid; GI = gastrointestinal; SLE = systemic lupus erythematosus

Study Questions

Choose the ONE best answer.

15.1 A nine-year-old boy is sent for neurologic evaluation because of episodes of confusion. Over the past year, the child has experienced episodes during which he develops a blank look on his face and fails to respond to questions. However, it appears to take several minutes before the boy recovers from the episodes. Which one the following best describes this patient's seizures?

A. Simple partial.
B. Complex partial.
C. Tonic-clonic.
D. Absence.
E. Myoclonic.

Correct answer = B. The patient is exhibiting episodes of complex partial seizures. Complex partial seizures impair consciousness and can occur in all age groups. Typically, staring is accompanied by impaired consciousness and recall. If asked a question, the patient might respond with an inappropriate or unintelligible answer. Automatic movements are associated with most complex partial seizures and involve the mouth and face (lip-smacking, chewing, tasting, and swallowing movements), upper extremities (fumbling, picking, tapping, or clasping movements), vocal apparatus (grunts or repetition of words or phrases), or more complex acts (such as walking or mixing foods in a bowl), although subtle lateralizing signs (such as an asymmetric smile) may be present.

15.2 Which one of the following therapies would be appropriate for the patient described in the above question?

A. Ethosuximide.
B. Carbamazepine.
C. Diazepam.
D. Carbamazepine plus primidone.
E. Watchful waiting.

Correct answer = B. The patient has had many seizures, and the risks of not starting drug therapy would be substantially greater than the risks of treating his seizures. Because the child has impaired consciousness during the seizure, he is at risk for injury during an attack. Monotherapy with primary agents is preferred for most patients. The advantages of monotherapy include reduced frequency of adverse effects, absence of interactions between antiepileptic drugs, lower cost, and improved compliance. Ethosuximide and diazepam are not indicated for complex partial seizures.

15.3 The patient described in Question 15.1 was treated for six months with carbamazepine but, recently, has been experiencing breakthrough seizures on a more frequent basis. You are considering adding a second drug to this patient's antiseizure regimen. Which of the following drugs is least likely to have a pharmacokinetic interaction with carbamazepine?

A. Topiramate.
B. Tiagabine.
C. Levetiracetam.
D. Lamotrigine.
E. Zonisamide.

Correct answer = C. Of the drugs listed, all of which are approved as adjunct therapy for refractory complex partial seizures, only levetiracetam does not affect the pharmacokinetics of other antiepileptic drugs, and neither are its pharmacokinetic properties significantly altered by other drugs. While the point is to review the drug interactions, any of the listed drugs could be added depending on the plan and the patient characteristics. It may be best to consider discontinuing carbamazepine in favor of adding lamotrigine in case there is any possibility the patient has primary generalized epilepsy because no electroencephalographic (EEG) report is present in Question 15.1. Treatment of epilepsy is complex, and diagnosis is based on history and may need to be reevaluated when drug therapy fails or seizures increase.

Heart Failure

16

I. OVERVIEW

Heart failure (HF) is a complex, progressive disorder in which the heart is unable to pump sufficient blood to meet the needs of the body. Its cardinal symptoms are dyspnea, fatigue, and fluid retention. HF is due to an impaired ability of the heart to adequately fill with and/or eject blood. It is often accompanied by abnormal increases in blood volume and interstitial fluid, hence the term "congestive" HF because symptoms include dyspnea from pulmonary congestion in left HF, and peripheral edema in right HF. Underlying causes of HF include arteriosclerotic heart disease, myocardial infarction, hypertensive heart disease, valvular heart disease, dilated cardiomyopathy, and congenital heart disease. Left systolic dysfunction secondary to coronary artery disease is the most common cause of HF, accounting for nearly 70 percent of all cases. The number of newly diagnosed patients with HF is increasing, because more individuals now survive acute myocardial infarction.

A. Role of physiologic compensatory mechanisms in the progression of HF

Chronic activation of the sympathetic nervous system and the renin-angiotensin-aldosterone axis is associated with remodeling of cardiac tissue, characterized by loss of myocytes, hypertrophy, and fibrosis. The geometry of the heart becomes less elliptical and more spherical, interfering with its ability to efficiently function as a pump. This prompts additional neurohumoral activation, creating a vicious cycle that, if left untreated, leads to death.

B. Goals of pharmacologic intervention in HF

The goals are to alleviate symptoms, slow disease progression, and improve survival. Accordingly, six classes of drugs have been shown to be effective: 1) inhibitors of the renin-angiotensin system, 2) β-adrenoreceptor blockers, 3) diuretics, 4) inotropic agents, 5) direct vasodilators, and 6) aldosterone antagonists (Figure 16.1). Depending on the severity of cardiac failure and individual patient factors, one or more of these classes of drugs are administered. Beneficial effects of

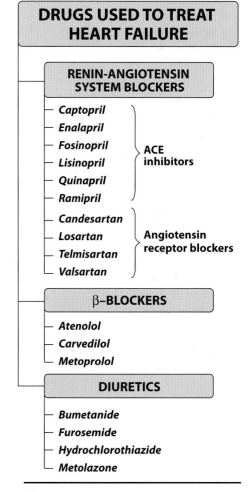

Figure 16.1
Summary of drugs used to treat heart failure. ACE = angiotensin-converting enzyme. (Continued on the next page.)

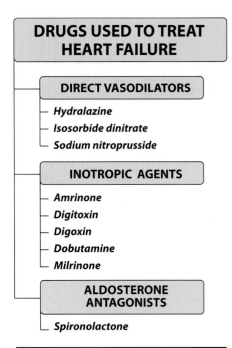

DRUGS USED TO TREAT HEART FAILURE

DIRECT VASODILATORS
— *Hydralazine*
— *Isosorbide dinitrate*
— *Sodium nitroprusside*

INOTROPIC AGENTS
— *Amrinone*
— *Digitoxin*
— *Digoxin*
— *Dobutamine*
— *Milrinone*

ALDOSTERONE ANTAGONISTS
— *Spironolactone*

Figure 16.1 (continued) Summary of drugs used to treat heart failure.

pharmacologic intervention include reduction of the load on the myocardium, decreased extracellular fluid volume, improved cardiac contractility, and slowing of the rate of cardiac remodeling. Knowledge of the physiology of cardiac muscle contraction is essential to understanding the compensatory responses evoked by the failing heart as well as the actions of drugs used to treat HF.

II. PHYSIOLOGY OF MUSCLE CONTRACTION

The myocardium, like smooth and skeletal muscle, responds to stimulation by depolarization of the membrane, which is followed by shortening of the contractile proteins and ends with relaxation and return to the resting state. However, unlike skeletal muscle, which shows graded contractions depending on the number of muscle cells that are stimulated, the cardiac muscle cells are interconnected in groups that respond to stimuli as a unit, contracting together whenever a single cell is stimulated.

A. Action potential

Cardiac muscle cells are electrically excitable. However, unlike the cells of other muscles and nerves, the cells of cardiac muscle show a spontaneous, intrinsic rhythm generated by specialized "pacemaker" cells located in the sinoatrial and atrioventricular nodes. The cardiac cells also have an unusually long action potential, which can be divided into five phases (0–4). Figure 16.2 illustrates the major ions contributing to depolarization and polarization of cardiac cells. These ions pass through channels in the sarcolemmal membrane and, thus, create a current. The channels open and close at different times during the action potential. Some respond primarily to changes in ion concentration, whereas others are sensitive to adenosine triphosphate, or to membrane voltage.

B. Cardiac contraction

The contractile machinery of the myocardial cell is essentially the same as that in striated muscle. The force of contraction of the cardiac muscle is directly related to the concentration of free (unbound) cytosolic calcium. Therefore, agents that increase these calcium levels (or that increase the sensitivity of the contractile machinery to calcium) result in an increased force of contraction (inotropic effect). [Note: The inotropic agents increase the contractility of the heart by directly or indirectly altering the mechanisms that control the concentration of intracellular calcium.]

1. **Sources of free intracellular calcium:** Calcium comes from several sources. The first is from outside the cell, where opening of voltage-sensitive calcium channels causes an immediate rise in free cytosolic calcium. Calcium may aslo enter by exchange with sodium. Calcium is also released from the sarcoplasmic reticulum and mitochondria, which further increases the cytosolic level of calcium (Figure 16.3).

2. **Removal of free cytosolic calcium:** If free cytosolic calcium levels were to remain high, the cardiac muscle would be in a constant state of contraction rather than showing a periodic contraction. Mechanisms of removal include two alternatives.

   a. **Sodium/calcium exchange:** Calcium is removed by a sodium/calcium exchange reaction that reversibly exchanges calcium ions for sodium ions across the cell membrane (see Figure 16.3).

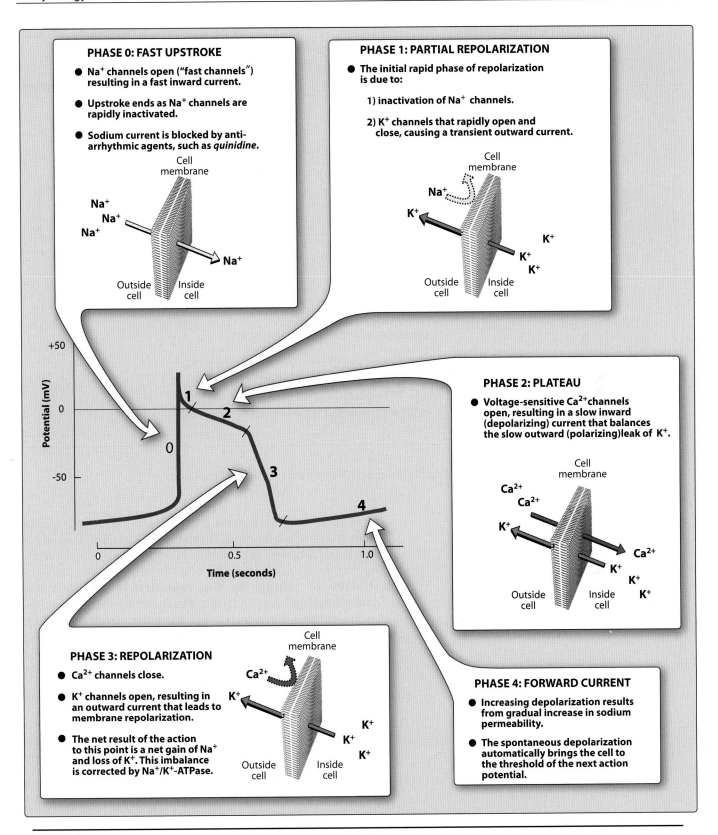

PHASE 0: FAST UPSTROKE

- Na⁺ channels open ("fast channels") resulting in a fast inward current.

- Upstroke ends as Na⁺ channels are rapidly inactivated.

- Sodium current is blocked by anti-arrhythmic agents, such as *quinidine*.

PHASE 1: PARTIAL REPOLARIZATION

- The initial rapid phase of repolarization is due to:

  1) inactivation of Na⁺ channels.

  2) K⁺ channels that rapidly open and close, causing a transient outward current.

PHASE 2: PLATEAU

- Voltage-sensitive Ca²⁺ channels open, resulting in a slow inward (depolarizing) current that balances the slow outward (polarizing) leak of K⁺.

PHASE 3: REPOLARIZATION

- Ca²⁺ channels close.

- K⁺ channels open, resulting in an outward current that leads to membrane repolarization.

- The net result of the action to this point is a net gain of Na⁺ and loss of K⁺. This imbalance is corrected by Na⁺/K⁺-ATPase.

PHASE 4: FORWARD CURRENT

- Increasing depolarization results from gradual increase in sodium permeability.

- The spontaneous depolarization automatically brings the cell to the threshold of the next action potential.

Figure 16.2
Action potential of a Purkinje fiber. ATPase = adenosine triphosphatase.

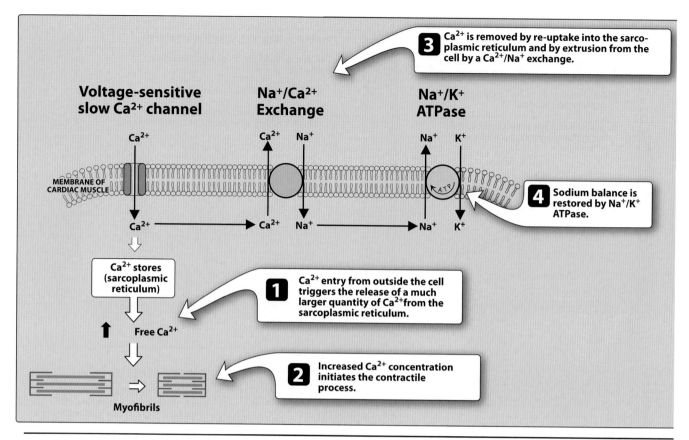

Figure 16.3
Ion movements during the contraction of cardiac muscle. ATPase = adenosine triphosphatase.

This interaction between the movement of calcium and sodium ions is significant, because changes in intracellular sodium can affect cellular levels of calcium.

    b. **Uptake of calcium by the sarcoplasmic reticulum and mitochondria:** Calcium is also recaptured by the sarcoplasmic reticulum and the mitochondria. More than 99 percent of the intracellular calcium is located in these organelles, and even a modest shift between these stores and free calcium can lead to large changes in the concentration of free cytosolic calcium.

C. Compensatory physiological responses in HF

The failing heart evokes three major compensatory mechanisms to enhance cardiac output (Figure 16.4). Although initially beneficial, these alterations ultimately result in further deterioration of cardiac function.

    1. **Increased sympathetic activity:** Baroreceptors sense a decrease in blood pressure and activate the sympathetic nervous system, which stimulates β-adrenergic receptors in the heart. This results in an increased heart rate and a greater force of contraction of the heart muscle (see Figure 16.4). In addition, vasoconstriction (α_1-mediated) enhances venous return and increases cardiac preload. These compensatory responses increase the work of the heart and, therefore, can contribute to further decline in cardiac function.

2. **Activation of the renin-angiotensin system:** A fall in cardiac output decreases blood flow to the kidney, prompting the release of renin, with a resulting increase in the formation of angiotensin II and release of aldosterone. This results in increased peripheral resistance and retention of sodium and water. Blood volume increases, and more blood is returned to the heart. If the heart is unable to pump this extra volume, venous pressure increases and peripheral edema and pulmonary edema occur (see Figure 16.4). These compensatory responses increase the work of the heart and, therefore, can contribute to further decline in cardiac function.

3. **Myocardial hypertrophy:** The heart increases in size, and the chambers dilate and become more globular. Initially, stretching of the heart muscle leads to a stronger contraction of the heart. However, excessive elongation of the fibers results in weaker contractions, and the geometry diminishes the ability to eject blood. This type of failure is termed systolic failure and is the result of a ventricle being unable to pump effectively. Less commonly, patients with HF may have diastolic dysfunction—a term applied when the ability of the ventricles to relax and accept blood is impaired by structural changes, such as hypertrophy. The thickening of the ventricular wall and subsequent decrease in ventricular volume decrease the ability of heart muscle to relax. In this case, the ventricle does not fill adequately, and the inadequacy of cardiac output is termed diastolic HF—a particularly common feature of HF in elderly women. Diastolic dysfunction in its pure form is characterized by signs and symptoms of HF in the presence of a normal function of the left ventricle. However, both systolic and diastolic dysfunction commonly coexist in HF.

D. Decompensated HF

If the mechanisms listed above adequately restore cardiac output, the HF is said to be compensated. However, these compensations increase the work of the heart and contribute to further decline in cardiac performance. If the adaptive mechanisms fail to maintain cardiac output, the HF is termed decompensated.

E. Therapeutic strategies in HF

Chronic HF is typically managed by a reduction in physical activity, low dietary intake of sodium (<1500 mg/day), treatment of comorbid conditions, and judicious use of diuretics, inhibitors of the renin-angiotensin system, and inotropic agents. Drugs that may precipitate or exacerbate HF, such as nonsteroidal anti-inflammatory drugs, alcohol, calcium-channel blockers, and some antiarrhythmic drugs, should be avoided if possible. Patients with HF complain of dyspnea on exertion, orthopnea, paroxysmal nocturnal dyspnea, fatigue, and dependent edema.

III. INHIBITORS OF THE RENIN-ANGIOTENSIN SYSTEM

HF leads to activation of the renin-angiotensin system via two mechanisms: 1) Increased renin release by juxtaglomerular cells in renal afferent arterioles occurs in response to the diminished renal perfusion pressure produced by the failing heart, and 2) renin release by the juxtaglomerular cells is promoted by sympathetic stimulation. The production of angiotensin II—a potent vasoconstrictor—and the subsequent stimulation of aldosterone release that causes salt and water retention lead to the increases in

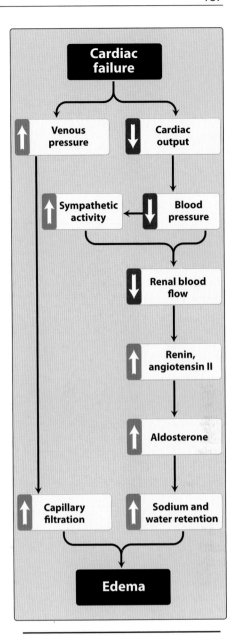

Figure 16.4
Cardiovascular consequences of heart failure.

both preload and afterload that are characteristic of the failing heart. In addition, high levels of angiotensin II and of aldosterone have direct detrimental effects on the cardiac muscle, favoring remodeling, fibrosis, and inflammatory changes.

A. Angiotensin-converting enzyme inhibitors

Angiotensin-converting enzyme (ACE) inhibitors are the agents of choice in HF. These drugs block the enzyme that cleaves angiotensin I to form the potent vasoconstrictor angiotensin II (Figure 16.5). These agents also diminish the rate of bradykinin inactivation. [Note: Vasodilation occurs as a result of the combined effects of lower vasoconstriction caused by diminished levels of angiotensin II and the potent vasodilating effect of increased bradykinin.] By reducing circulating angiotensin II levels, ACE inhibitors also decrease the secretion of aldosterone, resulting in decreased sodium and water retention.

1. **Actions on the heart:** ACE inhibitors decrease vascular resistance, venous tone, and blood pressure, resulting in an increased cardiac output (see Figure 16.5). ACE inhibitors also blunt the usual angiotensin II–mediated increase in epinephrine and aldosterone seen in HF. ACE inhibitors improve clinical signs and symptoms in patients also receiving thiazide or loop diuretics and/or *digoxin*. The use of ACE inhibitors in the treatment of HF has significantly decreased both morbidity and mortality. For example, Figure 16.6 shows that the ACE inhibitor *enalapril* [e-NAL-a-pril] decreases the cumulative mortality in patients with congestive HF. [Note: Reduction in mortality is due primarily to a decrease in deaths caused by progressive HF.] Treatment with *enalapril* also reduces arrhythmic death, myocardial infarction, and strokes. Similar data have been obtained with other ACE inhibitors.

2. **Indications:** ACE inhibitors may be considered for single-agent therapy in patients who present with mild dyspnea on exertion and do not show signs or symptoms of volume overload. ACE inhibitors are useful in decreasing HF in asymptomatic patients with an ejection fraction of less than 35 percent (left ventricular dysfunction). Patients who have had a recent myocardial infarction also benefit from long-term ACE inhibitor therapy. Patients with the lowest ejec-

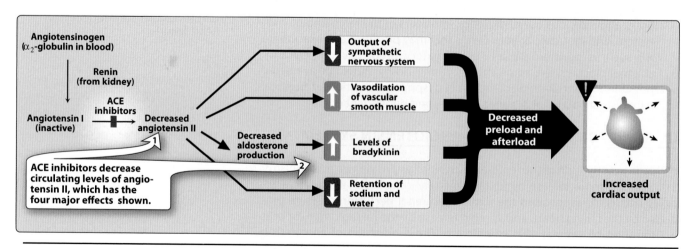

Figure 16.5
Effects of angiotensin-converting enzyme (ACE) inhibitors.

tion fraction show the greatest benefit. Early use of ACE inhibitors is indicated in patients with all stages of left ventricular failure, with and without symptoms, and therapy should be initiated immediately after myocardial infarction. (See p. 221 for the use of ACE inhibitors in the treatment of hypertension.)

3. **Pharmacokinetics:** All ACE inhibitors are adequately but incompletely absorbed following oral administration. The presence of food may decrease absorption, so they should be taken on an empty stomach. Except for *captopril* [CAP-toe-pril], ACE inhibitors are prodrugs that require activation by hydrolysis via hepatic enzymes. Renal elimination of the active moiety is important for most ACE inhibitors, an exception being *fosinopril* [foe-SIH-no-pril]. Plasma half-lives of active compounds vary from 2 to 12 hours, although the inhibition of ACE may be much longer. The newer compounds such as *ramipril* [RA-mi-pril] and *fosinopril* require only once-a-day dosing.

4. **Adverse effects:** These include postural hypotension, renal insufficiency, hyperkalemia, angioedema, and a persistent dry cough. The potential for symptomatic hypotension with ACE inhibitor therapy requires careful monitoring. ACE inhibitors should not be used in pregnant women, because they are fetotoxic.

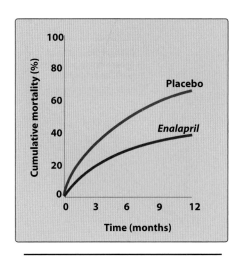

Figure 16.6
Effect of *enalapril* on the mortality of patients with congestive heart failure.

B. Angiotensin-receptor blockers

Angiotensin-receptor blockers (ARBs) are nonpeptide, orally active compounds that are extremely potent competitive antagonists of the angiotensin type 1 receptor. *Losartan* [loe-SAR-tan] is the prototype drug. ARBs have the advantage of more complete blockade of angiotensin action, because ACE inhibitors inhibit only one enzyme responsible for the production of angiotensin II. Further, the ARBs do not affect bradykinin levels. Although ARBs have actions similar to those of ACE inhibitors, they are not therapeutically identical. Even so, ARBs are a substitute for ACE inhibitors in those patients who cannot tolerate the latter.

1. **Actions on the cardiovascular system:** All the ARBs are approved for treatment of hypertension based on their clinical efficacy in lowering blood pressure and reducing the morbidity and mortality associated with hypertension. As indicated above, their use in HF is as a substitute for ACE inhibitors in those patients with severe cough or angioedema.

2. **Pharmacokinetics:** All the drugs are orally active and require only once-a-day dosing. *Losartan*, the first approved member of the class, differs from the others in that it undergoes extensive first-pass hepatic metabolism, including conversion to its active metabolite. The other drugs have inactive metabolites. Elimination of metabolites and parent compounds occurs in the urine and feces; the proportion is dependent on the individual drug. All are highly plasma protein–bound (greater than 90 percent) and, except for *candesartan* [kan-des-AR-tan], have large volumes of distribution.

3. **Adverse effects:** ARBs have an adverse effect profile similar to that of ACE inhibitors. However, ARBs do not produce cough. ARBs are contraindicated in pregnancy.

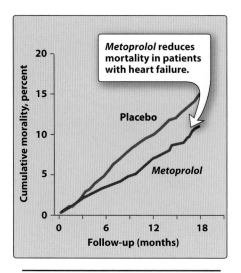

Figure 16.7
Cumulative mortality in patients with heart failure treated using placebo or *metoprolol*.

IV. β-BLOCKERS

Although it may seem counterintuitive to administer drugs with negative inotropic activity to a patient with HF, several clinical studies have clearly demonstrated improved systolic functioning and reverse cardiac remodeling in patients receiving β-blockers. These benefits arise in spite of occasional initial exacerbation of symptoms. The benefit of β-blockers is attributed, in part, to their ability to prevent the changes that occur because of the chronic activation of the sympathetic nervous system, including decreasing the heart rate and inhibiting the release of renin. In addition, β-blockers also prevent the direct deleterious effects of norepinephrine on the cardiac muscle fibers, decreasing remodeling, hypertrophy and cell death. Two β-blockers have been approved for use in HF: *carvedilol* [KAR-ve-dil-ol], and long-acting *metoprolol* [me-TOE-proe-lol]. *Carvedilol* is a nonselective β-adrenoreceptor antagonist that also blocks α-adrenoreceptors, whereas *metoprolol* is a β_1-selective antagonist. [Note: The pharmacology of β-blockers is described in detail in Chapter 7.] β-Blockade is recommended for all patients with heart disease except those who are at high risk but have no symptoms or those who are in acute HF. *Carvedilol* and *metoprolol* reduce morbidity and mortality associated with HF. Treatment should be started at low doses and gradually titrated to effective doses based on patient tolerance. Obviously, the patient who also is hypertensive will obtain additional benefit from the β-blocker. Figure 16.7 shows the beneficial effect of *metoprolol* treatment in patients with HF.

V. DIURETICS

Diuretics relieve pulmonary congestion and peripheral edema. These agents are also useful in reducing the symptoms of volume overload, including orthopnea and paroxysmal nocturnal dyspnea. Diuretics decrease plasma volume and, subsequently, decrease venous return to the heart (preload). This decreases the cardiac workload and the oxygen demand. Diuretics may also decrease afterload by reducing plasma volume, thus decreasing blood pressure. Thiazide diuretics are relatively mild diuretics and lose efficacy if patient creatinine clearance is less than 50 mL/min. Loop diuretics are used for patients who require extensive diuresis and those with renal insufficiency. [Note: Overdoses of loop diuretics can lead to profound hypovolemia.]

VI. DIRECT VASODILATORS

Dilation of venous blood vessels leads to a decrease in cardiac preload by increasing the venous capacitance; arterial dilators reduce systemic arteriolar resistance and decrease afterload. Nitrates are commonly employed venous dilators for patients with congestive HF. If the patient is intolerant of ACE inhibitors or β-blockers, the combination of *hydralazine* and *isosorbide dinitrate* is most commonly used. [Note: Calcium-channel blockers should be avoided in patients with HF.]

VII. INOTROPIC DRUGS

Positive inotropic agents enhance cardiac muscle contractility and, thus, increase cardiac output. Although these drugs act by different mechanisms, in each case the inotropic action is the result of an increased cytoplasmic calcium concentration that enhances the contractility of cardiac muscle.

A. Digitalis

The cardiac glycosides are often called *digitalis* or digitalis glycosides, because most of the drugs come from the digitalis (foxglove) plant. They are a group of chemically similar compounds that can increase the contractility of the heart muscle and, therefore, are widely used in treating HF. Like the antiarrhythmic drugs described in Chapter 17, the cardiac glycosides influence the sodium and calcium ion flows in the cardiac muscle, thereby increasing contraction of the atrial and ventricular myocardium (positive inotropic action). The digitalis glycosides show only a small difference between a therapeutically effective dose and doses that are toxic or even fatal. Therefore, the drugs have a low therapeutic index. The most widely used agent is *digoxin* [di-JOX-in].

1. Mechanism of action:

a. Regulation of cytosolic calcium concentration: Free cytosolic calcium concentrations at the end of contraction must be lowered for cardiac muscle to relax. The Na^+/Ca^{2+}-exchanger plays an important role in this process by extruding Ca^{2+} from the myocyte in exchange for Na^+ (Figure 16.8). The concentration gradient for both ions is a major determinant of the net movement of ions. By inhibiting the ability of the myocyte to actively pump Na^+ from the cell, cardiac glycosides decrease the Na^+ concentration gradient and, consequently, the ability of the Na^+/Ca^{2+}-exchanger to move calcium out of the cell. Further, the higher cellular Na^+ is exchanged by extracellular Ca^{2+} by the Na^+/Ca^{2+}-exchanger increasing intracellular Ca^{2+}. Because more Ca^{2+} is retained intracellularly, a small but physiologically important increase occurs in the free Ca^{2+} that is available at the next contraction cycle of the cardiac muscle. It follows that if the Na^+/K^+–adenosine triphosphatase is extensively inhibited, the ionic gradient becomes so disturbed that dysrhythmias can occur.

b. Increased contractility of the cardiac muscle: Administration of digitalis glycosides increases the force of cardiac contraction, causing the cardiac output to more closely resemble that of the

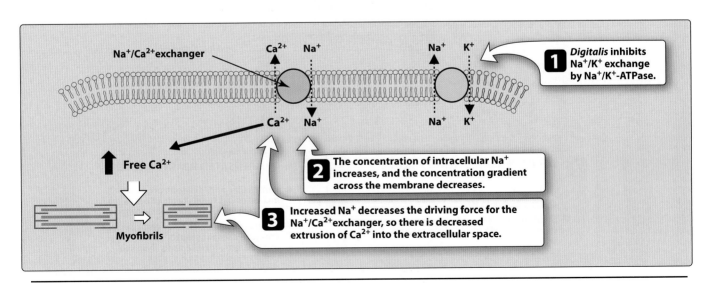

Figure 16.8
Mechanism of action of cardiac glycosides, or *digitalis*. ATPase = adenosine triphosphatase.

normal heart (Figure 16.9). Increased myocardial contraction leads to a decrease in end-diastolic volume, thus increasing the efficiency of contraction (increased ejection fraction). The resulting improved circulation leads to reduced sympathetic activity, which then reduces peripheral resistance. Together, these effects cause a reduction in heart rate. Vagal tone is also enhanced, so the heart rate decreases and myocardial oxygen demand diminishes. [Note: In the normal heart, the positive inotropic effect of *digitalis* is counteracted by compensatory autonomic reflexes.]

2. **Therapeutic uses:** *Digoxin* therapy is indicated in patients with severe left ventricular systolic dysfunction after initiation of ACE inhibitor and diuretic therapy. *Digoxin* is not indicated in patients with diastolic or right-sided HF. *Digoxin's* major indication is HF with atrial fibrillation. *Dobutamine* [doe-BYOO-ta-meen], another inotropic agent, can be given intravenously in the hospital, but at present, no effective oral inotropic agents exist other than *digoxin*. Patients with mild to moderate HF will often respond to treatment with ACE inhibitors and diuretics, and they do not require *digoxin*.

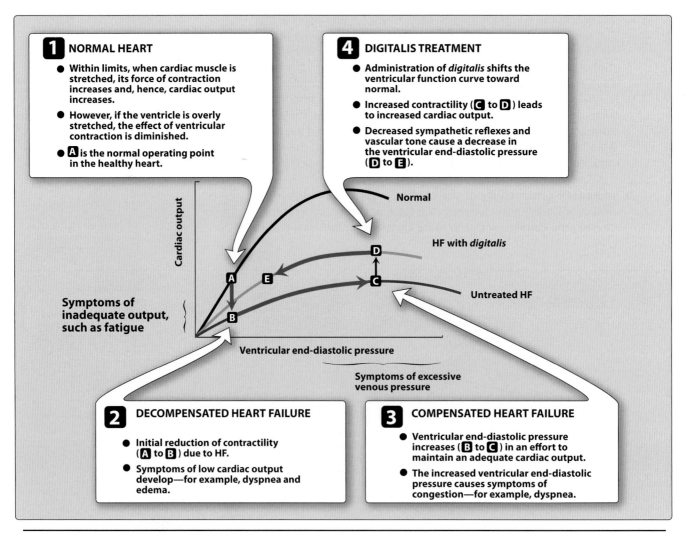

Figure 16.9
Ventricular function curves in the normal heart, in heart failure (HF), and in HF treated with *digitalis*.

3. **Pharmacokinetics:** All digitalis glycosides possess the same pharmacologic actions, but they vary in potency and pharmacokinetics (Figure 16.10). *Digoxin* is the only digitalis available in the United States. *Digoxin* is very potent, with a narrow margin of safety and long half-life of around 36 hours. *Digoxin* is mainly eliminated intact by the kidney, requiring dose adjustment based on creatinine clearance. *Digoxin* has a large volume of distribution, because it accumulates in muscle. A loading dose regimen is employed when acute digitalization is needed. *Digitoxin* [DIJ-i-tox-in] has a much longer half-life and is extensively metabolized by the liver before excretion in the feces, and patients with hepatic disease may require decreased doses.

4. **Adverse effects:** *Digitalis* toxicity is one of the most commonly encountered adverse drug reactions. Side effects often can be managed by discontinuing cardiac glycoside therapy, determining serum potassium levels (decreased K+ enhances potential for cardiotoxicity), and if indicated, giving potassium supplements. In general, decreased serum levels of potassium predispose a patient to *digoxin* toxicity. *Digoxin* levels must be closely monitored in the presence of renal insufficiency, and dosage adjustment may be necessary. Severe toxicity resulting in ventricular tachycardia may require administration of antiarrhythmic drugs and the use of antibodies to *digoxin* (digoxin immune Fab), which bind and inactivate the drug. Types of adverse effects include:

   a. **Cardiac effects:** The common cardiac side effect is arrhythmia, characterized by slowing of atrioventricular conduction associated with atrial arrhythmias. A decrease in intracellular potassium is the primary predisposing factor in these effects.

   b. **Gastrointestinal effects:** Anorexia, nausea, and vomiting are commonly encountered adverse effects.

   c. **Central nervous system effects:** These include headache, fatigue, confusion, blurred vision, alteration of color perception, and halos on dark objects.

5. **Factors predisposing to digitalis toxicity:**

   a. **Electrolytic disturbances:** Hypokalemia can precipitate serious arrhythmia. Reduction of serum potassium levels is most frequently observed in patients receiving thiazide or loop diuretics, and this usually can be prevented by use of a potassium-sparing diuretic or supplementation with potassium chloride. Hypercalcemia and hypomagnesemia also predispose to *digitalis* toxicity.

   b. **Drugs:** *Quinidine*, *verapamil*, and *amiodarone*, to name a few, can cause *digoxin* intoxication, both by displacing *digoxin* from tissue protein-binding sites and by competing with *digoxin* for renal excretion. As a consequence, *digoxin* plasma levels may increase by 70 to 100 percent, requiring dosage reduction. Potassium-depleting diuretics, corticosteroids, and a variety of other drugs can also increase *digoxin* toxicity (Figure 16.11). Hypothyroidism, hypoxia, renal failure, and myocarditis are also predisposing factors to *digoxin* toxicity.

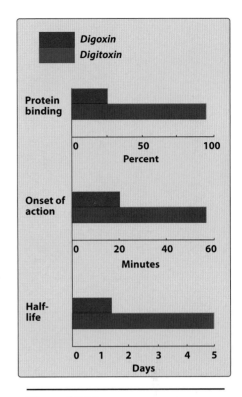

Figure 16.10
A comparison of the properties of *digoxin* and *digitoxin*.

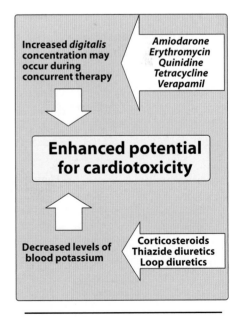

Figure 16.11
Drugs interacting with *digoxin* and other digitalis glycosides.

B. β-Adrenergic agonists

β-Adrenergic stimulation improves cardiac performance by causing positive inotropic effects and vasodilation. *Dobutamine* is the most commonly used inotropic agent other than *digitalis*. *Dobutamine* leads to an increase in intracellular cyclic adenosine monophosphate (cAMP), which results in the activation of protein kinase. Slow calcium channels are one important site of phosphorylation by protein kinase. When phosphorylated, the entry of calcium ion into the myocardial cells increases, thus enhancing contraction (Figure 16.12). *Dobutamine* must be given by intravenous infusion and is primarily used in the treatment of acute HF in a hospital setting.

C. Phosphodiesterase inhibitors

Amrinone [AM-ri-none] and *milrinone* [MIL-ri-none] are phosphodiesterase inhibitors that increase the intracellular concentration of cAMP (see Figure 16.12). This results in an increase of intracellular calcium and, therefore, cardiac contractility, as discussed above for the β-adrenergic agonists. Long-term *amrinone* or *milrinone* therapy may be associated with a substantial increase in the risk of mortality. However, short-term use of intravenous *milrinone* is not associated with increased mortality, and some symptomatic benefit may be obtained when it is used in patients with refractory HF.

VIII. SPIRONOLACTONE

Patients with advanced heart disease have elevated levels of aldosterone due to angiotensin II stimulation and reduced hepatic clearance of the hor-

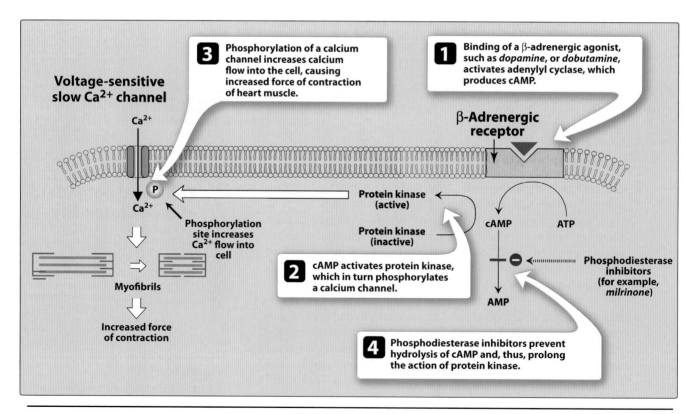

Figure 16.12
Sites of action by β-adrenergic agonists on heart muscle. AMP = adenosine monophosphate; ATP = adenosine triphospha
cAMP = cyclic adenosine monophosphate; P = phosphate.

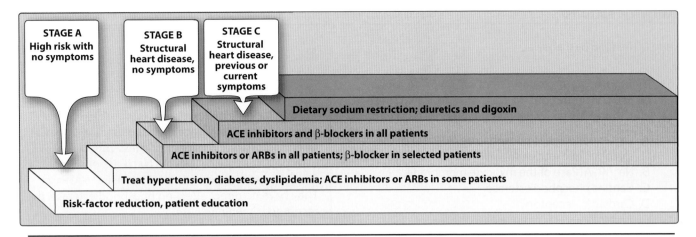

Figure 16.13
Treatment options for various stages of heart failure. ACE = Angiotensin-converting enzyme; ARB = angiotensin-receptor blockers. Stage D (refractory symptoms requiring special interventions) is not shown.

mone. *Spironolactone* is a direct antagonist of aldosterone, thereby preventing salt retention, myocardial hypertrophy, and hypokalemia. *Spironolactone* therapy should be reserved for the most advanced cases of HF. Because *spironolactone* promotes potassium retention, patients should not be taking potassium supplements. Adverse effects include gastric disturbances, such as gastritis and peptic ulcer; central nervous system effects, such as lethargy and confusion; and endocrine abnormalities, such as gynecomastia, decreased libido, and menstrual irregularities.

IX. ORDER OF THERAPY

Experts have classified HF into four stages, from least severe to most severe. Figure 16.13 shows a treatment strategy using this classification and the drugs described in this chapter. Note that as the disease progresses, polytherapy is initiated.

In patients with overt heart failure, loop diuretics are often introduced first for relief of signs or symptoms of volume overload, such as dyspnea and peripheral edema. ACE inhibitors, or if not tolerated, ARBs are added after the optimization of diuretic therapy. Gradually titrate the dosage to that which is maximally tolerated and/or produces optimal cardiac output. β Blockers are initiated after the patient is stable on ACE inhibitors, again beginning at low doses with titration to optimal levels. *Digoxin* is initiated in patients who continue to have symptoms of heart failure despite the multiple drug therapy. For example, Figure 16.14 shows that treatment with *digoxin* plus a diuretic plus an ACE inhibitor in patients with HF is superior to treatment with diuretics alone or a diuretic plus either *digoxin* or an ACE inhibitor.

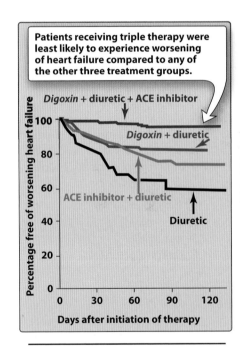

Figure 16.14
Use of multiple drugs in the treatment of heart failure. ACE = angiotensin-converting enzyme.

Study Questions

Choose the ONE best answer.

16.1 Digitalis has a profound effect on myocyte intracellular concentrations of Na^+, K^+, and Ca^{2+}. These effects are caused by digitalis inhibiting:

    A. Ca^{2+}–adenosine triphosphatose (ATPase) of the sarcoplasmic reticulum.
    B. Na^+/K^+-ATPase of the myocyte membrane.
    C. Cardiac phosphodiesterase.
    D. Cardiac β_1 receptors.
    E. Juxtaglomerular renin release.

Correct answer = B. The cardiac glycosides bind to and block the action of the Na^+/K^+-ATPase. This leads to increased intracellular sodium. The diminished sodium gradient results in less Ca^{2+} being extruded from the cell via the Na^+/Ca^{2+}-exchanger. Cardiac glycosides do not bind to the Ca^{2+}-ATPase. They have no direct effect on phosphodiesterase, β_1 receptors, or renin release.

16.2 Compensatory increases in heart rate and renin release that occur in heart failure may be alleviated by which of the following drugs?

    A. Milrinone.
    B. Digoxin.
    C. Dobutamine.
    D. Enalapril.
    E. Metoprolol.

Correct answer = E. Metoprolol, a β_1-selective antagonist, prevents the increased heart rate and renin release that result from sympathetic stimulation, which occurs as compensation for reduced cardiac output of heart failure. Enalapril is an ACE inhibitor that actually increases renin release. Dobutamine increases cardiac contractility but does not slow the heart rate or interfere with renin release. Digoxin decreases the heart rate because of its vagomimetic effects, but it does not decrease renin release.

16.3 A 58-year-old man is admitted to the hospital with acute heart failure and pulmonary edema. Which one of the following drugs would be most useful in treating the pulmonary edema?

    A. Digoxin.
    B. Dobutamine.
    C. Furosemide.
    D. Minoxidil.
    E. Spironolactone.

Correct answer = C. Furosemide has the ability to dilate vessels in the context of acute heart failure. It also mobilizes the edematous fluid and promotes its excretion. Dobutamine increases contractility but does not appreciably improve pulmonary edema. Digoxin acts too slowly and has no vasodilating effects. Minoxidil decreases arterial pressure and causes reflex tachycardia. Spironolactone does not alleviate acute pulmonary edema.

16.4 A 46-year-old man is admitted to the emergency department. He has taken more than 90 digoxin tablets (0.25 mg each), ingesting them about 3 hours before admission. His pulse is 50 to 60 beats per minute, and the electrocardiogram shows third-degree heart block. Which one of the following is the most important therapy to initiate in this patient?

    A. Digoxin immune Fab.
    B. Potassium salts.
    C. Lidocaine.
    D. Phenytoin.
    E. DC cardioversion.

Correct answer = A. In the severely poisoned patient, reduction of digoxin plasma concentrations is paramount and can be accomplished with administration of antidigoxin antibodies. Potassium concentrations, if low, can be increased, but not much greater than 4 mM. Antiarrhythmics are useful if there is need, but not in this case. DC cardioversion is used only if ventricular fibrillation occurs.

Antiarrhythmics

17

I. OVERVIEW

In contrast to skeletal muscle, which contracts only when it receives a stimulus, the heart contains specialized cells that exhibit automaticity; that is, they can intrinsically generate rhythmic action potentials in the absence of external stimuli. These "pacemaker" cells differ from other myocardial cells in showing a slow, spontaneous depolarization during diastole (Phase 4), caused by an inward positive current carried by sodium- and calcium-ion flows. This depolarization is fastest in the sinoatrial (SA) node (the normal initiation site of the action potential), and it decreases throughout the normal conduction pathway through the atrioventricular (AV) node to the bundle of His and the Purkinje system. Dysfunction of impulse generation or conduction at any of a number of sites in the heart can cause an abnormality in cardiac rhythm. Figure 17.1 summarizes the drugs used to treat cardiac arrhythmias.

II. INTRODUCTION TO THE ARRHYTHMIAS

The arrhythmias are conceptually simple—dysfunctions cause abnormalities in impulse formation and conduction in the myocardium. However, in the clinic, arrhythmias present as a complex family of disorders that show a variety of symptoms. For example, cardiac arrhythmias may cause the heart to beat too slowly (bradycardia) or to beat too rapidly (tachycardia), and to beat regularly (sinus tachycardia or sinus bradycardia) or irregularly (atrial fibrillation). The heart cavity from which the arrhythmia originates gives the name to the arrhythmia—atrial tachycardia for a rapid arrhythmia originating in the atria. Impulses originating from sites other than the SA node, or impulses traveling along accessory (extra) pathways that lead to deviant depolarizations (AV reentry, Wolff-Parkinson-White syndrome), may also trigger arrhythmias. To make sense of this large group of disorders, it is useful to organize the arrhythmias into groups according to the anatomic site of the abnormality—the atria, the AV node, or the ventricles. Figure 17.2 summarizes several commonly occurring atrial, AV junction, or ventricular arrhythmias. Although not shown here, each of these abnormalities can be further divided into subgroups depending on the electrocardiogram findings.

A. Causes of arrhythmias

Most arrhythmias arise either from aberrations in impulse generation (abnormal automaticity) or from a defect in impulse conduction.

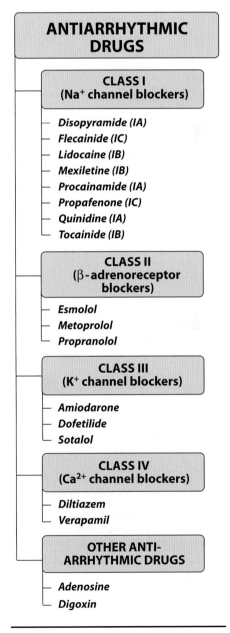

Figure 17.1
Summary of antiarrhythmic drugs.

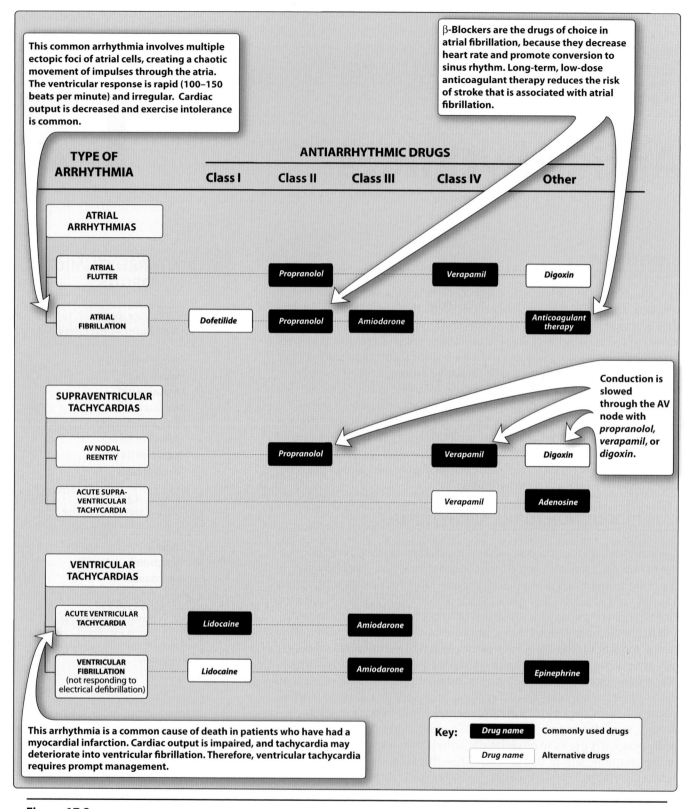

Figure 17.2
Therapeutic indications for some commonly encountered arrhythmias. AV = atrioventricular.

1. **Abnormal automaticity:** The SA node shows the fastest rate of Phase 4 depolarization and, therefore, exhibits a higher rate of discharge than that occurring in other pacemaker cells exhibiting automaticity. Thus, the SA node normally sets the pace of contraction for the myocardium, and latent pacemakers are depolarized by impulses coming from the SA node. However, if cardiac sites other than the SA node show enhanced automaticity, they may generate competing stimuli, and arrhythmias may arise. Abnormal automaticity may also occur if the myocardial cells are damaged (for example, by hypoxia or potassium imbalance). These cells may remain partially depolarized during diastole and, therefore, can reach the firing threshold earlier than normal cells. Abnormal automatic discharges may thus be induced.

2. **Effect of drugs on automaticity:** Most of the antiarrhythmic agents suppress automaticity by blocking either Na^+ or Ca^{2+} channels to reduce the ratio of these ions to K^+. This decreases the slope of Phase 4 (diastolic) depolarization and/or raises the threshold of discharge to a less negative voltage. Such drugs cause the frequency of discharge to decrease—an effect that is more pronounced in cells with ectopic pacemaker activity than in normal cells.

3. **Abnormalities in impulse conduction:** Impulses from higher pacemaker centers are normally conducted down pathways that bifurcate to activate the entire ventricular surface (Figure 17.3). A phenomenon called reentry can occur if a unidirectional block caused by myocardial injury or a prolonged refractory period results in an abnormal conduction pathway. Reentry is the most common cause of arrhythmias, and it can occur at any level of the cardiac conduction system. For example, consider a single Purkinje fiber with two conduction pathways to ventricular muscle. An impulse normally travels down both limbs of the conduction path. However, if myocardial injury results in a unidirectional block, the impulse may only be conducted down Pathway 1 (see Figure 17.3). If the block in Pathway 2 is in the forward direction only, the impulse may travel in a retrograde fashion through Pathway 2 and reenter the point of bifurcation. This short-circuit pathway results in reexcitation of the ventricular muscle, causing premature contraction or sustained ventricular arrhythmia.

4. **Effects of drugs on conduction abnormalities:** Antiarrhythmic agents prevent reentry by slowing conduction and/or increasing the refractory period, thereby converting a unidirectional block into a bidirectional block.

B. Antiarrhythmic drugs

As noted above, the antiarrhythmic drugs can modify impulse generation and conduction. More than a dozen such drugs that are potentially useful in treating arrhythmias are currently available. However, only a limited number of these agents are clinically beneficial in the treatment of selected arrhythmias. For example, the acute termination of ventricular tachycardia by *lidocaine* or of supraventricular tachycardia by *adenosine* or *verapamil* are examples in which antiarrhythmic therapy results in decreased morbidity. In contrast, many of the antiarrhythmic agents are now known to have dangerous proarrhythmic actions—that is, to cause

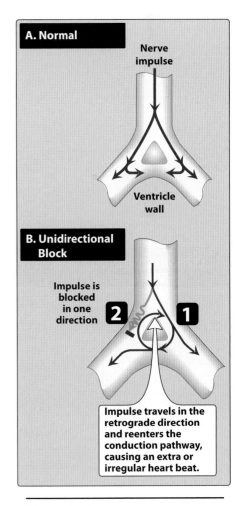

A. Normal
Nerve impulse
Ventricle wall

B. Unidirectional Block
Impulse is blocked in one direction
2   1
Impulse travels in the retrograde direction and reenters the conduction pathway, causing an extra or irregular heart beat.

Figure 17.3
Schematic representation of reentry.

arrhythmias. The efficacy of many antiarrhythmic agents remains unproven in placebo-controlled, random trials. [Note: Implantable cardioverter defibrillators are becoming more widely used to manage this condition.]

III. CLASS I ANTIARRHYTHMIC DRUGS

The antiarrhythmic drugs can be classified according to their predominant effects on the action potential (Figure 17.4). Although this classification is convenient, it is not entirely clear-cut, because many of the drugs have actions relating to more than one class or may have active metabolites with a different class of action. Class I antiarrhythmic drugs act by blocking voltage-sensitive sodium channels via the same mechanism as local anesthetics. The decreased rate of entry of sodium slows the rate of rise of Phase 0 of the action potential. [Note: At therapeutic doses, these drugs have little effect on the resting, fully polarized membrane because of their higher affinity for the active and inactive channels rather than for the resting channel.] Class I antiarrhythmic drugs, therefore, generally cause a decrease in excitability and conduction velocity. The use of sodium channel blockers has been declining continuously due to their possible proarrhythmic effects, particularly in patients with reduced left ventricular function and ischemic heart disease.

A. Use-dependence

Class I drugs bind more rapidly to open or inactivated sodium channels than to channels that are fully repolarized following recovery from the previous depolarization cycle. Therefore, these drugs show a greater degree of blockade in tissues that are frequently depolarizing (for example, during tachycardia, when the sodium channels open often). This property is called use-dependence (or state-dependence), and it enables these drugs to block cells that are discharging at an abnormally high frequency without interfering with the normal, low-frequency beating of the heart. The Class I drugs have been subdivided into three groups according to their effect on the duration of the action potential. Class IA agents slow the rate of rise of the action potential (thus slowing conduction), prolong the action potential, and increase the ventricular effective refractory period. They have an intermediate speed of asso-

CLASSIFICATION OF DRUG	MECHANISM OF ACTION	COMMENT
IA	Na⁺ channel blocker	Slows Phase 0 depolarization in ventricular muscle fibers
IB	Na⁺ channel blocker	Shortens Phase 3 repolarization in ventricular muscle fibers
IC	Na⁺ channel blocker	Markedly slows Phase 0 depolarization in ventricular muscle fibers
II	β-Adrenoreceptor blocker	Inhibits Phase 4 depolarization in SA and AV nodes
III	K⁺ channel blocker	Prolongs Phase 3 repolarization in ventricular muscle fibers
IV	Ca²⁺ channel blocker	Inhibits action potential in SA and AV nodes

Figure 17.4
Actions of antiarrhythmic drugs.

ciation with activated/inactivated sodium-channels and an intermediate rate of dissociation from resting channels. Prolongation of duration of the action potential and increased ventricular effective period are due to concomitant Class III activity. Class IB drugs have little effect on the rate of depolarization; rather, they decrease the duration of the action potential by shortening repolarization. They rapidly interact with sodium channels. Class IC agents markedly depress the rate of rise of the membrane action potential. Therefore, they cause marked slowing of conduction but have little effect on the duration of the membrane action potential or the ventricular effective refractory period. They bind slowly to sodium channels.

B. Arrhythmias

Inhibition of potassium channels (Class III activity) widens the action potential, leading to a prolonged QT interval on the electrocardiogram. Such an effect is associated with increased risk of developing life-threatening ventricular tachyarrhythmias (torsades de pointes). The most common cause of QT prolongation is drug-induced, although it may also be genetic. QT prolongation is not only seen with Class III antiarrhythmics. Drugs such as *cisapride, grepafloxacin, terfenadine,* and *astemizole* were withdrawn from the market because of severe and fatal arrhythmias. *Erythromycin, clarithromycin, pentamidine, moxifloxacin, levofloxacin, imipramine, desipramine, amitriptyline, doxepin, thioridazine, mesoridazine, haloperidol, risperidone, ziprasidone,* and *quetiapine* are some of the drugs known to prolong the QT interval. Caution should be exerted when combining several drugs with effects on the QT interval (for example, *quinidine* with *levofloxacin*) or when giving these drugs combined with azole antifungals (*fluconazole* and *itraconazole*). The latter are known to inhibit drug metabolism, leading to large increases in plasma drug concentrations.

C. Quinidine

Quinidine [KWIN-i-deen] is the prototype Class IA drug. Because of its concomitant Class III activity, it can actually precipitate arrhythmias such as polymorphic ventricular tachycardia (torsades de pointes), which can degenerate into ventricular fibrillation. Because of the toxic potential of *quinidine,* calcium antagonists, such as *amiodarone* and *verapamil,* are increasingly replacing this drug in clinical use.

1. **Mechanism of action:** *Quinidine* binds to open and inactivated sodium channels and prevents sodium influx, thus slowing the rapid upstroke during Phase 0 (Figure 17.5). It also decreases the slope of Phase 4 spontaneous depolarization and inhibits potassium channels.

2. **Therapeutic uses:** *Quinidine* is used in the treatment of a wide variety of arrhythmias, including atrial, AV-junctional, and ventricular tachyarrhythmias. *Quinidine* is used to maintain sinus rhythm after direct-current cardioversion of atrial flutter or fibrillation and to prevent frequent ventricular tachycardia.

3. **Pharmacokinetics:** *Quinidine sulfate* is rapidly and almost completely absorbed after oral administration. It undergoes extensive metabolism by the hepatic cytochrome P450 enzymes, forming active metabolites.

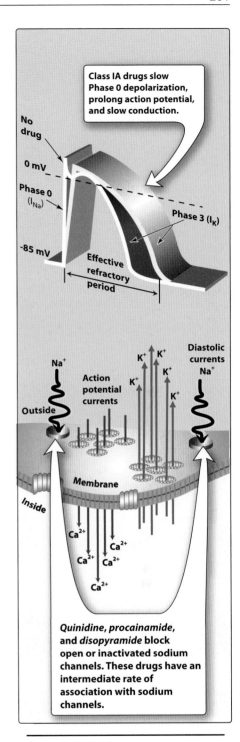

Figure 17.5
Schematic diagram of the effects of Class IA agents. I_{Na} and I_K are transmembrane currents due to the movement of Na^+ and K^+, respectively.

4. **Adverse effects:** A potential adverse effect of *quinidine* (or of any antiarrhythmic drug) is development of arrhythmia (torsades de pointes). *Quinidine* may cause SA and AV block or asystole. At toxic levels, the drug may induce ventricular tachycardia. Cardiotoxic effects are exacerbated by hyperkalemia. Nausea, vomiting, and diarrhea are commonly observed. Large doses of *quinidine* may induce the symptoms of cinchonism (for example, blurred vision, tinnitus, headache, disorientation, and psychosis). The drug has a mild α-adrenergic blocking action as well as an *atropine*-like effect. *Quinidine* can increase the steady-state concentration of *digoxin* by displacement of *digoxin* from tissue-binding sites (minor effect) and by decreasing *digoxin* renal clearance (major effect).

D. Procainamide

1. **Actions:** This Class IA drug, a derivative of the local anesthetic *procaine*, shows actions similar to those of *quinidine*.

2. **Pharmacokinetics:** *Procainamide* [proe-KANE-a-mide] is well-absorbed following oral administration. [Note: The intravenous route is rarely used, because hypotension occurs if the drug is infused too rapidly.] *Procainamide* has a relatively short half-life of 2 to 3 hours. A portion of the drug is acetylated in the liver to N-acetylprocainamide (NAPA), which has little effect on the maximum polarization of Purkinje fibers but prolongs the duration of the action potential. Thus, NAPA has properties of a Class III drug. NAPA is eliminated via the kidney, and dosages of *procainamide* may need to be adjusted in patients with renal failure.

3. **Adverse effects:** With chronic use, *procainamide* causes a high incidence of side effects, including a reversible lupus erythematosus–like syndrome that develops in 25 to 30 percent of patients. Toxic concentrations of *procainamide* may cause asystole or induction of ventricular arrhythmias. Central nervous system (CNS) side effects include depression, hallucination, and psychosis. With this drug, gastrointestinal intolerance is less frequent than with *quinidine*.

E. Disopyramide

1. **Actions:** This Class IA drug shows actions similar to those of *quinidine*. *Disopyramide* [dye-soe-PEER-a-mide] produces a negative inotropic effect that is greater than the weak effect exerted by *quinidine* and *procainamide*, and unlike the latter drugs, *disopyramide* causes peripheral vasoconstriction. The drug may produce a clinically important decrease in myocardial contractility in patients with preexisting impairment of left ventricular function. *Disopyramide* is used in the treatment of ventricular arrhythmias as an alternative to *procainamide* or *quinidine*. Like *procainamide* and *quinidine*, it also has Class III activity.

2. **Pharmacokinetics:** Approximately half of the orally ingested drug is excreted unchanged by the kidneys. Approximately 30 percent of the drug is converted by the liver to the less active mono-N-dealkylated metabolite.

3. **Adverse effects:** *Disopyramide* shows effects of anticholinergic activity (for example, dry mouth, urinary retention, blurred vision, and constipation).

F. Lidocaine

Lidocaine [LYE-doe-kane] is a Class IB drug. The Class IB agents rapidly associate and dissociate from sodium channels. Thus, the actions of Class IB agents are manifested when the cardiac cell is depolarized or firing rapidly. Class IB drugs are particularly useful in treating ventricular arrhythmias. *Lidocaine* was the drug of choice for emergency treatment of cardiac arrhythmias.

1. **Actions:** *Lidocaine*, a local anesthetic, shortens Phase 3 repolarization and decreases the duration of the action potential (Figure 17.6).

2. **Therapeutic uses:** *Lidocaine* is useful in treating ventricular arrhythmias arising during myocardial ischemia, such as that experienced during a myocardial infarction. The drug does not markedly slow conduction and, thus, has little effect on atrial or AV junction arrhythmias.

3. **Pharmacokinetics:** *Lidocaine* is given intravenously because of extensive first-pass transformation by the liver, which precludes oral administration. The drug is dealkylated and eliminated almost entirely by the liver; consequently, dosage adjustment may be necessary in patients with liver dysfunction or those taking drugs that lower hepatic blood flow, such as *propranolol*.

4. **Adverse effects:** *Lidocaine* has a fairly wide toxic-to-therapeutic ratio. It shows little impairment of left ventricular function and has no negative inotropic effect. CNS effects include drowsiness, slurred speech, paresthesia, agitation, confusion, and convulsions. Cardiac arrhythmias may also occur.

G. Mexiletine and tocainide

These Class IB drugs have actions similar to those of *lidocaine*, and they can be administered orally. *Mexiletine* [MEX-i-le-teen] is used for chronic treatment of ventricular arrhythmias associated with previous myocardial infarction. *Tocainide* [toe-KAY-nide] is used for treatment of ventricular tachyarrhythmias. *Tocainide* has pulmonary toxicity, which may lead to pulmonary fibrosis.

H. Flecainide

Flecainide [FLEK-a-nide] is a Class IC drug. These drugs slowly dissociate from resting sodium channels, and they show prominent effects even at normal heart rates. They are approved for refractory ventricular arrhythmias and for the prevention of paroxysmal atrial fibrillation/flutter associated with disabling symptoms and paroxysmal supraventricular tachycardia. However, recent data have cast serious doubts on the safety of the Class IC drugs.

1. **Actions:** *Flecainide* suppresses Phase 0 upstroke in Purkinje and myocardial fibers (Figure 17.7). This causes marked slowing of con-

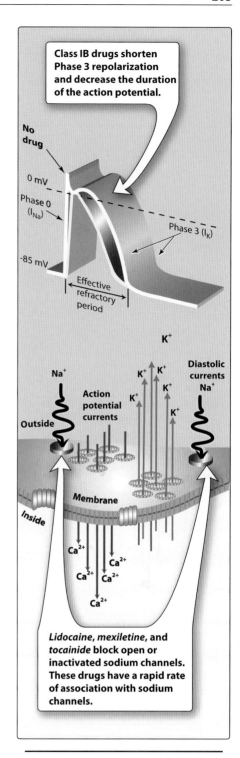

Figure 17.6
Schematic diagram of the effects of Class IB agents. I_{Na} and I_K are transmembrane currents due to the movement of Na^+ and K^+, respectively.

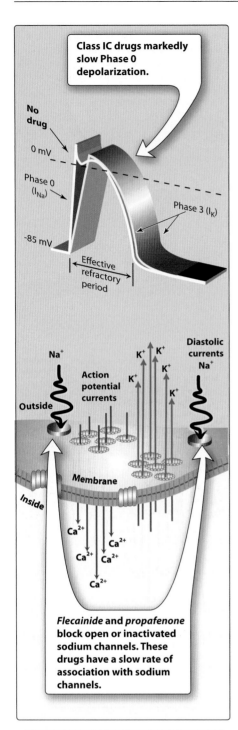

Class IC drugs markedly slow Phase 0 depolarization.

No drug

0 mV

Phase 0 (I$_{Na}$)

Phase 3 (I$_K$)

−85 mV

Effective refractory period

Na$^+$

K$^+$ K$^+$

K$^+$

Diastolic currents Na$^+$

Action potential currents

K$^+$

Outside

K$^+$

Membrane

Inside

Ca^{2+}

Ca^{2+}

Ca^{2+} Ca^{2+}

Ca^{2+}

Flecainide and *propafenone* block open or inactivated sodium channels. These drugs have a slow rate of association with sodium channels.

Figure 17.7
Schematic diagram of the effects of Class IC agents. I$_{Na}$ and I$_K$ are transmembrane currents due to the movement of Na$^+$ and K$^+$, respectively.

duction in all cardiac tissue, with a minor effect on the duration of the action potential and refractoriness. Automaticity is reduced by an increase in the threshold potential rather than a decrease in the slope of Phase 4 depolarization.

2. **Therapeutic uses:** *Flecainide* is useful in treating refractory ventricular arrhythmias. It is particularly useful in suppressing premature ventricular contraction. *Flecainide* has a negative inotropic effect and can aggravate congestive heart failure.

3. **Pharmacokinetics:** *Flecainide* is absorbed orally, undergoes minimal biotransformation, and has a half-life of 16 to 20 hours.

4. **Adverse effects:** *Flecainide* can cause dizziness, blurred vision, headache, and nausea. Like other Class IC drugs, *flecainide* can aggravate preexisting arrhythmias or induce life-threatening ventricular tachycardia that is resistant to treatment.

I. Propafenone

This Class IC drug shows actions similar to those of *flecainide*. *Propafenone* [proe-pa-FEEN-one], like *flecainide*, slows conduction in all cardiac tissues and is considered to be a broad-spectrum antiarrhythmic agent.

IV. CLASS II ANTIARRHYTHMIC DRUGS

Class II agents are β-adrenergic antagonists. These drugs diminish Phase 4 depolarization, thus depressing automaticity, prolonging AV conduction, and decreasing heart rate and contractility. Class II agents are useful in treating tachyarrhythmias caused by increased sympathetic activity. They are also used for atrial flutter and fibrillation and for AV-nodal reentrant tachycardia. [Note: In contrast to the sodium-channel blockers, β-blockers and Class III compounds, such as *sotalol* and *amiodarone*, are increasing in use.]

A. Propranolol

Propranolol [pro-PRAN-oh-lol] reduces the incidence of sudden arrhythmic death after myocardial infarction (the most common cause of death in this group of patients). The mortality rate in the first year after a heart attack is significantly reduced by *propranolol*, partly because of its ability to prevent ventricular arrhythmias.

B. Metoprolol

Metoprolol [me-TOE-pro-lol] is the β-adrenergic antagonist most widely used in the treatment of cardiac arrhythmias. Compared to propranolol, it reduces the risk of bronchospasm.

C. Esmolol

Esmolol [ESS-moe-lol] is a very short-acting β-blocker used for intravenous administration in acute arrhythmias that occur during surgery or emergency situations.

V. CLASS III ANTIARRHYTHMIC DRUGS

Class III agents block potassium channels and, thus, diminish the outward potassium current during repolarization of cardiac cells. These agents prolong the duration of the action potential without altering Phase 0 of depolarization or the resting membrane potential (Figure 17.8). Instead, they prolong the effective refractory period. All Class III drugs have the potential to induce arrhythmias.

A. Amiodarone

1. **Actions:** *Amiodarone* [a-MEE-oh-da-rone] contains iodine and is related structurally to thyroxine. It has complex effects, showing Class I, II, III, and IV actions. Its dominant effect is prolongation of the action potential duration and the refractory period. *Amiodarone* has antianginal as well as antiarrhythmic activity.

2. **Therapeutic uses:** *Amiodarone* is effective in the treatment of severe refractory supraventricular and ventricular tachyarrhythmias. Despite its side-effect profile, *amiodarone* is the most commonly employed antiarrhythmic.

3. **Pharmacokinetics:** *Amiodarone* is incompletely absorbed after oral administration. The drug is unusual in having a prolonged half-life of several weeks, and it distributes extensively in adipose issue. Full clinical effects may not be achieved until 6 weeks after initiation of treatment.

4. **Adverse effects:** *Amiodarone* shows a variety of toxic effects. After long-term use, more than half of patients receiving the drug show side effects that are severe enough to prompt its discontinuation. However, use of low doses reduces toxicity, while retaining clinical efficacy. Some of the more common effects include interstitial pulmonary fibrosis, gastrointestinal tract intolerance, tremor, ataxia, dizziness, hyper- or hypothyroidism, liver toxicity, photosensitivity, neuropathy, muscle weakness, and blue skin discoloration caused by iodine accumulation in the skin. As noted earlier, recent clinical trials have shown that *amiodarone* does not reduce the incidence of sudden death or prolong survival in patients with congestive heart failure.

B. Sotalol

Sotalol [SOE-ta-lol], although a class III antiarrhythmic agent, also has potent nonselective β-blocker activity. It is well established that β-blockers reduce mortality associated with acute myocardial infarction.

1. **Actions:** *Sotalol* blocks a rapid outward potassium current, known as the delayed rectifier. This blockade prolongs both repolarization and duration of the action potential, thus lengthening the effective refractory period.

2. **Therapeutic uses:** β-Blockers are used for long-term therapy to decrease the rate of sudden death following an acute myocardial infarction. β-Blockers have a modest ability to suppress ectopic beats and to reduce myocardial oxygen demand. They have strong antifibrillatory effects, particularly in the ischemic myocardium. *Sotalol* was more effective in preventing recurrence of arrhythmia and in decreasing mortality than *imipramine*, *mexiletine*, *procainamide*, *propafenone*, and *quinidine* in patients with sustained ventricular tachycardia (Figure 17.9).

3. **Adverse effects:** This drug also has the lowest rate of acute or long-term adverse effects. As with all drugs that prolong the QT interval,

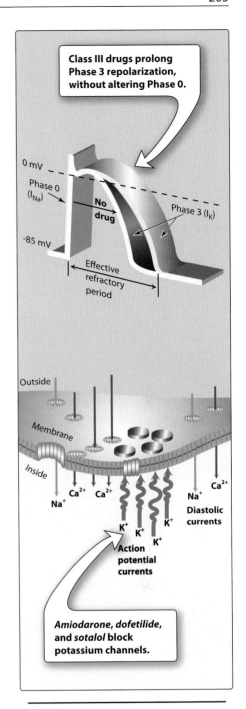

Figure 17.8
Schematic diagram of the effects of Class III agents. I_{Na} and I_K are transmembrane currents due to the movement of Na^+ and K^+, respectively.

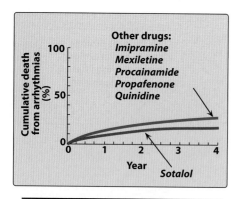

Figure 17.9
Comparison of *sotalol* with six other drugs with respect to deaths due to cardiac arrhythmias.

the syndrome of torsade de pointes is a serious potential adverse effect, typically seen in three to four percent of patients.

C. Dofetilide

Dofetilide [doh-FET-il-ide] can be used as a first-line antiarrhythmic agent in patients with persistent atrial fibrillation and heart failure or in those with coronary artery disease with impaired left ventricular function. Because of the risk of proarrhythmia, *dofetilide* initiation is limited to the inpatient setting and is restricted to prescribers who have completed a specific manufacturer's training session. Along with *amiodarone* and β-blockers, *dofetilide* is the only antiarrhythmic drug that is recommended by experts for the treatment of atrial fibrillation in a wide range of patients. The half-life is 10 hours. Excretion is in the urine, with 80 percent as unchanged drug and 20 percent as inactive or minimally active metabolites.

VI. CLASS IV ANTIARRHYTHMIC DRUGS

Class IV drugs are calcium-channel blockers (see p. 223). They decrease the inward current carried by calcium, resulting in a decreased rate of Phase 4 spontaneous depolarization. They also slow conduction in tissues that are dependent on calcium currents, such as the AV node (Figure 17.10). Although voltage-sensitive calcium channels occur in many different tissues, the major effect of calcium-channel blockers is on vascular smooth muscle and the heart.

A. Verapamil and diltiazem

Verapamil [ver-AP-a-mil] shows greater action on the heart than on vascular smooth muscle, whereas *nifedipine*, a calcium-channel blocker used to treat hypertension (see p. 223), exerts a stronger effect on the vascular smooth muscle than on the heart. *Diltiazem* [dil-TYE-a-zem] is intermediate in its actions.

1. **Actions:** Calcium enters cells by voltage-sensitive channels and by receptor-operated channels that are controlled by the binding of agonists, such as catecholamines, to membrane receptors. Calcium-channel blockers, such as *verapamil* and *diltiazem*, are more effective against the voltage-sensitive channels, causing a decrease in the slow inward current that triggers cardiac contraction. *Verapamil* and *diltiazem* bind only to open, depolarized channels, thus preventing repolarization until the drug dissociates from the channel. These drugs are therefore use-dependent; that is, they block most effectively when the heart is beating rapidly, because in a normally paced heart, the calcium channels have time to repolarize and the bound drug dissociates from the channel before the next conduction pulse. By decreasing the inward current carried by calcium, *verapamil* and *diltiazem* slow conduction and prolong the effective refractory period in tissues that are dependent on calcium currents, such as the AV node. These drugs are therefore effective in treating arrhythmias that must traverse calcium-dependent cardiac tissues.

2. **Therapeutic uses:** *Verapamil* and *diltiazem* are more effective against atrial than against ventricular arrhythmias. They are useful in treating reentrant supraventricular tachycardia and in reducing

the ventricular rate in atrial flutter and fibrillation. In addition, these drugs are used to treat hypertension and angina.

3. **Pharmacokinetics:** *Verapamil* and *diltiazem* are absorbed after oral administration. *Verapamil* is extensively metabolized by the liver; thus, care should be taken when administering this drug to patients with hepatic dysfunction.

4. **Adverse effects:** *Verapamil* and *diltiazem* have negative inotropic properties and, therefore, may be contraindicated in patients with preexisting depressed cardiac function. Both drugs can also produce a decrease in blood pressure because of peripheral vasodilation—an effect that is actually beneficial in treating hypertension.

VII. OTHER ANTIARRHYTHMIC DRUGS

A. Digoxin

Digoxin [di-JOX-in] shortens the refractory period in atrial and ventricular myocardial cells while prolonging the effective refractory period and diminishing conduction velocity in the AV node. *Digoxin* is used to control the ventricular response rate in atrial fibrillation and flutter. At toxic concentrations, *digoxin* causes ectopic ventricular beats that may result in ventricular tachycardia and fibrillation. [Note: This arrhythmia is usually treated with *lidocaine* or *phenytoin*.]

B. Adenosine

Adenosine [ah-DEN-oh-zeen] is a naturally occurring nucleoside, but at high doses, the drug decreases conduction velocity, prolongs the refractory period, and decreases automaticity in the AV node. Intravenous *adenosine* is the drug of choice for abolishing acute supraventricular tachycardia. It has low toxicity but causes flushing, chest pain, and hypotension. *Adenosine* has an extremely short duration of action (approximately 15 seconds).

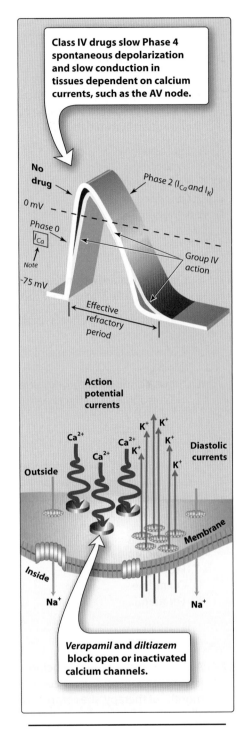

Figure 17.10
Schematic diagram of the effects of Class IV agents. I_{Ca} and I_K are transmembrane currents due to the movement of Ca^{2+} and K^+, respectively.

Study Questions

Choose the ONE best answer.

17.1 A 66-year-old man had a myocardial infarct. Which one of the following would be appropriate prophylactic antiarrhythmic therapy?

A. Lidocaine.
B. Metoprolol.
C. Procainamide.
D. Quinidine.
E. Verapamil.

Correct answer = B. β-Blockers, such as metoprolol, prevent cardiac arrhythmias that occur subsequent to a myocardial infarction. None of the other drugs has been shown to be particularly effective in preventing postinfarct arrhythmias.

17.2 Suppression of arrhythmias resulting from a reentry focus is most likely to occur if the drug:

A. Has vagomimetic effects on the AV node.
B. Is a β-blocker.
C. Converts a unidirectional block to a bidirectional block.
D. Slows conduction through the atria.
E. Has atropine-like effects on the AV node.

Correct answer = C. Current theory holds that a reentrant arrhythmia is caused by damaged heart muscle so that conduction is slowed through the damaged area in only one direction. A drug that prevents conduction in either direction through the damaged area interrupts the reentrant arrhythmia. Class I antiarrhythmics, such as lidocaine, are capable of producing bidirectional block. The other choices do not have any direct effects on the direction of blockade of conduction through damaged cardiac muscle.

17.3 A 57-year-old man is being treated for an atrial arrhythmia. He complains of headache, dizziness, and tinnitus. Which one of the following antiarrhythmic drugs is the most likely cause?

A. Amiodarone.
B. Procainamide.
C. Propranolol.
D. Quinidine.
E. Verapamil.

Correct answer = D. The clustered symptoms of headache, dizziness, and tinnitus are characteristic of cinchonism, which is caused by quinidine. The other drugs have characteristic adverse effects, but not this particular group of effects.

17.4 A 58-year-old woman is being treated for chronic suppression of a ventricular arrhythmia. After 2 months of therapy, she complains about feeling tired all the time. Examination reveals a resting heart rate of 10 beats per minute lower than her previous rate. Her skin is cool and clammy. Laboratory test results indicate low thyroxin and elevated thyroid-stimulating hormone levels. Which of the following antiarrhythmic drugs is the likely cause of these signs and symptoms?

A. Amiodarone.
B. Procainamide.
C. Propranolol.
D. Quinidine.
E. Verapamil.

Correct answer = A. The patient is exhibiting symptoms of hypothyroidism, which is often associated with amiodarone therapy. Propranolol could slow the heart but would not produce the changes in thyroid function. None of the other antiarrhythmics is likely to cause hypothyroidism.

Antianginal Drugs

18

I. OVERVIEW

Angina pectoris is a characteristic sudden, severe, pressing chest pain radiating to the neck, jaw, back, and arms. It is caused by coronary blood flow that is insufficient to meet the oxygen demands of the myocardium, leading to ischemia. The imbalance between oxygen delivery and utilization may result during exertion, from a spasm of the vascular smooth muscle, or from obstruction of blood vessels caused by atherosclerotic lesions. These transient episodes (15 seconds to 15 minutes) of myocardial ischemia do not cause cellular death, such as occurs in myocardial infarction. Three classes of drugs, used either alone or in combination, are effective in treating patients with stable angina: organic nitrates, β-blockers, and calcium-channel blockers (Figure 18.1). These agents lower the oxygen demand of the heart by affecting blood pressure, venous return, heart rate, and contractility. Lifestyle and risk factor modifications, especially cessation of smoking, are also important in the treatment of angina. [Note: Options other than medications for treating angina include angioplasty and coronary artery bypass surgery.]

II. TYPES OF ANGINA

Angina pectoris has three overlapping patterns: 1) stable or typical angina, 2) unstable angina, and 3) Prinzmetal's or variant angina. They are caused by varying combinations of increased myocardial demand and decreased myocardial perfusion.

A. Stable angina

Stable angina is the most common form of angina and, therefore, is called typical angina pectoris. It is characterized by a burning, heavy, or squeezing feeling in the chest. It is caused by the reduction of coronary perfusion due to a fixed obstruction produced by coronary atherosclerosis. The heart becomes vulnerable to ischemia whenever there is increased demand, such as that produced by physical activity, emotional excitement, or any other cause of increased cardiac workload. Typical angina pectoris is promptly relieved by rest or *nitroglycerin* (a vasodilator).

B. Unstable angina

Unstable angina lies between stable angina on the one hand and myocardial infarction on the other. In unstable angina, chest pains occur with increased frequency and are precipitated by progres-

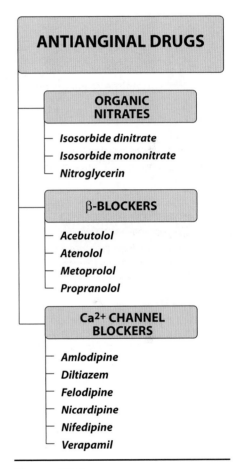

Figure 18.1
Summary of antianginal drugs.

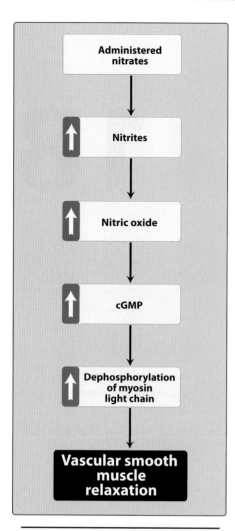

Figure 18.2
Effects of nitrates and nitrites on smooth muscle. cGMP = cyclic guanosine 3', 5'-monophosphate.

sively less effort. The symptoms are not relieved by rest or *nitroglycerin*. Unstable angina requires hospital admission and more aggressive therapy to prevent death and progression to myocardial infarction.

C. Prinzmetal's or variant or vasospastic angina

Prinzmetal's angina is an uncommon pattern of episodic angina that occurs at rest and is due to coronary artery spasm. Symptoms are caused by decreased blood flow to the heart muscle due to spasm of the coronary artery. Although individuals with this form of angina may have significant coronary atherosclerosis, the angina attacks are unrelated to physical activity, heart rate, or blood pressure. Prinzmetal's angina generally responds promptly to coronary vasodilators, such as *nitroglycerin* and calcium-channel blockers.

D. Mixed forms of angina

Patients with advanced coronary artery disease may present with angina episodes during effort as well as at rest, suggesting the presence of a fixed obstruction associated with endothelial dysfunction.

III. ORGANIC NITRATES

Organic nitrates (and nitrites) used in the treatment of angina pectoris are simple nitric and nitrous acid esters of glycerol. They differ in their volatility. For example, *isosorbide dinitrate* and *isosorbide mononitrate* are solids at room temperature, *nitroglycerin* is only moderately volatile, and *amyl nitrite* is extremely volatile. These compounds cause a rapid reduction in myocardial oxygen demand, followed by rapid relief of symptoms. They are effective in stable and unstable angina as well as in variant angina pectoris.

A. Mechanism of action

Nitrates decrease coronary vasoconstriction or spasm and increase perfusion of the myocardium by relaxing coronary arteries. In addition, they relax veins, decreasing preload and myocardial oxygen consumption. Organic nitrates, such as *nitroglycerin* [nye-troe-GLIS-er-in], which is also known as *glyceryl trinitrate*, are thought to relax vascular smooth muscle by their intracellular conversion to nitrite ions, and then to nitric oxide, which in turn activates guanylate cyclase and increases the cells' cyclic guanosine monophosphate (GMP).[1] Elevated cGMP ultimately leads to dephosphorylation of the myosin light chain, resulting in vascular smooth muscle relaxation (Figure 18.2).

B. Effects on the cardiovascular system

All these agents are effective, but they differ in their onset of action and rate of elimination. For prompt relief of an ongoing attack of angina precipitated by exercise or emotional stress, sublingual (or spray form) *nitroglycerin* is the drug of choice. At therapeutic doses, *nitroglycerin* has two major effects. First, it causes dilation of the large veins, resulting in pooling of blood in the veins. This diminishes preload (venous return to the heart) and reduces the work of the heart. Second, *nitroglycerin* dilates the coronary vasculature, providing an increased blood supply to the heart muscle. *Nitroglycerin* decreases myocardial oxygen consumption because of decreased cardiac work.

 [1]See p. 150 in *Lippincott's Illustrated Reviews: Biochemistry* (4th ed.) for a discussion of the role of nitric oxide in cyclic GMP production.

C. Pharmacokinetics

The time to onset of action varies from 1 minute for *nitroglycerin* to more than 1 hour for *isosorbide mononitrate* (Figure 18.3). Significant first-pass metabolism of *nitroglycerin* occurs in the liver. Therefore, it is common to take the drug either sublingually or via a transdermal patch, thereby avoiding this route of elimination. *Isosorbide mononitrate* owes its improved bioavailability and long duration of action to its stability against hepatic breakdown. Oral *isosorbide dinitrate* undergoes denitration to two mononitrates, both of which possess antianginal activity.

D. Adverse effects

The most common adverse effect of *nitroglycerin*, as well as of the other nitrates, is headache. From 30 to 60 percent of patients receiving intermittent nitrate therapy with long-acting agents develop headaches. High doses of organic nitrates can also cause postural hypotension, facial flushing, and tachycardia. *Sildenafil* potentiates the action of the nitrates. To preclude the dangerous hypotension that may occur, this combination is contraindicated.

E. Tolerance

Tolerance to the actions of nitrates develops rapidly. The blood vessels become desensitized to vasodilation. Tolerance can be overcome by providing a daily "nitrate-free interval" to restore sensitivity to the drug. This interval is typically 10 to 12 hours, usually at night, because demand on the heart is decreased at that time. *Nitroglycerin* patches are worn for 12 hours then removed for 12 hours. However, variant angina worsens early in the morning, perhaps due to circadian catecholamine surges. Therefore, the nitrate-free interval in these patients should occur in the late afternoon. Patients who continue to have angina despite nitrate therapy may benefit by addition of another class of agent.

IV. β-ADRENERGIC BLOCKERS

The β-adrenergic–blocking agents decrease the oxygen demands of the myocardium by lowering both the rate and the force of contraction of the heart (see p. 86). They suppress the activation of the heart by blocking β₁ receptors, and they reduce the work of the heart by decreasing heart rate, contractility, cardiac output, and blood pressure. With β-blockers, the demand for oxygen by the myocardium is reduced both during exertion and at rest. *Propranolol* is the prototype for this class of compounds, but it is not cardioselective. Thus, other β-blockers, such as *metoprolol* or *atenolol*, are preferred. [Note: All β-blockers are nonselective at high doses and can inhibit β₂ receptors. This is particularly important to remember in the case of asthmatics.] Agents with intrinsic sympathomimetic activity (for example, *pindolol*) are less effective and should be avoided in angina. The β-blockers reduce the frequency and severity of angina attacks. These agents are particularly useful in the treatment of patients with myocardial infarction and have been shown to prolong survival. The β-blockers can be used with nitrates to increase exercise duration and tolerance. They are, however, contraindicated in patients with asthma, diabetes, severe bradycardia, peripheral vascular disease, or chronic obstructive pulmonary disease. [Note: It is important not to discontinue β-blocker therapy abruptly. The dose should be gradually tapered off over 5 to 10 days to avoid rebound angina or hypertension.]

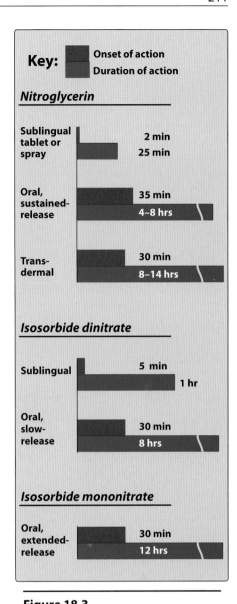

Figure 18.3
Time to peak effect and duration of action for some common organic nitrate preparations.

V. CALCIUM-CHANNEL BLOCKERS

Calcium is essential for muscular contraction. Calcium influx is increased in ischemia because of the membrane depolarization that hypoxia produces. In turn, this promotes the activity of several adenosine triphosphate–consuming enzymes, thereby depleting energy stores and worsening the ischemia. The calcium-channel blockers protect the tissue by inhibiting the entrance of calcium into cardiac and smooth muscle cells of the coronary and systemic arterial beds. All calcium-channel blockers are therefore arteriolar vasodilators that cause a decrease in smooth muscle tone and vascular resistance. (See p. 206 for a description of the mechanism of action for this group of drugs.) At clinical doses, these agents affect primarily the resistance of vascular smooth muscle and the myocardium. [Note: *Verapamil* mainly affects the myocardium, whereas *nifedipine* exerts a greater effect on smooth muscle in the peripheral vasculature. *Diltiazem* is intermediate in its actions.] All calcium-channel blockers lower blood pressure. They may worsen heart failure due to their negative inotropic effect. [Note: Variant angina caused by spontaneous coronary spasm (either at work or at rest; Figure 18.4) rather than by increased myocardial oxygen requirement is controlled by organic nitrates or calcium-channel blockers; β-blockers are contraindicated.]

A. Nifedipine

Nifedipine [nye-FED-i-peen], a dihydropyridine derivative, functions mainly as an arteriolar vasodilator. This drug has minimal effect on cardiac conduction or heart rate. Other members of this class, *amlodipine*, *nicardipine*, and *felodipine*, have similar cardiovascular characteristics except for *amlodipine*, which does not affect heart rate or cardiac output. *Nifedipine* is administered orally, usually as extended-release tablets. It undergoes hepatic metabolism to products that are eliminated in both urine and the feces. The vasodilation effect of *nifedipine* is useful in the treatment of variant angina caused by spontaneous coronary spasm. *Nifedipine* can cause flushing, headache, hypotension, and peripheral edema as side effects of its vasodilation activity. As with all calcium-channel blockers, constipation is a problem. Because it has little to no sympathetic antagonistic action, *nifedipine* may cause reflex tachycardia if peripheral vasodilation is marked. [Note: The general consensus is that short-acting dihydropyridines should be avoided in coronary artery disease.]

B. Verapamil

The diphenylalkylamine *verapamil* [ver-AP-a-mil] slows cardiac atrioventricular (AV) conduction directly, and decreases heart rate, contractility, blood pressure, and oxygen demand. *Verapamil* causes greater negative inotropic effects than *nifedipine*, but it is a weaker vasodilator. The drug is extensively metabolized by the liver; therefore, care must be taken to adjust the dose in patients with liver dysfunction. *Verapamil* is contraindicated in patients with preexisting depressed cardiac function or AV conduction abnormalities. It also causes constipation. *Verapamil* should be used with caution in patients taking *digoxin*, because *verapamil* increases *digoxin* levels.

C. Diltiazem

Diltiazem [dil-TYE-a-zem] has cardiovascular effects that are similar to those of *verapamil*. Both drugs slow AV conduction and decrease the rate of firing of the sinus node pacemaker. *Diltiazem* reduces the heart

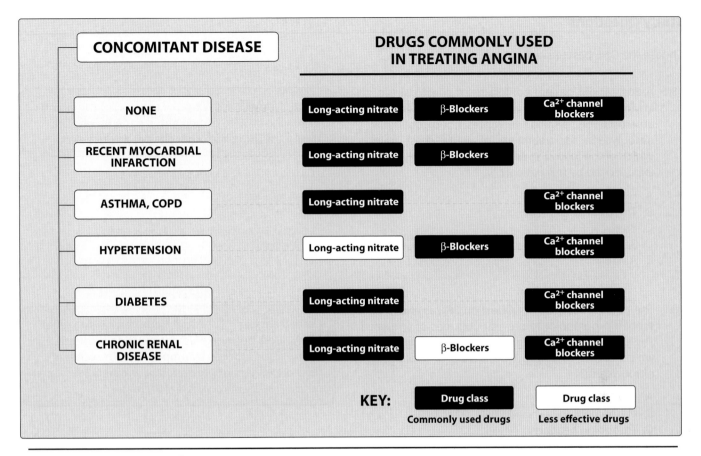

Figure 18.5
Treatment of angina in patients with concomitant diseases. COPD = chronic obstructive pulmonary disease.

rate, although to a lesser extent than *verapamil*, and also decreases blood pressure. In addition, *diltiazem* can relieve coronary artery spasm and, therefore, is particularly useful in patients with variant angina. It is extensively metabolized by the liver. The incidence of adverse side effects is low (the same as those for other calcium-channel blockers). Interactions with other drugs are the same as those indicated for *verapamil*.

Figure 18.5 summarizes the treatment of angina in patients with concomitant diseases.

Study Questions

Choose the ONE best answer.

18.1 A 56-year-old patient complains of chest pain fol-
      lowing any sustained exercise. He is diagnosed with
      atherosclerotic angina. He is prescribed sublingual
      nitroglycerin for treatment of acute chest pain.
      Which of the following adverse effects is likely to be
      experienced by this patient?

      A. Hypertension.
      B. Throbbing headache.
      C. Bradycardia.
      D. Sexual dysfunction.
      E. Anemia.

> Correct answer = B. Nitroglycerin causes throbbing
> headache in 30 to 60 percent of patients who are
> taking the drug. The other choices are incorrect.

18.2 The patient described in Question 18.1 is also pre-
      scribed propranolol to prevent episodes of angina.
      The β-blocker has the added benefit of preventing
      which of the following side effects of sublingual
      nitroglycerin?

      A. Dizziness.
      B. Methemoglobinemia.
      C. Throbbing headache.
      D. Reflex tachycardia.
      E. Edema.

> Correct answer = D. Nitroglycerin can cause a reflex
> tachycardia because of its vasodilating properties.
> This reflex is blocked by propranolol. The other ef-
> fects are either not prevented by propranolol or are
> not caused by nitroglycerin (edema).

18.3 A 68-year-old man has been successfully treated for
      exercise-induced angina for several years. He recent-
      ly has been complaining about being awakened at
      night with chest pain. Which of the following drugs
      would be useful in preventing this patient's noctur-
      nal angina?

      A. Amyl nitrite.
      B. Nitroglycerin (sublingual).
      C. Nitroglycerin (transdermal).
      D. Esmolol.
      E. Hydralazine.

> Correct answer = C. Transdermal nitroglycerin can
> sustain blood levels for as long as 24 hours. Because
> tolerance occurs, however, it is recommended that
> the patch be removed after 8 to 10 hours to al-
> low recovery of sensitivity. Amyl nitrite, sublingual
> nitroglycerin, and esmolol all have short durations
> of actions. Hydralazine may actually precipitate an
> angina attack.

Antihypertensives 19

I. OVERVIEW

Hypertension is defined as either a sustained systolic blood pressure (SBP) of greater than 140 mm Hg or a sustained diastolic blood pressure (DBP) of greater than 90 mm Hg. Hypertension results from increased peripheral vascular smooth muscle tone, which leads to increased arteriolar resistance and reduced capacitance of the venous system. In most cases, the cause of the increased vascular tone is unknown. Elevated blood pressure is an extremely common disorder, affecting approximately 15 percent of the population of the United States (60 million people). Although many of these individuals have no symptoms, chronic hypertension—either systolic or diastolic—can lead to cerebrovascular accidents (strokes), congestive heart failure, myocardial infarction, and renal damage. The incidence of morbidity and mortality significantly decreases when hypertension is diagnosed early and is properly treated. In recognition of the progressive nature of hypertension, the Seventh Report of the Joint National Committee classifies hypertension into four categories for the purpose of treatment management. The categories are normal (SBP/DBP, <120/<80), prehypertension (SBP/DBP, 120–139/80–89), stage 1 hypertension (SBP/DBP, 140–159/90 –99), and stage 2 hypertension (SBP/DBP ≥160/≥100).

II. ETIOLOGY OF HYPERTENSION

Although hypertension may occur secondary to other disease processes, more than 90 percent of patients have essential hypertension, a disorder of unknown origin affecting the blood pressure regulating mechanism. A family history of hypertension increases the likelihood that an individual will develop hypertensive disease. The incidence of essential hypertension is four-fold more frequent among blacks than among whites. It occurs more often among middle-aged males than among middle-aged females, and its prevalence increases with age and obesity. Environmental factors, such as a stressful lifestyle, high dietary intake of sodium, and smoking, further predispose an individual to the occurrence of hypertension. Figure 19.1 summarizes the drugs used to treat hypertension.]

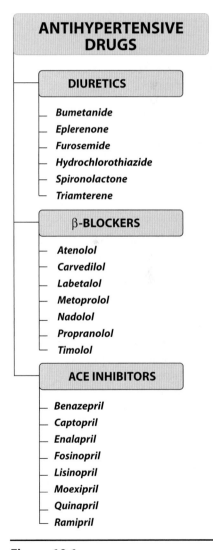

ANTIHYPERTENSIVE DRUGS

DIURETICS
- *Bumetanide*
- *Eplerenone*
- *Furosemide*
- *Hydrochlorothiazide*
- *Spironolactone*
- *Triamterene*

β-BLOCKERS
- *Atenolol*
- *Carvedilol*
- *Labetalol*
- *Metoprolol*
- *Nadolol*
- *Propranolol*
- *Timolol*

ACE INHIBITORS
- *Benazepril*
- *Captopril*
- *Enalapril*
- *Fosinopril*
- *Lisinopril*
- *Moexipril*
- *Quinapril*
- *Ramipril*

Figure 19.1
Summary of antihypertensive drugs. ACE = angiotensin-converting enzyme. (Continued on next page.)

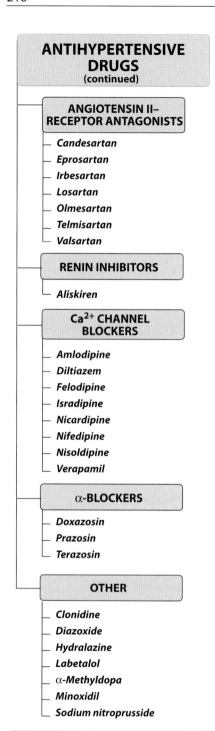

ANTIHYPERTENSIVE DRUGS
(continued)

ANGIOTENSIN II–RECEPTOR ANTAGONISTS

— *Candesartan*
— *Eprosartan*
— *Irbesartan*
— *Losartan*
— *Olmesartan*
— *Telmisartan*
— *Valsartan*

RENIN INHIBITORS

— *Aliskiren*

Ca²⁺ CHANNEL BLOCKERS

— *Amlodipine*
— *Diltiazem*
— *Felodipine*
— *Isradipine*
— *Nicardipine*
— *Nifedipine*
— *Nisoldipine*
— *Verapamil*

α-BLOCKERS

— *Doxazosin*
— *Prazosin*
— *Terazosin*

OTHER

— *Clonidine*
— *Diazoxide*
— *Hydralazine*
— *Labetalol*
— *α-Methyldopa*
— *Minoxidil*
— *Sodium nitroprusside*

Figure 19.1
Summary of antihypertensive drugs.

III. MECHANISMS FOR CONTROLLING BLOOD PRESSURE

Arterial blood pressure is regulated within a narrow range to provide adequate perfusion of the tissues without causing damage to the vascular system, particularly the arterial intima (endothelium). Arterial blood pressure is directly proportional to the product of the cardiac output and the peripheral vascular resistance (Figure 19.2). Cardiac output and peripheral resistance are controlled mainly by two overlapping control mechanisms: the baroreflexes, which are mediated by the sympathetic nervous system, and the renin-angiotensin-aldosterone system (Figure 19.3). Most antihypertensive drugs lower blood pressure by reducing cardiac output and/or decreasing peripheral resistance.

A. Baroreceptors and the sympathetic nervous system

Baroreflexes involving the sympathetic nervous system are responsible for the rapid, moment-to-moment regulation of blood pressure. A fall in blood pressure causes pressure-sensitive neurons (baroreceptors in the aortic arch and carotid sinuses) to send fewer impulses to cardiovascular centers in the spinal cord. This prompts a reflex response of increased sympathetic and decreased parasympathetic output to the heart and vasculature, resulting in vasoconstriction and increased cardiac output. These changes result in a compensatory rise in blood pressure (see Figure 19.3).

B. Renin-angiotensin-aldosterone system

The kidney provides for the long-term control of blood pressure by altering the blood volume. Baroreceptors in the kidney respond to reduced arterial pressure (and to sympathetic stimulation of β-adrenoceptors) by releasing the enzyme renin (see Figure 19.3). Low sodium intake and greater sodium loss also increase renin release. This peptidase converts angiotensinogen to angiotensin I, which is converted in turn to angiotensin II in the presence of angiotensin-converting enzyme (ACE). Angiotensin II is the body's most potent circulating vasoconstrictor, constricting both arterioles and veins, causing an increase in blood pressure. Angiotensin II exerts a preferential vasoconstrictor action on the efferent arterioles of the renal glomerulus, increasing glomerular filtration. Furthermore, angiotensin II stimulates aldosterone secretion, leading to increased renal sodium reabsorption and increased blood volume, which contribute to a further increase in blood pressure. These effects of angiotensin II are mediated by stimulation of angiotensin II–AT1 receptors.

IV. TREATMENT STRATEGIES

The goal of antihypertensive therapy is to reduce cardiovascular and renal morbidity and mortality. The relationship between blood pressure and the risk of a cardiovascular event is continuous, and thus lowering of even moderately elevated blood pressure significantly reduces cardiovascular disease. The newly added classification of "prehypertension" recognizes this relationship and emphasizes the need for decreasing blood pressure in the general population by education and adoption of blood pressure–lowering behaviors. Mild hypertension can often be controlled with a single drug; however, most patients require more than one drug to achieve blood pressure control. Current recommendations are to initiate therapy with a thiazide diuretic unless there are compelling reasons to employ other drug classes (Figure 19.4). If blood pressure is inadequately controlled, a second

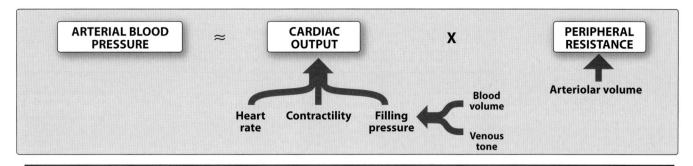

Figure 19.2
Major factors influencing blood pressure.

drug is added, with the selection based on minimizing the adverse effects of the combined regimen. A β-blocker is usually added if the initial drug was a diuretic, or a diuretic is usually added if the first drug was a β-blocker. A vasodilator can be added as a third step for those patients who still fail to respond. However, angiotensin II–converting enzyme inhibitors, angiotensin II–AT1 receptor blockers, and calcium-channel blockers can also be used to initiate therapy.

A. Individualized care

Certain subsets of the hypertensive population respond better to one class of drug than they do to another. For example, black patients

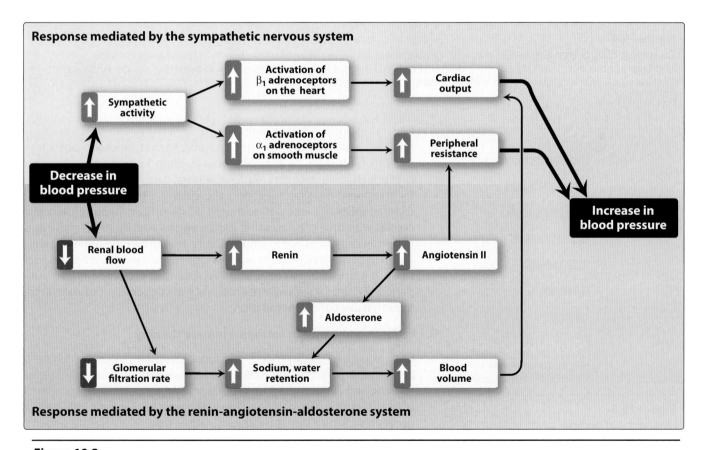

Figure 19.3
Response of the autonomic nervous system and the renin-angiotensin-aldosterone system to a decrease in blood pressure.

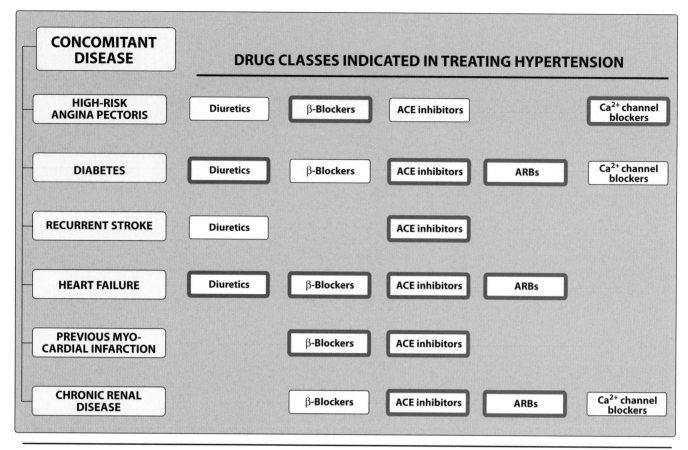

Figure 19.4
Treatment of hypertension in patients with concomitant diseases. Drug classes shown in blue boxes provide improvement in outcome (for example diabetes or renal disease) independent of blood pressure . [Note: ARBs are an alternative to ACE inhibitors.] ACE = angiotensin-converting enzyme; ARB = angiotensin receptor blocker.

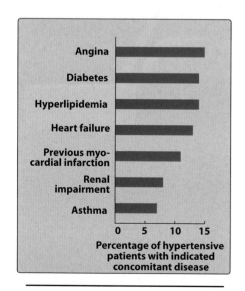

Figure 19.5
Frequency of occurrence of concomitant disease among the hypertensive patient population.

respond well to diuretics and calcium-channel blockers, but therapy with β-blockers or ACE inhibitors is often less effective. Similarly, calcium-channel blockers, ACE inhibitors, and diuretics are favored for treatment of hypertension in the elderly, whereas β-blockers and α-antagonists are less well tolerated. Furthermore, hypertension may coexist with other diseases that can be aggravated by some of the antihypertensive drugs. For example, Figure 19.4 shows the preferred therapy in hypertensive patients with various concomitant diseases. In such cases, it is important to match antihypertensive drugs to the particular patient. Figure 19.5 shows the frequency of concomitant disease in the hypertensive patient population.

B. Patient compliance in antihypertensive therapy

Lack of patient compliance is the most common reason for failure of antihypertensive therapy. The hypertensive patient is usually asymptomatic and is diagnosed by routine screening before the occurrence of overt end-organ damage. Thus, therapy is generally directed at preventing future disease sequelae rather than relieving the patient's present discomfort. The adverse effects associated with the hypertensive therapy may influence the patient more than the future benefits.

For example, β-blockers can decrease libido and induce impotence in males, particularly middle-aged and elderly men. This drug-induced sexual dysfunction may prompt the patient to discontinue therapy. Thus, it is important to enhance compliance by carefully selecting a drug regimen that both reduces adverse effects and minimizes the number of doses required daily.

V. DIURETICS

Diuretics can be used as first-line drug therapy for hypertension unless there are compelling reasons to choose another agent. Low-dose diuretic therapy is safe, inexpensive, and effective in preventing stroke, myocardial infarction, and congestive heart failure, all of which can cause mortality. Recent data suggest that diuretics are superior to β-blockers for treating hypertesnion in older adults.

A. Thiazide diuretics

All oral diuretic drugs are effective in the treatment of hypertension, but the thiazides have found the most widespread use.

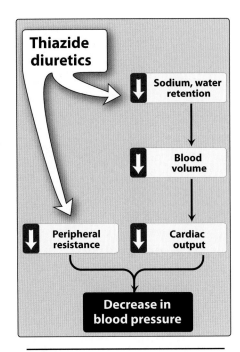

Figure 19.6
Actions of thiazide diuretics.

1. **Actions:** Thiazide diuretics, such as *hydrochlorothiazide* [hye-droe-klor-oh-THYE-a-zide], lower blood pressure initially by increasing sodium and water excretion. This causes a decrease in extracellular volume, resulting in a decrease in cardiac output and renal blood flow (Figure 19.6). With long-term treatment, plasma volume approaches a normal value, but peripheral resistance decreases. Potassium-sparing diuretics are often used combined with thiazides.

2. **Therapeutic uses:** Thiazide diuretics decrease blood pressure in both the supine and standing positions, and postural hypotension is rarely observed except in elderly, volume-depleted patients. These agents counteract the sodium and water retention observed with other agents used in the treatment of hypertension (for example, *hydralazine*). Thiazides are therefore useful in combination therapy with a variety of other antihypertensive agents, including β-blockers, ACE inhibitors, angiotensin-receptor blockers, and potassium-sparing diuretics. Thiazide diuretics are particularly useful in the treatment of black or elderly patients. They are not effective in patients with inadequate kidney function (creatinine clearance, <50 mL/min). Loop diuretics may be required in these patients.

3. **Pharmacokinetics:** Thiazide diuretics are orally active. Absorption and elimination rates vary considerably, although no clear advantage is present for one agent over another. All thiazides are ligands for the organic acid secretory system of the nephron, and as such, they may compete with uric acid for elimination.

4. **Adverse effects:** Thiazide diuretics induce hypokalemia and hyperuricemia in 70 percent of patients and hyperglycemia in 10 percent of patients. Hypomagnesemia may also occur. Serum potassium levels should be monitored closely in patients who are predisposed to cardiac arrhythmias (particularly individuals with left ventricular hypertrophy, ischemic heart disease, or chronic heart failure) and who are concurrently being treated with both thiazide diuretics and *digoxin*.

B. Loop diuretics

The loop diuretics act promptly, even in patients with poor renal function or who have not responded to thiazides or other diuretics. Loop diuretics cause decreased renal vascular resistance and increased renal blood flow. [Note: Loop diuretics increase the Ca^{2+} content of urine, whereas thiazide diuretics decrease it.]

C. Potassium-sparing diuretics.

Amiloride [a-MIL-oh-ride] and *triamterene* [tri-AM-ter-een] (inhibitors of epithelial sodium transport at the late distal and collecting ducts) as well as *spironolactone* [speer-on-oh-LAK-tone] and *eplerenone* [eh-PLEH-reh-none](aldosterone-receptor antagonists) reduce potassium loss in the urine. *Spironolactone* has the additional benefit of diminishing the cardiac remodeling that occurs in heart failure. (A complete discussion of diuretics is found in Chapter 22, p. 257.)

VI. β-ADRENOCEPTOR BLOCKING AGENTS

β-Blockers are currently recommended as first-line drug therapy for hypertension when when concomitant disease is present (see Figure 19.4)—for example, with heart failure. These drugs are efficacious but have some contraindications.

A. Actions

The β-blockers reduce blood pressure primarily by decreasing cardiac output (Figure 19.7). They may also decrease sympathetic outflow from the central nervous system (CNS) and inhibit the release of renin from the kidneys, thus decreasing the formation of angiotensin II and the secretion of aldosterone. The prototype β-blocker is *propranolol* [proe PRAN-oh-lol], which acts at both β_1 and β_2 receptors. Selective blockers of β_1 receptors, such as *metoprolol* [met-OH-pro-lol] and *atenolol* [ah-TEN-oh-lol], are among the most commonly prescribed β-blockers. The selective β-blockers may be administered cautiously to hypertensive patients who also have asthma, for which *propranolol* is contraindicated due to its blockade of β_2-mediated bronchodilation. (See p. 220 for a

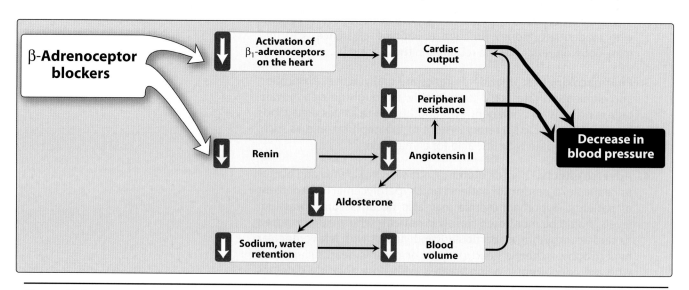

Figure 19.7
Actions of β-adrenoceptor blocking agents.

discussion of the β-blockers). The β-blockers should be employed cautiously in the treatment of patients with acute heart failure or peripheral vascular disease.

B. Therapeutic uses

1. **Subsets of the hypertensive population:** The β-blockers are more effective for treating hypertension in white than in black patients and in young compared to elderly patients. [Note: Conditions that discourage the use of β-blockers (for example, severe chronic obstructive lung disease, chronic congestive heart failure, or severe symptomatic occlusive peripheral vascular disease) are more commonly found in the elderly and in diabetics.]

2. **Hypertensive patients with concomitant diseases:** The β-blockers are useful in treating conditions that may coexist with hypertension, such as supraventricular tachyarrhythmia, previous myocardial infarction, angina pectoris, chronic heart failure, and migraine headache.

C. Pharmacokinetics

The β-blockers are orally active. *Propranolol* undergoes extensive and highly variable first-pass metabolism. The β-blockers may take several weeks to develop their full effects.

D. Adverse effects

1. **Common effects:** The β-blockers may cause bradycardia and CNS side effects such as fatigue, lethargy, insomnia, and hallucinations; these drugs can also cause hypotension (Figure 19.8). The β-blockers may decrease libido and cause impotence. [Note: Drug-induced sexual dysfunction can severely reduce patient compliance.]

2. **Alterations in serum lipid patterns:** The β-blockers may disturb lipid metabolism, decreasing high-density lipoprotein cholesterol and increasing plasma triacylglycerol.

3. **Drug withdrawal:** Abrupt withdrawal may induce angina, myocardial infarction, or even sudden death in patients with ischemic heart disease. Therefore, the dose of these drugs must be tapered over 2 to 3 weeks in patients with hypertension and ischemic heart disease.

VII. ACE INHIBITORS

The ACE inhibitors, such as *enalapril* [e-NAL-ah-pril] or *lisinopril* [lye-SIN-oh-pril], are recommended when the preferred first-line agents (diuretics or β-blockers) are contraindicated or ineffective. Despite their widespread use, it is not clear if antihypertensive therapy with ACE inhibitors increases the risk of other major diseases.

A. Actions

The ACE inhibitors lower blood pressure by reducing peripheral vascular resistance without reflexively increasing cardiac output, rate, or contractility. These drugs block the ACE that cleaves angiotensin I to form the potent vasoconstrictor angiotensin II (Figure 19.9). The converting enzyme is also responsible for the breakdown of bradykinin. ACE inhibitors decrease angiotensin II and increase bradykinin levels. Vasodilation

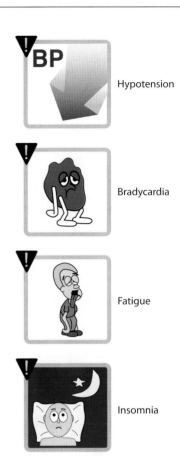

Hypotension

Bradycardia

Fatigue

Insomnia

Sexual dysfunction

Figure 19.8
Some adverse effects of β-blockers.

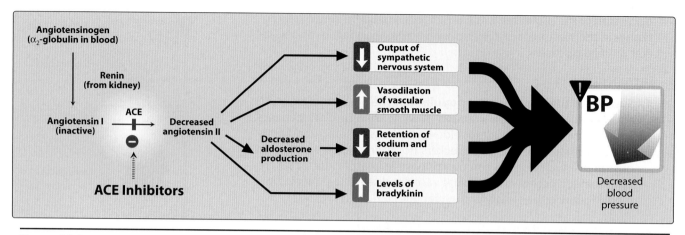

Figure 19.9
Effects of angiotensin-converting enzyme (ACE) inhibitors.

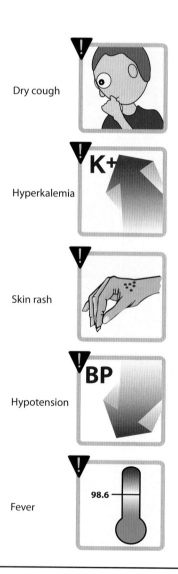

Dry cough

Hyperkalemia

Skin rash

Hypotension

Fever

Figure 19.10
Some common adverse effects of the ACE inhibitors.

occurs as a result of the combined effects of lower vasoconstriction caused by diminished levels of angiotensin II and the potent vasodilating effect of increased bradykinin. By reducing circulating angiotensin II levels, ACE inhibitors also decrease the secretion of aldosterone, resulting in decreased sodium and water retention.

B. Therapeutic uses

Like β-blockers, ACE inhibitors are most effective in hypertensive patients who are white and young. However, when used in combination with a diuretic, the effectiveness of ACE inhibitors is similar in white and black patients with hypertension. Along with the angiotensin-receptor blockers, ACE inhibitors slow the progression of diabetic nephropathy and decrease albuminuria. ACE inhibitors are also effective in the management of patients with chronic heart failure. ACE inhibitors are a standard in the care of a patient following a myocardial infarction. Therapy is started 24 hours after the end of the infarction.

C. Adverse effects

Common side effects include dry cough, rash, fever, altered taste, hypotension (in hypovolemic states), and hyperkalemia (Figure 19.10). The dry cough, which occurs in about 10 percent of patients, is thought to be due to increased levels of bradykinin in the pulmonary tree. Potassium levels must be monitored, and potassium supplements (or a high postasium diets) or potassium-sparing diuretics are contraindicated. Angioedema is a rare but potentially life-threatening reaction and may also be due to increased levels of bradykinin. Because of the risk of angioedema and first-dose syncope, ACE inhibitors may be first administered in the physician's office with close observation. Reversible renal failure can occur in patients with severe bilateral renal artery stenosis. ACE inhibitors are fetotoxic and should not be used by women who are pregnant.

VIII. ANGIOTENSIN II–RECEPTOR ANTAGONISTS

The angiotensin II–receptor blockers (ARBs) are alternatives to the ACE inhibitors. These drugs block the AT1 receptors. *Losartan* [LOW-sar-tan], is the prototypic ARB; currently, there are six additional ARBs. Their pharmacologic effects are similar to those of ACE inhibitors in that they produce arteriolar and venous dilation and block aldosterone secretion, thus lowering blood pressure and decreasing salt and water retention. ARBs do not increase bradykinin levels. ARBs decrease the nephrotoxicity of diabetes, making them an attractive therapy in hypertensive diabetics. Their adverse effects are similar to those of ACE inhibitors, although the risks of cough and angioedema are significantly decreased. ARBs are also fetotoxic. [Note: The ARBs are discussed more fully in Chapter 16.]

IX. RENIN INHIBITORS

A selective renin inhibitor, *aliskiren* [a-LIS-ke-rin] has been released for the treatment of hypertension. *Aliskiren* directly inhibits renin and, thus, acts earlier in the renin-angiotensin-aldosterone system than ACE inhibitors or ARBs. It lowers blood pressure about as effectively as ARBs, ACE inhibitors, and thiazides. It can also be combined other antihypertensives, such diuretics, ACE inhibitors, ARBs, or calcium-channel blockers. *Aliskiren* can cause diarrhea, especially at the higher doses. *Aliskiren* can also cause cough and angioedema but probably less often than ACE inhibitors. The drug is contraindicated during pregnancy. The combination of maximum doses of *aliskiren* and *valsartan* decreased blood pressure more than maximum doses of either agent alone but not more than would be expected with dual therapy consisting of agents of different classes. Hyperkalemia was significantly more common in patients who received both *valsartan* and *aliskiren*.

X. CALCIUM-CHANNEL BLOCKERS

Calcium-channel blockers are recommended when the preferred first-line agents are contraindicated or ineffective. They are effective in treating hypertension in patients with angina or diabetes. High doses of short-acting calcium-channel blockers should be avoided because of increased risk of myocardial infarction due to excessive vasodilation and marked reflex cardiac stimulation.

A. Classes of calcium-channel blockers

The calcium-channel blockers are divided into three chemical classes, each with different pharmacokinetic properties and clinical indications (Figure 19.11).

1. **Diphenylalkylamines:** *Verapamil* [ver-AP-ah-mil] is the only member of this class that is currently approved in the United States. *Verapamil* is the least selective of any calcium-channel blocker and has significant effects on both cardiac and vascular smooth muscle cells. It is used to treat angina, supraventricular tachyarrhythmias, and migraine headache.

2. **Benzothiazepines:** *Diltiazem* [dil-TYE-ah-zem] is the only member of this class that is currently approved in the United States. Like *verapamil*, *diltiazem* affects both cardiac and vascular smooth muscle cells; however, it has a less pronounced negative inotropic effect on the heart compared to that of *verapamil*. *Diltiazem* has a favorable side-effect profile.

3. **Dihydropyridines:** This rapidly expanding class of calcium-channel blockers includes the first-generation *nifedipine* [ni-FED-i-peen] and five second-generation agents for treating cardiovascular disease: *amlodipine* [am-LOE-di-peen], *felodipine* [fe-LOE-di-peen], *isradipine*

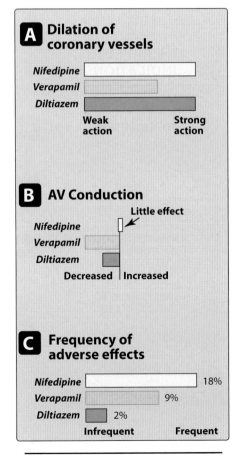

Figure 19.11
Actions of calcium-channel blockers.

[iz-RA-di-peen], *nicardipine* [nye-KAR-de-peen], and *nisoldipine* [ni-SOLD-i-peen]. These second-generation calcium-channel blockers differ in pharmacokinetics, approved uses, and drug interactions. All dihydropyridines have a much greater affinity for vascular calcium channels than for calcium channels in the heart. They are therefore particularly attractive in treating hypertension. Some of the newer agents, such as *amlodipine* and *nicardipine*, have the advantage that they show little interaction with other cardiovascular drugs, such as *digoxin* or *warfarin*, which are often used concomitantly with calcium-channel blockers.

B. Actions

The intracellular concentration of calcium plays an important role in maintaining the tone of smooth muscle and in the contraction of the myocardium. Calcium enters muscle cells through special voltage-sensitive calcium channels. This triggers release of calcium from the sarcoplasmic reticulum and mitochondria, which further increases the cytosolic level of calcium. Calcium-channel antagonists block the inward movement of calcium by binding to L-type calcium channels in the heart and in smooth muscle of the coronary and peripheral vasculature. This causes vascular smooth muscle to relax, dilating mainly arterioles.

C. Therapeutic uses

Calcium-channel blockers have an intrinsic natriuretic effect and, therefore, do not usually require the addition of a diuretic. These agents are

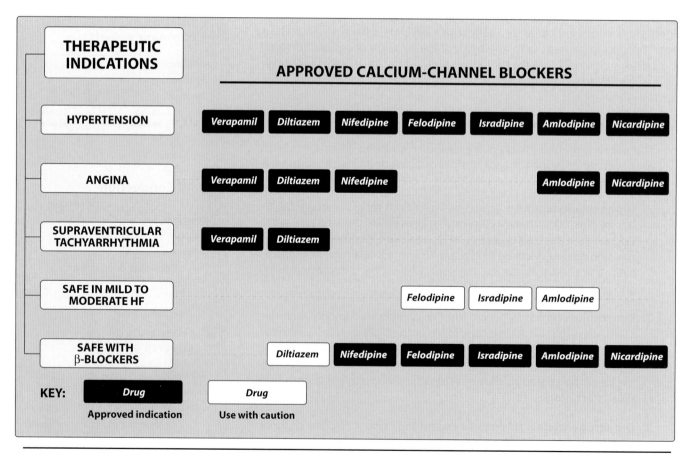

Figure 19.12
Some therapeutic applications of calcium channel blockers. HF = heart failure.

useful in the treatment of hypertensive patients who also have asthma, diabetes, angina, and/or peripheral vascular disease (Figure 19.12). Black hypertensives respond well to calcium-channel blockers.

D. Pharmacokinetics

Most of these agents have short half-lives (3–8 hours) following an oral dose. Treatment is required three times a day to maintain good control of hypertension. Sustained-release preparations are available and permit less frequent dosing. *Amlodipine* has a very long half-life and does not required a sustained-release formulation.

E. Adverse effects

Constipation occurs in 10 percent of patients treated with *verapamil*. Dizziness, headache, and a feeling of fatigue caused by a decrease in blood pressure are more frequent with dihydropyridines (Figure 19.13). *Verapamil* should be avoided in patients with congestive heart failure or with atrioventricular block due to its negative inotropic (force of cardiac muscle contraction) and dromotropic (velocity of conduction) effects.

XI. α-ADRENOCEPTOR BLOCKING AGENTS

Prazosin [PRAY-zo-sin], *doxazosin* [dox-AH-zoe-sin], and *terazosin* [ter-AH-zoe-sin] produce a competitive block of α_1-adrenoceptors. They decrease peripheral vascular resistance and lower arterial blood pressure by causing relaxation of both arterial and venous smooth muscle. These drugs cause only minimal changes in cardiac output, renal blood flow, and glomerular filtration rate. Therefore, long-term tachycardia does not occur, but salt and water retention does. Postural hypotension may occur in some individuals. *Prazosin* is used to treat mild to moderate hypertension and is prescribed in combination with *propranolol* or a diuretic for additive effects. Reflex tachycardia and first-dose syncope are almost universal adverse effects. Concomitant use of a β-blocker may be necessary to blunt the short-term effect of reflex tachycardia. An increased rate of congestive heart failure occurs in patients taking *doxazosin* alone compared to those taking a thiazide diuretic alone. Because of the side-effect profile, development of tolerance, and the advent of safer antihypertensives, α-blockers are seldom used in the treatment of hypertension. *Tamsulosin*, an α_1–blocker with greater selectivity for prostate muscle, has been used in the treatment of prostate hyperplasia.

XII. α- β- ADRENOCEPTOR BLOCKING AGENTS

Labetalol [la-BET-ah-lol] and *carvedilol* [kar-VEH-di-lol] block both α_1- and β_1- and β_2- receptors. *Carvedilol,* although an effective antihypertensive, is mainly used in the treatment of heart failure. *Carvedilol* has been shown to reduce mortality associated with heart failure.

XIII. CENTRALLY ACTING ADRENERGIC DRUGS

A. Clonidine

This α_2-agonist diminishes central adrenergic outflow. *Clonidine* [KLOE-ni-deen] is used primarily for the treatment of hypertension that has not responded adequately to treatment with two or more drugs. *Clonidine* does not decrease renal blood flow or glomerular filtration and, therefore, is useful in the treatment of hypertension complicated

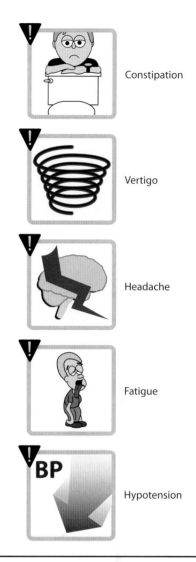

Constipation

Vertigo

Headache

Fatigue

Hypotension

Figure 19.13
Some common adverse effects of the calcium-channel blockers.

by renal disease. *Clonidine* is absorbed well after oral administration and is excreted by the kidney. Because it may cause sodium and water retention, *clonidine* may be administered in combination with a diuretic. Adverse effects are generally mild, but the drug can produce sedation and drying of the nasal mucosa. Rebound hypertension occurs following abrupt withdrawal of *clonidine*. The drug should therefore be withdrawn slowly if the clinician wishes to change agents.

B. α-Methyldopa

This α_2-agonist is converted to methylnorepinephrine centrally to diminish the adrenergic outflow from the CNS. This leads to reduced total peripheral resistance and a decreased blood pressure. Cardiac output is not decreased, and blood flow to vital organs is not diminished. Because blood flow to the kidney is not diminished by its use, *α-methyldopa* [meth-ill-DOE-pa] is especially valuable in treating hypertensive patients with renal insufficiency. The most common side effects of *α-methyldopa* are sedation and drowsiness. It has been used in hypertensive pregnant patients.

XIV. VASODILATORS

The direct-acting smooth muscle relaxants, such as *hydralazine* and *minoxidil*, have traditionally not been used as primary drugs to treat hypertension. Vasodilators act by producing relaxation of vascular smooth muscle, which decreases resistance and, therefore, blood pressure. These agents produce reflex stimulation of the heart, resulting in the competing reflexes of increased myocardial contractility, heart rate, and oxygen consumption. These actions may prompt angina pectoris, myocardial infarction, or cardiac failure in predisposed individuals. Vasodilators also increase plasma renin concentration, resulting in sodium and water retention. These undesirable side effects can be blocked by concomitant use of a diuretic and a β-blocker.

A. Hydralazine

This drug causes direct vasodilation, acting primarily on arteries and arterioles. This results in a decreased peripheral resistance, which in turn prompts a reflex elevation in heart rate and cardiac output. *Hydralazine* [hye-DRAL-ah-zeen] is used to treat moderately severe hypertension. It is almost always administered in combination with a β-blocker, such as *propranolol* (to balance the reflex tachycardia), and a diuretic (to decrease sodium retention). Together, the three drugs decrease cardiac output, plasma volume, and peripheral vascular resistance. *Hydralazine* monotherapy is an accepted method of controlling blood pressure in pregnancy-induced hypertension. Adverse effects of *hydralazine* therapy include headache, tachycardia, nausea, sweating, arrhythmia, and precipitation of angina. A lupus-like syndrome can occur with high dosage, but it is reversible on discontinuation of the drug.

B. Minoxidil

This drug causes dilation of resistance vessels (arterioles) but not of capacitance vessels (venules). *Minoxidil* [mi-NOX-i-dill] is administered orally for treatment of severe to malignant hypertension that is refractory to other drugs. Reflex tachycardia and fluid retention may be severe and require the concomitant use of a loop diuretic and a β-blocker.

Minoxidil causes serious sodium and water retention, leading to volume overload, edema, and congestive heart failure. [Note: *Minoxidil* treatment also causes hypertrichosis (the growth of body hair). This drug is now used topically to treat male pattern baldness.]

XV. HYPERTENSIVE EMERGENCY

Hypertensive emergency is a rare but life-threatening situation in which the DBP is either >150 mm Hg (with SBP >210 mm Hg) in an otherwise healthy person or >130 mm Hg in an individual with preexisting complications, such as encephalopathy, cerebral hemorrhage, left ventricular failure, or aortic stenosis. The therapeutic goal is to rapidly reduce blood pressure.

A. Sodium nitroprusside

Nitroprusside [nye-troe-PRUSS-ide] is administered intravenously and causes prompt vasodilation with reflex tachycardia. It is capable of reducing blood pressure in all patients regardless of the cause of hypertension (Figure 19.14). The drug has little effect outside the vascular system, acting equally on arterial and venous smooth muscle. [Note: Because *nitroprusside* also acts on the veins, it can reduce cardiac preload.] *Nitroprusside* is metabolized rapidly (half-life of minutes) and requires continuous infusion to maintain its hypotensive action. *Sodium nitroprusside* exerts few adverse effects except for those of hypotension caused by overdose. *Nitroprusside* metabolism results in cyanide ion production. Although cyanide toxicity is rare, it can be effectively treated with an infusion of *sodium thiosulfate* to produce thiocyanate, which is less toxic and is eliminated by the kidneys. [Note: *Nitroprusside* is poisonous if given orally because of its hydrolysis to cyanide.] Nitroprusside is light sensitive, and when in solution, it should be protected from light.

B. Labetalol

Labetalol [lah-BET-a-lole] is both an α- and a β-blocker and is given as an intravenous bolus or infusion in hypertensive emergencies. *Labetalol* does not cause reflex tachycardia. *Labetalol* carries the contraindications of a nonselective β-blocker. The major limitation is a longer half-life, which precludes rapid titration (see Figure 19.14)

C. Fenoldopam

Fenoldopam [feh-NOL-doh-pam] is a peripheral dopamine-1 receptor agonist that is given as an intravenous infusion. Unlike other parenteral antihypertensive agents, *fenoldopam* maintains or increases renal perfusion while it lowers blood pressure. *Fenoldopam* can be safely used in all hypertensive emergencies and may be particularly beneficial in patients with renal insufficiency. The drug is contraindicated in patients with glaucoma.

D. Nicardipine

Nicardipine, a calcium-channel blocker, can be given as an intravenous infusion. The initial dose is 5 mg/h and can be increased to a maximum of 15 mg/h. The major limitation of *nicardipine* in treating hypertensive emergency is its long half-time (approximately 8 hours), which precludes rapid titration.

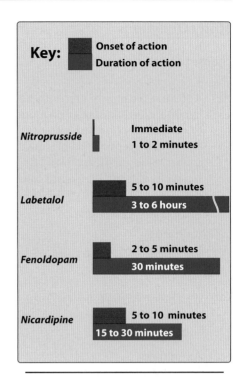

Key:
- Onset of action
- Duration of action

Nitroprusside — Immediate / 1 to 2 minutes

Labetalol — 5 to 10 minutes / 3 to 6 hours

Fenoldopam — 2 to 5 minutes / 30 minutes

Nicardipine — 5 to 10 minutes / 15 to 30 minutes

Figure 19.14
Time to peak effect and duration of action for some drugs used in hypertensive emergency.

Study Questions

Choose the ONE best answer.

19.1 A 45-year-old man has recently been diagnosed with hypertension and started on monotherapy designed to reduce peripheral resistance and prevent NaCl and water retention. He has developed a persistent cough. Which of the following drugs would have the same benefits but would not cause cough?

    A. Losartan.
    B. Nifedipine.
    C. Prazosin.
    D. Propranolol.

Correct answer = A. The cough is an adverse effect of an ACE inhibitor. Losartan is an ARB that will have the same beneficial effects as an ACE inhibitor but will not produce a cough. The other drugs also do not cause this side effect.

19.2 Which one of the following drugs may cause a precipitous fall in blood pressure and fainting on initial administration?

    A. Atenolol.
    B. Hydrochlorothiazide.
    C. Nifedipine.
    D. Prazosin.
    E. Verapamil.

Correct answer = D. Prazosin produces first-dose hypotension, presumably by blocking α_1-receptors. This effect is minimized by initially giving the drug in small, divided doses. The other agents do not have this adverse effect.

19.3 Which one of the following antihypertensive drugs can precipitate a hypertensive crisis following abrupt cessation of therapy?

    A. Clonidine.
    B. Diltiazem.
    C. Enalapril.
    D. Losartan.
    E. Hydrochlorothiazide.

Correct answer = A. Increased sympathetic nervous system activity occurs if clonidine therapy is abruptly stopped after prolonged administration. Uncontrolled elevation in blood pressure can occur. Patients should be slowly weaned from clonidine while other antihypertensive medications are initiated. The other drugs on the list do not produce this phenomenon.

19.4 A 48-year-old hypertensive patient has been successfully treated with a thiazide diuretic for the last 5 years. Over the last 3 months, his diastolic pressure has steadily increased, and he has been started on an additional antihypertensive medication. He complains of several instances of being unable to achieve an erection and that he is no longer able to complete three sets of tennis. The second antihypertensive medication is most likely which one of the following?

    A. Captopril.
    B. Losartan.
    C. Minoxidil.
    D. Metoprolol.
    E. Nifedipine.

Correct answer = D. The side effect profile of β-blockers, such as metoprolol, are characterized by interference with sexual performance and decreased exercise tolerance. None of the other drugs is likely to produce this combination of side effects.

Blood Drugs

20

I. OVERVIEW

This chapter describes drugs that are useful in treating three important dysfunctions of blood: thrombosis, bleeding, and anemia. Thrombosis—the formation of an unwanted clot within a blood vessel—is the most common abnormality of hemostasis. Thrombotic disorders include acute myocardial infarction, deep-vein thrombosis, pulmonary embolism, and acute ischemic stroke. These are treated with drugs such as anticoagulants and fibrinolytics. Bleeding disorders involving the failure of hemostasis are less common than thromboembolic diseases. These disorders include hemophilia, which is treated with transfusion of Factor VIII prepared by recombinant DNA techniques, and vitamin K deficiency, which is treated with dietary supplements of the vitamin. Anemias caused by nutritional deficiencies, such as the commonly encountered iron-deficiency anemia, can be treated with either dietary or pharmaceutical supplementation. However, individuals with anemias that have a genetic basis, such as sickle-cell disease, can benefit from additional treatment. See Figure 20.1 for a summary of drugs affecting the blood.

II. THROMBUS VS. EMBOLUS

First, a few definitions to clarify the discussion of undesirable blood clots: A clot that adheres to a vessel wall is called a thrombus, whereas an intravascular clot that floats in the blood is termed an embolus. Thus, a detached thrombus becomes an embolus. Both thrombi and emboli are dangerous, because they may occlude blood vessels and deprive tissues of oxygen and nutrients. Arterial thrombosis most often occurs in medium-sized vessels rendered thrombogenic by surface lesions on endothelial cells caused by atherosclerosis. Arterial thrombosis usually consists of a platelet-rich clot. In contrast, venous thrombosis is triggered by blood stasis or inappropriate activation of the coagulation cascade, frequently as a result of a defect in the normal hemostatic defense mechanisms. Venous thrombosis typically involves a clot that is rich in fibrin, with fewer platelets than are observed with arterial clots.

III. PLATELET RESPONSE TO VASCULAR INJURY

Physical trauma to the vascular system, such as a puncture or a cut, initiates a complex series of interactions between platelets, endothelial cells, and the coagulation cascade. This results in the formation of a platelet-fibrin plug (clot) at the site of the puncture. The creation of an unwant-

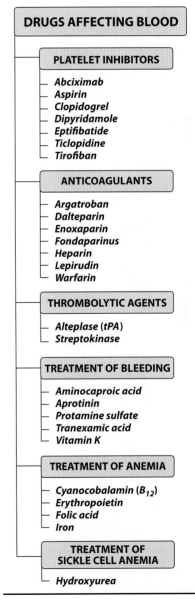

DRUGS AFFECTING BLOOD

PLATELET INHIBITORS
- *Abciximab*
- *Aspirin*
- *Clopidogrel*
- *Dipyridamole*
- *Eptifibatide*
- *Ticlopidine*
- *Tirofiban*

ANTICOAGULANTS
- *Argatroban*
- *Dalteparin*
- *Enoxaparin*
- *Fondaparinus*
- *Heparin*
- *Lepirudin*
- *Warfarin*

THROMBOLYTIC AGENTS
- *Alteplase (tPA)*
- *Streptokinase*

TREATMENT OF BLEEDING
- *Aminocaproic acid*
- *Aprotinin*
- *Protamine sulfate*
- *Tranexamic acid*
- *Vitamin K*

TREATMENT OF ANEMIA
- *Cyanocobalamin (B$_{12}$)*
- *Erythropoietin*
- *Folic acid*
- *Iron*

TREATMENT OF SICKLE CELL ANEMIA
- *Hydroxyurea*

Figure 20.1
Summary of drugs used in treating dysfunctions of the blood.

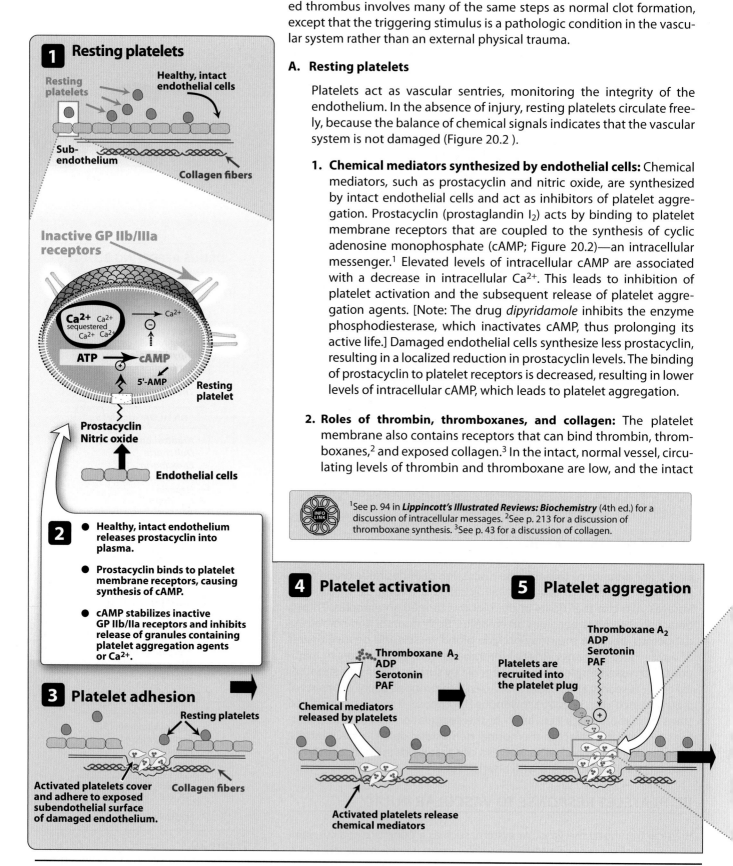

1 **Resting platelets**

Resting platelets

Healthy, intact endothelial cells

Sub-endothelium

Collagen fibers

Inactive GP IIb/IIIa receptors

Ca^{2+} Ca^{2+} sequestered Ca^{2+} Ca^{2+}

Ca^{2+}

ATP → cAMP

5'-AMP

Resting platelet

Prostacyclin
Nitric oxide

Endothelial cells

2
- Healthy, intact endothelium releases prostacyclin into plasma.
- Prostacyclin binds to platelet membrane receptors, causing synthesis of cAMP.
- cAMP stabilizes inactive GP IIb/IIa receptors and inhibits release of granules containing platelet aggregation agents or Ca^{2+}.

3 **Platelet adhesion**

Resting platelets

Activated platelets cover and adhere to exposed subendothelial surface of damaged endothelium.

Collagen fibers

4 **Platelet activation**

Thromboxane A_2
ADP
Serotonin
PAF

Chemical mediators released by platelets

Activated platelets release chemical mediators

5 **Platelet aggregation**

Thromboxane A_2
ADP
Serotonin
PAF

Platelets are recruited into the platelet plug

ed thrombus involves many of the same steps as normal clot formation, except that the triggering stimulus is a pathologic condition in the vascular system rather than an external physical trauma.

A. Resting platelets

Platelets act as vascular sentries, monitoring the integrity of the endothelium. In the absence of injury, resting platelets circulate freely, because the balance of chemical signals indicates that the vascular system is not damaged (Figure 20.2).

1. **Chemical mediators synthesized by endothelial cells:** Chemical mediators, such as prostacyclin and nitric oxide, are synthesized by intact endothelial cells and act as inhibitors of platelet aggregation. Prostacyclin (prostaglandin I_2) acts by binding to platelet membrane receptors that are coupled to the synthesis of cyclic adenosine monophosphate (cAMP; Figure 20.2)—an intracellular messenger.[1] Elevated levels of intracellular cAMP are associated with a decrease in intracellular Ca^{2+}. This leads to inhibition of platelet activation and the subsequent release of platelet aggregation agents. [Note: The drug *dipyridamole* inhibits the enzyme phosphodiesterase, which inactivates cAMP, thus prolonging its active life.] Damaged endothelial cells synthesize less prostacyclin, resulting in a localized reduction in prostacyclin levels. The binding of prostacyclin to platelet receptors is decreased, resulting in lower levels of intracellular cAMP, which leads to platelet aggregation.

2. **Roles of thrombin, thromboxanes, and collagen:** The platelet membrane also contains receptors that can bind thrombin, thromboxanes,[2] and exposed collagen.[3] In the intact, normal vessel, circulating levels of thrombin and thromboxane are low, and the intact

[1]See p. 94 in *Lippincott's Illustrated Reviews: Biochemistry* (4th ed.) for a discussion of intracellular messages. [2]See p. 213 for a discussion of thromboxane synthesis. [3]See p. 43 for a discussion of collagen.

Figure 20.2
Formation of a hemostatic plug. (Continued on facing page.)

endothelium covers the collagen in the subendothelial layers. The corresponding platelet receptors are thus unoccupied and remain inactive; as a result, platelet activation and aggregation are not initiated. However, when occupied, each of these receptor types triggers a series of reactions leading to the release into the circulation of intracellular granules by the platelets. This ultimately stimulates platelet aggregation.

B. Platelet adhesion

When the endothelium is injured, platelets adhere to and virtually cover the exposed collagen of the subendothelium (see Figure 20.2). This triggers a complex series of chemical reactions, resulting in platelet activation.

C. Platelet activation

Receptors on the surface of the adhering platelets are activated by the collagen of the underlying connective tissue. This causes morphologic changes in the platelets (Figure 20.3) and the release of platelet granules containing chemical mediators, such as adenosine diphosphate (ADP), thromboxane A_2, serotonin, platelet-activation factor, and thrombin (see Figure 20.2). These signaling molecules bind to receptors in the outer membrane of resting platelets circulating nearby. These receptors function as sensors that are activated by the signals sent from the adhering platelets. The previously dormant platelets become activated and start to aggregate—actions mediated by several messenger systems that ultimately result in elevated levels of Ca^{2+} and a decreased concentration of cAMP within the platelet.

D. Platelet aggregation

The increase in cytosolic Ca^{2+} accompanying activation is due to a release of sequestered stores within the platelet (see Figure 20.2). This leads to 1) the release of platelet granules containing mediators, such

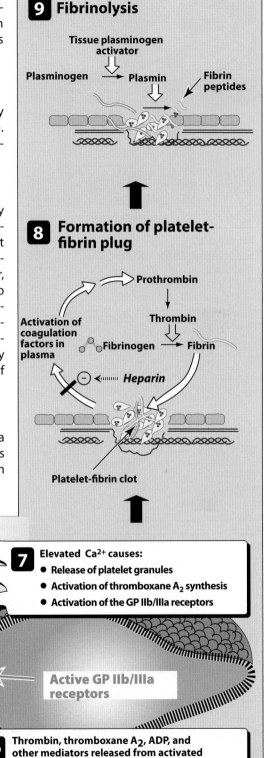

Figure 20.2 (continued)
Formation of a hemostatic plug. PAF = platelet-activation factor.

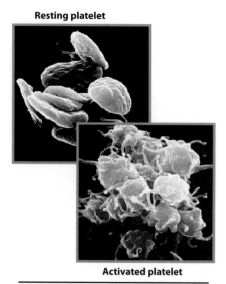

Figure 20.3
Scanning electron micrograph of platelets.

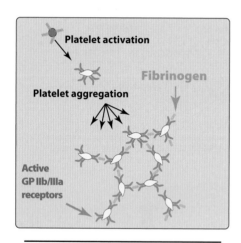

Figure 20.4
Activation and aggregation of platelets. GP = glycoprotein.

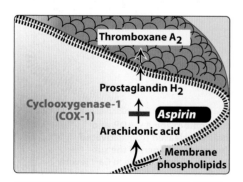

Figure 20.5
Aspirin irreversibly inhibits platelet cyclooxygenase-1.

as ADP and serotonin that activate other platelets; 2) activation of thromboxane A_2 synthesis; and 3) activation of the glycoprotein (GP) IIb/IIIa receptors that bind fibrinogen and, ultimately, regulate platelet-platelet interaction and thrombus formation (see Figure 20.2). Fibrinogen, a soluble plasma GP, simultaneously binds to GP IIb/IIIa receptors on two separate platelets, resulting in platelet cross-linking and platelet aggregation. This leads to an avalanche of platelet aggregation, because each activated platelet can recruit other platelets (Figure 20.4).

E. Formation of a clot

Local stimulation of the coagulation cascade by tissue factors released from the injured tissue and by mediators on the surface of platelets results in the formation of thrombin (Factor IIa). In turn, thrombin—a serine protease—catalyzes the hydrolysis of fibrinogen to fibrin, which is incorporated into the plug. Subsequent cross-linking of the fibrin strands stabilizes the clot and forms a hemostatic platelet-fibrin plug (see Figure 20.2).

F. Fibrinolysis

During plug formation, the fibrinolytic pathway is locally activated. Plasminogen is enzymatically processed to plasmin (fibrinolysin) by plasminogen activators in the tissue (see Figure 20.2). Plasmin limits the growth of the clot and dissolves the fibrin network as wounds heal. At present, a number of fibrinolytic enzymes are available for treatment of myocardial infarctions, pulmonary emboli, or ischemic stroke.

IV. PLATELET AGGREGATION INHIBITORS

Platelet aggregation inhibitors decrease the formation or the action of chemical signals that promote platelet aggregation. The last step in this response to vascular trauma depends on a family of membrane GP receptors that—after activation—can bind adhesive proteins, such as fibrinogen, von Willebrand factor, and fibronectin. The most important of these is the GP IIb/IIIa receptor that ultimately regulates platelet-platelet interaction and thrombus formation. Thus, platelet activation agents, such as thromboxane A_2, ADP, thrombin, serotonin, and collagen, all promote the conformational change necessary for the GP IIb/IIIa receptor to bind ligands, particularly fibrinogen. Fibrinogen simultaneously binds to GP IIb/IIIa receptors on two separate platelets, resulting in platelet cross-linking and aggregation (see Figure 20.4). The platelet aggregation inhibitors described below inhibit cyclooxygenase-1 (COX-1) or block GP IIb/IIIa or ADP receptors, thereby interfering in the signals that promote platelet aggregation. Since these agents have different mechanisms of actions, synergistic or additive effects may be achieved when agents from different classes are combined. These agents are beneficial in the prevention and treatment of occlusive cardiovascular diseases, in the maintenance of vascular grafts and arterial patency, and as adjuncts to thrombin inhibitors or thrombolytic therapy in myocardial infarction.

A. Aspirin

Stimulation of platelets by thrombin, collagen and ADP results in activation of platelet membrane phospholipases that liberate arachidonic acid from membrane phospholipids.[4] Arachidonic acid is first converted

[4]See p. 213 in *Lippincott's Illustrated Reviews: Biochemistry* (4th ed.) for a discussion of the function of membrane-bound phospholipase.

to prostaglandin H_2 by COX-1 (Figure 20.5); prostaglandin H_2 is further metabolized to thromboxane A_2, which is released into plasma. Thromboxane A_2 produced by the aggregating platelets further promotes the clumping process that is essential to the rapid formation of a hemostatic plug. *Aspirin* [AS-pir-in] inhibits thromboxane A_2 synthesis from arachidonic acid in platelets by irreversible acetylation of a serine, resulting in a blockade of arachidonate to the active site and, thus, inhibition of COX-1 (Figure 20.6). This shifts the balance of chemical mediators to favor the antiaggregatory effects of prostacyclin, thus impeding platelet aggregation. The inhibitory effect is rapid, apparently occurring in the portal circulation. The *aspirin*-induced suppression of thromboxane A_2 synthetase and the resulting suppression of platelet aggregation last for the life of the anucleate platelet—approximately 7 to 10 days. *Aspirin* is currently employed in the prophylactic treatment of transient cerebral ischemia, to reduce the incidence of recurrent myocardial infarction, and to decrease mortality in pre– and post–myocardial infarct patients. The recommended dose of *aspirin* ranges from 81 to 325 mg, with side effects determining the dose chosen. Bleeding time is prolonged by *aspirin* treatment, causing complications that include an increased incidence of hemorrhagic stroke as well as gastrointestinal bleeding, especially at higher doses of the drug. *Aspirin* is frequently used in combination with other drugs having anticlotting properties—for example, *heparin* or *clopidogrel*. Nonsteroidal anti-inflammatory drugs, such as *ibuprofen*, inhibit COX-1 by transiently competing at the catalytic site. *Ibuprofen*, if taken concomitantly with, or 2 hours prior to *aspirin*, can obstruct the access of *aspirin* to the serine residue and, thereby, antagonize the platelet inhibition by *aspirin*. Therefore, *aspirin* should be taken at least 30 minutes before *ibuprofen* or at least 8 hours after *ibuprofen*. Although *celecoxib* (a selective COX-2 inhibitor—see Chapter 39) does not interfere in the antiaggregation activity of *aspirin*, there is some evidence that it may contribute to cardiovascular events by shifting the balance of chemical mediators in favor of thromboxane A_2.

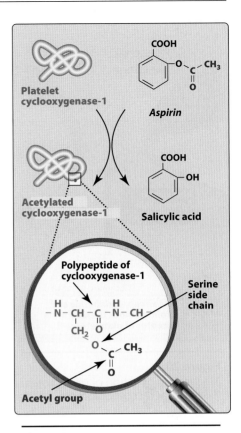

Figure 20.6
Acetylation of cyclooxygenase-1 by *aspirin*.

B. Ticlopidine and clopidogrel

Ticlopidine [ti-KLOE-pi-deen] and *clopidogrel* (kloh-PID-oh-grel) are closely related thienopyridines that also block platelet aggregation, but by a mechanism different from that of *aspirin*.

1. **Mechanism of action:** These drugs irreversibly inhibit the binding of ADP to its receptors on platelets and, thus, inhibit the activation of the GP IIb/IIIa receptors required for platelets to bind to fibrinogen and to each other (Figure 20.7).

2. **Therapeutic use:** Although *ticlopidine* and *clopidogrel* are similar in both structure and mechanism of action, their therapeutic uses are different. *Ticlopidine* is approved for the prevention of transient ischemic attacks and strokes for patients with prior cerebral thrombotic event. It is also used as adjunct therapy with *aspirin* following coronary stent implantation to decrease the incidence of stent thrombosis. However, due to its life-threatening hematologic adverse reactions, including neutropenia/agranulocytosis, thrombotic thrombocytopenic purpura (TTP), and aplastic anemia, it is generally reserved for patients who are intolerant to other therapies. *Clopidogrel* is approved for prevention of atherosclerotic events following recent myocardial infarction, stroke, or established peripheral arterial disease. It is also approved for prophylaxis of thrombotic events in acute coronary syndrome (unstable angina or non-Q-wave

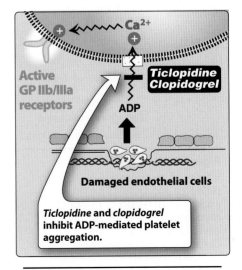

Figure 20.7
Mechanism of action of *ticlopidine* and *clopidogrel*. GP = glycoprotein.

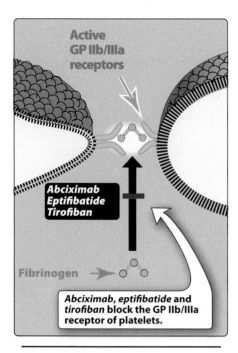

Figure 20.8
Mechanism of action of glycoprotein
(GP) IIb/IIIa–receptor blockers.

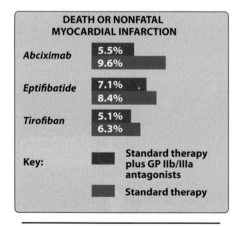

Figure 20.9
Effects of glycoprotein (GP) IIb/IIIa–
receptor antagonists on the
incidence of death or nonfatal
myocardial infarction following
percutaneous transluminal
coronary angioplasty. [Note: Data
are from several studies; thus,
reported incidence of complications
with standard therapy, such as
heparin, is not the same for each
drug.]

myocardial infarction). Additionally, *clopidogrel* is used to prevent thrombotic events associated with percutaneous coronary intervention with or without coronary stent. Compared to *ticlopidine*, *clopidogrel* is the preferred agent in ischemic heart disease events, because there is more data to support use of *clopidogrel* in these cardiac patients. Furthermore, *clopidogrel* has a better overall side-effect profile, although TTP may also occur with this agent.

3. **Pharmacokinetics:** Food interferes with the absorption of *ticlopidine* but not with *clopidogrel*. After oral ingestion, both drugs are extensively bound to plasma proteins. They undergo hepatic metabolism by the cytochrome P450 system to active metabolites that are yet to be identified. The maximum effect is achieved in 3 to 5 days; when treatment is suspended, the platelet system requires time to recover. Elimination of the drugs and metabolites occurs by both the renal and fecal routes. *Ticlopidine* has a black box warning due to the severe hematologic adverse reactions associated with its use. Both drugs can cause prolonged bleeding for which there is no antidote. Serious adverse effects of *ticlopidine* include neutropenia, TTP, and aplastic anemia requiring frequent blood monitoring, especially during the first 3 months of treatment. *Clopidogrel* causes fewer adverse reactions, and the incidence of neutropenia is lower. However, TTP has been reported as an adverse effect for both drugs. Because these drugs can inhibit cytochrome P450, they may interfere with the metabolism of drugs such as *phenytoin*, *tolbutamide*, *warfarin*, *fluvastatin*, and *tamoxifen* if taken concomitantly. Indeed, *phenytoin* toxicity has been reported when taken with *ticlopidine*.

C. Abciximab

The realization of the key role of the platelet GP IIb/IIIa receptor in stimulating platelet aggregation directed attempts to block this receptor on activated platelets. This led to the development of a chimeric monoclonal antibody, *abciximab* [ab-SIKS-eh-mab], which is composed of the constant regions of human immunoglobulin joined to the Fab fragments of a murine monoclonal antibody directed against the GP IIb/IIIa complex. By binding to GP IIb/IIIa, the antibody blocks the binding of fibrinogen and von Willebrand factor; consequently, aggregation does not occur (Figure 20.8). *Abciximab* is given intravenously along with *heparin* or *aspirin* as an adjunct to percutaneous coronary intervention for the prevention of cardiac ischemic complications. After cessation of infusion, platelet function gradually returns to normal, with the antiplatelet effect persisting for 24 to 48 hours. The major adverse effect of *abciximab* therapy is the potential for bleeding, especially if the drug is used with anticoagulants or if the patient has a clinical hemorrhagic condition. *Abciximab* is expensive, limiting its use in some settings.

D. Eptifibatide and tirofiban

These two antiplatelet drugs act similarly to *abciximab*—namely, blocking the GP IIb/IIIa receptor (see Figure 20.8). *Eptifibatide* [ep-ti-FIB-ih-tide] is a cyclic peptide that binds to GP IIb/IIIa at the site that interacts with the arginine-glycine-aspartic acid sequence of fibrinogen. *Tirofiban* [tye-roe-FYE-ban] is not a peptide, but it blocks the same site as *eptifibatide*. These compounds, like *abciximab*, can decrease the incidence of thrombotic complications associated with acute coronary syndromes. When intravenous infusion is stopped, these agents are rapidly cleared from the plasma, but their effect can persist for as long as 4 hours. [Note: Only intravenous formulations are available, because oral preparations of GP IIb/IIIa blockers are too toxic.] *Eptifibatide* and its metabolites are excreted by the kidney. *Tirofiban* is excreted unchanged by the kidney. The major adverse effect of both drugs is bleeding. Figure 20.9 summarizes the effects of the GP IIb/IIIa–receptor antagonists on death and myocardial infarction.

E. Dipyridamole

Dipyridamole [dye-peer-ID-a-mole], a coronary vasodilator, is employed prophylactically to treat angina pectoris. It is usually given in combination with *aspirin or warfarin*; it is ineffective when used alone. *Dipyridamole* increases intracellular levels of cAMP by inhibiting cyclic nucleotide phosphodiesterase, resulting in decreased thromboxane A_2 synthesis. It may potentiate the effect of prostacyclin to antagonize platelet stickiness and, therefore, decrease platelet adhesion to thrombogenic surfaces (see Figure 20.2). The meager data available suggest that *dipyridamole* makes only a marginal contribution to the antithrombotic action of *aspirin*. In combination with *warfarin*, however, *dipyridamole* is effective for inhibiting embolization from prosthetic heart valves.

V. BLOOD COAGULATION

The coagulation process that generates thrombin consists of two interrelated pathways—the extrinsic and the intrinsic systems. The extrinsic system, which is probably the more important system <u>in vivo</u>, is initiated by the activation of clotting Factor VII by tissue factor, or thromboplastin. Tissue factor is a lipoprotein that is expressed by activated endothelial cells, activated leukocytes, subendothelial fibroblasts, and subendothelial smooth muscle cells at the site of vascular injury. The intrinsic system is triggered by the activation of clotting Factor XII, following its contact <u>in vitro</u> with glass or highly charged surfaces. <u>In vivo</u>, this pathway may be initiated by Factor XII contact with charged cell surfaces containing phospholipids.

A. Formation of fibrin

Both systems involve a cascade of enzyme reactions that sequentially transform various plasma factors (proenzymes) to their active (enzymatic) forms. They ultimately produce Factor Xa, which converts prothrombin (Factor II) to thrombin (Factor IIa, Figure 20.10). Thrombin plays a key role in coagulation, because it is responsible for generation of fibrin, the GP that forms the mesh-like matrix of the blood clot. If thrombin is not formed or if its function is impeded (for example, by antithrombin III), coagulation is inhibited. Each step in the activation process is catalytic; for example, one unit of activated Factor X (Xa) can potentially generate 40 units of thrombin. This will result in the production of large amounts of fibrin at the site of injury.

B. Role of cell surfaces

Each reaction involved with the coagulation cascade takes place at a localized activated cell surface where a phospholipid-based protein-protein complex has formed. This complex consists of membrane surfaces provided by phospholipid (primarily phosphatidyl serine) of activated platelets or activated endothelial cells, an enzyme (an activated coagulation factor), a substrate (the proenzyme form of the downstream coagulation factor), and a cofactor. Ca^{2+} is essential in this process, bridging the anionic phospholipids and γ-carboxyglutamic acid residues of the clotting factors. [Note: Removal of Ca^{2+} with calcium chelators such as ethylenediamine tetra-acetic acid or citrate is used to prevent clotting in a test tube].

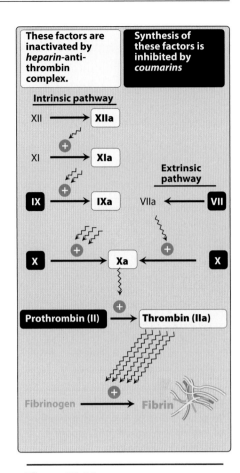

Figure 20.10
Formation of fibrin clot.

C. Inhibitors of coagulation

It is important that coagulation is restricted to the local site of vascular injury. Endogenously, there are several inhibitors of coagulation factors, including protein C, protein S, antithrombin III, and tissue factor pathway inhibitor. The mechanism of action of several anticoagulant agents, including *heparin* and *heparin*-related products, involves activation of these endogenous inhibitors (primarily antithrombin III).

VI. ANTICOAGULANTS

The anticoagulant drugs either inhibit the action of the coagulation factors (the thrombin inhibitors, such as *heparin* and *heparin*-related agents) or interfere with the synthesis of the coagulation factors (the vitamin K antagonists, such as *warfarin*).

A. Thrombin inhibitors: heparin and low-molecular-weight heparins (LMWHs)

Heparin [HEP-a-rin] is an injectable, rapidly acting anticoagulant that is often used acutely to interfere with the formation of thrombi. *Heparin* normally occurs as a macromolecule complexed with histamine in mast cells, where its physiologic role is unknown. It is extracted for commercial use from porcine intestine. Unfractionated *heparin* is a mixture of straight-chain, anionic glycosaminoglycans with a wide range of molecular weights (Figure 20.11). It is strongly acidic because of the presence of sulfate and carboxylic acid groups (Figure 20.12). [Note: In this discussion, the term *heparin* will indicate the unfractionated form of the drug.] The realization that low-molecular-weight forms of *heparin* (*LMWHs*) can also act as anticoagulants led to the isolation of *enoxaparin* [e-NOX-a-par-in], the first *LMWH* (<6000) available in the United States. The *LMWHs* are heterogeneous compounds (one-third the size of unfractionated *heparin*) produced by the chemical or enzymatic depolymerization of unfractionated *heparin*. Because they are free of some of the drawbacks associated with the polymer, they are replacing the use of *heparin* in many clinical situations. *Heparin* is used in the prevention of venous thrombosis and the treatment of a variety of thrombotic diseases, such as pulmonary embolism and acute myocardial infarction.

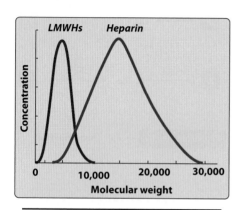

Figure 20.11
Typical molecular weight distributions of *low-molecular-weight heparins* (*LMWHs*) and *heparin*.

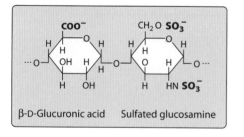

Figure 20.12
Disaccharide component of *heparin* showing negative charges due to carboxyl and sulfate groups.

1. **Mechanism of action:** *Heparin* acts at a number of molecular targets, but its anticoagulant effect is a consequence of binding to antithrombin III, with the subsequent rapid inactivation of coagulation factors (Figure 20.13). Antithrombin III is an α-globulin. It inhibits serine proteases, including several of the clotting factors—most importantly, thrombin (Factor IIa) and Factor Xa (see Figure 20.10). In the absence of *heparin*, antithrombin III interacts very slowly with thrombin and Factor Xa. *Heparin* molecules bind antithrombin III inducing a conformational change that accelerates its rate of action about 1000-fold. *Heparin* also serves as a catalytic template for the interaction of antithrombin III and the activated coagulation factors. *Heparin* serves as a true catalyst, allowing antithrombin III to rapidly combine with and inhibit circulating thrombin and Factor Xa (Figure 20.14). In contrast, *LMWHs* complex with antithrombin III and inactivate Factor Xa—including that located on platelet surfaces—but do not bind as avidly to thrombin. Indeed, *LMWHs* are less likely than *heparin* to activate resting platelets. [Note: A unique pentasaccharide sequence contained in *heparin* and *LMWHs* permits their binding to antithrombin III (see Figure 20.14).]

2. Therapeutic uses: *Heparin* and the *LMWHs* limit the expansion of thrombi by preventing fibrin formation. *Heparin* has been the major antithrombotic drug for the treatment of acute deep-vein thrombosis and pulmonary embolism. The incidence of recurrent thromboembolic episodes is also decreased. Clinically, *heparin* is used prophylactically to prevent postoperative venous thrombosis in patients undergoing elective surgery (for example, hip replacement) and those in the acute phase of myocardial infarction. Coronary artery rethrombosis after thrombolytic treatment is reduced with *heparin*. The drug is also used in extracorporeal devices (for example, dialysis machines) to prevent thrombosis. *Heparin* and *LMWHs* are the anticoagulants of choice for treating pregnant women with prosthetic heart valves or venous thromboembolism, because these agents do not cross the placenta (due to their large size and negative charge). *Heparin* has the advantage of speedy onset of action, which is rapidly terminated on suspension of therapy. However, it is being supplanted by the *LMWHs*, such as *enoxaparin* and *dalteparin*, because they can be conveniently injected subcutaneously on a patient weight–adjusted basis, have predictable therapeutic effects, and have a more predictable pharmacokinetic profile (Figure 20.15). Specifically, *LMWHs* do not require the same intense monitoring that *heparin* needs, subsequently saving laboratory costs as well as nursing time and costs. Therefore, these advantages make *LMWHs* useful for inpatient and outpatient therapy.

3. Pharmacokinetics:

a. Absorption: Whereas the anticoagulant effect with *heparin* occurs within minutes of intravenous administration (or 1 to 2 hours after subcutaneous injection), the maximum anti–Factor Xa activity of the *LMWHs* occurs about 4 hours after subcutaneous injection. (This is in comparison to the vitamin K–antagonist anticoagulants, such as *warfarin*, the activity of which requires 8 to 12 hours.) *Heparin* must be given parenterally, either in a deep subcutaneous site or intravenously,

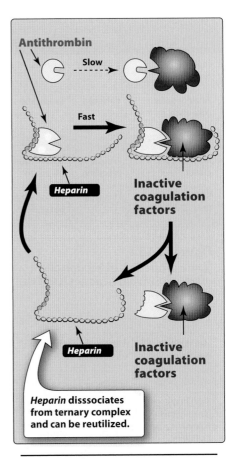

Figure 20.13
Heparin accelerates inactivation of coagulation factors by antithrombin.

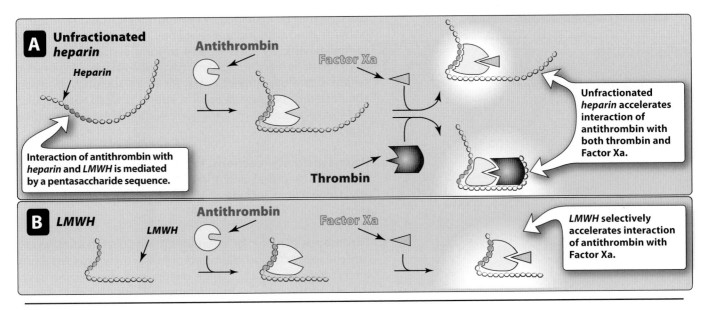

Figure 20.14
Heparin- and *low-molecular-weight heparin* (*LMWH*)–mediated inactivation of thrombin or Factor Xa.

DRUG CHARACTERISTIC	HEPARIN	LMWHs
Intravenous half-life	2 hours	4 hours
Anticoagulant response	Variable	Predicable
Bioavailability:	20%	90%
Major adverse effect	Frequent bleeding	Less frequent bleeding
Setting for therapy	Hospital	Hospital and outpatient

Figure 20.15
Some properties of *heparin* and *low-molecular-weight heparins* (*LMWHs*)

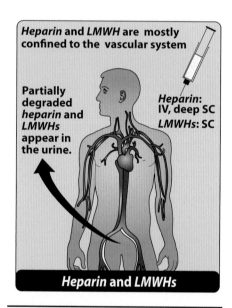

Figure 20.16
Administration and fate of *heparin* and *low-molecular-weight heparins* (*LMWHs*).

because the drug does not readily cross membranes (Figure 20.16). The *LMWHs* are administered subcutaneously. [Note: Intramuscular administration of either agent is contraindicated because of hematoma formation.] *Heparin* is often administered intravenously in a bolus to achieve immediate anticoagulation. This is followed by lower doses or continuous infusion of *heparin* for 7 to 10 days, titrating the dose so that the activated partial thromboplastin time (aPTT) is 1.5- to 2.5-fold that of the normal control. It is usually not necessary to obtain such an index with the *LMWHs* because the plasma levels and pharmacokinetics of these drugs are predictable, However, for those patients with renal impairment, the dose should be reduced to account for decreased renal function.

   b. **Fate:** In the blood, *heparin* binds to many proteins that neutralize its activity, thereby causing resistance to the drug. Although generally restricted to the circulation, *heparin* is taken up by the monocyte/macrophage system, and it undergoes depolymerization and desulfation to inactive products. [Note: *Heparin* therefore has a longer half-life in patients with hepatic cirrhosis.] The inactive metabolites as well as some of the parent *heparin* and *LMWHs* are excreted into the urine. Therefore, renal insufficiency also prolongs the half-life. Neither *heparin* nor the *LMWHs* cross the placental barrier. The half-life of *heparin* is approximately 1.5 hours, whereas the half-life of the *LMWHs* is two to four times longer than that of *heparin*, ranging from around 3 to 7 hours.

4. **Adverse effects:** Despite early hopes of fewer side effects with *LMWHs*, complications have proven to be similar to those seen with *heparin*. However, exceptions are thromboembolic problems, which are less common.

   a. **Bleeding complications:** The chief complication of *heparin* therapy is hemorrhage (Figure 20.17). Careful monitoring of the bleeding time is required to minimize this problem. Excessive bleeding may be managed by ceasing administration of the drug or by treating with *protamine sulfate*. Infused slowly, the latter combines ionically with *heparin* to form a stable, 1:1 inactive complex. It is very important that the dosage of *protamine sulfate* is carefully titrated (1 mg for every 100 units of *heparin* administered) because *heparin sulfate* is a weak anticoagulant and excess amounts may trigger bleeding episodes or worsen bleeding potential.

   b. **Hypersensitivity reactions:** *Heparin* preparations are obtained from porcine sources and, therefore, may be antigenic. Possible adverse reactions include chills, fever, urticaria, or anaphylactic shock.

   c. **Thrombosis:** Chronic or intermittent administration of *heparin* can lead to a reduction in antithrombin III activity, thus decreasing the inactivation of coagulation factors and, thereby, increasing the risk of thrombosis. To minimize this risk, low-dose *heparin* therapy is usually employed.

d. Thrombocytopenia: This condition, in which circulating blood contains an abnormally small number of platelets, is a common abnormality among hospital patients and can be caused by a variety of factors. One of these is associated with the use of *heparin* and is called *heparin*-induced thrombocytopenia (HIT). Two types of this abnormality have been identified. Type I is common and involves a mild decrease in platelet number due to nonimmunologic mechanisms. Type I usually occurs within the first 5 days of treatment and is not serious. In Type II, platelets are activated by an immunoglobulin G–mediated reaction with a *heparin*–platelet Factor 4 complex, causing platelet aggregation and release of platelet contents. This can result in thrombocytopenia and thrombosis—dangerous complications of *heparin* therapy occurring between the fifth and fourteenth days of treatment—that range from mild to life-threatening. Platelet counts can drop 50 percent or more, and thromboembolic complications can develop. Although Type II is relatively rare, the wide use of *heparin* has resulted in a greater recognition of its role in thrombocytopenia. It is imperative that *heparin* therapy be discontinued in such patients. *Heparin* can be replaced by another anticoagulant, such as *lepirudin* or *argatroban* (see below).

e. Heparin may produce abnormal liver function tests, and osteoporosis has been observed in patients on long term *heparin* therapy.

f. Contraindications: *Heparin* is contraindicated for patients who are hypersensitive to it, have bleeding disorders, are alcoholics, or are having or have had recent surgery of the brain, eye, or spinal cord.

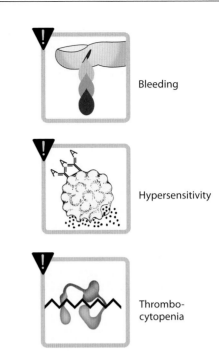

Bleeding

Hypersensitivity

Thrombo-cytopenia

Figure 20.17
Adverse effects of *heparin*.

B. Other parenteral anticoagulants

1. Lepirudin: A highly specific, direct thrombin antagonist, *lepirudin* [leh-PEE-roo-din] is a polypeptide that is closely related to *hirudin*—a thrombin inhibitor derived from medicinal leech saliva. *Lepirudin* is produced in yeast cells by recombinant DNA technology. One molecule of *lepirudin* binds to one molecule of thrombin, resulting in blockade of the thrombogenic activity of thrombin. It has little effect on platelet aggregation. Administered intravenously (Figure 20.18), *lepirudin* is effective in the treatment of HIT and other thromboembolic disorders, and it can prevent further thromboembolic complications. *Lepirudin* has a half-life of about 1 hour, and it undergoes hydrolysis. The parent drug and its fragments are eliminated in the urine. Bleeding is the major adverse effect of treatment with *lepirudin*, and it can be exacerbated by concomitant thrombolytic therapy, such as treatment with *streptokinase* or *alteplase*. About half the patients receiving *lepirudin* develop antibodies. However, the drug-antibody complex retains anticoagulant activity. Because renal elimination of the complex is slower than that of the free drug, the anticoagulant effect may be increased. It is important to monitor the aPTT and renal function when a patient is receiving *lepirudin*.

2. Argatroban: *Argatroban* [ar-GA-troh-ban] is a parenteral anticoagulant that is a small molecule that direct inhibits thrombin. *Argatroban*

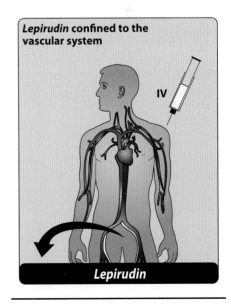

Lepirudin confined to the vascular system

IV

Lepirudin

Figure 20.18
Administration of *lepirudin*.

is used prophylactically for the treatment of thrombosis in patients with HIT, and it is also approved for use during percutaneous coronary interventions in patients who have or are at risk for developing HIT. *Argatroban* is metabolized in the liver and has a half life of about 50 minutes. It is monitored by aPTT. The patient's hemoglobin and hematocrit must also be monitored. Because *argatroban* is metabolized in the liver, it may be used in patients with renal dysfunction but it should be used cautiously in patients with hepatic impairment. As with other agents in this class, the major side effect is bleeding.

3. **Fondaparinux:** *Fondaparinux* [fawn-da-PEH-rih-nox] is the first in a new class of pentasaccharide anticoagulants that is purely synthetically, derived with no variable biologic activity. It has been recently approved by the U.S. Food and Drug Administration for use in the prophylaxis of deep-vein thrombosis that could lead to pulmonary embolism in patients undergoing hip fracture surgery, hip replacement surgery, and knee replacement surgery. This agent selectively inhibits only Factor Xa. By selectively binding to antithrombin III, *fondaparinux* potentiates (300- to 1000-fold) the innate neutralization of Factor Xa by antithrombin III. It is well absorbed from the subcutaneous route with a predictable pharmacokinetic profile. *Fondaparinux* requires less monitoring than *heparin*. *Fondaparinux* is eliminated in urine mainly as unchanged drug with an elimination half-life of 17 to 21 hours. It is contraindicated in patients with severe renal impairment (<30 mL/min). Bleeding episodes are the major side effect of *fondaparinux* therapy. Thrombocytopenia, in particular Type II thrombocytopenia, is not a problem, and this agent may be used in patients with HIT.

C. Vitamin K antagonists

The coumarin anticoagulants, which include *warfarin* [WAR-far-in], and *dicumarol* [dye-KOO-ma-role] (*bishydroxycoumarin*), owe their action to their ability to antagonize the cofactor functions of vitamin K. The only therapeutically relevant coumarin anticoagulant is *warfarin*. Initially used as a rodenticide, *warfarin* is now widely employed clinically as an oral anticoagulant. With the availability of the *LMWHs* and platelet aggregate inhibitors, however, use of the vitamin K antagonists is decreasing. The potential morbidity associated with the use of *warfarin* makes it important to identify those patients who are truly at risk for thrombosis. Even careful monitoring to keep the prothrombin time at 1.5- to 2.5-fold longer than normal values does not prevent bleeding complications in about 20 percent of the patients.

1. **Mechanism of action:** Several of the protein coagulation factors (including Factors II, VII, IX, and X; see Figure 20.10) require vitamin K as a cofactor for their synthesis by the liver. These factors undergo vitamin K–dependent posttranslational modification, whereby a number of their glutamic acid residues are carboxylated to form γ-carboxyglutamic acid residues (Figure 20.19). The γ-carboxyglutamyl residues bind calcium ions, which are essential for interaction between the coagulation factors and platelet mem-

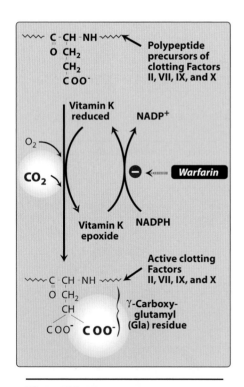

Figure 20.19
Mechanism of action of *warfarin*. $NADP^+$ = oxidized form of nicotinamide-adenine dinucleotide phosphate; NADPH = reduced form of nicotinamide-adenine dinucleotide phosphate.

[5]See p. 157 *Lippincott's Illustrated Reviews: Biochemistry* (4th ed.) for a discussion of the structure of heparin, dermatan and chondroitin.

branes. In the carboxylation reactions, the vitamin K–dependent carboxylase fixes CO_2 to form the new COOH group on glutamic acid. The reduced vitamin K cofactor is converted to vitamin K epoxide during the reaction. Vitamin K is regenerated from the epoxide by vitamin K epoxide reductase—the enzyme that is inhibited by *warfarin*. *Warfarin* treatment results in the production of clotting factors with diminished activity (10%–40% of normal), because they lack sufficient γ-carboxyglutamyl side chains. Unlike *heparin*, the anticoagulant effects of *warfarin* are not observed until 8 to 12 hours after drug administration, but peak effects may be delayed for 72 to 96 hours—the time required to deplete the pool of circulating clotting factors. The anticoagulant effects of *warfarin* can be overcome by the administration of vitamin K. However, reversal following administration of vitamin K takes approximately 24 hours (the time necessary for degradation of already synthesized clotting factors).

2. **Therapeutic uses:** *Warfarin* is used to prevent the progression or recurrence of acute deep-vein thrombosis or pulmonary embolism after initial *heparin* treatment. It is also used for the prevention of venous thromboembolism during orthopaedic or gynecologic surgery. Prophylactically, it is used in patients with acute myocardial infarction, prosthetic heart valves, or chronic atrial fibrillation.

3. **Pharmacokinetics:**

    a. **Absorption:** *Warfarin* is rapidly absorbed after oral administration (100% bioavailability with little individual patient variation). Although food may delay absorption, it does not affect the extent of absorption of the drug. *Warfarin* is 99 percent bound to plasma albumin, which prevents its diffusion into the cerebrospinal fluid, urine, and breast milk. However, drugs that have a greater affinity for the albumin binding site, such as sulfonamides, can displace the anticoagulant and lead to a transient, elevated activity. *Warfarin* readily crosses the placental barrier. The mean half life of *warfarin* is approximately 40 hours, but this value is highly variable among individuals. Prothrombin time, a measure of the extrinsic pathway, may be used to monitor *warfarin* therapy. In the 1990s, the international normalized ratio (INR) was adopted to monitor *warfarin* concentration. The INR corrects for variations that would occur with different thromboplastin reagents, between different hospitals, or when a single hospital gets a new lot of reagent. The goal of *warfarin* therapy is an INR of 2 to 3 for most indications and 2.5 to 3.5 in patients with mechanical heart valves.

    b. **Fate:** The products of *warfarin* metabolism, catalyzed by the cytochrome P450 system, are inactive. After conjugation to glucuronic acid, they are excreted in the urine and stool.

4. **Adverse effects :**

    a. **Bleeding disorders:** The principal untoward reaction caused by *warfarin* treatment is hemorrhage. Therefore, it is important to frequently monitor and adjust the anticoagulant effect. Minor bleeding may be treated by withdrawal of the drug and administration of oral vitamin K_1; severe bleeding requires that greater doses of the vitamin be given intravenously. Whole blood, frozen plasma, or plasma concentrates of the blood factors may also be employed to arrest hemorrhaging. Skin lesions

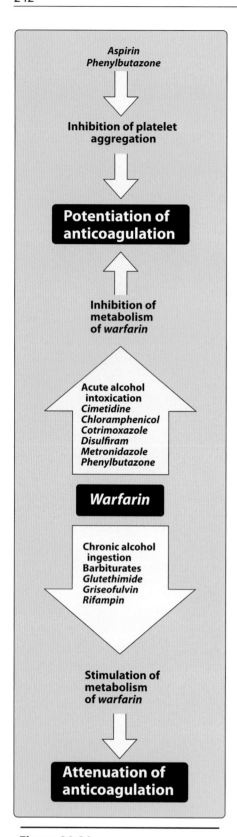

Figure 20.20
Drugs affecting the anticoagulant effect of *warfarin*.

and necrosis are rare complications of *warfarin* therapy and are observed primarily in women. Purple toe syndrome, a painful, blue-tinged discoloration of the toe caused by cholesterol emboli from plaques, has also been observed with *warfarin* therapy.

  b. Drug interactions: *Warfarin* has numerous drug interactions that may potentiate or attenuate its anticoagulant effect. The list of interacting drugs is extensive. A summary of some of the important interactions is shown in Figure 20.20.

  c. Disease states: Vitamin K deficiency, hepatic disease that impairs synthesis of the clotting factors or affects *warfarin* metabolism, and hypermetabolic states that increase catabolism of the vitamin K–dependent clotting factors can all influence the hypoprothrombinemic state of the patient and augment the response to the oral anticoagulants.

  d. Contraindications: *Warfarin* should never be used during pregnancy, because it is teratogenic and can cause abortion as well as birth defects.

VII. THROMBOLYTIC DRUGS

Acute thromboembolic disease in selected patients may be treated by the administration of agents that activate the conversion of plasminogen to plasmin—a serine protease that hydrolyzes fibrin and, thus, dissolves clots (Figure 20.21). *Streptokinase*, one of the first such agents to be approved, causes a systemic fibrinolytic state that can lead to bleeding problems. *Alteplase* acts more locally on the thrombotic fibrin to produce fibrinolysis. Figure 20.22 compares these commonly used thrombolytic agents. Clinical experience has shown nearly equal efficacy between *streptokinase* and *alteplase*. Unfortunately, thrombolytic therapy is unsuccessful in about 20 percent of infarcted arteries, and about 15 percent of the arteries that are opened will later close again. In the case of acute myocardial infarction, the thrombolytic drugs are reserved for those instances when angioplasty is not an option or until the patient can be taken to a facility that performs percutaneous coronary interventions. Fibrinolytic drugs may lyse both normal and pathologic thrombi.

A. Common characteristics of thrombolytic agents

  1. Mechanism of action: The thrombolytic agents share some common features. All act either directly or indirectly to convert plasminogen to plasmin, which in turn cleaves fibrin, thus lysing thrombi (see Figure 20.21). Clot dissolution and reperfusion occur with a higher frequency when therapy is initiated early after clot formation, because clots become more resistant to lysis as they age. Unfortunately, increased local thrombi may occur as the clot dissolves, leading to enhanced platelet aggregability and thrombosis. Strategies to prevent this include administration of antiplatelet drugs, such as *aspirin*, or antithrombotics, such as *heparin*.

  2. Therapeutic uses: Originally used for the treatment of deep-vein thrombosis and serious pulmonary embolism, thrombolytic drugs are now being used less frequently for these conditions. Their tendency to cause bleeding has also blunted their used in treating acute myocardial infarction or peripheral arterial thrombosis. However, thrombolytic agents are helpful in restoring catheter and shunt function, by lysing clots causing occlusions. Thrombolytic agents are also used to dissolve clots that result in strokes.

3. **Pharmacokinetics:** For myocardial infarction, intracoronary delivery of the drugs is the most reliable in terms of achieving recanalization. However, cardiac catheterization may not be possible in the 2- to 6-hour "therapeutic window," beyond which significant myocardial salvage becomes less likely. Thus, thrombolytic agents are usually administered intravenously, because this route is rapid, is inexpensive, and does not have the risks of catheterization.

4. **Adverse effects:** The thrombolytic agents do not distinguish between the fibrin of an unwanted thrombus and the fibrin of a beneficial hemostatic plug. Thus, hemorrhage is a major side effect. For example, a previously unsuspected lesion, such as a peptic ulcer, may hemorrhage following injection of a thrombolytic agent (Figure 20.23). These drugs are contraindicated in patients with healing wounds, pregnancy, history of cerebrovascular accident, or metastatic cancer. Continued presence of thrombogenic stimuli may cause rethrombosis after lysis of the initial clot.

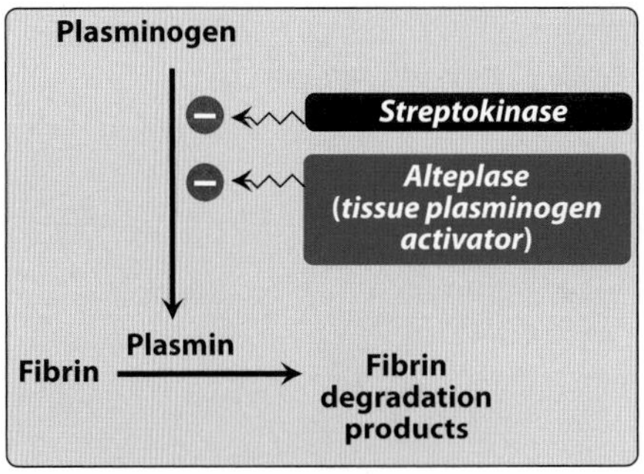

B. Alteplase

Alteplase [AL-te-place] (formerly known as *tissue plasminogen activator*, or *tPA*) is a serine protease originally derived from cultured human melanoma cells. It is now obtained as a product of recombinant DNA technology.

1. **Mechanism of action:** *Alteplase* has a low affinity for free plasminogen in the plasma, but it rapidly activates plasminogen that is bound to fibrin in a thrombus or a hemostatic plug. Thus, *alteplase* is said to be "fibrin selective," and at low doses, it has the advantage of lysing only fibrin, without unwanted degradation of other proteins—notably fibrinogen. This contrasts with *streptokinase*, which acts on free plasminogen and induces a general fibrinolytic state. [Note: At dose levels of *alteplase* currently in use clinically, circulating plasminogen may be activated, resulting in hemorrhage.]

2. **Therapeutic uses:** *Alteplase* is approved for the treatment of myocardial infarction, massive pulmonary embolism, and acute ischemic stroke. *Alteplase* seems to be superior to *streptokinase* in dissolving older clots and, ultimately, may be approved for other applications. *Alteplase,* administered within 3 hours of the onset of ischemic stroke, significantly improves clinical outcome—that is, the patient's ability to perform activities of daily living (Figure 20.24). *Reteplase* (*Retavase*) is similar to *alteplase* and can be used as an alternative.

3. **Pharmacokinetics:** *Alteplase* has a very short half-life (about 5 minutes) and, therefore, is administered as a total dose equal to 0.9 mg/ kg. Ten percent of the total dose injected intravenously as a bolus and the remaining drug is administered over 60 minutes.

4. **Adverse effects:** Bleeding complications, including gastrointestinal and cerebral hemorrhages, may occur.

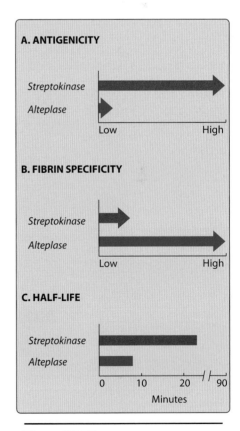

Figure 20.21
Activation of plasminogen by fibrinolytic agents.

Figure 20.22
A comparison of *streptokinase* and *alteplase*.

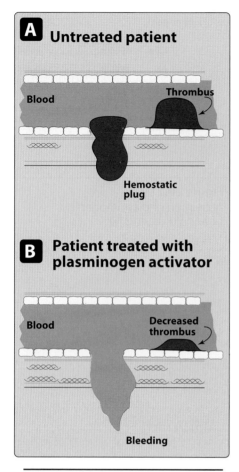

Figure 20.23
Degradation of an unwanted thrombus and a beneficial hemostatic plug by plasminogen activators.

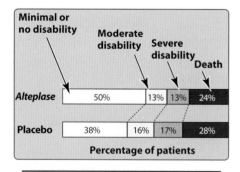

Figure 20.24
Outcome at 12 months of stroke patients treated with *alteplase* within 3 hours of the onset of symptoms compared to those treated with placebo.

C. Streptokinase

Streptokinase [strep-toe-KYE-nase] is an extracellular protein purified from culture broths of Group C β-hemolytic streptococci.[6]

1. **Mechanism of action:** *Streptokinase* has no enzymic activity. Instead, it forms an active one-to-one complex with plasminogen. This enzymatically active complex converts uncomplexed plasminogen to the active enzyme plasmin (Figure 20.25). In addition to the hydrolysis of fibrin plugs, the complex also catalyzes the degradation of fibrinogen as well as clotting Factors V and VII (Figure 20.26).

2. **Therapeutic uses:** *Streptokinase* is approved for use in acute pulmonary embolism, deep-vein thrombosis, acute myocardial infarction, arterial thrombosis, and occluded access shunts.

3. **Pharmacokinetics:** *Streptokinase* therapy is instituted within 4 hours of a myocardial infarction and is infused for 1 hour. Its half-life is less than half an hour. Thromboplastin time is monitored and maintained at two- to five-fold the control value. On discontinuation of treatment, either *heparin* or oral anticoagulants may be administered.

4. **Adverse effects:**

   a. **Bleeding disorders:** Activation of circulating plasminogen by *streptokinase* leads to elevated levels of plasmin, which may precipitate bleeding by dissolving hemostatic plugs (see Figure 20.23). In the rare instance of life-threatening hemorrhage, *aminocaproic acid* may be administered.

   b. **Hypersensitivity:** *Streptokinase* is a foreign protein and is antigenic. Rashes, fever, and rarely, anaphylaxis occur. Because most individuals have had a streptococcal infection sometime in their lives, circulating antibodies against *streptokinase* are likely to be present in most patients. These antibodies can combine with *streptokinase* and neutralize its fibrinolytic properties. Therefore, sufficient quantities of *streptokinase* must be administered to overwhelm the antibodies and provide a therapeutic concentration of plasmin. Fever, allergic reactions, and therapeutic failure may be associated with the presence of antistreptococcal antibodies in the patient. The incidence of allergic reactions is approximately 3 percent.

D. Anistreplase (anisoylated plasminogen streptokinase activator complex

Anistreplase is a preformed complex of *streptokinase* and plasminogen and it is considered to be a prodrug. *Streptokinase* must be released, and only plasminogen to which it was associated will get converted to plasmin.

[6]See p. 79 in ***Lippincott's Illustrated Reviews: Microbiology*** (2nd ed.) for a discussion of the streptococci.

VIII. DRUGS USED TO TREAT BLEEDING

Bleeding problems may have their origin in naturally occurring pathologic conditions, such as hemophilia, or as a result of fibrinolytic states that may arise after gastrointestinal surgery or prostatectomy. The use of anticoagulants may also give rise to hemorrhage. Certain natural proteins and vitamin K, as well as synthetic antagonists, are effective in controlling this bleeding. For example, hemophilia is a consequence of a deficiency in plasma coagulation factors, most frequently Factors VIII and IX. Concentrated preparations of these factors are available from human donors. However, these preparations carry the risk of transferring viral infections. Blood transfusion is also an option for treating severe hemorrhage.

A. Aminocaproic acid and tranexamic acid

Fibrinolytic states can be controlled by the administration of *aminocaproic* [a-mee-noe-ka-PROE-ic] *acid* or *tranexamic* [tran-ex-AM-ic] *acid*. Both agents are synthetic, inhibit plasminogen activation, are orally active, and are excreted in the urine. A potential side effect of treatment is intravascular thrombosis.

B. Protamine sulfate

Protamine [PROE-ta-meen] *sulfate* antagonizes the anticoagulant effects of *heparin*. This protein is derived from fish sperm or testes and is high in arginine content, which explains its basicity. The positively charged *protamine* interacts with the negatively charged *heparin*, forming a stable complex without anticoagulant activity. Adverse effects of drug administration include hypersensitivity as well as dyspnea, flushing, bradycardia, and hypotension when rapidly injected.

C. Vitamin K

That vitamin K_1 (*phytonadione*) administration can stem bleeding problems due to the oral anticoagulants is not surprising, because those substances act by interfering with the action of the vitamin (see Figure 20.19). The response to vitamin K is slow, requiring about 24 hours (time to synthesize new coagulation factors). Thus, if immediate hemostasis is required, fresh-frozen plasma should be infused.

D. Aprotinin

Aprotinin [ah-PRO-ti-nin] is a serine protease inhibitor that stops bleeding by blocking plasmin. It can inhibit *streptokinase*. It is approved for prophylactic use to reduce perioperative blood loss and the need for blood transfusion in patients undergoing cardiopulmonary bypass surgery. *Aprotinin* may cause renal dysfunction and hypersensitivity (anaphylactic) reactions. In addition, *aprotinin* should not be administered to patients who have already been exposed to the drug within the previous 12 months due to the possibility of anaphylactic reactions.

IX. AGENTS USED TO TREAT ANEMIA

Anemia is defined as a below-normal plasma hemoglobin concentration resulting from a decreased number of circulating red blood cells or an abnormally low total hemoglobin content per unit of blood volume. Anemia can be caused by chronic blood loss, bone marrow abnormalities, increased hemolysis, infections, malignancy, endocrine deficiencies, renal failure, and

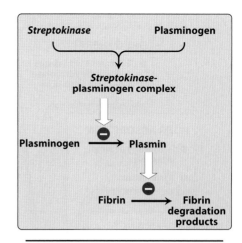

Figure 20.25
Mechanism of action of *streptokinase*.

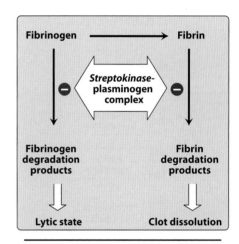

Figure 20.26
Streptokinase degrades both fibrin and fibrinogen.

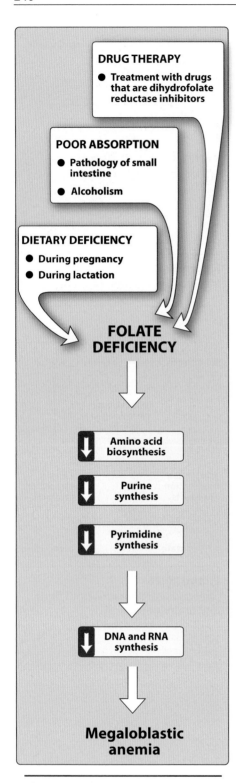

Figure 20.27
Causes and consequences of folic acid depletion.

a number of other disease states. Anemia can be at least temporarily corrected by transfusion of whole blood. A large number of drugs cause toxic effects on blood cells, hemoglobin production, or erythropoietic organs, which in turn may cause anemia. In addition, nutritional anemias are caused by dietary deficiencies of substances such as iron, folic acid, or vitamin B_{12} (cyanocobalamin) that are necessary for normal erythropoiesis.

A. Iron

Iron is stored in intestinal mucosal cells as ferritin (an iron-protein complex) until needed by the body. Iron deficiency results from acute or chronic blood loss, from insufficient intake during periods of accelerated growth in children, or in heavily menstruating or pregnant women. Thus, iron deficiency results from a negative iron balance due to depletion of iron stores and/or inadequate intake, culminating in hypochromic microcytic anemia (due to low iron and small-sized red blood cells). Supplementation with *ferrous sulfate* is required to correct the deficiency. Gastrointestinal disturbances caused by local irritation are the most common adverse effects of iron supplements.

B. Folic acid

The primary use of *folic acid* is in treating deficiency states that arise from inadequate levels of the vitamin. Folate deficiency may be caused by 1) increased demand (for example, pregnancy and lactation), 2) poor absorption caused by pathology of the small intestine, 3) alcoholism, or 4) treatment with drugs that are dihydrofolate reductase inhibitors (for example, *methotrexate* or *trimethoprim*). A primary result of folic acid deficiency is megaloblastic anemia (large-sized red blood cells), which is caused by diminished synthesis of purines and pyrimidines. This leads to an inability of erythropoietic tissue to make DNA and, thereby, proliferate[7] (Figure 20.27). [Note: To avoid neurological complications of vitamin B_{12} deficiency, it is important to evaluate the basis of the megaloblastic anemia prior to instituting therapy. Vitamin B_{12} and folate deficiency causes similar symptoms (see below).] *Folic acid* is well absorbed in the jejunum unless pathology is present. If excessive amounts of the vitamin are ingested, they are excreted in the urine and feces. Oral *folic acid* administered has no known toxicity.

C. Cyanocobalamin (vitamin B_{12})

Deficiencies of vitamin B_{12} can result from either low dietary levels or, more commonly, poor absorption of the vitamin due to the failure of gastric parietal cells to produce intrinsic factor (as in pernicious anemia) or a loss of activity of the receptor needed for intestinal uptake of the vitamin.[8] Intrinsic factor is a GP produced by the parietal cells of the stomach and it is required for vitamin B_{12} absorption. In patients with bariatric surgery (surgical gastrointestinal treatment for obesity), vitamin B_{12} supplementation is required in large oral doses, sublingually or once a month by the parenteral route. Nonspecific malabsorption syndromes or gastric resection can also cause vitamin B_{12} deficiency. The vitamin may be administered orally (for dietary deficiencies), intramus-

[7]See p. 374 in *Lippincott's Illustrated Reviews: Biochemistry* (4th ed.) for a discussion of folic acid deficiency and DNA replication.
[8]See p. 376 in *Lippincott's Illustrated Reviews: Biochemistry* (4th ed.) for a discussion of vitamin B_{12} and its deficiency state.

cularly, or deep subcutaneously (for pernicious anemia). [Note: *Folic acid* administration alone reverses the hematologic abnormality and, thus, masks the B_{12} deficiency, which can then proceed to severe neurologic dysfunction and disease. Therefore, megaloblastic anemia should not be treated with *folic acid* alone but, rather, with a combination of *folate* and vitamin B_{12}.] Therapy must be continued for the remainder of the life of a patient suffering from pernicious anemia. There are no known adverse effects of this vitamin.

D. Erythropoietin and darbepoetin

Erythropoietin [ee-rith-ro-POI-eh-tin] is a GP, normally made by the kidney, that regulates red blood cell proliferation and differentiation in bone marrow. Human *erythropoietin*, produced by recombinant DNA technology, is effective in the treatment of anemia caused by endstage renal disease, anemia associated with human immunodeficiency virus infection, and anemia in some cancer patients. *Darbepoetin* [dar-be-POE-e-tin] is a long-acting version of *erythropoietin* that differs from *erythropoietin* by the addition of two carbohydrate chains, which improves its biologic activity. Therefore, *darbepoetin* has decreased clearance and has a half life about three times that of *erythropoietin*. Due to its delayed onset of action, *darbepoetin* has no value in acute treatment of anemia. Supplementation with iron may be required to assure an adequate response. The protein is usually administered intravenously in renal dialysis patients, but the subcutaneous route is preferred. Side effects are generally well tolerated but may include elevation in blood pressure and arthralgia in some cases. [Note: The former may be due to increases in peripheral vascular resistance and/or blood viscosity.] When *erythropoietin* is used to target hemoglobin concentration >12 g/dL, serious and life-threatening cardiovascular events, increased risk of death, shortened time to tumor progression and/or decreased survival have been observed. The recommendations for all patients receiving *erythropoietin* include a minimum effective dose that does not exceed a hemoglobin level of 12 g/dL, and this should not rise more than 1 g/dL over a 2-week period.

X. AGENTS USED TO TREAT SICKLE-CELL DISEASE

Clinical trials have shown that *hydroxyurea* can relieve the painful clinical course of sickle-cell disease (Figure 20.28). *Hydroxyurea* is currently also being used to treat chronic myelogenous leukemia and polycythemia vera. In sickle-cell disease, the drug apparently increases fetal hemoglobin levels, thus diluting the abnormal hemoglobin S (HbS).[9] This process takes several months. Polymerization of HbS is delayed in the treated patients so that painful crises are not caused by sickled cells blocking capillaries and causing tissue anoxia. Important side effects of *hydroxyurea* include bone marrow suppression and cutaneous vasculitis. It is important that *hydroxyurea* is administered under the supervision of a physician experienced in the treatment of sickle-cell disease.

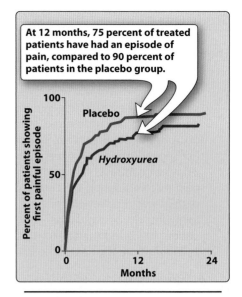

Figure 20.28
Effect of treatment with *hydroxyurea* on the percentage of sickle-cell patients experiencing first painful episode.

[9]See p. 35 in ***Lippincott's Illustrated Reviews: Biochemistry*** (4th ed.) for a discussion of sickle-cell diseases and hemoglobin.

Study Questions

Choose the ONE best answer.

20.1 A 22-year-old woman who experienced pain and swelling in her right leg presented at the emergency room. An ultrasound study showed thrombosis in the popliteal vein. The patient, who was in her second trimester of pregnancy, was treated for 7 days with intravenous unfractionated heparin. The pain resolved during the course of therapy, and the patient was discharged on Day 8. Which one of the following drugs would be most appropriate outpatient follow-up therapy for this patient, who lives 100 miles from the nearest hospital?

A. Warfarin.
B. Aspirin.
C. Alteplase.
D. Unfractionated heparin.
E. Low-molecular-weight heparin (LMWH).

Correct answer = E. LMWH has a reliable dose response and can be administered subcutaneously by selected patients who have been taught home injection technique. LMWH does not cross the placenta and shows no teratogenic effects. By contrast, warfarin is teratogenic and is contraindicated in pregnant patients. Aspirin, which inhibits platelet aggregation, has little effect on venous thrombosis, which is composed of fibrin with only a few platelets. Alteplase is not indicated for deep-vein thrombosis.

20.2 A 60-year-old man is diagnosed with deep-vein thrombosis. The patient was treated with a bolus of heparin, and a heparin drip was started. One hour later, he was bleeding profusely from the intravenous site. The heparin therapy was suspended, but the bleeding continued. Protamine was administered intravenously, and the bleeding resolved. The protamine:

A. Degraded the heparin.
B. Inactivates antithrombin.
C. Activates the coagulation cascade.
D. Activates tissue-plasminogen activator.
E. Ionically combines with heparin.

Correct answer = E. Excessive bleeding may be managed by ceasing administration of the drug or by treating with protamine sulfate. Infused slowly, protamine combines ionically with heparin to form a stable, inactive complex.

20.3 A 54-year-old male with a prosthetic aortic valve replacement complained to his family physician of black and tarry stools. Physical examination and vital signs were unremarkable except for subconjunctival hemorrhages and bleeding gums. Stools tested positive for heme, and hematuria was observed. The patient has been receiving oral warfarin since his valve replacement 1 year earlier. Prothrombin time was found to be significantly elevated. Which one of the following therapies would provide the most rapid recovery from the observed bleeding secondary to warfarin treatment?

A. Intravenous vitamin K.
B. Transfusion of fresh-frozen plasma.
C. Intravenous protamine.
D. Immediate withdrawal of warfarin treatment.
E. Intravenous administration of anti-warfarin antibodies.

Correct answer = B. Whole blood, frozen plasma, or plasma concentrates of the blood factors may be employed to rapidly arrest hemorrhaging. Minor bleeding may be treated by withdrawal of the drug and administration of oral vitamin K_1; severe bleeding requires greater doses of the vitamin given intravenously. However, reversal following administration of vitamin K takes approximately 24 hours. Protamine is used to neutralize an overdose of heparin, not an overdose of warfarin. Immediate withdrawal of warfarin treatment will not have an immediate effect, because the anticoagulant effects of warfarin last between 5 and 7 days.

Hyperlipidemias

21

I. OVERVIEW

Coronary heart disease (CHD) is the cause of about half of all deaths in the United States. The incidence of CHD is correlated with elevated levels of low-density lipoprotein (LDL) cholesterol and triacylglycerols and with low levels of high-density lipoprotein (HDL) cholesterol. Other risk factors for CHD include cigarette smoking, hypertension, obesity, and diabetes. Cholesterol levels may be elevated as a result of an individual's lifestyle (for example, by lack of exercise and consumption of a diet containing excess saturated fatty acids). Hyperlipidemias can also result from a single inherited gene defect in lipoprotein metabolism or, more commonly, from a combination of genetic and lifestyle factors. Appropriate lifestyle changes in combination with drug therapy can lead to a decline in the progression of coronary plaque, regression of preexisting lesions, and reduction in mortality due to CHD by 30 to 40 percent. Antihyperlipidemic drugs must be taken indefinitely; when therapy is terminated, plasma lipid levels return to pretreatment levels. The lipid-lowering drugs are listed in Figure 21.1. Figure 21.2 illustrates the normal metabolism of serum lipoproteins and the characteristics of the major genetic hyperlipidemias.

II. TREATMENT GOALS

Plasma lipids consist mostly of lipoproteins—spherical macromolecular complexes of lipids and specific proteins (apolipoproteins). The clinically important lipoproteins, listed in decreasing order of atherogenicity, are LDL, very-low-density lipoprotein (VLDL) and chylomicrons, and HDL. The occurrence of CHD is positively associated with high total cholesterol, and even more strongly with elevated LDL cholesterol in the blood. In contrast to LDL cholesterol, high levels of HDL cholesterol have been associated with a decreased risk for heart disease (Figure 21.3). Reduction of the LDL level is the primary goal of cholesterol-lowering therapy. Figure 21.4 shows the current goals in the treatment of hyperlipidemia. Recommendations for the reduction of LDL cholesterol to specific target levels are influenced by the coexistence of CHD and the number of other cardiac risk factors. The higher the overall risk of heart disease, the more aggressive the recommended LDL-lowering therapy.

A. Treatment options for hypercholesterolemia

In patients with moderate hyperlipidemia, lifestyle changes, such as diet, exercise, and weight reduction, can lead to modest decreases in LDL levels and increases in HDL levels. However, most patients are

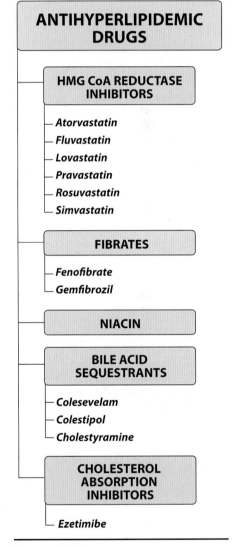

ANTIHYPERLIPIDEMIC DRUGS

HMG CoA REDUCTASE INHIBITORS
- *Atorvastatin*
- *Fluvastatin*
- *Lovastatin*
- *Pravastatin*
- *Rosuvastatin*
- *Simvastatin*

FIBRATES
- *Fenofibrate*
- *Gemfibrozil*

NIACIN

BILE ACID SEQUESTRANTS
- *Colesevelam*
- *Colestipol*
- *Cholestyramine*

CHOLESTEROL ABSORPTION INHIBITORS
- *Ezetimibe*

Figure 21.1
Summary of antihyperlipidemic drugs. HMG CoA = 3-hydroxy-3-methylglutaryl coenzyme A.

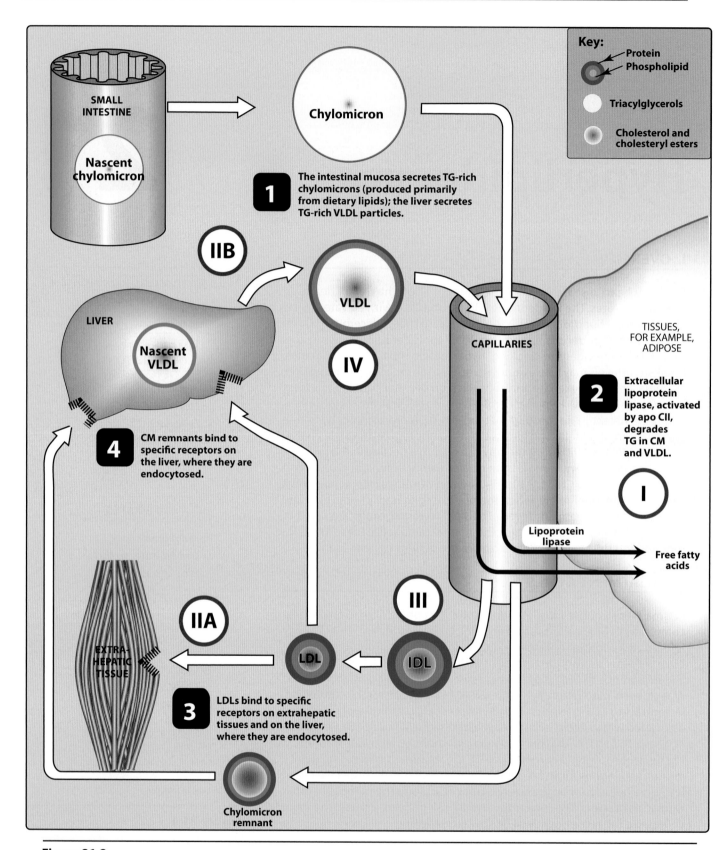

Figure 21.2

Metabolism of plasma lipoproteins and related genetic diseases. Roman numerals in the white circles refer to specific genetic types of hyperlipidemias summarized on the facing page. CM = chylomicron, TG = triacylglycerol; VLDL = very-low density lipoprotein, LDL = low-density lipoprotein, IDL = intermediate-density lipoprotein, apo CII = apolipoprotein CII found in chylomicrons and VLDL.

Type I [FAMILIAL HYPERCHYLOMICRONEMIA]

- Massive fasting hyperchylomicronemia, even following normal dietary fat intake, resulting in greatly elevated serum TG levels.
- Deficiency of lipoprotein lipase or deficiency of normal apolipoprotein CII (rare).
- Type I is not associated with an increase in coronary heart disease.
- Treatment: Low-fat diet. No drug therapy is effective for Type I hyperlipidemia.

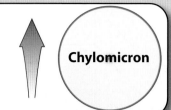

Type IIA [FAMILIAL HYPERCHOLESTEROLEMIA]

- Elevated LDL with normal VLDL levels due to a block in LDL degradation. This results in increased serum cholesterol but normal TG levels.
- Caused by defects in the synthesis or processing of LDL receptors.
- Ischemic heart disease is greatly accelerated.
- Treatment: Diet. Heterozygotes: *Cholestyramine* and *niacin*, or a statin.

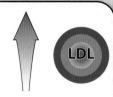

Type IIB [FAMILIAL COMBINED (MIXED) HYPERLIPIDEMIA]

- Similar to Type IIA except that VLDL is also increased, resulting in elevated serum TG as well as cholesterol levels.
- Caused by overproduction of VLDL by the liver.
- Relatively common.
- Treatment: Diet. Drug therapy is similar to that for Type IIA .

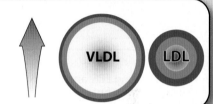

Type III [FAMILIAL DYSBETALIPOPROTEINEMIA]

- Serum concentrations of IDL are increased, resulting in increased TG and cholesterol levels.
- Cause is either overproduction or underutilization of IDL due to mutant apolipoprotein E.
- Xanthomas and accelerated vascular disease develop in patients by middle age.
- Treatment: Diet. Drug therapy includes *niacin* and *fenofibrate*, or a statin.

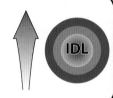

Type IV [FAMILIAL HYPERTRIGLYCERIDEMIA]

- VLDL levels are increased, whereas LDL levels are normal or decreased, resulting in normal to elevated cholesterol, and greatly elevated circulating TG levels.
- Cause is overproduction and/or decreased removal of VLDL TG in serum.
- This is a relatively common disease. It has few clinical manifestations other than accelerated ischemic heart disease. Patients with this disorder are frequently obese, diabetic, and hyperuricemic.
- Treatment: Diet. If necessary, drug therapy includes *niacin* and/or *fenofibrate*.

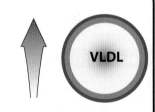

Type V [FAMILIAL MIXED HYPERTRIGLYCERIDEMIA]

- Serum VLDL and chylomicrons are elevated. LDL is normal or decreased. This results in elevated cholesterol and greatly elevated TG levels.
- Cause is either increased production or decreased clearance of VLDL and chylomicrons. Usually, it is a genetic defect.
- Occurs most commonly in adults who are obese and/or diabetic.
- Treatment: Diet. If necessary, drug therapy includes *niacin*, and/or *fenofibrate*, or a statin.

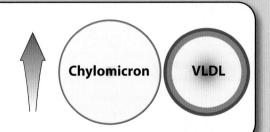

Figure 21.2 (continued).

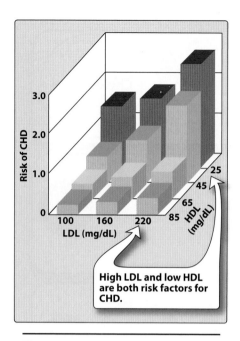

Figure 21.3
Effect of circulating LDL and HDL on the risk of coronary heart disease (CHD).

unwilling to modify their lifestyle sufficiently to achieve LDL treatment goals, and drug therapy may be required. Patients with LDL levels higher than 160 mg/dL and with one other major risk factor, such as hypertension, diabetes, smoking, or a family history of early CHD, are candidates for drug therapy. Patients with two or more additional risk factors should be treated aggressively, with the aim of reducing their LDL level to less than 100 mg/dL and, in some patients, to as low as 70 mg/dL.

B. Treatment options for hypertriacylglycerolemia

Elevated triacylglycerol (triglyceride) levels are independently associated with increased risk of CHD. Diet and exercise are the primary modes of treating hypertriacylglycerolemia. If indicated, *niacin* and *fibric acid* derivatives are the most efficacious in lowering triacylglycerol levels. Triacylglycerol reduction is a secondary benefit of the statin drugs (the primary benefit being LDL cholesterol reduction). [Note: The major lipid component of VLDL is composed of triacylglycerol.]

III. DRUGS THAT LOWER THE SERUM LIPOPROTEIN CONCENTRATION

Antihyperlipidemic drugs target the problem of elevated serum lipids with complementary strategies. Some of these agents decrease production of the lipoprotein carriers of cholesterol and triglyceride, whereas others increase the degradation of lipoprotein. Still others decrease cholesterol absorption or directly increase cholesterol removal from the body. These drugs may be used singly or in combination. However, they are always accompanied by the requirement that dietary saturated and transfats[1] be low, and the caloric content of the diet must be closely monitored.

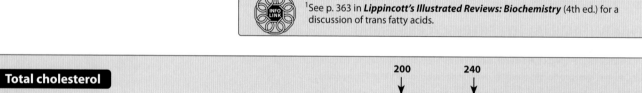

[1] See p. 363 in *Lippincott's Illustrated Reviews: Biochemistry* (4th ed.) for a discussion of trans fatty acids.

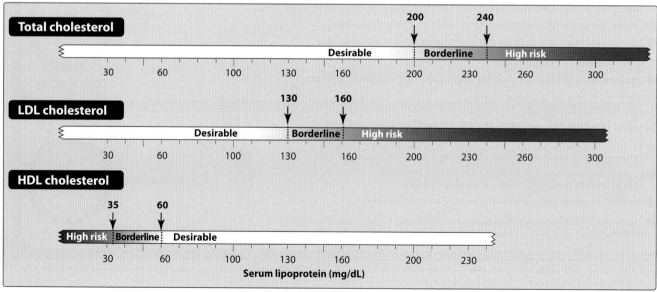

Figure 21.4
Goal lipoprotein levels achieved with dietary or drug therapy for the prevention of coronary heart disease. [Note: Lower goals for total and LDL cholesterol are recommended for patients with a history of heart disease.]

A. HMG CoA reductase inhibitors

3-Hydroxy-3-methylglutaryl (HMG) coenzyme A (COA) reductase inhibitors (commonly known as statins) lower elevated LDL cholesterol levels, resulting in a substantial reduction in coronary events and death from CHD. This group of antihyperlipidemic agents inhibits the first committed enzymatic step of cholesterol synthesis, and they are the first-line and more effective treatment for patients with elevated LDL cholesterol. Therapeutic benefits include plaque stabilization, improvement of coronary endothelial function, inhibition of platelet thrombus formation, and anti-inflammatory activity. The value of lowering the level of cholesterol with statin drugs has now been demonstrated in 1) patients with CHD with or without hyperlipidemia, 2) men with hyperlipidemia but no known CHD, and 3) men and women with average total and LDL cholesterol levels and no known CHD.

1. **Mechanism of action:**

   a. **Inhibition of HMG CoA reductase:** *Lovastatin* [LOE-vah-statin] *simvastatin* [sim-vah-STAT-in], *pravastatin* [PRAH-vah-stat-in], *atorvastatin* (a-TOR-vah-stat-in), *fluvastatin* [FLOO-vah-stat-in], and *rosuvastatin* [roe-SOO-va-sta-tin] are analogs of HMG, the precursor of cholesterol. *Lovastatin* and *simvastatin* are lactones that are hydrolyzed to the active drug. *Pravastatin* and *fluvastatin* are active as such. Because of their strong affinity for the enzyme, all compete effectively to inhibit HMG CoA reductase, the rate-limiting step in cholesterol synthesis. By inhibiting de novo cholesterol synthesis, they deplete the intracellular supply of cholesterol (Figure 21.5). *Rosuvastatin* and *atorvastatin* are the most potent LDL cholesterol–lowering statin drugs, followed by *simvastatin*, *pravastatin* and then *lovastatin* and *fluvastatin*.

   b. **Increase in LDL receptors:** Depletion of intracellular cholesterol causes the cell to increase the number of specific cell-surface LDL receptors that can bind and internalize circulating LDLs. Thus, the end result is a reduction in plasma cholesterol, both by lowered cholesterol synthesis and by increased catabolism of LDL. [Note: Because these agents undergo a marked first-pass extraction by the liver, their dominant effect is on that organ.] The HMG CoA reductase inhibitors, like the bile acid sequestrant *cholestyramine*, can increase plasma HDL levels in some patients, resulting in an additional lowering of risk for CHD. Decreases in triglyceride also occur.

2. **Therapeutic uses:** These drugs are effective in lowering plasma cholesterol levels in all types of hyperlipidemias (Figure 21.6). However, patients who are homozygous for familial hypercholesterolemia lack LDL receptors and, therefore, benefit much less from treatment with these drugs. [Note: These drugs are often given in combination with other antihyperlipidemic drugs; see below.] It should be noted that in spite of the protection afforded by cholesterol lowering, about one-fourth of the patients treated with these drugs still present with coronary events. Thus, additional strategies, such as diet, exercise, or additional agents, may be warranted.

3. **Pharmacokinetics:** *Pravastatin* and *fluvastatin* are almost completely absorbed after oral administration; oral doses of *lovastatin* and *simvastatin* are from 30 to 50 percent absorbed. Similarly, *pravastatin*

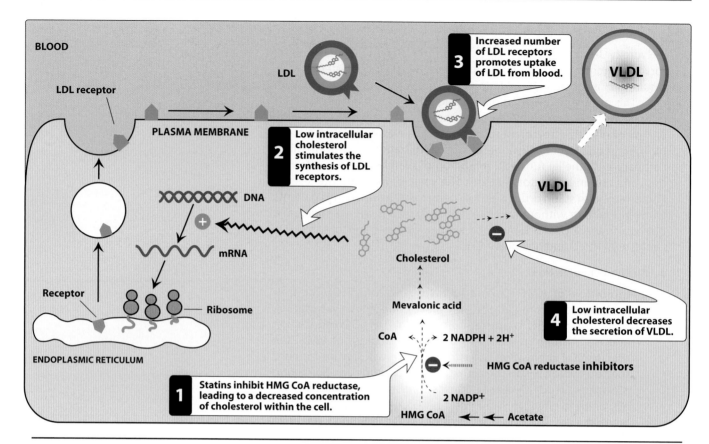

Figure 21.5
Inhibition of HMG CoA reductase by the statin drugs.

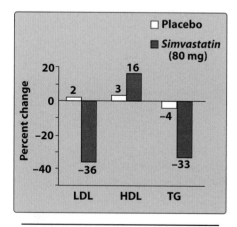

Figure 21.6
Effect of *simvastatin* on serum lipids of 130 patients with Type 2 diabetes treated for 6 weeks. HDL = high-density lipoprotein; LDL = low-density lipoprotein; TG = triacylglycerol.

and *fluvastatin* are active as such, whereas *lovastatin* and *simvastatin* must be hydrolyzed to their acid forms. Due to first-pass extraction, the primary action of these drugs is on the liver. All are biotransformed, with some of the products retaining activity. Excretion takes place principally through the bile and feces, but some urinary elimination also occurs. Their half-lives range from 1.5 to 2 hours. Some characteristics of the statins are summarized in Figure 21.7.

4. **Adverse effects:** It is noteworthy that during the 5-year trials of *simvastatin* and *lovastatin*, only a few adverse effects, related to liver and muscle function, were reported (Figure 21.8).

   a. **Liver:** Biochemical abnormalities in liver function have occurred with the HMG CoA reductase inhibitors. Therefore, it is prudent to evaluate liver function and measure serum transaminase levels periodically. These return to normal on suspension of the drug. [Note: Hepatic insufficiency can cause drug accumulation.]

   b. **Muscle:** Myopathy and rhabdomyolysis (disintegration or dissolution of muscle) have been reported only rarely. In most of these cases, patients usually suffered from renal insufficiency or were taking drugs such as *cyclosporine, itraconazole, erythromycin, gemfibrozil,* or *niacin*. Plasma creatine kinase levels should be determined regularly.

Characteristic	Atorvastatin	Fluvastatin	Lovastatin	Pravastatin	Rosuvastatin	Simvastatin
Serum LDL cholesterol reduction produced (%)	50	24	34	34	50	41
Serum triacylglycerol reduction produced (%)	29	10	16	24	18	18
Serum HDL cholesterol increase produced (%)	6	8	9	12	8	12
Plasma half-life (hr)	14	1–2	2	1–2	19	1–2
Penetration of central nervous system	No	No	Yes	No	No	Yes
Renal excretion of absorbed dose (%)	2	<6	10	20	10	13

Figure 21.7
Summary of 3-hydroxy-3-methylglutaryl coenzyme (HMG CoA) reductase inhibitors.

   c. Drug interactions: The HMG CoA reductase inhibitors may also increase *warfarin* levels. Thus, it is important to evaluate INR times frequently.

   d. Contraindications: These drugs are contraindicated during pregnancy and in nursing mothers. They should not be used in children or teenagers.

B. Niacin (nicotinic acid)

Niacin[2] [NYE-a-sin] can reduce LDL (the "bad" cholesterol carrier) levels by 10 to 20 percent and is the most effective agent for increasing HDL (the "good" cholesterol carrier) levels. *Niacin* can be used in combination with statins, and a fixed-dose combination of *lovastatin* and long-acting *niacin* is available.

1. **Mechanism of action:** At gram doses, *niacin* strongly inhibits lipolysis in adipose tissue—the primary producer of circulating free fatty acids. The liver normally utilizes these circulating fatty acids as a major precursor for triacylglycerol synthesis. Thus, *niacin* causes a decrease in liver triacylglycerol synthesis, which is required for VLDL production (Figure 21.9). LDL (the cholesterol-rich lipoprotein) is derived from VLDL in the plasma. Therefore, a reduction in the VLDL concentration also results in a decreased plasma LDL concentration. Thus, both plasma triacylglycerol (in VLDL) and cholesterol (in VLDL and LDL) are lowered (Figure 21.10). Furthermore, *niacin* treatment increases HDL cholesterol levels. Moreover, by boosting secretion of tissue plasminogen activator and lowering the level of plasma fibrinogen, *niacin* can reverse some of the endothelial cell dysfunction contributing to thrombosis associated with hypercholesterolemia and atherosclerosis.

 [2]See p. 379 in *Lippincott's Illustrated Reviews: Biochemistry* (4th ed.) for a discussion of niacin as a vitamin.

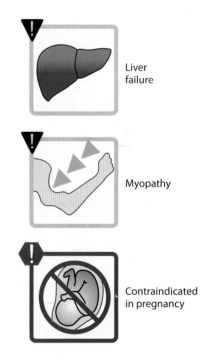

Liver failure

Myopathy

Contraindicated in pregnancy

Figure 21.8
Some adverse effects and precautions associated with 3-hydroxy-3-methylglutaryl coenzyme (HMG CoA) reductase inhibitors.

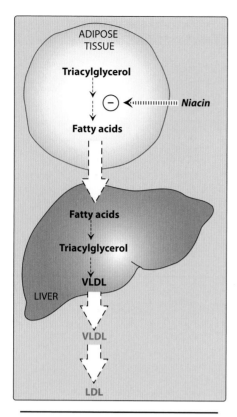

Figure 21.9
Niacin inhibits lipolysis in adipose tissue, resulting in decreased hepatic VLDL synthesis and production of LDLs in the plasma.

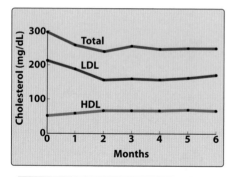

Figure 21.10
Plasma levels of cholesterol in hyperlipidemic patients during treatment with *niacin*.

2. **Therapeutic uses:** *Niacin* lowers plasma levels of both cholesterol and triacylglycerol. Therefore, it is particularly useful in the treatment of familial hyperlipidemias. *Niacin* is also used to treat other severe hypercholesterolemias, often in combination with other antihyperlipidemic agents. In addition, it is the most potent antihyperlipidemic agent for raising plasma HDL levels, which is the most common indication for its clinical use.

3. **Pharmacokinetics:** *Niacin* is administered orally. It is converted in the body to nicotinamide, which is incorporated into the cofactor nicotinamide-adenine dinucleotide (NAD$^+$). *Niacin*, its nicotinamide derivative, and other metabolites are excreted in the urine. [Note: Nicotinamide alone does not decrease plasma lipid levels.]

4. **Adverse effects:** The most common side effects of *niacin* therapy are an intense cutaneous flush (accompanied by an uncomfortable feeling of warmth) and pruritus. Administration of *aspirin* prior to taking *niacin* decreases the flush, which is prostaglandin mediated. The sustained-release formulation of *niacin*, which is taken once daily at bedtime, reduces bothersome initial adverse effects. Some patients also experience nausea and abdominal pain. *Niacin* inhibits tubular secretion of uric acid and, thus, predisposes to hyperuricemia and gout. Impaired glucose tolerance and hepatotoxicity have also been reported.

C. The fibrates: Fenofibrate and gemfibrozil

Fenofibrate [fen-oh-FIH-brate] and *gemfibrozil* [jem-FI-broh-zill] are derivatives of fibric acid that lower serum triacylglycerols and increase HDL levels. Both have the same mechanism of action. However, *fenofibrate* is more effective than *gemfibrozil* in lowering plasma LDL cholesterol and triglyceride levels.

1. **Mechanism of action:** The peroxisome proliferator–activated receptors (PPARs) are members of the nuclear receptor supergene family that regulates lipid metabolism. PPARs functions as a ligand-activated transcription factor. Upon binding to its natural ligand (fatty acids or eicosanoids) or hypolipidemic drugs, PPARs are activated. They then bind to peroxisome proliferator response elements, which are localized in numerous gene promoters. In particular, PPARs regulates the expression of genes encoding for proteins involved in lipoprotein structure and function. Fibrate-mediated gene expression ultimately leads to decreased triacylglycerol concentrations by increasing the expression of lipoprotein lipase (Figure 22.11) and decreasing apo CII concentration. Fibrates also increase the level of HDL cholesterol by increasing the expression of apo AI and apo AII. *Fenofibrate* is a prodrug, producing an active metabolite, fenofibric acid, which is responsible for the primary effects of the drug.

2. **Therapeutic uses:** The fibrates are used in the treatment of hypertriacylglycerolemias, causing a significant decrease in plasma triacylglycerol levels. *Fenofibrate* and *gemfibrozil* are particularly useful in treating Type III hyperlipidemia (dysbetalipoproteinemia), in which

 ^{3}See p. 449 in ***Lippincott's Illustrated Reviews: Biochemistry*** (4th ed.) for a discussion of the regulation of gene expression.

intermediate-density lipoprotein particles accumulate. Patients with hypertriacylglycerolemia [Type IV (elevated VLDL) or Type V (elevated VLDL plus chylomicron) disease] who do not respond to diet or other drugs may also benefit from treatment with these agents.

3. **Pharmacokinetics:** Both drugs are completely absorbed after an oral dose. *Gemfibrozil* and *fenofibrate* distribute widely, bound to albumin. Both drugs undergo extensive biotransformation and are excreted in the urine as their glucuronide conjugates.

4. **Adverse effects:**

   a. **Gastrointestinal effects:** The most common adverse effects are mild gastrointestinal disturbances. These lessen as the therapy progresses.

   b. **Lithiasis:** Because these drugs increase biliary cholesterol excretion, there is a predisposition to the formation of gallstones.

   c. **Muscle:** Myositis (inflammation of a voluntary muscle) can occur with both drugs; thus, muscle weakness or tenderness should be evaluated. Patients with renal insufficiency may be at risk. Myopathy and rhabdomyolysis have been reported in a few patients taking *gemfibrozil* and *lovastatin* together.

   d. **Drug interactions:** Both fibrates compete with the coumarin anticoagulants for binding sites on plasma proteins, thus transiently potentiating anticoagulant activity. INR times should therefore be monitored when a patient is taking both drugs. Similarly, these drugs may transiently elevate the levels of sulfonylureas.

   e. **Contraindications:** The safety of these agents in pregnant or lactating women has not been established. They should not be used in patients with severe hepatic and renal dysfunction or in patients with preexisting gallbladder disease.

D. Bile acid–binding resins

Bile acid sequestrants (resins) have significant LDL cholesterol–lowering effects, although the benefits are less than those observed with statins.

1. **Mechanism of action:** *Cholestyramine* [koe-LES-tir-a-meen], *colestipol* [koe-LES-tih-pole], and *colesevelam* [koh-le-SEV-e-lam] are anion-exchange resins that bind negatively charged bile acids and bile salts in the small intestine (Figure 21.12). The resin/bile acid complex is excreted in the feces, thus preventing the bile acids from returning to the liver by the enterohepatic circulation. Lowering the bile acid concentration causes hepatocytes to increase conversion of cholesterol to bile acids, resulting in a replenished supply of these compounds, which are essential components of the bile. Consequently, the intracellular cholesterol concentration decreases, which activates an increased hepatic uptake of cholesterol-containing LDL particles, leading to a fall in plasma LDL. [Note: This

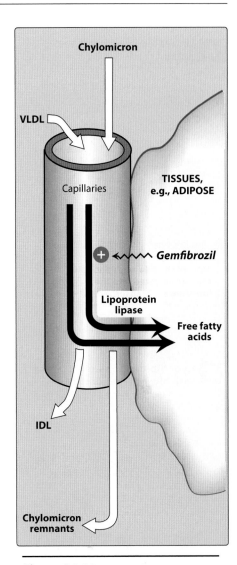

Figure 21.11
Activation of lipoprotein lipase by *gemfibrozil*.

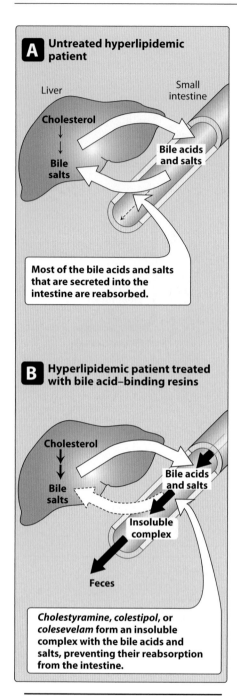

Figure 21.12
Mechanism of bile acid–binding resins.

increased uptake is mediated by an up-regulation of cell-surface LDL receptors.] In some patients, a modest rise in plasma HDL levels is also observed. The final outcome of this sequence of events is a decreased total plasma cholesterol concentration.

2. **Therapeutic uses:** The bile acid–binding resins are the drugs of choice (often in combination with diet or *niacin*) in treating Type IIa and Type IIb hyperlipidemias. [Note: In those rare individuals who are homozygous for Type IIa—that is, for whom functional LDL receptors are totally lacking—these drugs have little effect on plasma LDL levels.] *Cholestyramine* can also relieve pruritus caused by accumulation of bile acids in patients with biliary obstruction.

3. **Pharmacokinetics:** *Cholestyramine*, *colestipol*, and *colesevelam* are taken orally. Because they are insoluble in water and are very large (molecular weights are greater than 10^6), they are neither absorbed nor metabolically altered by the intestine. Instead, they are totally excreted in the feces.

4. **Adverse effects:**

   a. **Gastrointestinal effects:** The most common side effects are gastrointestinal disturbances, such as constipation, nausea, and flatulence. *Colesevelam* has fewer gastrointestinal side effects than other bile acid sequestrants.

   b. **Impaired absorptions:** At high doses, *cholestyramine* and *colestipol* (but not *colesevelam*) impair the absorption of the fat-soluble vitamins (A, D, E, and K).

   c. **Drug interactions:** *Cholestyramine* and *colestipol* interfere with the intestinal absorption of many drugs—for example, *tetracycline*, *phenobarbital*, *digoxin*, *warfarin*, *pravastatin*, *fluvastatin*, *aspirin*, and thiazide diuretics. Therefore, drugs should be taken at least 1 to 2 hours before, or 4 to 6 hours after, the bile acid–binding resins.

E. Cholesterol absorption inhibitors

Ezetimibe [eh-ZEH-teh-mib] selectively inhibits intestinal absorption of dietary and biliary cholesterol in the small intestine, leading to a decrease in the delivery of intestinal cholesterol to the liver. This causes a reduction of hepatic cholesterol stores and an increase in clearance of cholesterol from the blood. *Ezetimibe* lowers LDL cholesterol by 17 percent and triacylglycerols by 6 percent, and it increases HDL cholesterol by 1.3 percent. *Ezetimibe* is primarily metabolized in the small intestine and liver via glucuronide conjugation (a Phase II reaction), with subsequent biliary and renal excretion. Both *ezetimibe* and *ezetimibe*-glucuronide are slowly eliminated from plasma, with a half-life of approximately 22 hours. *Ezetimibe* has no clinically meaningful effect on the plasma concentrations of the fat-soluble vitamins A, D, and E. Patients with moderate to severe hepatic insufficiency should not be treated with *ezetimibe*. [Note: A formulation of *ezetimibe* and *simvastatin* has been shown to lower LDL levels more effectively than the statin alone.]

F. Combination drug therapy

It is often necessary to employ two antihyperlipidemic drugs to achieve treatment goals in plasma lipid levels. For example, in Type II hyperlipidemias, patients are commonly treated with a combination of *niacin* plus a bile acid–binding agent, such as *cholestyramine*. [Note: Remember that *cholestyramine* causes an increase in LDL receptors that clears the plasma of circulating LDL, whereas *niacin* decreases synthesis of VLDL and, therefore, also the synthesis of LDL.] The combination of an HMG CoA reductase inhibitor with a bile acid–binding agent has also been shown to be very useful in lowering LDL cholesterol levels (Figure 21.13). A low dose statin in combination with *ezetimibe* achieves comparable or even greater LDL cholesterol reduction than a very-high-dose statin. *Simvastatin* and *ezetimibe* are currently available combined in one pill to treat elevated LDL cholesterol.

However, the clinical value of *ezetimibe* either alone or in combination with statins is uncertain. For example, in the ENHANCE study, patients with familial hypercholesterolemia were randomized to *simvastatin* plus either *ezetimibe* or placebo. At 2 years, patients who received *ezetimibe* had significantly greater reductions in LDL cholesterol, triglycerides, and C-reactive protein than did those on placebo. However, there were no significant differences between groups in HDL cholesterol, cardiovascular events, adverse events, or the primary endpoint—change in carotid-artery intima–media thickness

This study contradicts previous results in which clinical benefits correlated with the concurrent reduction in LDL cholesterol. Until this discrepancy is resolved, many experts recommend clinicians maximize statin dosages and use *niacin*, fibrates, and resins before considering *ezetimibe*,

Figure 21.14 summarizes some actions of the antihyperlipidemic drugs.

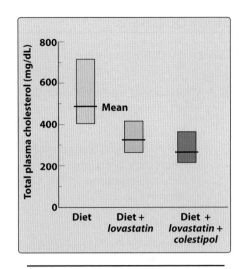

Figure 21.13
Response of total plasma cholesterol in patients with heterozygous familial hypercholesterolemia to a diet (low in cholesterol, low in saturated fat) and antihyperlipidemic drugs.

TYPE OF DRUG	EFFECT ON LDL	EFFECT ON HDL	EFFECT ON TRIACYLGLYCEROLS
HMG CoA reducatase inhibitors (statins)	↓↓↓↓	↑↑	↓↓
Fibrates	↓	↑↑↑	↓↓↓↓
Niacin	↓↓	↑↑↑↑	↓↓↓
Bile acid sequestrants	↓↓↓	↑	Minimal
Cholesterol absorption inhibitor	↓	↑	↓

Figure 21.14
Characteristics of antihyperlipidemic drug families. HDL = high-density lipoprotein; HMG-CoA = 3-hydroxy-3-methylglutaryl coenzyme A; LDL = low-density lipoprotein.

Study Questions

Choose the ONE best answer.

21.1 Which one of the following is the most common side effect of antihyperlipidemic drug therapy?

A. Elevated blood pressure.
B. Gastrointestinal disturbance.
C. Neurologic problems.
D. Heart palpitations.
E. Migraine headaches.

Correct answer = B. Gastrointestinal disturbances frequently occur as a side effect of antihyperlipidemic drug therapy.

21.2 Which one of the following hyperlipidemias is characterized by elevated plasma levels of chylomicrons and has no drug therapy available to lower the plasma lipoprotein levels?

A. Type I.
B. Type II.
C. Type III.
D. Type IV.
E. Type V.

Correct answer = A. Type I hyperlipidemia (hyperchylomicronemia) is treated with a low-fat diet. No drug therapy is effective for this disorder.

21.3 Which one of the following drugs decreases de novo cholesterol synthesis by inhibiting the enzyme 3-hydroxy-3-methylglutaryl coenzyme A reductase?

A. Fenofibrate.
B. Niacin.
C. Cholestyramine.
D. Lovastatin.
E. Gemfibrozil.

Correct answer = D. Fenofibrate and gemfibrozil increase the activity of lipoprotein lipase, thereby increasing the removal of VLDL from plasma. Niacin inhibits lipolysis in adipose tissue, thus eliminating the building blocks needed by the liver to produce triacylglycerol and, therefore, very-low-density lipoprotein (VLDL). Cholestyramine lowers the amount of bile acids returning to the liver via the enterohepatic circulation.

21.4 Which one of the following drugs causes a decrease in liver triacylglycerol synthesis by limiting available free fatty acids needed as building blocks for this pathway?

A. Niacin.
B. Fenofibrate.
C. Cholestyramine.
D. Gemfibrozil.
E. Lovastatin.

Correct answer = A. At gram doses, niacin strongly inhibits lipolysis in adipose tissue—the primary producer of circulating free fatty acids. The liver normally utilizes these circulating fatty acids as a major precursor for triacylglycerol synthesis. Thus, niacin causes a decrease in liver triacylglycerol synthesis, which is required for VLDL production.

21.5 Which one of the following drugs binds bile acids in the intestine, thus preventing their return to the liver via the enterohepatic circulation?

A. Niacin.
B. Fenofibrate.
C. Cholestyramine.
D. Fluvastatin.
E. Lovastatin.

Correct answer = C. Cholestyramine is anion-exchange resins that bind negatively charged bile acids and bile salts in the small intestine. The resin/bile acid complex is excreted in the feces, thus preventing the bile acids from returning to the liver by the enterohepatic circulation.

Diuretics

22

I. OVERVIEW

Drugs inducing a state of increased urine flow are called diuretics. These agents are inhibitors of renal ion transporters that decrease the reabsorption of Na^+ at different sites in the nephron. As a result, Na^+ and other ions, such as Cl^-, enter the urine in greater than normal amounts along with water, which is carried passively to maintain osmotic equilibrium. Diuretics thus increase the volume of urine and often change its pH as well as the ionic composition of the urine and blood. The efficacy of the different classes of diuretics varies considerably, with the increase in Na^+ secretion varying from less than two percent for the weak, potassium-sparing diuretics to over 20 percent for the potent loop diuretics. In addition to these ion-transport inhibitors, there are osmotic diuretics that prevent water reabsorption, as well as aldosterone antagonists and a carbonic anhydrase inhibitor. The major clinical uses of diuretics are in managing disorders involving abnormal fluid retention (edema) or treating hypertension in which their diuretic action causes a decreased blood volume, leading to reduced blood pressure. In this chapter, the diuretic drugs (Figure 22.1) are discussed according to the frequency of their use.

II. NORMAL REGULATION OF FLUID AND ELECTROLYTES BY THE KIDNEYS

Approximately 16 to 20 percent of the blood plasma entering the kidneys is filtered from the glomerular capillaries into the Bowman's capsule. The filtrate, although normally free of proteins and blood cells, does contain most low-molecular-weight plasma components in approximately the same concentrations as are found in the plasma. These include glucose, sodium bicarbonate, amino acids, and other organic solutes as well as electrolytes, such as Na^+, K^+, and Cl^-. The kidney regulates the ionic composition and volume of urine by the active reabsorption or secretion of ions and/or the passive reabsorption of water at five functional zones along the nephron—namely, the proximal convoluted tubule, the descending loop of Henle, the ascending loop of Henle, the distal convoluted tubule, and the collecting tubule and duct (Figure 22.2).

A. Proximal convoluted tubule

In the extensively convoluted proximal tubule located in the cortex of the kidney, almost all the glucose, bicarbonate, amino acids, and other metabolites are reabsorbed. Approximately two-thirds of the Na^+ is also reabsorbed. Chloride enters the lumen of the tubule in

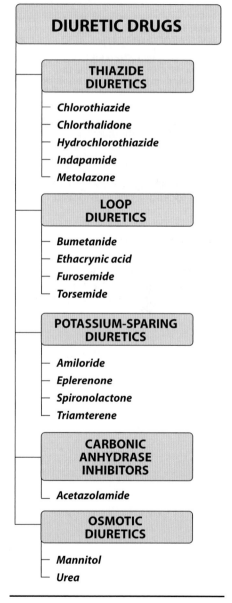

DIURETIC DRUGS

THIAZIDE DIURETICS
- Chlorothiazide
- Chlorthalidone
- Hydrochlorothiazide
- Indapamide
- Metolazone

LOOP DIURETICS
- Bumetanide
- Ethacrynic acid
- Furosemide
- Torsemide

POTASSIUM-SPARING DIURETICS
- Amiloride
- Eplerenone
- Spironolactone
- Triamterene

CARBONIC ANHYDRASE INHIBITORS
- Acetazolamide

OSMOTIC DIURETICS
- Mannitol
- Urea

Figure 22.1
Summary of diuretic drugs.

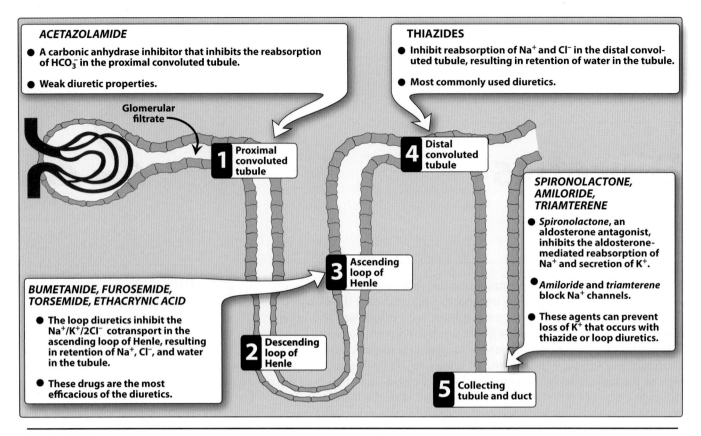

Figure 22.2
Major locations of ion and water exchange in the nephron, showing sites of action of the diuretic drugs.

exchange for a base anion, such as formate or oxalate, as well as paracellularly through the lumen. Water follows passively from the lumen to the blood to maintain osmolar equality. If not for the extensive reabsorption of solutes and water in the proximal tubule, the mammalian organism would rapidly become dehydrated and lose its normal osmolarity. The Na^+ that is reabsorbed is pumped into the interstitium by Na^+/K^+–adenosine triphosphatase (ATPase), thereby maintaining normal levels of Na^+ and K^+ in the cell. Carbonic anhydrase in the luminal membrane and cell of the proximal tubule modulates the reabsorption of bicarbonate (see *acetazolamide* below). Water follows salt reabsorption; thus, the presence of substances like mannitol and glucose would tend to become concentrated. This condition results in a higher osmolarity of the tubular fluid and prevents further water reabsorption, resulting in osmotic diuresis.

1. **Acid and base secretory systems:** The proximal tubule is the site of the organic acid and base secretory systems (Figure 22.3). The organic acid secretory system, located in the middle-third segment, secretes a variety of organic acids, such as uric acid, some antibiotics, and diuretics, from the bloodstream into the proximal tubule's lumen. Most diuretic drugs are delivered to the tubular fluid via this system. The organic acid secretory system is saturable, and diuretic drugs in the bloodstream compete for transfer with endogenous organic acids, such as uric acid. This explains the hyperuricemia seen with certain of the diuretic drugs, such as *furosemide* or *hydrochlorothiazide*. A number of other interactions can also occur; for exam-

ple, *probenecid* interferes with *penicillin* secretion. The organic base secretory system is responsible for the secretion of creatinine, choline, and so on, and it is found in the upper and middle segments of the proximal tubule.

B. Descending loop of Henle

The remaining filtrate, which is isotonic, next enters the descending limb of the loop of Henle and passes into the medulla of the kidney. The osmolarity increases along the descending portion of the loop of Henle because of the countercurrent mechanism that is responsible for water reabsorption. This results in a tubular fluid with a three-fold increase in salt concentration. Osmotic diuretics exert part of their action in this region (see Figure 22.2).

C. Ascending loop of Henle

The cells of the ascending tubular epithelium are unique in being impermeable to water. Active reabsorption of Na^+, K^+, and Cl^- is mediated by a $Na^+/K^+/2Cl^-$ cotransporter. Both Mg^{2+} and Ca^{2+} enter the interstitial fluid via the paracellular pathway. The ascending loop is thus a diluting region of the nephron. Approximately 25 to 30 percent of the tubular sodium chloride returns to the interstitial fluid, thus helping to maintain the fluid's high osmolarity. Because the ascending loop of Henle is a major site for salt reabsorption, drugs affecting this site, such as loop diuretics (see Figure 22.2), are the most efficacious of all the diuretic classes.

D. Distal convoluted tubule

The cells of the distal convoluted tubule are also impermeable to water. About 10 percent of the filtered sodium chloride is reabsorbed via a Na^+/Cl^- transporter that is sensitive to thiazide diuretics. Calcium reabsorption is mediated by passage through a channel and then transported by a Na^+/Ca^{2+}-exchanger into the interstitial fluid. The mechanism thus differs from that in the loop of Henle. Additionally, Ca^{2+} excretion is regulated by parathyroid hormone in this portion of the tubule.

E. Collecting tubule and duct

The principal cells of the collecting tubule and duct are responsible for Na^+, K^+, and water transport, whereas the intercalated cells affect H^+ secretion. The sodium enters the principal cells through channels but relies on a Na^+/K^+-ATPase to be transported into the blood. Aldosterone receptors in the principal cells influence Na^+ reabsorption and K^+ secretion. Antidiuretic hormone (ADH; vasopressin) receptors promote the reabsorption of water from the collecting tubules and ducts (see Figure 22.3). This action is mediated by cyclic adenosine monophosphate.

III. KIDNEY FUNCTION IN DISEASE

A. Edematous states

In many diseases, the amount of sodium chloride reabsorbed by the kidney tubules is abnormally high. This leads to the retention of water, an increase in blood volume, and expansion of the extravascular fluid compartment, resulting in edema of the tissues. Several commonly encountered causes of edema include the following.

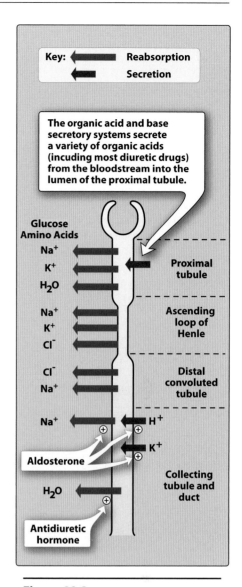

Figure 22.3
Sites of transport of solutes and water along the nephron.

1. **Heart failure:** The decreased ability of the failing heart to sustain adequate cardiac output causes the kidney to respond as if there were a decrease in blood volume (hypovolemia). The kidney, as part of the normal compensatory mechanism, retains more salt and water as a means of raising blood volume and increasing the amount of blood that is returned to the heart. However, the diseased heart cannot increase its output, and the increased vascular volume results in edema (see p. 183 for causes and treatment of heart failure). Loop diuretics are commonly used.

2. **Hepatic ascites:** Ascites, the accumulation of fluid in the abdominal cavity, is a common complication of cirrhosis of the liver.

   a. **Increased portal blood pressure:** Blood flow in the portal system is often obstructed in cirrhosis, resulting in an increased portal blood pressure. Furthermore, the colloidal osmotic pressure of the blood is decreased as a result of impaired synthesis of plasma proteins by the diseased liver. Increased portal blood pressure and low osmolarity of the blood cause fluid to escape from the portal vascular system and collect in the abdomen.

   b. **Secondary hyperaldosteronism:** Fluid retention is also promoted by elevated levels of circulating aldosterone due to decreased blood volume. This secondary hyperaldosteronism results from the decreased ability of the liver to inactivate the steroid hormone and leads to increased Na^+ and water reabsorption, increased vascular volume, and exacerbation of fluid accumulation (see Figure 22.3). The potassium-sparing diuretic *spironolactone* is effective in this condition, but the loop diuretics are usually not.

3. **Nephrotic syndrome:** When damaged by disease, the glomerular membranes allow plasma proteins to enter the glomerular ultra-filtrate. The loss of protein from the plasma reduces the colloidal osmotic pressure, resulting in edema. The low plasma volume stimulates aldosterone secretion through the renin-angiotensin-aldosterone system. This leads to retention of Na^+ and fluid, further aggravating the edema.

4. **Premenstrual edema:** Edema associated with menstruation is the result of imbalances in hormones, such as estrogen excess, which facilitates the loss of fluid into the extracellular space. Diuretics can reduce the edema.

B. **Nonedematous states**

Diuretics also find wide usage in the treatment of nonedematous diseases.

1. **Hypertension:** Thiazides have been widely used in the treatment of hypertension, because of their ability not only to reduce blood volume but also to dilate arterioles (see p. 219).

2. **Hypercalcemia:** The seriousness of this condition requires a fast response. Usually, loop diuretics are employed, because they promote calcium excretion. However, it is important to understand that hypovolemia may counteract the desired effect; therefore, normal saline must also be infused to maintain blood volume.

3. **Diabetes insipidus:** When patients suffer from polyuria and polydipsia associated with this condition, they usually respond to thiazide diuretics. This seemingly paradoxic treatment depends on the
ability of the thiazide to reduce plasma volume, thus causing a drop
in glomerular filtration rate and promoting the reabsorption of Na^+
and water. The volume of urine entering the diluting segment and
the subsequent urine flow are both decreased.

IV. THIAZIDES AND RELATED AGENTS

The thiazides are the most widely used of the diuretic drugs. They are sulfonamide derivatives and, as such, are related in structure to the carbonic anhydrase inhibitors. However, the thiazides have significantly greater diuretic
activity than *acetazolamide* (see below), and they act on the kidney by different mechanisms. All thiazides affect the distal tubule, and all have equal maximum diuretic effects, differing only in potency (expressed on a per milligram
basis). [Note: They are sometimes called "ceiling diuretics," because increasing the dose above normal does not promote a further diuretic response.]
Like the actions of the loop diuretics, the thiazides partly depend on renal
prostaglandin synthesis by a mechanism that is not yet understood.

A. Thiazides

Chlorothiazide [klor-oh-THYE-ah-zide] was the first modern diuretic that
was active orally, and was capable of affecting the severe edema of cirrhosis and heart failure with a minimum of side effects. Its properties are
representative of the thiazide group, although newer derivatives, such
as *hydrochlorothiazide* [hi-dro-klor-oh-THYE-ah-zide] or *chlorthalidone*,
are now used more commonly. *Hydrochlorothiazide* has far less ability to inhibit carbonic anhydrase compared to *chlorothiazide*. It is also
more potent, so that the required dose is considerably lower than that
of *chlorothiazide*. On the other hand, the efficacy is exactly the same as
that of the parent drug. In all other aspects it resembles *chlorothiazide*.
[Note: *Chlorthalidone*, *indapamide*, and *metolazone* are referred to as
thiazide-like diuretics, because they contain the sulfonamide residue
in their chemical structures and their mechanism of action is similar.
However, they are not truly thiazides.]

1. **Mechanism of action:** The thiazide derivatives act mainly in the
distal tubule to decrease the reabsorption of Na^+—apparently by
inhibition of a Na^+/Cl^- cotransporter on the luminal membrane of
the distal convoluted tubule (see Figure 22.2). They have a lesser
effect in the proximal tubule. As a result, these drugs increase the
concentration of Na^+ and Cl^- in the tubular fluid. The acid-base balance is not usually affected. [Note: Because the site of action of the
thiazide derivatives is on the luminal membrane, these drugs must
be excreted into the tubular lumen to be effective. Therefore, with
decreased renal function, thiazide diuretics lose efficacy.]

2. **Actions:**

   a. **Increased excretion of Na^+ and Cl^-:** *Chlorothiazide* causes
   diuresis with increased Na^+ and Cl^- excretion, which can result
   in the excretion of a very hyperosmolar urine. This latter effect
   is unique; the other diuretic classes are unlikely to produce a
   hyperosmolar urine. The diuretic action is not affected by the
   acid-base status of the body, nor does *chlorothiazide* change the

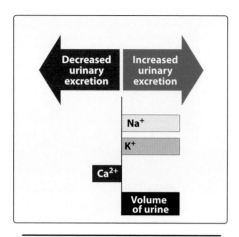

Figure 22.4
Relative changes in the composition of
urine induced by thiazide diuretics.

acid-base status of the blood. The relative changes in the ionic composition of the urine during therapy with thiazide diuretics are given in Figure 22.4.

b. Loss of K⁺: Because thiazides increase the Na⁺ in the filtrate arriving at the distal tubule, more K⁺ is also exchanged for Na⁺, resulting in a continual loss of K⁺ from the body with prolonged use of these drugs. Therefore, it is imperative to measure serum K⁺ often (more frequently at the beginning of therapy) to assure that hypokalemia does not develop.

c. Loss of Mg²⁺: Magnesium deficiency requiring supplementation can occur with chronic use of thiazide diuretics, particularly in the elderly. The mechanism for the magnesuria is not understood.

d. Decreased urinary calcium excretion: Thiazide diuretics decrease the Ca²⁺ content of urine by promoting the reabsorption of Ca²⁺. This contrasts with the loop diuretics, which increase the Ca²⁺ concentration of the urine. [Note: There is evidence from epidemiologic studies that use of thiazides preserves bone mineral density at the hip and spine and that the risk for hip fracture is reduced by a third.]

e. Reduced peripheral vascular resistance: An initial reduction in blood pressure results from a decrease in blood volume and, therefore, a decrease in cardiac output. With continued therapy, volume recovery occurs. However, there are continued hypotensive effects, resulting from reduced peripheral vascular resistance caused by relaxation of arteriolar smooth muscle.

3. Therapeutic uses:

a. Hypertension: Clinically, the thiazides have long been the mainstay of antihypertensive medication, because they are inexpensive, convenient to administer, and well tolerated. They are effective in reducing systolic and diastolic blood pressure for extended periods in the majority of patients with mild to moderate essential hypertension (see p. 215 for details on the treatment of hypertension). After 3 to 7 days of treatment, the blood pressure stabilizes at a lower level and can be maintained indefinitely by a daily-dosage level of the drug, which causes lower peripheral resistance without having a major diuretic effect. Many patients can be continued for years on the thiazides alone, although a small percentage of patients require additional medication, such as β-adrenergic blockers. [Note: The hypotensive actions of angiotensin-converting enzyme inhibitors are enhanced when given in combination with the thiazides.]

b. Heart failure: Thiazides can be the diuretic of choice in reducing extracellular volume in mild to moderate heart failure. If the thiazide fails, loop diuretics may be useful.

c. Hypercalciuria: The thiazides can be useful in treating idiopathic hypercalciuria, because they inhibit urinary Ca²⁺ excretion. This is particularly beneficial for patients with calcium oxalate stones in the urinary tract.

d. Diabetes insipidus: Thiazides have the unique ability to produce a hyperosmolar urine. Thiazides can substitute for antidiuretic hormone in the treatment of nephrogenic diabetes insipidus. The urine volume of such individuals may drop from 11 L/day to about 3 L/day when treated with the drug.

4. **Pharmacokinetics:** The drugs are effective orally. Most thiazides take 1 to 3 weeks to produce a stable reduction in blood pressure, and they exhibit a prolonged biologic half-life (40 hours). All thiazides are secreted by the organic acid secretory system of the kidney (see Figure 22.3).

5. **Adverse effects:** Most of the adverse effects involve problems in fluid and electrolyte balance.

   a. Potassium depletion: Hypokalemia is the most frequent problem encountered with the thiazide diuretics, and it can predispose patients who are taking digitalis to ventricular arrhythmias (Figure 22.5). Often, K+ can be supplemented by diet alone, such as by increasing the intake of citrus fruits, bananas, and prunes. In some cases, K+ salt supplementation may be necessary. Activation of the renin-angiotensin-aldosterone system by the decrease in intravascular volume contributes significantly to urinary K+ losses. Under these circumstances, the K+ deficiency can be overcome by *spironolactone*, which interferes with aldosterone action, or by administering *triamterene*, which acts to retain K+. Low-sodium diets blunt the potassium depletion caused by thiazide diuretics.

   b. Hyponatremia: This serious adverse effect may develop due to elevation of ADH as a result of hypovolemia, as well as diminished diluting capacity of the kidney and increased thirst. Limiting water intake and lowering the dose of diuretic can prevent this condition.

   c. Hyperuricemia: Thiazides increase serum uric acid by decreasing the amount of acid excreted by the organic acid secretory system. Being insoluble, the uric acid deposits in the joints, and a full-blown attack of gout may result in individuals who are predisposed to gouty attacks. It is important, therefore, to perform periodic blood tests for uric acid levels. [Note: *Probenecid*, a drug sometimes used in the treatment of gout, can interfere in the excretion of the thiazides and increase serum uric acid levels.]

   d. Volume depletion: This can cause orthostatic hypotension or light-headedness.

   e. Hypercalcemia: The thiazides inhibit the secretion of Ca^{2+}, sometimes leading to elevated levels of Ca^{2+} in the blood.

   f. Hyperglycemia: Patients with diabetes mellitus who are taking thiazides for hypertension may become hyperglycemic and have difficulty in maintaining appropriate blood sugar levels. This is due to impaired release of insulin and tissue uptake of glucose.

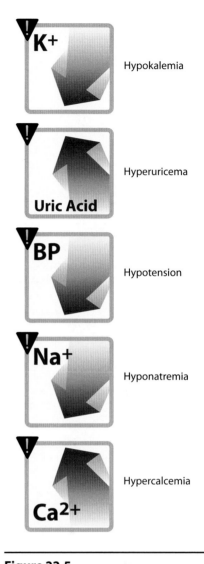

K+ — Hypokalemia

Uric Acid — Hyperuricema

BP — Hypotension

Na+ — Hyponatremia

Ca2+ — Hypercalcemia

Figure 22.5
Summary of some adverse effects commonly observed with thiazide diuretics.

g. Hyperlipidemia: The thiazides can cause a 5- to 15-percent increase in serum cholesterol as well as increased serum low-density lipoproteins. Lipid levels, however, may return to normal with long-term therapy.

h. Hypersensitivity: Bone marrow suppression, dermatitis, necrotizing vasculitis, and interstitial nephritis are very rare. Individuals who are hypersensitive to sulfa drugs may also be allergic to the thiazide diuretics.

B. Thiazide-like analogs

These compounds lack the thiazide structure, but like the thiazides, they have the unsubstituted sulfonamide group and share their mechanism of action.

1. **Chlorthalidone:** *Chlorthalidone* [klor-THAL-i-done] is a nonthiazide derivative that behaves pharmacologically like *hydrochlorothiazide*. It has a very long duration of action and, therefore, is often used to treat hypertension. It is given once per day for this indication.

2. **Metolazone:** *Metolazone* [me-TOL-ah-zone] is more potent than the thiazides and, unlike the thiazides, causes Na^+ excretion in advanced renal failure.

3. **Indapamide:** *Indapamide* [in-DAP-a-mide] is a lipid-soluble, non-thiazide diuretic that has a long duration of action. At low doses, it shows significant antihypertensive action with minimal diuretic effects. *Indapamide* is metabolized and excreted by the gastrointestinal tract and the kidneys. It is therefore less likely to accumulate in patients with renal failure and may be useful in their treatment.

V. LOOP OR HIGH-CEILING DIURETICS

Bumetanide [byoo-MET-ah-nide], *furosemide* [fu-RO-se-mide], *torsemide* [TOR-se-myde], and *ethacrynic* [eth-a-KRIN-ik] *acid* are four diuretics that have their major action on the ascending limb of the loop of Henle (see Figure 22.2). Compared to all other classes of diuretics, these drugs have the highest efficacy in mobilizing Na^+ and Cl^- from the body. They produce copious amounts of urine. *Furosemide* is the most commonly used of these drugs. *Ethacrynic acid* has a steeper dose-response curve than *furosemide*, but it shows greater side effects than those seen with the other loop diuretics and its use is therefore limited. *Bumetanide* is much more potent than *furosemide*, and its use is increasing. *Bumetanide* and *furosemide* are sulfonamide derivatives.

A. Bumetanide, furosemide, torsemide, and ethacrynic acid

1. **Mechanism of action:** Loop diuretics inhibit the cotransport of Na^+/K^+/$2Cl^-$ in the luminal membrane in the ascending limb of the loop of Henle. Therefore, reabsorption of these ions is decreased (Figure 22.6). The loop diuretics are the most efficacious of the diuretic drugs, because the ascending limb accounts for the reabsorption of 25 to 30 percent of filtered NaCl and downstream sites are not able to compensate for this increased Na^+ load.

2. **Actions:** The loop diuretics act promptly, even among patients who have poor renal function or have not responded to thiazides or other

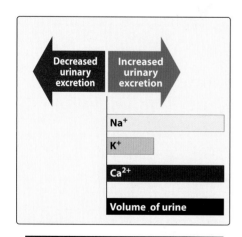

Figure 22.6
Relative changes in the composition of urine induced by loop diuretics.

diuretics. Changes in the composition of the urine induced by loop diuretics are shown in Figure 22.6. [Note: Loop diuretics increase the Ca^{2+} content of urine, whereas thiazide diuretics decrease the Ca^{2+} concentration of the urine. In patients with normal serum Ca^{2+} concentrations, hypocalcemia does not result, because Ca^{2+} is reabsorbed in the distal convoluted tubule. However, hypomagnesemia can occur due to loss of Mg^{2+}.] The loop diuretics cause decreased renal vascular resistance and increased renal blood flow. In addition, loop diuretics increase prostaglandin synthesis. The prostaglandins have a role in their diuretic action, and substances such as *indomethacin* that interfere in prostaglandin synthesis can reduce the diuretic action of these agents.

3. **Therapeutic uses:** The loop diuretics are the drugs of choice for reducing the acute pulmonary edema of heart failure. Because of their rapid onset of action, particularly when given intravenously, the drugs are useful in emergency situations, such as acute pulmonary edema, which calls for a rapid, intense diuresis. Loop diuretics (along with hydration) are also useful in treating hypercalcemia, because they stimulate tubular Ca^{2+} excretion. They also are useful in the treatment of hyperkalemia.

4. **Pharmacokinetics:** Loop diuretics are administered orally or parenterally. Their duration of action is relatively brief—2 to 4 hours. They are secreted into the urine.

5. **Adverse effects:** The adverse effects of the loop diuretics are summarized in Figure 22.7.

   a. **Ototoxicity:** Hearing can be affected adversely by the loop diuretics, particularly when used in conjunction with the aminoglycoside antibiotics. Permanent damage may result with continued treatment. *Ethacrynic acid* is the most likely to cause deafness. Vestibular function is less likely to be disturbed, but it, too, may be affected by combined treatment with the antibiotic.

   b. **Hyperuricemia:** *Furosemide* and *ethacrynic acid* compete with uric acid for the renal and biliary secretory systems, thus blocking its secretion and, thereby, causing or exacerbating gouty attacks.

   c. **Acute hypovolemia:** Loop diuretics can cause a severe and rapid reduction in blood volume, with the possibility of hypotension, shock, and cardiac arrhythmias. Hypercalcemia may occur under these conditions.

   d. **Potassium depletion:** The heavy load of Na^+ presented to the collecting tubule results in increased exchange of tubular Na^+ for K^+, with the possibility of inducing hypokalemia. The loss of K^+ from cells in exchange for H^+ leads to hypokalemic alkalosis. Potassium depletion can be averted by use of potassium-sparing diuretics or dietary supplementation with K^+.

   e. **Hypomagnesemia:** A combination of chronic use of loop diuretics and low dietary intake of Mg^{2+} can lead to hypomagnesemia, particularly in the elderly. This can be corrected by oral supplementation.

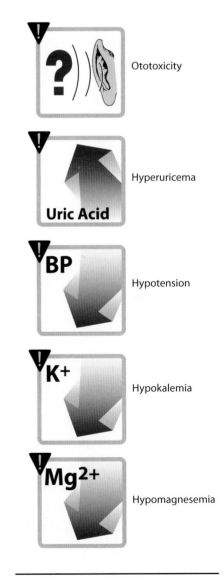

Figure 22.7
Summary of some adverse effects commonly observed with loop diuretics.

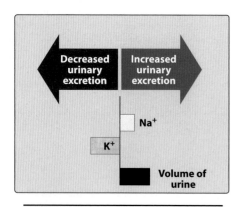

Figure 22.8
Relative changes in the composition of urine induced by potassium-sparing diuretics.

VI. POTASSIUM-SPARING DIURETICS

Potassium-sparing diuretics act in the collecting tubule to inhibit Na^+ reabsorption and K^+ excretion (Figure 22.8). Potassium-sparing diuretics are used alone primarily when aldosterone is present in excess. The major use of potassium-sparing agents is in the treatment of hypertension, most often in combination with a thiazide. It is extremely important that patients who are treated with any potassium-sparing diuretic be closely monitored for potassium levels. Exogenous potassium supplementation is usually discontinued when potassium-sparing diuretic therapy is instituted.

A. Aldosterone antagonists: Spironolactone and eplerenone

1. **Mechanism of action:** *Spironolactone* [spear-oh-no-LAK-tone] is a synthetic steroid that antagonizes aldosterone at intracellular cytoplasmic receptor sites. The *spironolactone*-receptor complex is inactive. That is, it prevents translocation of the receptor complex into the nucleus of the target cell; thus, it cannot bind to DNA. This results in a failure to produce proteins that are normally synthesized in response to aldosterone. These mediator proteins normally stimulate the Na^+/K^+-exchange sites of the collecting tubule. Thus, a lack of mediator proteins prevents Na^+ reabsorption and, therefore, K^+ and H^+ secretion.

2. **Actions:** In most edematous states, blood levels of aldosterone are high, which is instrumental in retaining Na^+. When *spironolactone* is given to a patient with elevated circulating levels of aldosterone, the drug antagonizes the activity of the hormone, resulting in retention of K^+ and excretion of Na^+ (see Figure 22.8). In patients who have no significant circulating levels of aldosterone, such as those with Addison's disease (primary adrenal insufficiency), no diuretic effect of the drug occurs. In common with the thiazides and loop diuretics, the effect of *spironolactone* depends on renal prostaglandin synthesis. *Eplerenone* [eh-PLEH-reh-none] is a new aldosterone-receptor antagonist, with actions comparable to those of *spironolactone*. *Eplerenone* may have less endocrine effects than *spironolactone*.

3. **Therapeutic uses:**

   a. **Diuretic:** Although *spironolactone* has a low efficacy in mobilizing Na^+ from the body in comparison with the other drugs, it has the useful property of causing the retention of K^+. Because of this latter action, *spironolactone* is often given in conjunction with a thiazide or loop diuretic to prevent the K^+ excretion that would otherwise occur with these drugs. It is the diuretic of choice in patients with hepatic cirrhosis.

   b. **Secondary hyperaldosteronism:** *Spironolactone* is the only potassium-sparing diuretic that is routinely used alone to induce a net negative salt balance. It is particularly effective in clinical situations associated with secondary hyperaldosteronism.

   c. **Heart failure:** *Spironolactone* prevents the remodeling that occurs as compensation for the progressive failure of the heart.

4. **Pharmacokinetics:** *Spironolactone* is completely absorbed orally and is strongly bound to proteins. It is rapidly converted to an active metabolite, canrenone. The action of *spironolactone* is largely due

to the effect of canrenone, which has mineralocorticoid-blocking activity. *Spironolactone* induces hepatic cytochrome P450.

5. **Adverse effects:** *Spironolactone* frequently causes gastric upsets and can cause peptic ulcers. Because it chemically resembles some of the sex steroids, *spironolactone* may act at receptors in other organs to induce gynecomastia in males and menstrual irregularities in females; therefore, the drug should not be given at high doses on a chronic basis. It is most effectively employed in mild edematous states, for which it is given for a few days at a time. At low doses, *spironolactone* can be used chronically with few side effects. Hyperkalemia, nausea, lethargy, and mental confusion can occur.

B. Triamterene and amiloride

Triamterene [trye-AM-ter-een] and *amiloride* [a-MIL-oh-ride] block Na$^+$ transport channels, resulting in a decrease in Na$^+$/K$^+$ exchange. Although they have a K$^+$-sparing diuretic action similar to that of *spironolactone*, their ability to block the Na$^+$/K$^+$-exchange site in the collecting tubule does not depend on the presence of aldosterone. Thus, they have diuretic activity even in individuals with Addison's disease. Like *spironolactone*, they are not very efficacious diuretics. Both *triamterene* and *amiloride* are frequently used in combination with other diuretics, usually for their potassium-sparing properties. For example, much like *spironolactone*, they prevent the loss of K$^+$ that occurs with thiazides and *furosemide*. The side effects of *triamterene* are leg cramps and the possibility of increased blood urea nitrogen as well as uric acid and K$^+$ retention.

VII. CARBONIC ANHYDRASE INHIBITORS

Acetazolamide [ah-set-a-ZOLE-a-mide] inhibits the enzyme carbonic anhydrase in the proximal tubular epithelial cells. Carbonic anhydrase inhibitors are more often used for their other pharmacologic actions rather than for their diuretic effect, because they are much less efficacious than the thiazides or loop diuretics.

A. Acetazolamide

1. **Mechanism of action:** *Acetazolamide* inhibits carbonic anhydrase located intracellularly (cytoplasm) and on the apical membrane of the proximal tubular epithelium (Figure 22.9). [Note: Carbonic anhydrase catalyzes the reaction of CO$_2$ and H$_2$O, leading to H$_2$CO$_3$, which spontaneously ionizes to H$^+$ and HCO$_3^-$ (bicarbonate)]. The decreased ability to exchange Na$^+$ for H$^+$ in the presence of *acetazolamide* results in a mild diuresis. Additionally, HCO$_3^-$ is retained in the lumen, with marked elevation in urinary pH. The loss of HCO$_3^-$ causes a hyperchloremic metabolic acidosis and decreased diuretic efficacy following several days of therapy. Changes in the composition of urinary electrolytes induced by *acetazolamide* are summarized in Figure 22.10. Phosphate excretion is increased by an unknown mechanism.

2. **Therapeutic uses:**

   a. **Treatment of glaucoma:** The most common use of *acetazolamide* is to reduce the elevated intraocular pressure of open-angle glaucoma. *Acetazolamide* decreases the production of aqueous humor, probably by blocking carbonic anhydrase in the ciliary

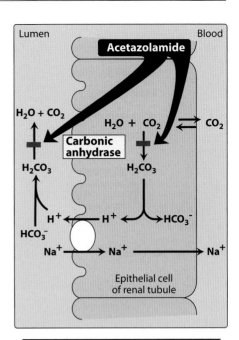

Figure 22.9
Role of carbonic anhydrase in sodium retention by epithelial cells of renal tubule.

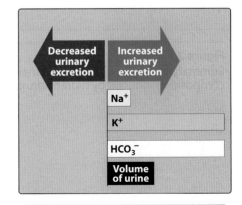

Figure 22.10
Relative changes in the composition of urine induced by *acetazolamide*.

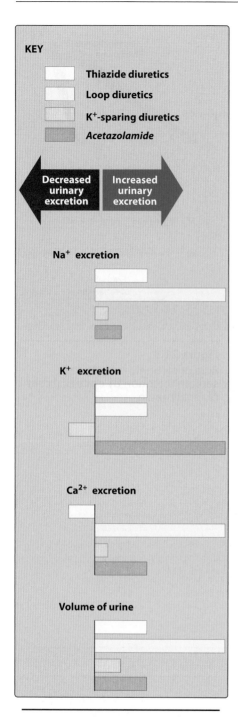

Figure 22.11
Summary of relative changes in urinary composition induced by diuretic drugs.

body of the eye. It is useful in the chronic treatment of glaucoma but should not be used for an acute attack; *pilocarpine* is preferred for an acute attack because of its immediate action. Topical carbonic anhydrase inhibitors, such as *dorzolamide* and *brinzolamide*, have the advantage of not causing any systemic effects.

  b. **Mountain sickness:** Less commonly, *acetazolamide* can be used in the prophylaxis of acute mountain sickness among healthy, physically active individuals who rapidly ascend above 10,000 feet. *Acetazolamide* given nightly for 5 days before the ascent prevents the weakness, breathlessness, dizziness, nausea, and cerebral as well as pulmonary edema characteristic of the syndrome.

3. **Pharmacokinetics:** *Acetazolamide* is given orally once to four times daily. It is secreted by the proximal tubule.

4. **Adverse effects:** Metabolic acidosis (mild), potassium depletion, renal stone formation, drowsiness, and paresthesia may occur. The drug should be avoided in patients with hepatic cirrhosis, because it could lead to a decreased excretion of NH_4^+.

VIII. OSMOTIC DIURETICS

A number of simple, hydrophilic chemical substances that are filtered through the glomerulus, such as *mannitol* [MAN-i-tol] and *urea* [yu-REE-ah], result in some degree of diuresis. This is due to their ability to carry water with them into the tubular fluid. If the substance that is filtered subsequently undergoes little or no reabsorption, then the filtered substance will cause an increase in urinary output. Only a small amount of additional salt may also be excreted. Because osmotic diuretics are used to effect increased water excretion rather than Na^+ excretion, they are not useful for treating conditions in which Na^+ retention occurs. They are used to maintain urine flow following acute toxic ingestion of substances capable of producing acute renal failure. Osmotic diuretics are a mainstay of treatment for patients with increased intracranial pressure or acute renal failure due to shock, drug toxicities, and trauma. Maintaining urine flow preserves long-term kidney function and may save the patient from dialysis. [Note: *Mannitol* is not absorbed when given orally and should only be given intravenously.] Adverse effects include extracellular water expansion and dehydration as well as hypo- or hypernatremia. The expansion of extracellular water results because the presence of *mannitol* in the extracellular fluid extracts water from the cells and causes hyponatremia until diuresis occurs. Dehydration, on the other hand, can occur if water is not replaced adequately.

Figure 22.11 summarizes the relative changes in urinary composition induced by diuretic drugs.

Study Questions

Choose the ONE best answer.

22.1 An elderly patient with a history of heart disease and who is having difficulty breathing is brought into the emergency room. Examination reveals that she has pulmonary edema. Which of the following treatments is indicated?

A. Spironolactone.
B. Furosemide.
C. Acetazolamide.
D. Chlorthalidone.
E. Hydrochlorothiazide.

Correct choice = B. This is a potentially fatal situation. It is important to administer a diuretic that will reduce fluid accumulation in the lungs and, thus, improve oxygenation and heart function. The loop diuretics are most effective in removing large fluid volumes from the body and are the treatment of choice in this situation. Furosemide is usually administered intravenously. The other choices are inappropriate.

22.2 A group of college students is planning a mountain climbing trip to the Andes. Which of the following drugs would be appropriate for them to take to prevent mountain sickness?

A. A thiazide diuretic.
B. An anticholinergic.
C. A carbonic anhydrase inhibitor.
D. A loop diuretic.
E. A β-blocker.

Correct choice = C. Acetazolamide is used prophylactically for several days before an ascent above 10,000 feet. This treatment prevents the cerebral and pulmonary problems associated with the syndrome as well as other difficulties, such as nausea.

22.3 An alcoholic male has developed hepatic cirrhosis. To control the ascites and edema, he is prescribed which one of the following?

A. Hydrochlorothiazide.
B. Acetazolamide.
C. Spironolactone.
D. Furosemide.
E. Chlorthalidone.

Correct choice = C. Spironolactone is very effective in the treatment of hepatic edema. These patients are frequently resistant to the diuretic action of loop diuretics, although a combination with spironolactone may be beneficial. The other agents are not indicated.

22.4 A 55-year-old male with kidney stones has been placed on a diuretic to decrease calcium excretion. However, after a few weeks, he develops an attack of gout. Which diuretic was he taking?

A. Furosemide.
B. Hydrochlorothiazide.
C. Spironolactone.
D. Triamterene.

Correct choice = B. Hydrochlorothiazide is effective in increasing calcium reabsorption, thus decreasing the amount of calcium excreted, and decreasing the formation kidney stones that contain calcium phosphate or calcium oxalate. However, hydrochlorothiazide can also inhibit the excretion of uric acid and cause its accumulation, leading to an attack of gout in some individuals. Furosemide increases the excretion of calcium, whereas the K^+-sparing diuretics, spironolactone and triamterene, do not have an effect.

22.5 A 75-year-old woman with hypertension is being treated with a thiazide. Her blood pressure responds and reads at 120/76 mm Hg. After several months on the medication, she complains of being tired and weak. An analysis of the blood indicates low values for which of the following ?

A. Calcium.
B. Uric acid.
C. Potassium.
D. Sodium.
E. Glucose

Correct choice = C. Hypokalemia is a common adverse effect of the thiazides and causes fatigue and lethargy in the patient. Supplementation with potassium chloride or with foods high in K+ corrects the problem. Alternatively, one may add a potassium-sparing diuretic like spironolactone. Calcium, uric acid, and glucose are usually elevated by thiazide diuretics. The sodium loss does not weaken the patient.

22.6 Which of the following drugs is contraindicated in a patient with hyperkalemia?

A. Acetazolamide
B. Chlorothiazide
C. Ethacrynic acid
D. Chlorthalidone
E. Spironolactone

Correct choice = E. Spironolactone acts in the collecting tubule to inhibit Na+ reabsorption and K+ excretion. It is extremely important that patients who are treated with any potassium-sparing diuretic be closely monitored for potassium levels. Exogenous potassium supplementation is usually discontinued when potassium-sparing diuretic therapy is instituted and the spironlactone is contraindicated in patients with hyperkalemia. The other drugs promote the excretion of potassium.

22.7 Which would be the initial treatment choice to manage the hypertension in an African-American woman with a past medical history of gout and severe hypokalemia?

A. Hydrochlorothiazide
B. Spironolactone
C. alsartan
D. Atenolol
E. Enalapril

Correct choice = B. African American patients with hypertension respond poorly to valsartan, atenolol and enalapril. Hydrochlorothiazide is generally consider the first-line drug. However, and because of the patient's medical history of hypokalemia and gout, spironalctone is the drug of choice. Additionally, the feminizing hormonal effects of spironolactone may be bothersome in men, but not in women.

Pituitary and Thyroid

23

I. OVERVIEW

The neuroendocrine system, which is controlled by the pituitary and hypothalamus, coordinates body functions by transmitting messages between individual cells and tissues. This contrasts with the nervous system which communicates locally by electrical impulses and neurotransmitters directed through neurons to other neurons or to specific target organs, such as muscle or glands. Nerve impulses generally act within milliseconds. The endocrine system releases hormones into the bloodstream, which carries these chemical messengers to target cells throughout the body. Hormones have a much broader range of response time than do nerve impulses, requiring from seconds to days, or longer, to cause a response that may last for weeks or months. The two regulatory systems are closely interrelated. For example, in several instances, the release of hormones is stimulated or inhibited by the nervous system, and some hormones can stimulate or inhibit nerve impulses. Chapters 24 to 26 focus on drugs that affect the synthesis and/or secretion of specific hormones and their actions. In this chapter, the central role of the hypothalamic and pituitary hormones in regulating body functions is briefly presented (Figure 23.1). In addition, drugs affecting thyroid hormone synthesis and/or secretion are discussed.

II. HYPOTHALAMIC AND ANTERIOR PITUITARY HORMONES

The hormones secreted by the hypothalamus and the pituitary are all peptides or low-molecular-weight proteins that act by binding to specific receptor sites on their target tissues. The hormones of the anterior pituitary are regulated by neuropeptides that are called either "releasing" or "inhibiting" factors or hormones. These are produced in cell bodies in the hypothalamus, and they reach the cells of the pituitary by the hypophysial portal system (Figure 23.2). The interaction of the releasing hormones with their receptors results in the activation of genes that promote the synthesis of protein precursors. These are then processed posttranslationally to the hormones and are released into the circulation. [Note: Unlike those of the posterior pituitary, the hormones of the anterior pituitary are not stored in granules prior to release.] Each hypothalamic regulatory hormone controls the release of a specific hor-

---

HYPOTHALAMIC AND ANTERIOR PITUITARY HORMONES

- *Chorionic gonadotropin*
- *Corticotropin*
- *Cosyntropin*
- *Follitropin beta*
- *Gonadorelin*
- *Goserelin*
- *Histrelin*
- *Leuprolide*
- *Menotropins*
- *Nafarelin*
- *Octreotide*
- *Pegvisomant*
- *Somatostatin*
- *Somatotropin*
- *Somatrem*
- *Urofollitropin*

HORMONES OF THE POSTERIOR PITUITARY

- *Desmopressin*
- *Oxytocin*
- *Vasopressin (ADH)*

DRUGS AFFECTING THE THYROID

- *Iodide*
- *Levothyroxine*
- *Methimazole*
- *Propylthiouracil*
- *Thyroxine*
- *Triiodothyronine*

Figure 23.1
Some of the hormones and drugs affecting the hypothalamus, pituitary, and thyroid.

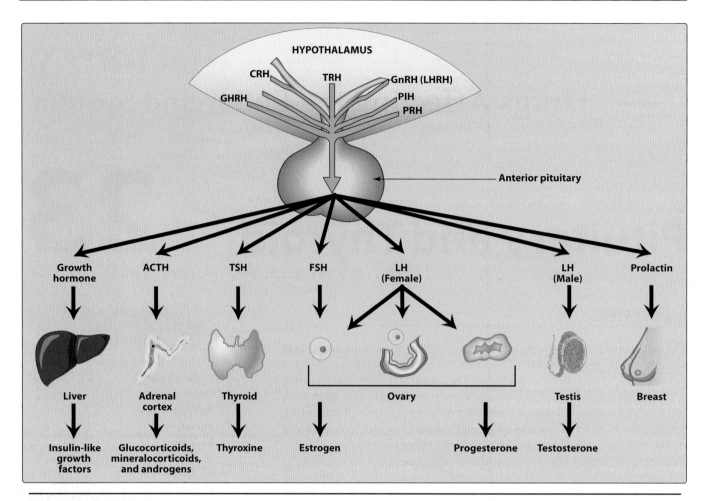

Figure 23.2
Hypothalamic-releasing hormones and actions of anterior pituitary hormones. GHRH = growth hormone-releasing hormone; TRH = thyrotropin-releasing hormone; CRH= corticotropin-releasing hormone; GnRH (LHRH) = gonadotropin-releasing hormone (luteinizing hormone-releasing hormone); PIH = prolactin-inhibiting hormone (dopamine); and PRH = prolactin-releasing hormone; ACTH = adrenocorticotropic hormone; TSH = thyrotropin-stimulating hormone; FSH = follicle-stimulating hormone; LH = luteinizing hormone

mone from the anterior pituitary. The hypothalamic-releasing hormones are primarily used for diagnostic purposes (that is, to determine pituitary insufficiency). [Note: The hypothalamus also synthesizes the precursor proteins of the hormones vasopressin and oxytocin, which are transported to the posterior pituitary, where they are stored until released.] Although a number of pituitary hormone preparations are currently used therapeutically for specific hormonal deficiencies (examples of which follow), most of these agents have limited therapeutic applications. Hormones of the anterior and posterior pituitary are administered either intramuscularly (IM), subcutaneously, or intranasally, but not orally, because their peptidyl nature makes them susceptible to destruction by the proteolytic enzymes of the digestive tract.

A. Adrenocorticotropic hormone (corticotropin)

Corticotropin-releasing hormone (CRH) is responsible for the synthesis and release of the peptide proopiomelanocortin by the hypothalamus (Figure 23.3). Adrenocorticotropic hormone (ACTH), or *corticotropin* [kor-ti-koe-TROE-pin] is a product of the posttranslational processing of this precursor polypeptide. [Note: CRH is used diagnostically to differentiate between Cushing's syndrome and ectopic ACTH-producing cells.] Other products of proopiomelanocortin are γ-melanocyte stimulating hormone and β-lipotropin, the latter being the precursor of the endorphins. Normally, ACTH is released from the pituitary in pulses with an overriding diurnal rhythm, with the highest concentration occurring at approximately 6 AM and the lowest in the evening. Stress stimulates its secretion, whereas cortisol acting via negative feedback suppresses its release.

1. **Mechanism of action:** The target organ of ACTH is the adrenal cortex, where it binds to specific receptors on the cell surfaces. The occupied receptors activate G protein–coupled processes to increase cyclic adenosine monophosphate (cAMP), which in turn stimulates the rate-limiting step in the adrenocorticosteroid synthetic pathway (cholesterol to pregnenolone). This pathway ends with the synthesis and release of the adrenocorticosteroids and the adrenal androgens (see Figure 23.3).

2. **Therapeutic uses:** The availability of synthetic adrenocorticosteroids with specific properties has limited the use of *corticotropin* mainly to serving as a diagnostic tool for differentiating between primary adrenal insufficiency (Addison's disease, associated with adrenal atrophy) and secondary adrenal insufficiency (caused by the inadequate secretion of ACTH by the pituitary). Therapeutic *corticotropin* preparations are extracts from the anterior pituitaries of domestic animals or synthetic human ACTH. The latter, *cosyntropin* [ko-sin-TROE-pin], which consists of the amino-terminal 24 amino acids of the hormone, is preferred for the diagnosis of adrenal insufficiency. ACTH is used in the treatment of infantile spasm (West Syndrome).

3. **Adverse effects:** Toxicities are similar to those of glucocorticoids. Antibodies can form against ACTH derived from animal sources.

B. Growth hormone (somatotropin)

Somatotropin [soe-mah-toe-TROE pin] is a large polypeptide that is released by the anterior pituitary in response to growth hormone (GH)–releasing hormone produced by the hypothalamus (see Figure 23.2). Secretion of GH is inhibited by another pituitary hormone, *somatostatin* (see below). GH is released in a pulsatile manner, with the highest levels occurring during sleep. With increasing age, GH secretion decreases, being accompanied by a decrease in lean muscle mass. Human GH is produced synthetically by recombinant DNA technology. GH from animal sources is ineffective in humans. *Somatotropin* influences a wide variety of biochemical processes; for example, through stimulation of protein synthetic processes, cell proliferation and bone growth are promoted. Increased formation of hydroxyproline from proline boosts cartilage synthesis.

1. **Mechanism of action:** Although many physiologic effects of GH are exerted directly at its targets, others are mediated through the somatomedins—insulin-like growth factors I and II (IGF-I and IGF-II). [Note: In acromegaly, IGF-I levels are consistently high, reflecting elevated GH.]

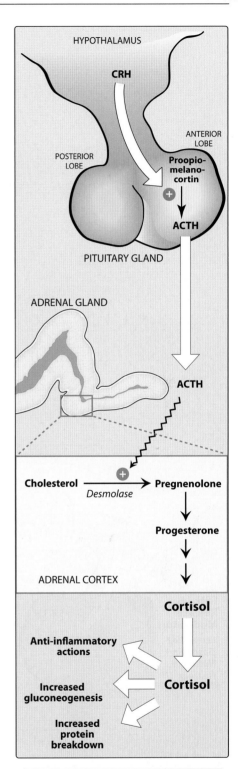

Figure 23.3
Secretion and actions of adrenocorticotropic hormone (ACTH). CRH = corticotropin-releasing hormone.

2. Therapeutic uses: *Somatotropin* is used in the treatment of GH deficiency in children. It is important to establish whether the GH deficit is actually due to hypopituitarism, because other factors, such as normal thyroid status, are essential for successful *somatotropin* therapy. [Note: After a study published in 1990 indicated that GH administered to men over 60 years of age for 6 months increased their lean body mass, bone density, and skin thickness, whereas adipose tissue mass decreased, many started to call GH the anti-aging hormone. This has led to abuse by some athletes seeking to enhance their performance. GH is not approved for this purpose, and some who have taken it have developed diabetes.] A therapeutically equivalent drug, *somatrem* [SOE-ma-trem], contains an extra terminal methionyl residue not found in *somatotropin*. Although the half-lives of these drugs are short (approximately 25 minutes), they induce the release from the liver of IGF-I (formerly somatomedin C), which is responsible for subsequent GH-like actions. *Somatotropin* and *somatrem* should not be used in individuals with closed epiphyses or an enlarging intracranial mass.

C. Growth hormone–inhibiting hormone (somatostatin)

In the pituitary, *somatostatin* [soe-ma-toe-STAT in] binds to distinct receptors, SSTR2 and SSTR5, which suppress GH and thyroid-stimulating hormone release. Originally isolated from the hypothalamus, *somatostatin* is a small polypeptide that is also found in neurons throughout the body as well as in the intestine and pancreas. *Somatostatin* therefore has a number of actions. For example, it not only inhibits the release of GH but, also, that of insulin, glucagon, and gastrin. *Octreotide* [ok-TREE-oh-tide] is a synthetic octapeptide analog of *somatostatin*. Its half-life is longer than that of the natural compound, and a depot form is also available. The two forms suppress GH and IGF-I for 12 hours and 6 weeks, respectively. They have found use in the treatment of acromegaly caused by hormone-secreting tumors and in secretory diarrhea associated with tumors producing vasoactive intestinal peptide (VIPomas). Adverse effects of *octreotide* treatment are flatulence, nausea, and steatorrhea. Gallbladder emptying is delayed, and asymptomatic cholesterol gallstones can occur with long-term treatment. [Note: An analog of human GH that has polyethylene glycol polymers attached, *pegvisomant* [peg-VI-soe-mant], is being employed in the treatment of acromegaly that is refractory to other modes of surgical, radiologic, or pharmacologic intervention. It acts as an antagonist at one of the GH receptors and results in the normalization of IGF-I levels.

D. Gonadotropin-releasing hormone/luteinizing hormone–releasing hormone

Gonadotropin-releasing hormone (GnRH), also called *gonadorelin* [go-nad-oh-RELL-in], is a decapeptide obtained from the hypothalamus. Pulsatile secretion of GnRH is essential for the release of *follicle-stimulating hormone* (*FSH*) and *luteinizing hormone* (*LH*) from the pituitary, whereas continuous administration inhibits gonadotropin release. GnRH is employed to stimulate gonadal hormone production in hypogonadism. A number of synthetic analogs, such as *leuprolide* [loo-PROE-lide], *goserelin* [GOE-se-rel-in], *nafarelin* [naf-A-rel-in], and *histrelin* [his-TREL-in], act as agonists at GnRH receptors (Figure 23.4). These are effective in suppressing production of the gonadal hormones and, thus, are effective in the treatment of prostatic cancer,

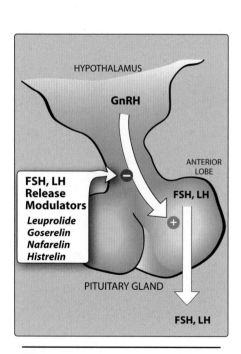

Figure 23.4
Secretion of follicle-stimulating hormone (FSH) and luteinizing hormone (LH). GnRH = gonadotropin-releasing hormone.

endometriosis, and precocious puberty. Adverse effects of *gonadorelin* include hypersensitivity, dermatitis, and headache. In women, the analogs may cause hot flushes and sweating as well as diminished libido, depression, and ovarian cysts. They are contraindicated in pregnancy and breast-feeding. In men, they initially cause a rise in testosterone that can result in bone pain; hot flushes, edema, gynecomastia, and diminished libido also occur.

E. Gonadotropins: Human menopausal gonadotropin, follicle-stimulating hormone, and human chorionic gonadotropin

The gonadotropins are glycoproteins that are produced in the anterior pituitary. The regulation of gonadal steroid hormones depends on these agents. They find use in the treatment of infertility in men and women. *Menotropins* [men-oh-TROE-pin] (*human menopausal gonadotropins*, or *hMG*) are obtained from the urine of menopausal women and contain *FSH* and *luteinizing hormone LH*. *Chorionic gonadotropin* (*hCG*) is a placental hormone and an *LH* agonist, to which it is structurally related. It is also excreted in the urine. *Urofollitropin* [yoor-oh-fol-li-TROE-pin] is *FSH* obtained from menopausal women and is devoid of *LH*. *Follitropin beta* [fol-ih-TROE-pin] is human *FSH* manufactured by recombinant DNA technology. All of these hormones are injected IM. Injection of *hMG* or *FSH* over a period of 5 to 12 days causes ovarian follicular growth and maturation, and with subsequent injection of *hCG*, ovulation occurs. In men who are lacking gonadotropins, treatment with *hCG* causes external sexual maturation, and with the subsequent injection of *hMG*, spermatogenesis occurs. Adverse effects include ovarian enlargement and possible hypovolemia. Multiple births are not uncommon. Men may develop gynecomastia.

F. Prolactin

Prolactin is a peptide hormone similar in structure to GH, and is also secreted by the anterior pituitary. Its secretion is inhibited by dopamine acting at D_2 receptors. Its primary function is to stimulate and maintain lactation. In addition, it decreases sexual drive and reproductive function. The hormone enters a cell, where it activates a tyrosine kinase to promote tyrosine phosphorylation and gene activation. There is no preparation available for hypoprolactinemic conditions. On the other hand, hyperprolactinemia, which is associated with galactorrhea and hypogonadism, is usually treated with D_2-receptor agonists, such as *bromocriptine* and *cabergoline*. Both of these agents also find use in the treatment of microadenomas and macroprolactinomas. They not only act at the D_2 receptor to inhibit prolactin secretion but also cause increased hypothalamic dopamine by decreasing its turnover. Among their adverse effects are nausea, headache, and sometimes, psychiatric problems.

III. HORMONES OF THE POSTERIOR PITUITARY

In contrast to the hormones of the anterior lobe of the pituitary, those of the posterior lobe, *vasopressin* and *oxytocin*, are not regulated by releasing hormones. Instead, they are synthesized in the hypothalamus, transported to the posterior pituitary, and released in response to specific physiologic signals, such as high plasma osmolarity or parturition. Each is a nonapeptide with a circular structure due to a disulfide bridge. Reduction of the disulfide inactivates these hormones. They are susceptible to proteolytic

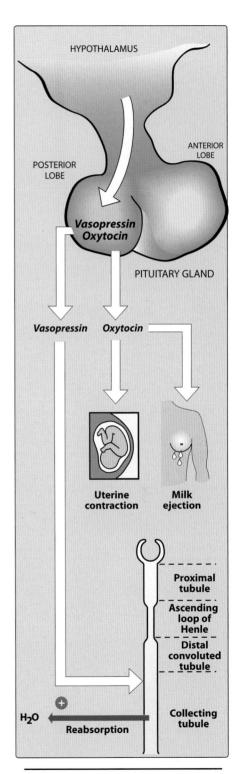

Figure 23.5
Actions of oxytocin and vasopressin. ACTH = adrenocorticotropic hormone.

cleavage and, thus, are given parenterally. Both hormones have very short half-lives. Their actions are summarized in Figure 23.5.

A. Oxytocin

Oxytocin [ok-se-TOE-sin], originally extracted from animal posterior pituitaries, is now chemically synthesized. Its only use is in obstetrics, where it is employed to stimulate uterine contraction to induce or reinforce labor or to promote ejection of breast milk. [Note: The sensitivity of the uterus to *oxytocin* increases with the duration of pregnancy when it is under estrogenic dominance.] To induce labor, the drug is administered intravenously. However, when used to induce "milk letdown," it is given as a nasal spray. *Oxytocin* causes milk ejection by contracting the myoepithelial cells around the mammary alveoli. Although toxicities are uncommon when the drug is used properly, hypertensive crises, uterine rupture, water retention, and fetal death have been reported. Its antidiuretic and pressor activities are very much lower than those of *vasopressin*. [Note: *Oxytocin* is contraindicated in abnormal fetal presentation, fetal distress, and premature births.]

B. Vasopressin

Vasopressin [vas-oh-PRESS-in] (antidiuretic hormone), is structurally related to *oxytocin*. The chemically synthesized nonapeptide has replaced that extracted from animal posterior pituitaries. *Vasopressin* has both antidiuretic and vasopressor effects (see Figure 23.5). In the kidney, it binds to the V_2 receptor to increase water permeability and resorption in the collecting tubules. Thus, the major use of *vasopressin* is to treat diabetes insipidus. It also finds use in controlling bleeding due to esophageal varices or colonic diverticula. Other effects of *vasopressin* are mediated by the V_1 receptor, which is found in liver, vascular smooth muscle (where it causes constriction), and other tissues. As might be expected, the major toxicities are water intoxication and hyponatremia. Headache, bronchoconstriction, and tremor can also occur. Caution must be used when treating patients with coronary artery disease, epilepsy, and asthma.

C. Desmopressin

Because of its pressor properties, *vasopressin* has been modified to *desmopressin* [des-moe-PRESS-in] (1-desamino-8-d-arginine vasopressin), which has minimal activity at the V_1 receptor, making it largely free of pressor effects. This analog is now preferred for diabetes insipidus and nocturnal enuresis and is longer-acting than *vasopressin*. *Desmopressin* is conveniently administered intranasally. However, local irritation may occur.

IV. THYROID HORMONES

The thyroid gland facilitates normal growth and maturation by maintaining a level of metabolism in the tissues that is optimal for their normal function. The two major thyroid hormones are *triiodothyronine* (T_3; the most active form) and *thyroxine* (T_4). Although the thyroid gland is not essential for life, inadequate secretion of thyroid hormone (hypothyroidism) results in bradycardia, poor resistance to cold, and mental and physical slowing (in children, this can cause mental retardation and dwarfism). If, however, an excess of thyroid hormones is secreted (hyperthyroidism), then tachycardia and cardiac arrhythmias, body wasting, nervousness, tremor, and excess

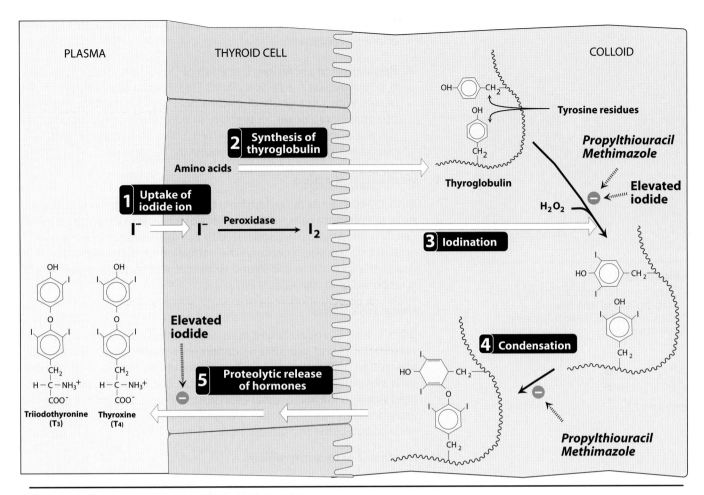

Figure 23.6
Biosynthesis of thyroid hormones.

heat production can occur. [Note: The thyroid gland also secretes the hormone calcitonin—a serum calcium-lowering hormone.]

A. Thyroid hormone synthesis and secretion

The thyroid gland is made up of multiple follicles that consist of a single layer of epithelial cells surrounding a lumen filled with colloid (thyroglobulin), which is the storage form of thyroid hormone. A summary of the steps in thyroid hormone synthesis and secretion is shown in Figure 23.6.

1. **Regulation of synthesis:** Thyroid function is controlled by a tropic hormone, thyroid-stimulating hormone (TSH; thyrotropin). TSH is a glycoprotein, structurally related to *LH* and *FSH*, which is synthesized by the anterior pituitary (see Figure 23.2). TSH generation is governed by the hypothalamic thyrotropin-releasing hormone (TRH). TSH action is mediated by cAMP and leads to stimulation of *iodide* (I^-) uptake. Oxidation to iodine (I_2) by a peroxidase is followed by iodination of tyrosines on thyroglobulin. [Note: Antibodies to thyroid peroxidase are diagnostic for Hashimoto's thyroiditis.] Condensation of two diiodotyrosine residues gives rise to T_4, whereas condensation of a monoiodotyrosine residue with a diiodotyrosine residue generates T_3, which is still bound to the

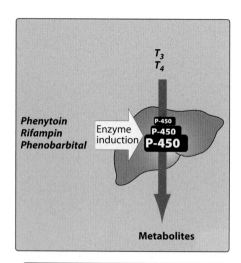

Figure 23.7
Enzyme induction can increase the
metabolism of the thyroid
hormones. T_3 = triiodothyronine;
T_4 = thyroxine.

protein. The hormones are released following proteolytic cleavage of the thyroglobulin.

2. **Regulation of secretion:** Secretion of TSH by the anterior pituitary is stimulated by the hypothalamic TRH. Feedback inhibition of TRH occurs with high levels of circulating thyroid hormone. [Note: At pharmacologic doses, *dopamine*, *somatostatin*, or glucocorticoids can also suppress TSH secretion.] Most of the hormone (T_3 and T_4) is bound to thyroxine-binding globulin in the plasma.

B. **Mechanism of action**

Both T_4 and T_3 must dissociate from thyroxine-binding plasma proteins prior to entry into cells, either by diffusion or by active transport. In the cell, T_4 is enzymatically deiodinated to T_3, which enters the nucleus and attaches to specific receptors. The activation of these receptors promotes the formation of RNA and subsequent protein synthesis, which is responsible for the effects of T_4.

C. **Pharmacokinetics**

Both T_4 and T_3 are absorbed after oral administration. Food, calcium preparations, and aluminum-containing antacids can decrease the absorption of T_4 but not of T_3. T_4 is converted to T_3 by one of two distinct deiodinases, depending on the tissue. The hormones are metabolized through the microsomal P450 system. Drugs that induce the P450 enzymes, such as *phenytoin*, *rifampin*, and *phenobarbital*, accelerate metabolism of the thyroid hormones (Figure 23.7).

D. **Treatment of hypothyroidism**

Hypothyroidism usually results from autoimmune destruction of the gland or the peroxidase and is diagnosed by elevated TSH. It is treated with *levothyroxine* (T_4) [leh-vo-thye-ROK-sin]. The drug is given once daily because of its long half-life. Steady state is achieved in 6 to 8 weeks. Toxicity is directly related to T_4 levels and manifests itself as nervousness, heart palpitations and tachycardia, intolerance to heat, and unexplained weight loss.

E. **Treatment of hyperthyroidism (thyrotoxicosis)**

Excessive amounts of thyroid hormones in the circulation are associated with a number of disease states, including Graves' disease, toxic adenoma, and goiter. In these situations, TSH levels are reduced. The goal of therapy is to decrease synthesis and/or release of additional hormone. This can be accomplished by removing part or all of the thyroid gland, by inhibiting synthesis of the hormones, or by blocking release of the hormones from the follicle.

1. **Removal of part or all of the thyroid:** This can be accomplished either surgically or by destruction of the gland by beta particles emitted by radioactive iodine (^{131}I), which is selectively taken up by the thyroid follicular cells. Younger patients are treated with the isotope without prior pretreatment with *methimazole* (see below), whereas the opposite is the case in elderly patients. Most patients become hypothyroid as a result of this drug and require treatment with *levothyroxine*.

2. **Inhibition of thyroid hormone synthesis:** The thioamides, *propylthiouracil* [proe-pil-thye-oh-YOOR-ah-sil] *(PTU)* and *methimazole* [meth-IM-ah-zole], are concentrated in the thyroid, where they inhibit both the oxidative processes required for iodination of tyrosyl groups and the coupling of iodotyrosines to form T_3 and T_4 (see Figure 23.6). *PTU* can also block the conversion of T_4 to T_3 [Note: These drugs have no effect on the thyroglobulin already stored in the gland; therefore, observation of any clinical effects of these drugs may be delayed until thyroglobulin stores are depleted.] The thioamides are well absorbed from the gastrointestinal tract, but they have short half-lives. Several doses of *PTU* are required per day, whereas a single dose of *methimazole* suffices due to the duration of its antithyroid effect. The effects of these drugs are slow in onset; thus, they are not effective in the treatment of thyroid storm (see below). Relapse may occur. Relatively rare adverse effects include agranulocytosis, rash, and edema.

3. **Thyroid storm:** β-Blockers that lack sympathomimetic activity, such as *propranolol*, are effective in blunting the widespread sympathetic stimulation that occurs in hyperthyroidism. Intravenous administration is effective in treating thyroid storm. An alternative in patients suffering from severe heart failure or asthma is the calcium-channel blocker, *diltiazem*. Other agents used in the treatment of thyroid storm include *PTU* (because it inhibits the peripheral conversion of T_4 to T_3 but *methimazole* does not), *iodides*, and glucocorticoids (to protect against shock).

4. **Blockade of hormone release:** A pharmacologic dose of *iodide* inhibits the iodination of tyrosines (the so-called "acute Wolff-Chaikoff effect"), but this effect lasts only a few days. What is more important, *iodide* inhibits the release of thyroid hormones from thyroglobulin by mechanisms not yet understood. Today, *iodide* is rarely used as the sole therapy. However, it is employed to treat potentially fatal thyrotoxic crisis (thyroid storm) or prior to surgery, because it decreases the vascularity of the thyroid gland. *Iodide* is not useful for long-term therapy, because the thyroid ceases to respond to the drug after a few weeks. *Iodide* is administered orally. Adverse effects are relatively minor and include sore mouth and throat, swelling of the tongue or larynx, rashes, ulcerations of mucous membranes, and a metallic taste in the mouth.

Study Questions

Choose the ONE best answer.

23.1 Symptoms of hyperthyroidism include all of following except:

A. Tachycardia.
B. Nervousness.
C. Poor resistance to cold.
D. Body wasting.
E. Tremor.

Correct answer = C. An individual with hyperthyroidism often experiences excess heat production.

23.2 Which of the following best describes the effect of propylthiouracil on thyroid hormone production?

A. It blocks the release of thyrotropin-releasing hormone.
B. It inhibits uptake of iodide by thyroid cells.
C. It prevents the release of thyroid hormone from thyroglobulin.
D. It blocks iodination and coupling of tyrosines in thyroglobulin to form thyroid hormones.
E. It blocks the release of hormones from the thyroid gland.

Correct answer = D. Propylthiouracil blocks the synthesis of the thyroid hormones, but it does not affect the uptake of iodide, proteolytic cleavage of thyroglobulin, or release of hormones from the thyroid gland. The thyroid hormones inhibit the secretion of thyroid-stimulating hormone from the anterior pituitary.

23.3 Hyperthyroidism can be treated by all but which one of the following?

A. Triiodothyronine.
B. Surgical removal of the thyroid gland.
C. Iodide.
D. Propylthiouracil.
E. Methimazole.

Correct answer = A. Triiodothyronine is a thyroid hormone that is overproduced in hyperthyroidism.

23.4 Which one of the following hormones is a non-peptide, allowing oral administration?

A. ACTH
B. Growth hormone
C. GnRH
D. Thyroxine
E. CRH

Correct answer = D. Although thyroxine is derived from the amino acid, tyrosine, it is not a pepetide and is stable to stomach acid.

23.5 Which one of the following agents is INCORRECTLY paired to a clinical use of the drug?

A. Desmopressin: treatment of diabetes insipidis
B. Octreotide: treatment of diarrhea associated with vasoactive intestinal peptide tumors
C. Oxytocin: induction of labor
D. hCG: treatment of infertility in men and women
E. Pegvisoment: treatment of short stature in men and women

Correct answer = E. Pegvisoment is an antagonist at growth hormone receptors and is used to treat acromegaly.

Insulin and Oral Hypoglycemic Drugs

24

I. OVERVIEW

The pancreas is both an endocrine gland that produces the peptide hormones *insulin*, glucagon, and somatostatin and an exocrine gland that produces digestive enzymes. The peptide hormones are secreted from cells located in the islets of Langerhans (β cells produce *insulin*, α cells produce glucagon, and δ cells produce somatostatin). These hormones play an important role in regulating the metabolic activities of the body, particularly the homeostasis of blood glucose.[1] Hyperinsulinemia (due, for example, to an insulinoma) can cause severe hypoglycemia. More commonly, a relative or absolute lack of *insulin*, such as in diabetes mellitus, can cause serious hyperglycemia, which, if left untreated, can result in retinopathy, nephropathy, neuropathy, and cardiovascular complications. Administration of *insulin* preparations or oral hypoglycemic agents (Figure 24.1) can prevent morbidity and reduce mortality associated with diabetes.

II. DIABETES MELLITUS

The incidence of diabetes is growing rapidly both in the United States and worldwide. For example, it is estimated that more than 180 million people worldwide are afflicted with diabetes, and the prevalence is expected to more than double by the year 2030. In the United States, approximately 21 million people are estimated to suffer from diabetes, and it is a major cause of morbidity and mortality. Diabetes is not a single disease. Rather, it is a heterogeneous group of syndromes characterized by an elevation of blood glucose caused by a relative or absolute deficiency of *insulin*. [Note: Frequently, the inadequate release of *insulin* is aggravated by an excess of glucagon.] The American Diabetes Association (ADA) recognizes four clinical classifications of diabetes: Type 1 diabetes (formerly *insulin*-dependent diabetes mellitus), Type 2 diabetes (formerly non–*insulin* dependent diabetes mellitus), gestational diabetes, and diabetes due to other causes (e.g., genetic defects or medication induced).[2] Figure 24.2 summarizes the characteristics of Type 1 and Type 2 diabetes. Gestational diabetes is defined as carbohydrate intolerance with onset or first recognition during pregnancy. It is important to maintain adequate glycemic control during pregnancy, because uncontrolled gestational diabetes

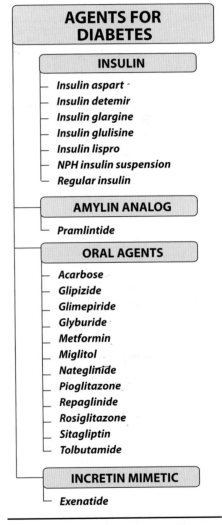

Figure 24.1
Summary of drugs used in the treatment of diabetes.

AGENTS FOR DIABETES

INSULIN
- *Insulin aspart*
- *Insulin detemir*
- *Insulin glargine*
- *Insulin glulisine*
- *Insulin lispro*
- *NPH insulin suspension*
- *Regular insulin*

AMYLIN ANALOG
- *Pramlintide*

ORAL AGENTS
- *Acarbose*
- *Glipizide*
- *Glimepiride*
- *Glyburide*
- *Metformin*
- *Miglitol*
- *Nateglinide*
- *Pioglitazone*
- *Repaglinide*
- *Rosiglitazone*
- *Sitagliptin*
- *Tolbutamide*

INCRETIN MIMETIC
- *Exenatide*

[1]See p. 310 in ***Lippincott's Illustrated Reviews: Biochemistry*** (4th ed.) for a discussion of insulin in glucose homeostasis.
[2]See p. 337 in ***Lippincott's Illustrated Reviews: Biochemistry*** (4th ed.) for a discussion of Type 1 and Type 2 diabetes.

	Type 1	Type 2
Age of onset	Usually during childhood or puberty	Frequently over age 35
Nutritional status at time of onset	Frequently undernourished	Obesity usually present
Prevalence	5 to 10 percent of diagnosed diabetics	90 to 95 percent of diagnosed diabetics
Genetic predisposition	Moderate	Very strong
Defect or deficiency	β Cells are destroyed, eliminating the production of insulin	Inability of β cells to produce appropriate quantities of insulin; insulin resistance; other defects

Figure 24.2
Comparison of Type 1 and Type 2 diabetes.

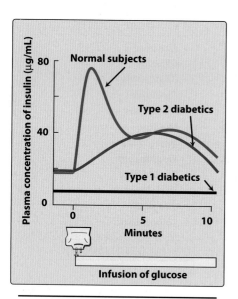

Figure 24.3
Release of insulin that occurs in response to an IV glucose load in normal subjects and diabetic patients.

can lead to fetal macrosomia (overly large body) and shoulder dystocia (difficult delivery), as well as neonatal hypoglycemia. Diet, exercise, and/ or *insulin* administration are effective in this condition. *Glyburide* may be a reasonably safe alternative to *insulin* therapy for gestational diabetes. However, larger randomized studies are needed to fully assess neonatal outcomes and optimal dosing regimens.

A. Type 1 diabetes

Type 1 diabetes most commonly afflicts individuals in puberty or early adulthood, but some latent forms can occur later in life. The disease is characterized by an absolute deficiency of *insulin* caused by massive β-cell necrosis. Loss of β-cell function is usually ascribed to autoimmune-mediated processes directed against the β cell, and it may be triggered by an invasion of viruses or the action of chemical toxins. As a result of the destruction of these cells, the pancreas fails to respond to glucose, and the Type 1 diabetic shows classic symptoms of *insulin* deficiency (polydipsia, polyphagia, polyuria, and weight loss). Type 1 diabetics require exogenous *insulin* to avoid the catabolic state that results from and is characterized by hyperglycemia and life-threatening ketoacidosis.

1. **Cause of Type 1 diabetes:** In the postabsorptive period of a normal individual, low, basal levels of circulating *insulin* are maintained through constant β-cell secretion. This suppresses lipolysis, proteolysis, and glycogenolysis. A burst of *insulin* secretion occurs within 2 minutes after ingesting a meal, in response to transient increases in the levels of circulating glucose and amino acids. This lasts for up to 15 minutes, and, is followed by the postprandial secretion of *insulin*. However, having virtually no functional β cells, the Type 1 diabetic can neither maintain a basal secretion level of *insulin* nor respond to variations in circulating fuels (Figure 24.3). The development and progression of neuropathy, nephropathy, and retinopathy are directly related to the extent of glycemic control (measured as blood levels of glucose and/or hemoglobin A_{1c} [HbA_{1c}]).[3]

2. **Treatment:** A Type 1 diabetic must rely on exogenous (injected) *insulin* to control hyperglycemia, avoid ketoacidosis, and maintain acceptable levels of glycosylated hemoglobin (HbA_{1c}). [Note: The rate of formation of HbA_{1c} is proportional to the average blood glucose concentration over the previous 3 months; thus, HbA_{1c} provides a measure of how well treatment has normalized blood glucose in diabetics.] The goal in administering *insulin* to Type 1 diabetics is to maintain blood glucose concentrations as close to normal as possible and to avoid wide swings in glucose levels that may contribute to long-term complications. The use of home blood glucose monitors facilitates frequent self-monitoring and treatment with *insulin* injections. Continuous subcutaneous *insulin* infusion—also called the *insulin* pump—is another method of *insulin* delivery. This method of administration may be more convenient for some patients, eliminating the multiple daily injections of *insulin*. The pump is programmed to deliver a basal rate

 [3]See p. 34 in ***Lippincott's Illustrated Reviews: Biochemistry*** (4th ed.) for a discussion of hemoglobin A_{1c}.

of *insulin* secretion, and it also allows the patient to control delivery of a bolus of *insulin* to compensate for high blood glucose or in anticipation of postprandial needs. Other methods of *insulin* delivery, such as transdermal, buccal, and intranasal, are currently under investigation. Amylin is a hormone that is cosecreted with *insulin* from pancreatic β cells following food intake. *Pramlintide* [PRAM-len-tide], a synthetic analog of amylin, may be used as an adjunct to *insulin* therapy.

B. Type 2 diabetes

Most diabetics are Type 2. The disease is influenced by genetic factors, aging, obesity, and peripheral *insulin* resistance rather than by autoimmune processes or viruses. The metabolic alterations observed are milder than those described for Type 1 (for example, Type 2 patients typically are not ketotic), but the long-term clinical consequences can be just as devastating (for example, vascular complications and subsequent infection can lead to amputation of the lower limbs).

1. **Cause:** In Type 2 diabetes, the pancreas retains some β-cell function, but variable *insulin* secretion is insufficient to maintain glucose homeostasis (see Figure 24.3). The β-cell mass may become gradually reduced in Type 2 diabetes. In contrast to patients with Type 1, those with Type 2 diabetes are often obese. [Note: Not all obese individuals become diabetic.] Type 2 diabetes is frequently accompanied by the lack of sensitivity of target organs to either endogenous or exogenous *insulin* (Figure 24.4). This resistance to *insulin* is considered to be a major cause of this type of diabetes .

2. **Treatment:** The goal in treating Type 2 diabetes is to maintain blood glucose concentrations within normal limits and to prevent the development of long-term complications of the disease. Weight reduction, exercise, and dietary modification decrease *insulin* resistance and correct the hyperglycemia of Type 2 diabetes in some patients. However, most patients are dependent on pharmacologic intervention with oral hypoglycemic agents. As the disease progresses, β-cell function declines, and *insulin* therapy is often required to achieve satisfactory serum glucose levels (Figure 24.5).

III. INSULIN AND ITS ANALOGS

Insulin [IN-su-lin] is a polypeptide hormone consisting of two peptide chains that are connected by disulfide bonds. It is synthesized as a precursor (proinsulin) that undergoes proteolytic cleavage to form *insulin* and C peptide, both of which are secreted by the β cells of the pancreas.[4] [Note: Type 2 patients secrete high levels of proinsulin. Because radioimmunoassays do not distinguish between proinsulin and *insulin*, Type 2 patients may have lower levels of the active hormone than the assay indicates. Thus, measurement of circulating C peptide provides a better index of *insulin* levels.]

A. Insulin secretion

Insulin secretion is regulated not only by blood glucose levels but also by certain amino acids, other hormones (see gastrointestinal hormones

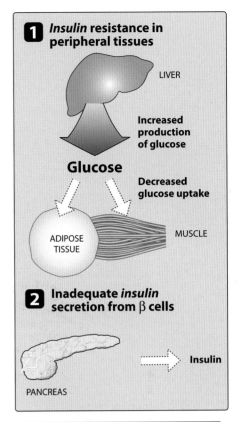

Figure 24.4
Major factors contributing to hyperglycemia observed in Type 2 diabetes.

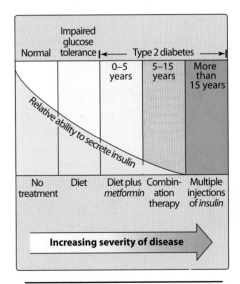

Figure 24.5
Duration of Type 2 diabetes mellitus, sufficiency of endogenous insulin, and recommended sequence of therapy.

[4]See p. 308 in ***Lippincott's Illustrated Reviews: Biochemistry*** (4th ed.) for a discussion of insulin synthesis and secretion.

below), and autonomic mediators. Secretion is most commonly triggered by high blood glucose, which is taken up by the glucose transporter into the β cells of the pancreas. There, it is phosphorylated by glucokinase, which acts as a glucose sensor. The products of glucose metabolism enter the mitochondrial respiratory chain and generate adenosine triphosphate (ATP). The rise in ATP levels causes a block of K^+ channels, leading to membrane depolarization and an influx of Ca^{2+}, which results in pulsatile *insulin* exocytosis. The sulfonylureas and meglitinides owe their hypoglycemic effect to the inhibition of the K^+ channels. [Note: Glucose given by injection has a weaker effect on *insulin* secretion than does glucose taken orally, because when given orally, glucose stimulates production of digestive hormones by the gut, which in turn stimulate *insulin* secretion by the pancreas.]

B. Sources of insulin

Human *insulin* is produced by recombinant DNA technology using special strains of Escherichia coli or yeast that have been genetically altered to contain the gene for human *insulin*. Modifications of the amino acid sequence of human *insulin* have produced *insulins* with different pharmacokinetic properties. For example, three such *insulins*—*lispro, aspart,* and *glulisine*—have a faster onset and shorter duration of action than regular *insulin*, because they do not aggregate or form complexes. On the other hand, *glargine* and *detemir* are long-acting *insulins* and show prolonged, flat levels of the hormone following injection.

C. Insulin administration

Because *insulin* is a polypeptide, it is degraded in the gastrointestinal tract if taken orally. It therefore is generally administered by subcutaneous injection. [Note: In a hyperglycemic emergency, regular *insulin* is injected intravenously.] Continuous subcutaneous *insulin* infusion has become popular, because it does not require multiple daily injections. *Insulin* preparations vary primarily in their times of onset of activity and in their durations of activity. This is due to differences in the amino acid sequences of the polypeptides. Dose, site of injection, blood supply, temperature, and physical activity can affect the duration of action of the various preparations. *Insulin* is inactivated by *insulin*-degrading enzyme (also called *insulin* protease), which is found mainly in the liver and kidney.

D. Adverse reactions to insulin

The symptoms of hypoglycemia are the most serious and common adverse reactions to an overdose of *insulin* (Figure 24.6). Long-term diabetics often do not produce adequate amounts of the counter-regulatory hormones (glucagon, epinephrine, cortisol, and growth hormone), which normally provide an effective defense against hypoglycemia. Other adverse reactions include weight gain, lipodystrophy (less common with human *insulin*), allergic reactions, and local injection site reactions. Diabetics with renal insufficiency may require adjustment of the *insulin* dose.

IV. INSULIN PREPARATIONS AND TREATMENT

It is important that any change in *insulin* treatment be made cautiously by the clinician, with strict attention paid to the dose. Figure 24.7 summarizes onset of action, timing of peak level, and duration of action for the various types of *insulins* that are currently in use.

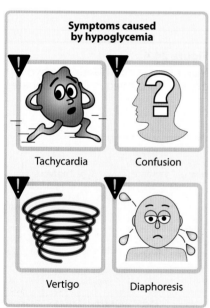

Symptoms caused by hypoglycemia

Tachycardia

Confusion

Vertigo

Diaphoresis

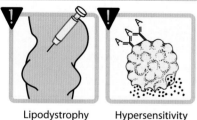

Lipodystrophy

Hypersensitivity

Figure 24.6
Adverse effects observed with *insulin*. [Note: Lipodystrophy is a local atrophy or hypertrophy of subcutaneous fatty tissue at the site of injections.]

handwritten note: Short acting insulins all contain "s" lispro aspart glulisine

A. Rapid-acting and short-acting insulin preparations

Four *insulin* preparations fall into this category: regular *insulin, insulin lispro, insulin aspart,* and *insulin glulisine*. Regular *insulin* is a short-acting, soluble, crystalline *zinc insulin*. Regular *insulin* is usually given subcutaneously (or intravenously in emergencies), and it rapidly lowers blood glucose (Figure 24.8). Regular *insulin, insulin lispro,* and *insulin aspart* are pregnancy category B. *Insulin glulisine* has not been studied in pregnancy. Because of their rapid onset and short duration of action, the *lispro* [LIS-proe], *aspart* [AS-part], and *glulisine* [gloo-LYSE-een] forms of *insulin* are classified as rapid-acting *insulins.* These agents offer more flexible treatment regimens and may lower the risk of hypoglycemia. *Insulin lispro* differs from regular *insulin* in that lysine and proline at positions 28 and 29 in the B chain are reversed. This results in more rapid absorption after subcutaneous injection than is seen with regular *insulin;* as a consequence, *insulin lispro* acts more rapidly. Peak levels of *insulin lispro* are seen at 30 to 90 minutes after injection, as compared with 50 to 120 minutes for regular *insulin. Insulin lispro* also has a shorter duration of activity. *Insulin aspart* and *insulin glulisine* have pharmacokinetic and pharmacodynamic properties similar to those of *insulin lispro.* They are administered to mimic the prandial (mealtime) release of *insulin,* and they are usually not used alone but, rather, along with a longer-acting *insulin* to assure proper glucose control. Like regular *insulin,* they are administered subcutaneously. *Insulin lispro* is usually administered 15 minutes prior to a meal or immediately following a meal, whereas *glulisine* can be taken either 15 minutes before a meal or within 20 minutes after starting a meal. *Insulin aspart* must be administered just prior to the meal. All of the rapid-acting formulations are suitable for intravenous administration, although regular *insulin* is most commonly used when the intravenous route is needed. *Insulin lispro, insulin aspart,* and *insulin glulisine* may also be used in external *insulin* pumps.

B. Intermediate-acting insulin

Neutral protamine Hagedorn (NPH) *insulin* is a suspension of crystalline *zinc insulin* combined at neutral pH with a positively charged polypeptide, protamine. [Note: Another name for this preparation is *insulin isophane.*] Its duration of action is intermediate. This is due to delayed absorption of the *insulin* because of its conjugation with protamine, forming a less-soluble complex. NPH *insulin* should only be given subcutaneously (never intravenously) and is useful in treating all forms of

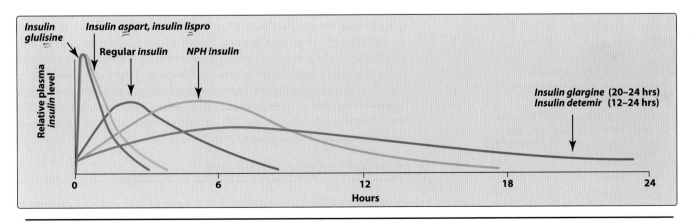

Figure 24.7
Onset and duration of action of human *insulin* and *insulin* analogs. NPH = Neutral Protamine Hagedorn.

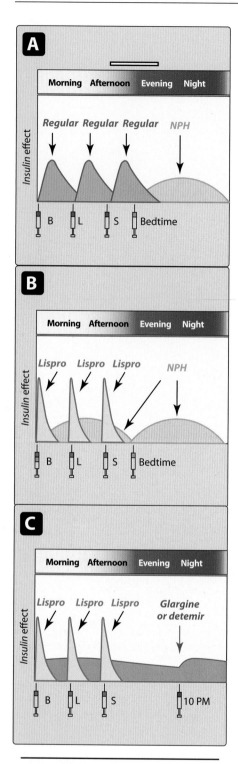

Figure 24.8
Examples of three regimens that provide both prandial and basal *insulin* replacement. B = breakfast; L = lunch; S = supper.

diabetes except diabetic ketoacidosis or emergency hyperglycemia. It is used for basal control and is usually given along with rapid- or short-acting *insulin* for mealtime control. [Note: A similar compound called *neutral protamine lispro* (NPL) *insulin,* has been prepared that is used only in combination with *insulin lispro* (see below).] Figure 24.8 shows three of many regimens that use combinations of *insulins.*

C. Long-acting insulin preparations

1. **Insulin glargine:** The isoelectric point of *insulin glargine* (GLAR-geen) is lower than that of human *insulin,* leading to precipitation at the injection site, thereby extending its action. It is slower in onset than *NPH insulin* and has a flat, prolonged hypoglycemic effect—that is, it has no peak (see Figure 24.7). Like the other *insulins,* it must be given subcutaneously.

2. **Insulin detemir:** *Insulin detemir* (deh-TEE-meer) has a fatty-acid side chain. The addition of the fatty-acid side chain enhances association to albumin. Slow dissociation from albumin results in long-acting properties similar to those of *insulin glargine.*

D. Insulin combinations

Various premixed combinations of human *insulins,* such as 70-percent *NPH insulin* plus 30-percent regular *insulin,* 50 percent of each of these, or 75 percent *NPL insulin* plus 25 percent *insulin lispro,* are also available.

E. Standard treatment versus intensive treatment

Standard treatment of patients with diabetes mellitus involves injection of *insulin* twice daily. In contrast, intensive treatment seeks to normalize blood glucose through more frequent injections of *insulin* (three or more times daily in response to monitoring blood glucose levels). Mean blood glucose levels of 170 mg/dL or less can be achieved with intensive treatment, with an HbA_{1c} content of approximately seven percent or less of total hemoglobin. [Note: Normal mean blood glucose is approximately 135 mg/dL or less, with an HbA_{1c} content of six percent or less.] Thus, the frequency of hypoglycemic episodes, coma, and seizures due to excessive *insulin* is particularly high with intensive treatment regimens (Figure 24.9A). Nonetheless, patients on intensive therapy show a significant reduction in the long-term complications of diabetes—retinopathy, nephropathy, and neuropathy— compared to patients receiving standard care (Figure 24.9B). However, the commonly used treatment algorithm of normalizing blood glucose in diabetics has recently been challenged. The ACCORD trial found that among adults with Type 2 diabetes who are at especially high risk of cardiovascular disease, a medical treatment strategy to intensively lower their blood glucose levels below the current guidelines increased the risk of death compared to standard blood glucose-lowering treatment. The intensive therapy arm of the trial, including those patients treated with intensive insulin therapy, was halted.

V. SYNTHETIC AMYLIN ANALOG

Pramlintide [PRAM-lin-tide] is a synthetic amylin analog that is indicated as an adjunct to mealtime *insulin* therapy in patients with Type 1 or Type 2 diabetes. By acting as an amylinomimetic, *pramlintide* delays gastric emptying, decreases postprandial glucagon secretion, and improves satiety.

Pramlintide is administered by subcutaneous injection and should be injected immediately prior to meals. When *pramlintide* is initiated, the dose of rapid- or short-acting *insulin* should be decreased by 50% prior to meals to avoid a risk of severe hypoglycemia. *Pramlintide* may not be mixed in the same syringe with any *insulin* preparation. Adverse effects are mainly gastrointestinal and consist of nausea, anorexia, and vomiting. *Pramlintide* should not be given to patients with diabetic gastroparesis (delayed stomach emptying)or a history of hypoglycemic unawareness.

VI. ORAL AGENTS: INSULIN SECRETAGOGUES

These agents are useful in the treatment of patients who have Type 2 diabetes but who cannot be managed by diet alone. The patient most likely to respond well to oral hypoglycemic agents is one who develops diabetes after age 40 and has had diabetes less than 5 years. Patients with long-standing disease may require a combination of hypoglycemic drugs with or without *insulin* to control their hyperglycemia. *Insulin* is added because of the progressive decline in β cells that occurs due to the disease or aging. Oral hypoglycemic agents should not be given to patients with Type 1 diabetes. Figure 24.10 summarizes the duration of action of some of the oral hypoglycemic drugs, and Figure 24.11 illustrates some of the common adverse effects of these agents.

A. Sulfonylureas

These agents are classified as *insulin* secretagogues, because they promote *insulin* release from the β cells of the pancreas. The primary drugs used today are *tolbutamide* [tole-BYOO-ta-mide] and the second-generation derivatives, *glyburide* [GLYE-byoor-ide], *glipizide* [GLIP-i-ih-zide], and *glimepiride* [GLYE-me-pih-ride].

1. **Mechanisms of action of the sulfonylureas:** These include 1) stimulation of *insulin* release from the β cells of the pancreas by blocking the ATP-sensitive K+ channels, resulting in depolarization and Ca2+ influx; 2) reduction in hepatic glucose production; and 3) increase in peripheral *insulin* sensitivity.

2. **Pharmacokinetics and fate:** Given orally, these drugs bind to serum proteins, are metabolized by the liver, and are excreted by the liver or kidney. *Tolbutamide* has the shortest duration of action (6–12 hours), whereas the second-generation agents last about 24 hours.

3. **Adverse effects:** Shortcomings of the sulfonylureas are their propensity to cause weight gain, hyperinsulinemia, and hypoglycemia. These drugs should be used with caution in patients with hepatic or renal insufficiency, because delayed excretion of the drug—resulting in its accumulation—may cause hypoglycemia. Renal impairment is a particular problem in the case of those agents that are metabolized to active compounds, such as *glyburide*. *Glyburide* has minimal transfer across the placenta and may be a reasonably safe alternative to *insulin* therapy for diabetes in pregnancy. Figure 24.12 summarizes some of the interactions of the sulfonylureas with other drugs.

B. Meglitinide analogs

This class of agents includes *repaglinide* [re-PAG-lin-ide] and *nateglinide* [nuh-TAY-gli-nide]. Although they are not sulfonylureas, they have common actions.

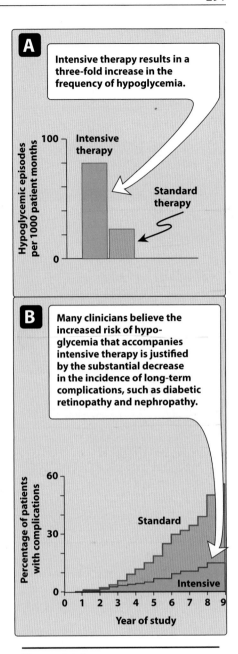

A Intensive therapy results in a three-fold increase in the frequency of hypoglycemia.

Hypoglycemic episodes per 1000 patient months

Intensive therapy

Standard therapy

B Many clinicians believe the increased risk of hypoglycemia that accompanies intensive therapy is justified by the substantial decrease in the incidence of long-term complications, such as diabetic retinopathy and nephropathy.

Percentage of patients with complications

Standard

Intensive

Year of study

Figure 24.9
A. Effect of tight glucose control on hypoglycemic episodes in a population of patients with Type 1 diabetes receiving intensive or standard therapy.
B. Effect of standard and intensive care on the long-term complications of diabetes.

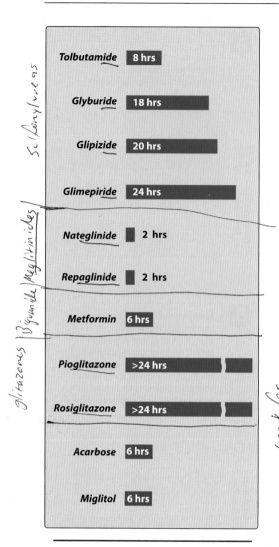

Figure 24.10
Duration of action of some oral hypoglycemic agents.

1. **Mechanism of action:** Like the sulfonylureas, their action is dependent on functioning pancreatic β cells. They bind to a distinct site on the sulfonylurea receptor of ATP-sensitive potassium channels, thereby initiating a series of reactions culminating in the release of *insulin*. However, in contrast to the sulfonylureas, the meglitinides have a rapid onset and a short duration of action. They are particularly effective in the early release of *insulin* that occurs after a meal and, thus, are categorized as postprandial glucose regulators. Combined therapy of these agents with *metformin* or the glitazones has been shown to be better than monotherapy with either agent in improving glycemic control. Meglitinides should not be used in combination with sulfonylureas due to overlapping mechanisms of action.

2. **Pharmacokinetics and fate:** These drugs are well absorbed orally after being taken 1 to 30 minutes before meals. Both meglitinides are metabolized to inactive products by CYP3A4 (see p. 14) in the liver and are excreted through the bile.

3. **Adverse effects:** Although these drugs can cause hypoglycemia, the incidence of this adverse effect appears to be lower than that with the sulfonylureas. [Note: Drugs that inhibit CYP3A4, like *ketoconazole, itraconazole, fluconazole, erythromycin,* and *clarithromycin,* may enhance the glucose-lowering effect of *repaglinide,* whereas drugs that increase levels of this enzyme, such as barbiturates, *carbamazepine,* and *rifampin,* may have the opposite effect.] *Repaglinide* has been reported to cause severe hypoglycemia in patients who are also taking the lipid-lowering drug *gemfibrozil.* Weight gain is less of a problem with the meglitinides than with the sulfonylureas. These agents must be used with caution in patients with hepatic impairment.

VII. ORAL AGENTS: INSULIN SENSITIZERS

Two classes of oral agents—the biguanides and thiazolidinediones—improve *insulin* action. These agents lower blood sugar by improving target-cell response to *insulin* without increasing pancreatic *insulin* secretion.

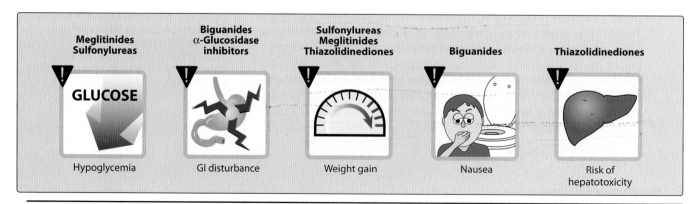

Figure 24.11
Some adverse effects observed with oral hypoglycemic agents.

A. Biguanides

Metformin [met-FOR-min], the only currently available biguanide, is classed as an *insulin* sensitizer; that is, it increases glucose uptake and utilization by target tissues, thereby decreasing *insulin* resistance. Like the sulfonylureas, *metformin* requires *insulin* for its action, but it differs from the sulfonylureas in that it does not promote *insulin* secretion. Hyperinsulinemia is not a problem. Thus, the risk of hypoglycemia is far less than that with sulfonylurea agents, and it may only occur if caloric intake is not adequate or exercise is not compensated for calorically.

1. **Mechanism of action:** The main mechanism of action of *metformin* is reduction of hepatic glucose output, largely by inhibiting hepatic gluconeogenesis. [Note: Excess glucose produced by the liver is the major source of high blood glucose in Type 2 diabetic, accounting for the high blood glucose on waking in the morning.] *Metformin* also slows intestinal absorption of sugars and improves peripheral glucose uptake and utilization. A very important property of this drug is its ability to modestly reduce hyperlipidemia (low-density lipoprotein [LDL] and very-low-density lipoprotein [VLDL] choles- terol concentrations fall, and high-density lipoprotein [HDL] cho- lesterol rises). These effects may not be apparent until 4 to 6 weeks of use. The patient often loses weight because of loss of appetite. The ADA treatment algorithm recommends *metformin* as the drug of choice for newly diagnosed Type 2 diabetics. *Metformin* may be used alone or in combination with one of the other agents, as well as with *insulin*. Hypoglycemia has occurred when *metformin* was taken in combination. [Note: If used with *insulin*, the dose of *insulin* may require adjustment, because *metformin* decreases the production of glucose by the liver.]

2. **Pharmacokinetics and fate:** *Metformin* is well absorbed orally, is not bound to serum proteins, and is not metabolized. Excretion is via the urine.

3. **Adverse effects:** These are largely gastrointestinal. *Metformin* is contraindicated in diabetics with renal and/or hepatic disease, acute myocardial infarction, severe infection, or diabetic ketoacidosis. It should be used with caution in patients greater than 80 years of age or in those with a history of congestive heart failure or alcohol abuse. [Note: Diabetics being treated with heart-failure medications should not be given *metformin* because of an increased risk of lactic acidosis.] *Metformin* should be temporarily discontinued in patients undergoing diagnosis requiring intravenous radiographic contrast agents. Rarely, potentially fatal lactic acidosis has occurred. Long- term use may interfere with vitamin B_{12} absorption.

4. **Other uses:** In addition to the treatment of Type 2 diabetes, *met- formin* is effective in the treatment of polycystic ovary disease. Its ability to lower *insulin* resistance in these women can result in ovula- tion and, possibly, pregnancy.

B. Thiazolidinediones or glitazones

Another group of agents that are *insulin* sensitizers are the thiazoli- dinediones (TZDs) or, more familiarly the glitazones. Although *insu- lin* is required for their action, these drugs do not promote its release from the pancreatic β cells; thus, hyperinsulinemia does not result.

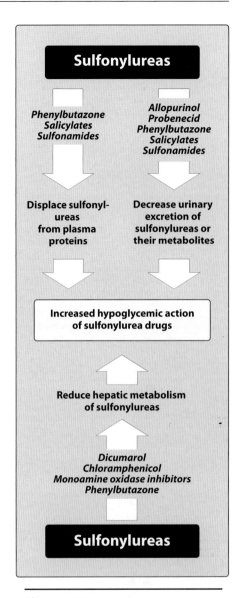

Figure 24.12
Drugs interacting with sulfonyl- urea drugs.

Troglitazone [TROE-glit-a-zone] was the first of these to be approved for the treatment of Type 2 diabetic, but was withdrawn after a number of deaths due to hepatotoxicity were reported. Presently, two members of this class are available, *pioglitazone* [pye-oh-GLI-ta-zone] and *rosiglitazone* [roe-si-GLIH-ta-zone].

1. **Mechanism of action:** Although the exact mechanism by which the TZDs lower *insulin* resistance remains to be elucidated, they are known to target the peroxisome proliferator–activated receptor-γ (PPARγ)—a nuclear hormone receptor. Ligands for PPARγ regulate adipocyte production and secretion of fatty acids as well as glucose metabolism, resulting in increased *insulin* sensitivity in adipose tissue, liver, and skeletal muscle. Hyperglycemia, hyperinsulinemia, hypertriacylglycerolemia, and elevated HbA$_{1c}$ levels are improved. Interestingly, LDL levels are not affected by *pioglitazone* monotherapy or when the drug is used in combination with other agents, whereas LDL levels have increased with *rosiglitazone*. HDL levels increase with both drugs. The TZDs lead to a favorable redistribution of fat from visceral to subcutaneous tissues. [Note: Whether the adipogenic effects can be separated from those of increased *insulin* sensitivity is the subject of much research, particularly because of the role of obesity in this disease.] *Pioglitazone* and *rosiglitazone* can be used as monotherapy or in combination with other hypoglycemics or with *insulin*. The dose of *insulin* required for adequate glucose control in these circumstances may have to be lowered. The glitazones are recommended as a second-line alternative for patients who fail or have contraindications to metformin therapy.

2. **Pharmacokinetics and fate:** Both *pioglitazone* and *rosiglitazone* are absorbed very well after oral administration and are extensively bound to serum albumin. Both undergo extensive metabolism by different cytochrome P450 isozymes (see p. 14). Some metabolites of *pioglitazone* have activity. Renal elimination of *pioglitazone* is negligible, with the majority of the active drug and metabolites excreted in the bile and eliminated in the feces. The metabolites of *rosiglitazone* are primarily excreted in the urine. No dosage adjustment is required in renal impairment. It is recommended that these agents not be used in nursing mothers.

3. **Adverse effects:** Because there have been deaths from hepatotoxicity in patients taking *troglitazone*, it is recommended that liver enzyme levels of patients on these medications be measured initially and periodically thereafter. Very few cases of liver toxicity have been reported with *rosiglitazone* or *pioglitazone*. Weight increase can occur, possibly through the ability of TZDs to increase subcutaneous fat or due to fluid retention. [Note: The latter can lead to or worsen heart failure.] Glitazones have been associated with osteopenia and increased fracture risk. A recent retrospective meta-analysis found that *rosiglitazone* was associated with an increased risk of myocardial infarction and death from cardiovascular causes; however, future prospective studies are needed to better ascertain the cardiovascular risks associated with rosiglitazone. Other adverse effects include headache and anemia. Women taking oral contraceptives and TZDs may become pregnant, because the latter have been shown to reduce plasma concentrations of the estrogen-containing contraceptives.

4. **Other uses:** As with *metformin*, the relief of *insulin* resistance with the TZDs can cause ovulation to resume in premenopausal women with polycystic ovary syndrome.

VIII. ORAL AGENTS: α-GLUCOSIDASE INHIBITORS

Acarbose [AY-car-bose] and *miglitol* [MIG-li-tol] are orally active drugs used for the treatment of patients with Type 2 diabetes.

A. Mechanism of action

These drugs are taken at the beginning of meals. They act by delaying the digestion of carbohydrates, thereby resulting in lower postprandial glucose levels. Both drugs exert their effects by reversibly inhibiting membrane-bound α-glucosidase in the intestinal brush border. This enzyme is responsible for the hydrolysis of oligosaccharides to glucose and other sugars. [Note: *Acarbose* also inhibits pancreatic α-amylase, thus interfering with the breakdown of starch to oligosaccharides.] Consequently, the postprandial rise of blood glucose is blunted. Unlike the other oral hypoglycemic agents, these drugs do not stimulate *insulin* release, nor do they increase *insulin* action in target tissues. Thus, as monotherapy, they do not cause hypoglycemia. However, when used in combination with the sulfonylureas or with *insulin*, hypoglycemia may develop. [Note: It is important that the hypoglycemic patient be treated with glucose rather than sucrose, because sucrase is also inhibited by these drugs.]

B. Pharmacokinetics

Acarbose is poorly absorbed. It is metabolized primarily by intestinal bacteria, and some of the metabolites are absorbed and excreted into the urine. On the other hand, *miglitol* is very well absorbed but has no systemic effects. It is excreted unchanged by the kidney.

C. Adverse effects

The major side effects are flatulence, diarrhea, and abdominal cramping. *→ creating osmotic diarrhea* Patients with inflammatory bowel disease, colonic ulceration, or intestinal obstruction should not use these drugs.

IX. ORAL AGENTS: DIPEPTIDYL PEPTIDASE-IV INHIBITORS

Sitagliptin [si-ta-GLIP-tin] is an orally active dipeptidyl peptidase-IV (DPP-IV) inhibitor used for the treatment of patients with Type 2 diabetes. Other agents in this category are currently in development.

A. Mechanism of action

Sitagliptin inhibits the enzyme DPP-IV, which is responsible for the inactivation of incretin hormones, such as glucagon-like peptide-1 (GLP-1). Prolonging the activity of incretin hormones results in increased *insulin* release in response to meals and a reduction in inappropriate secretion of glucagon. *Sitagliptin* may be used as monotherapy or in combination with a sulfonylurea, *metformin* or a *glitazone*.

B. Pharmacokinetics and fate

Sitagliptin is well absorbed after oral administration. Food does not affect the extent of absorption. The majority of *sitagliptin* is excreted unchanged in the urine. Dosage adjustments are recommended for patients with renal dysfunction.

C. Adverse effects

In general, *sitagliptin* is well tolerated, with the most common adverse effects being nasopharyngitis and headache. Rates of hypoglycemia are comparable to those with placebo when *sitagliptin* is used as monotherapy or in combination with *metformin* or *pioglitazone*.

X. INCRETIN MIMETICS

Oral glucose results in a higher secretion of *insulin* than occurs when an equal load of glucose is given intravenously. This effect is referred to as the "incretin effect" and is apparently reduced in Type 2 diabetes. It demonstrates the important role of the gastrointestinal hormones—notably GLP-1 and gastric inhibitory polypeptide—in the digestion and absorption of nutrients, including glucose. *Exenatide* [EX-e-nah-tide] is an incretin mimetic with a polypeptide sequence about 50-percent homologous to GLP-1. *Exenatide* not only improves glucose-dependent *insulin* secretion but also slows gastric emptying time, decreases food intake, decreases postprandial glucagon secretion, and promotes β-cell proliferation. Consequently, weight gain and postprandial hyperglycemia are reduced, and HbA$_{1c}$ levels decline. Being a polypeptide, *exenatide* must be administered subcutaneously. A drawback to its use is its short duration of action, requiring frequent injections. A once-weekly preparation is under investigation. *Exenatide* may be used as an adjunct to therapy in patients with Type 2 diabetes who have failed to achieve adequate glycemic control on a sulfonylurea, *metformin*, *glitazone*, or combination thereof. Similar to *pramlintide*, the main adverse effects consist of nausea, vomiting, and diarrhea.

A summary of the oral antidiabetic agents is presented in Figure 24.13.

DRUG CLASS	MECHANISM OF ACTION	EFFECT ON PLASMA INSULIN	RISK OF HYPO-GLYCEMIA	COMMENTS
First-generation sulfonylureas				
Tolbutamide	Stimulates insulin secretion	⬆	Yes	Well-established history of effectiveness. Weight gain can occur.
Second-generation sulfonylureas				
Glipizide *Glyburide* *Glimepiride*	Stimulates insulin secretion	⬆	Yes	Well-established history of effectiveness. Weight gain can occur.
Meglitinides				
Nateglinide *Repaglinide*	Stimulates insulin secretion	⬆	Yes (rarely)	Short action with less hypoglycemia either at night or with missed meal. Post-prandial effect.
Biguanides				
Metformin	Decreases endogenous hepatic production of glucose	⬇	No	Preferred agent for Type 2 diabetes. Well-established history of effectiveness. Weight loss may occur. Convenient daily dosing. Many contraindications. Monitor renal function.
Thiazolidinediones (glitazones)				
Pioglitazone *Rosiglitazone*	Binds to peroxisome proliferator–activated receptor-γ in muscle, fat and liver to decrease insulin resistance.	⬇⬇	No	Effective in highly insulin-resistant patients. Once-daily dosing for *pioglitazone* Monitor liver function.
α-Glucosidase inhibitors				
Acarbose *Miglitol*	Decreases glucose absorption	⬌	No	Taken with meals. Adverse gastro-intestinal effects.
DPP-IV inhibitors				
Sitagliptin	Increases glucose-dependent insulin release, decreases secretion of glucagon	⬆	No	Once-daily dosing. May be taken with or without food. Well tolerated.

Figure 24.13
Summary of oral agents used to treat diabetes. ⬌ = little or no change.

Study Questions

Choose the ONE best answer.

24.1 A 50-year-old woman has just been diagnosed as a Type 2 diabetic and given a prescription for metformin. Which of the following statements is characteristic of this medication?

A. Hypoglycemia is a common adverse effect.
B. Metformin undergoes metabolism to an active compound.
C. Many drug-drug interactions have been identified.
D. It decreases hepatic glucose production.
E. The patient often gains weight.

Correct answer = D. Metformin is classified as an insulin sensitizer. Hypoglycemia is not a problem with metformin, because it does not release insulin from the pancreas. Choices B and C are incorrect, because metformin is not metabolized and no significant drug-drug interactions occur. Unlike the sulfonylureas and thiazolidinediones, metformin causes the patient to lose appetite and, thus, to lose weight.

24.2 Which of the following statements is true for therapy with insulin glargine?

A. It is primarily used to control prandial hyperglycemia.
B. It should not be combined with any other insulin.
C. It is now used preferentially in Type 1 diabetics who are pregnant.
D. Pharmacokinetically, there is no peak activity, and the activity lasts about 24 hours.
E. It is effective by inhalation.

Correct answer = D. Insulin glargine is a long-acting insulin. It is slowly released from subcutaneous sites and exhibits no peak. Because of its low levels and prolonged action, insulin glargine best mimics basal secretion of insulin. It is used in combination with other insulins—for example, lispro. It is not used in the treatment of pregnant diabetics, because insulin-like growth factor-I increases—a change that has been implicated in some tumors.

24.3 The ability to reduce insulin resistance is associated with which one of the following classes of hypoglycemic agents?

A. Meglitinides.
B. Sulfonylureas.
C. α-Glucosidase inhibitors.
D. Thiazolidinediones.
E. Gastrointestinal hormones.

Correct answer = D. Insulin resistance is lowered by insulin sensitizers, which include the thiazolidinediones as well as metformin. The other agents do not have an effect.

24.4 A 64-year-old woman with a history of Type 2 diabetes is diagnosed with heart failure. Which of the following drugs would be a poor choice in controlling her diabetes?

A. Sitagliptin.
B. Exenatide.
C. Glyburide.
D. Glipizide.
E. Pioglitazone.

Correct answer = E. Edema is an adverse effect of pioglitazone, and so it would not be a good choice. Sitagliptin, glyburide and glipizide could be used. Exenatide is a new agent that acts as an analog of GLP-1. It has the ability to improve insulin secretion, lowers postprandial hyperglycemia, decreases body weight, and is well tolerated.

Estrogens and Androgens

25

I. OVERVIEW

Sex hormones produced by the gonads are necessary for conception, embryonic maturation, and development of primary and secondary sexual characteristics at puberty. Their activity in target cells is modulated by receptors. The gonadal hormones are used therapeutically in replacement therapy, for contraception, and in management of menopausal symptoms. Several antagonists are effective in cancer chemotherapy. All gonadal hormones are synthesized from the precursor, cholesterol, in a series of steps that includes shortening of the hydrocarbon side chain and hydroxylation of the steroid nucleus. Aromatization is the last step in estrogen synthesis.[1] Figure 25.1 lists the steroid hormones referred to in this chapter.

II. ESTROGENS

Estradiol [ess-tra-DYE-ole], also known as *17 β-estradiol*, is the most potent estrogen produced and secreted by the ovary. It is the principle estrogen in the premenopausal woman. *Estrone* [ESS-trone] is a metabolite of estradiol that has approximately one-third the estrogenic potency of *estradiol*. *Estrone* is the primary circulating estrogen after menopause, and it is generated mainly from conversion of androstenedione in peripheral tissues. *Estriol* [ess-TRI-ole], another metabolite of *estradiol*, is significantly less potent than *estradiol*. It is present in significant amounts during pregnancy, because it is the principal estrogen produced by the placenta. A preparation of conjugated estrogens containing sulfate esters of *estrone* and *equilin*—obtained from pregnant mare's urine—is a widely used oral preparation for hormone replacement therapy. Plant-derived conjugated estrogen products are also available. Synthetic estrogens, such as *ethinyl estradiol* [ETH-ih-nil-ess-tra-DYE-ole], undergo less first-pass metabolism than naturally occurring steroids and, thus, are effective when administered orally at lower doses. Nonsteroidal compounds that bind to estrogen receptors and exert either estrogenic or antiestrogenic effects on target tissues are called selective estrogen-receptor modulators. These include *tamoxifen* and *raloxifene*, among others.

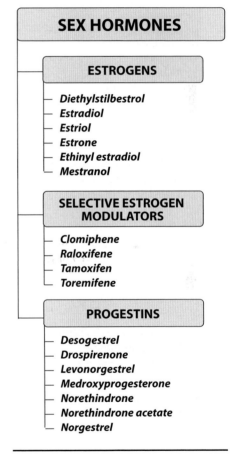

SEX HORMONES

ESTROGENS
- Diethylstilbestrol
- Estradiol
- Estriol
- Estrone
- Ethinyl estradiol
- Mestranol

SELECTIVE ESTROGEN MODULATORS
- Clomiphene
- Raloxifene
- Tamoxifen
- Toremifene

PROGESTINS
- Desogestrel
- Drospirenone
- Levonorgestrel
- Medroxyprogesterone
- Norethindrone
- Norethindrone acetate
- Norgestrel

Figure 25.1
Summary of sex hormones.
(Figure continues on next page.)

[1]See p. 237 in **Lippincott's Illustrated Reviews: Biochemistry** (4th ed.) for a discussion of steroid hormone synthesis.

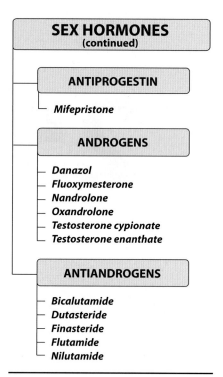

Figure 25.1 (continued)
Summary of sex hormones.

A. Mechanism of action

After dissociation from their binding sites on sex hormone–binding globulin or albumin in the plasma, steroid hormones diffuse across the cell membrane and bind with high affinity to specific nuclear-receptor proteins. [Note: These receptors belong to a large, nuclear hormone–receptor family that includes those for thyroid hormones and vitamin D.] Two estrogen-receptor subtypes, α and β, mediate the effects of the hormone. The α receptor may be considered as the classic estrogen receptor; the β receptor is highly homologous to the α receptor. However, the N-terminal portion of the α receptor contains a region that promotes transcription activation, whereas the β receptor contains a repressor domain. As a result, the transcriptional properties of the α and β estrogen receptors are different. Affinity for the receptor type varies with the particular estrogen. These receptor isoforms vary in structure, chromosomal location, and tissue distribution. The activated steroid-receptor complex interacts with nuclear chromatin to initiate hormone-specific RNA synthesis. The attachment of two estrogen-linked receptors (estrogen receptor dimer) to the genome is required for a response. This results in the synthesis of specific proteins that mediate a number of physiologic functions. [Note: The steroid hormones may elicit the synthesis of different RNA species in diverse target tissues and, therefore, are both receptor and tissue specific.] Other pathways that require these hormones have been identified that lead to more rapid results. For example, activation of an estrogen receptor in the membranes of hypothalamic cells has been shown to couple to a G protein, thereby initiating a second-messenger cascade.[2] In addition, estrogen-mediated dilation of coronary arteries occurs by the increased formation and release of nitric oxide and prostacyclin in endothelial cells.

B. Therapeutic uses of estrogens

The most frequent uses of estrogens are for contraception and post-menopausal hormone therapy, also called estrogen-progestogen therapy (EPT). Due to recent concerns over the risks of EPT, the National American Menopause Society recommends that EPT be prescribed at the lowest effective dose for the shortest possible time to relieve vasomotor symptoms and vaginal atrophy. Women that have only urogenital symptoms should be treated with vaginal rather than systemic estrogen. Estrogens were previously widely used for prevention and treatment of osteoporosis, but current guidelines recommend use of other therapies over estrogen. Estrogens are also used extensively for replacement therapy in premenopausal patients who are deficient in this hormone. Such a deficiency can be due to lack of development of the ovaries, premature menopause, or surgical menopause.

1. **Postmenopausal hormone therapy:** The primary indication for estrogen therapy is menopausal symptoms such as vasomotor instability (for example, "hot flashes" or "hot flushes") and vaginal atrophy. (Figure 25.2). For women who have not undergone a hysterectomy, a progestin is always included with the estrogen therapy, because the combination reduces the risk of endometrial carcinoma associated with unopposed estrogen. For women whose uterus

[2]See p. 93 in *Lippincott's Illustrated Reviews: Biochemistry* (4th ed.) for a discussion of the role of G-proteins and second messengers.
[3]See p. 360 in *Lippincott's Illustrated Reviews: Biochemistry* (4th ed.) for a discussion of LDLs, HDLs, and health.

has been surgically removed, unopposed estrogen therapy is recommended, because progestins may unfavorably alter the beneficial effects of estrogen on lipid parameters. [Note: The amount of estrogen used in replacement therapy is substantially less than the doses used in oral contraception. Thus, the adverse effects of estrogen r eplacement therapy tend to be less severe than the adverse effects seen in women who are taking estrogen for contraceptive purposes.] Delivery of *estradiol* by transdermal patch is also effective in treating postmenopausal symptoms. Osteoporosis is effectively treated with estrogen; however, other drugs, such as *alendronate*, should be considered first-line therapy over estrogen. (See p. 343 for a summary of some of the agents that are useful in the treatment of osteoporosis.)

2. **Primary hypogonadism:** Estrogen therapy mimicking the natural cyclic pattern, and usually in combination with progestins, is instituted to stimulate development of secondary sex characteristics in young women (11–13 years of age) with hypogonadism. Continued treatment is required after growth is completed.

C. Pharmacokinetics

1. **Naturally occurring estrogens:** These agents and their esterified or conjugated derivatives are readily absorbed through the gastrointestinal tract, skin, and mucous membranes. Taken orally, *estradiol* is rapidly metabolized (and partially inactivated) by the microsomal enzymes of the liver. Micronized *estradiol* is available and has better bioavailability. Although there is some first-pass metabolism, it is not sufficient to lessen the effectiveness when taken orally.

2. **Synthetic estrogen analogs:** These compounds, such as *ethinyl estradiol* and *mestranol* [MES-trah-nole]), are well absorbed after oral administration or through the skin or mucous membranes. *Mestranol* is quickly demethylated to *ethinyl estradiol*, which is metabolized more slowly than the naturally occurring estrogens by the liver and peripheral tissues. Being fat soluble, they are stored in adipose tissue, from which they are slowly released. Therefore, the synthetic estrogen analogs have a prolonged action and a higher potency compared to those of natural estrogens.

3. **Metabolism:** Estrogens are transported in the blood while bound to serum albumin or sex hormone–binding globulin. As mentioned above, bioavailability of *estrogen* taken orally is low due to first-pass metabolism in the liver. To reduce first-pass metabolism, the drugs may be administered by transdermal patch, topical gel or emulsion, intravaginally, or by injection. They are hydroxylated in the liver to derivatives that are subsequently glucuronidated or sulfated. The parent drugs and their metabolites undergo excretion into the bile and are then reabsorbed through the enterohepatic circulation. Inactive products are excreted in the urine. [Note: In individuals with liver damage, serum estrogen levels may increase due to reduced metabolism, causing feminization in males or signs of estrogen excess in females.]

D. Adverse effects

Nausea and breast tenderness are among the most common adverse effects of *estrogen* therapy. Postmenopausal uterine bleeding can occur.

OSTEOPOROSIS

- Estrogen decreases the resorption of bone but has no effect on bone formation.

- Estrogen decreases the frequency of hip fracture. [Note: Dietary calcium (1200 mg daily) and weight-bearing exercise also slow loss of bone.]

- Treatment with estrogens must begin within 2 or 3 years of menopause —and earlier if possible.

VASOMOTOR

- Estrogen treatment reestablishes feedback on hypothalamic control of norepinephrine secretion, leading to decreased frequency of "hot flashes."

UROGENITAL TRACT

- Estrogen treatment reverses postmenopausal atrophy of the vulva, vagina, urethra, and trigone of the bladder.

Figure 25.2
Benefits associated with postmenopausal estrogen replacement.

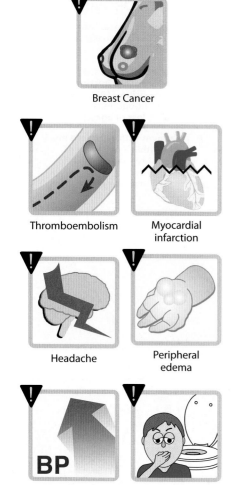

Figure 25.3
Some adverse effects associated with estrogen therapy.

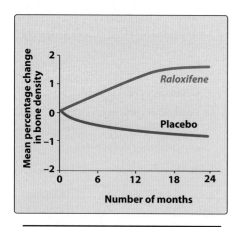

Figure 25.4
Hip bone density increases with *raloxifene* in postmenopausal women.

In addition, the risk of thromboembolic events, myocardial infarction, and breast and endometrial cancer is increased with use of estrogen therapy. [Note: The increased risk of endometrial cancer can be offset by including a progestin along with the estrogen therapy.] Other effects of *estrogen* therapy are shown in Figure 25.3. The synthetic nonsteroidal estrogen *diethylstilbestrol* has been implicated as the possible cause of a rare, clear-cell cervical or vaginal adenocarcinoma observed among the daughters of women who took the drug during pregnancy.

III. SELECTIVE ESTROGEN-RECEPTOR MODULATORS

Selective estrogen-receptor modulators (SERMs) are a new class of estrogen-related compounds. In the past, a number of these agents had been categorized as antiestrogens, and consequently, there is some confusion. The term SERM is now reserved for compounds that interact at estrogen receptors but have different effects on different tissues; that is, they display selective agonism or antagonism according to the tissue type. For example, *tamoxifen* is an estrogen antagonist in breast cancer tissue but can cause endometrial hyperplasia by acting as a partial agonist in the uterus. Other SERMs are *toremifene* and *raloxifene*. *Clomiphene* is also sometimes designated as a SERM.

A. Tamoxifen

Considered to be the first SERM, *tamoxifen* [tah-MOKS-ih-fen] competes with estrogen for binding to the estrogen receptor in breast tissue and is currently used in the palliative treatment of metastatic breast cancer in postmenopausal women. It may also be used as adjuvant therapy following mastectomy or radiation and to reduce the risk of breast cancer in high-risk patients. [Note: Normal breast growth is stimulated by estrogens. It is therefore not surprising that some breast tumors regress following treatment with *tamoxifen*.] The most frequent adverse effects of *tamoxifen* treatment are hot flashes and nausea. Menstrual irregularities and vaginal bleeding can also occur. Due to its estrogenic activity in the endometrium, hyperplasia and malignancies have been reported in women who have been maintained on *tamoxifen*. This has led to recommendations for limiting the length of time on the drug for some indications.

B. Raloxifene

Raloxifene [rah-LOX-ih-feen] is a second-generation SERM that is related to *tamoxifen*. Its clinical use is based on its ability to decrease bone resorption and overall bone turnover. Bone density is increased, and vertebral fractures are decreased (Figure 25.4). Unlike *estrogen* and *tamoxifen*, it apparently has little to no effect on the endometrium and, therefore, may not predispose to uterine cancer. *Raloxifene* lowers total cholesterol and low-density lipoprotein (LDL) in the serum, but it has no effect on high-density lipoprotein (HDL) or triacylglycerol levels. To date, clinical trials have not shown any significant reduction in coronary events with *raloxifene*. The drug is currently approved only for the prevention and treatment of osteoporosis in postmenopausal women. *Raloxifene* has been shown to reduce the incidence of invasive breast cancer in postmenopausal women. [Note: At present, an U.S. Food and Drug Administration advisory panel has recommended that *raloxifene* be approved for the prevention of breast cancer in high-risk postmenopausal women.]

1. **Pharmacokinetics:** The drug is readily absorbed orally and is rapidly converted to glucuronide conjugates through first-pass metabolism. More than 95 percent of *raloxifene* is bound to plasma proteins. Both the parent drug and the conjugates undergo enterohepatic cycling. The primary route of excretion is through the bile into the feces.

2. **Adverse effects:** Hot flashes and leg cramps are common adverse effects with *raloxifene*. As with the estrogens and *tamoxifen*, the use of *raloxifene* has an increased risk of deep-vein thrombosis, pulmonary embolism, and retinal-vein thrombosis. *Raloxifene* should be avoided in women who are or may become pregnant. In addition, women who have a past or active history of venous thromboembolic events should not take the drug. Coadministration with *cholestyramine* can reduce the absorption of *raloxifene* by 60 percent; therefore, these drugs should not be taken together. In one study, *raloxifene* caused a 10 percent drop in prothrombin time in patients taking *warfarin*. Thus, it is prudent to monitor prothrombin time in these individuals.

C. Toremifene

Toremifene [tor-EH-mih-feen] is a SERM with properties and side effects similar to those of *tamoxifen*. Data on the risk of endometrial hyperplasia and cancer with *toremifene* are lacking. The use of *toremifene* is restricted to postmenopausal women with metastatic breast cancer.

D. Clomiphene

By acting as a partial estrogen agonist and interfering with the negative feedback of estrogens on the hypothalamus, *clomiphene* [KLOE-mi-feen] increases the secretion of gonadotropin-releasing hormone and gonadotropins, leading to a stimulation of ovulation. The drug has been used successfully to treat infertility associated with anovulatory cycles, but it is not effective in women with ovulatory dysfunction due to pituitary or ovarian failure. Adverse effects are dose related and include headache, nausea, vasomotor flushes, visual disturbances, and ovarian enlargement.

IV. PROGESTINS

Progesterone, the natural progestin, is produced in response to luteinizing hormone (LH) by both females (secreted by the corpus luteum, primarily during the second half of the menstrual cycle, and by the placenta) and by males (secreted by the testes). It is also synthesized by the adrenal cortex in both sexes. In females, progesterone promotes the development of a secretory endometrium that can accommodate implantation of a newly forming embryo. The high levels of progesterone that are released during the second half of the menstrual cycle (the luteal phase) inhibit the production of gonadotropin and, therefore, prevent further ovulation. If conception takes place, progesterone continues to be secreted, maintaining the endometrium in a favorable state for the continuation of the pregnancy and reducing uterine contractions. If conception does not take place, the release of progesterone from the corpus luteum ceases abruptly. This decline stimulates the onset of menstruation. (Figure 25.5 summarizes the hormones produced during the menstrual cycle.) Progestins exert their mechanism of action in a manner analogous to that of the other steroid hormones. They cause: 1) an increase in hepatic glycogen—probably through an insulin-mediated mechanism; 2) a decrease in Na$^+$ reabsorption in the kidney due to compe-

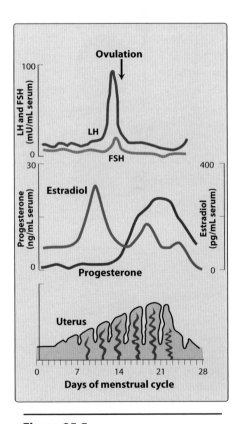

Figure 25.5
The menstrual cycle with plasma levels of pituitary and ovarian hormones and a schematic representation of changes in the morphology of the uterine lining. FSH = follicle-stimulating hormone; LH = luteinizing hormone.

tition with aldosterone at the mineralocorticoid receptor; 3) an increase in body temperature through an unknown mechanism; 4) a decrease in some plasma amino acids; and 5) an increase in excretion of urinary nitrogen.

A. Therapeutic uses of progestins

The major clinical uses of progestins are to rectify a hormonal deficiency and for contraception, in which they are generally used with estrogens, either in combination or in a sequential manner. Progesterone by itself is not used widely as a therapy because of its rapid metabolism, resulting in low bioavailability. Synthetic progestins used in contraception are more stable to first-pass metabolism, allowing lower doses when administered orally. These agents include *norethindrone* [nor-ETH-in-drone], *norethindrone acetate*, *norgestrel* [nor-JES-trel], *levonorgestrel* [lee-voe-nor-JES-trel], *desogestrel* [des-oh-JES-trel], *norgestimate* [nor-JES-tih-mate], and *drospirenone* [dro-SPY-re-none]. Most synthetic progestins used in oral contraceptives (for example, *norethindrone, norethindrone acetate, norgestrel, levonorgestrel*) are derived from 19-nortestosterone and possess some androgenic activity because of their structural similarity to *testosterone*. *Medroxyprogesterone* [me-DROK-see-proe-JES-ter-one] *acetate* is an injectable contraceptive, and the oral form is a common progestin component of postmenopausal EPT. Other clinical uses of the progestins are in the control of dysfunctional uterine bleeding, treatment of dysmenorrhea, and management of endometriosis.

B. Pharmacokinetics

A micronized preparation of *progesterone* is rapidly absorbed after oral administration. It has a short half-life in the plasma and is almost completely metabolized by the liver. The glucuronidated metabolite (pregnanediol glucuronide) is excreted primarily by the kidney. Synthetic progestins are less rapidly metabolized. *Medroxyprogesterone acetate* is injected intramuscularly or subcutaneously and has a duration of action of 3 months. The other progestins last from 1 to 3 days.

C. Adverse effects

The major adverse effects associated with the use of progestins are headache, depression, weight gain, and changes in libido (Figure 25.6). Some progestins, such as the 19-nortestosterone derivatives, have androgenic activity and can increase the ratio of LDL to HDL cholesterol and cause acne and hirsutism. Less androgenic progestins, such as *norgestimate* and *drospirenone,* may be preferred in women with acne. Injectable *medroxyprogesterone acetate* has been associated with an increased risk of osteoporosis, which has led to recommendations for limiting the duration of use.

D. Antiprogestin

Mifepristone [mih-feh-PRIH-stone] (also designated as RU 486) is a progesterone antagonist with partial agonist activity. [Note: *Mifepristone* also has potent antiglucocorticoid activity.] Administration of this drug to females early in pregnancy results, in most cases (up to 94 percent), in abortion of the fetus due to the interference with progesterone and the decline in human chorionic gonadotropin. The major adverse effects are significant uterine bleeding and the possibility of an incomplete abortion. However, administration of *misoprostol* orally or intravaginally after a single oral dose of *mifepristone* effectively terminates gestation. *Mifepristone* is being investigated as an oral contraceptive and an emergency contraceptive agent.

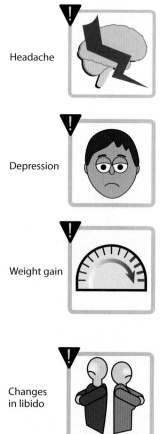

Headache

Depression

Weight gain

Changes in libido

Figure 25.6
Some adverse effects associated with progestin therapy.

V. CONTRACEPTIVES

Drugs are available that decrease fertility by a number of different mechanisms, such as preventing ovulation, impairing gametogenesis or gamete maturation, or interfering with gestation. Currently, interference with ovulation is the most common pharmacologic intervention for preventing pregnancy (Figure 25.7).

A. Major classes of contraceptives

1. **Combination oral contraceptives:** Products containing a combination of an estrogen and a progestin are the most common type of oral contraceptives. Monophasic combination pills contain a constant dose of estrogen and progestin given over 21 days. Triphasic oral contraceptive products attempt to mimic the natural female cycle and contain a constant dose of estrogen with increasing doses of progestin given over three successive 7-day periods. With either type of combination oral contraceptive, active pills are taken for 21 days followed by 7 days of placebo. Withdrawal bleeding occurs during the hormone-free interval. [Note: Estrogens that are commonly present in the combination pills are *ethinyl estradiol* and *mestranol*. The most common progestins are *norethindrone, norethindrone acetate, norgestrel, levonorgestrel, desogestrel, norgestimate,* and *drospirenone*.] These preparations are highly effective in achieving contraception (Figure 25.8). Use of extended-cycle contraception (84 active pills followed by 7 days of placebo) results in less frequent withdrawal bleeding. A continuous oral contraceptive product (active pills taken 365 days of the year) is also available.

2. **Transdermal patch:** An alternative to combination oral contraceptive pills is a transdermal contraceptive patch containing *ethinyl estradiol* and the progestin *norelgestromin*. One contraceptive patch is applied each week for 3 weeks to the abdomen, upper torso, or buttock. Week 4 is patch-free, and withdrawal bleeding occurs. The transdermal patch has efficacy comparable to that of the oral contraceptives; however, it has been shown to be less effective in women weighing greater than 90 kilograms. Contraindications and adverse effects for the patch are similar to those of oral contraceptives. Recent data have indicated that total estrogen exposure with the transdermal patch is up to 60 percent greater than that seen with a 35 µg estrogen oral contraceptive. Increased exposure to estrogen may increase the risk of adverse events such as thromboembolism.

3. **Vaginal ring:** An additional contraceptive option is a vaginal ring containing *ethinyl estradiol* and *etonogestrel*. The ring is inserted into the vagina and is left in place for 3 weeks. Week 4 is ring-free, and withdrawal bleeding occurs. The contraceptive vaginal ring has efficacy, contraindications, and adverse effects similar to those of oral contraceptives. One caveat with the vaginal ring is that it may occasionally slip or be expelled accidentally.

4. **Progestin-only pills:** Products containing a progestin only, usually *norethindrone* or *norgestrel* (called a "mini-pill"), are taken daily on a continuous schedule. Progestin-only pills deliver a low, continuous dosage of drug. These preparations are less effective than the combination pill (see Figure 25.8), and they may produce irregular menstrual cycles more frequently than the combination product. The progestin-only pill has limited patient acceptance because of

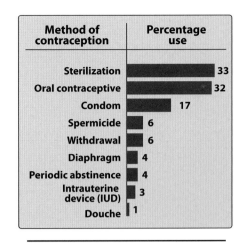

Figure 25.7
Comparison of contraceptive use among United States women ages 15 to 44 years.

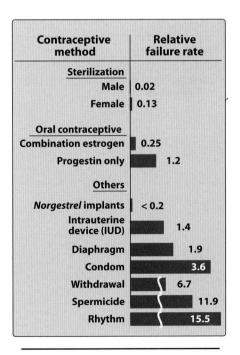

Figure 25.8
Comparison of failure rate for various methods of contraception. Longer bars indicate a higher failure rate—that is, more pregnancies.

anxiety over the increased possibility of pregnancy and the frequent occurrence of menstrual irregularities. The progestin-only pill may be used for patients who are breast-feeding (unlike estrogen, progestins do not have an effect on milk production), are intolerant to estrogen, or are smokers or have other contraindications to estrogen-containing products.

5. **Progestin implants:** A subdermal implant containing *etonogestrel* offers long-term contraception. One 4-cm capsule is placed subcutaneously in the upper arm and provides contraception for approximately 3 years. The implant is nearly as reliable as sterilization, and the effect is totally reversible when surgically removed. Once the progestin-containing capsule is implanted, this method of contraception does not rely on patient compliance. This may, in part, explain the low failure rate for this method. Principal side effects of the implants are irregular menstrual bleeding and headaches.

6. **Progestin intrauterine device:** A *levonorgestrel*-releasing intrauterine system offers a highly effective method of long-term contraception. This intrauterine device provides contraception for up to 5 years. It is a suitable method of contraception for women who already have at least one child and do not have a history of pelvic inflammatory disease or ectopic pregnancy.

7. **Postcoital contraception:** The overall risk of pregnancy after an episode of coitus without effective contraception is shown in the Figure 25.9. Postcoital or emergency contraception reduces the probability of pregnancy to between 0.2 and 3 percent. Emergency contraception uses high doses of progestin (for example, 0.75 mg of *levonorgestrel*) or high doses of estrogen (100 μg of *ethinyl estradiol*) plus progestin (0.5 mg of *levonorgestrel*) administered within 72 hours of unprotected intercourse (the "morning-after" pill). A second dose of emergency contraception should be taken 12 hours after the first dose. For maximum effectiveness, emergency contraception should be taken as soon as possible after unprotected intercourse. The progestin-only emergency contraceptive regimens are generally better tolerated than the estrogen-progestin combination regimens. A single dose of *mifepristone* has also been used for emergency contraception.

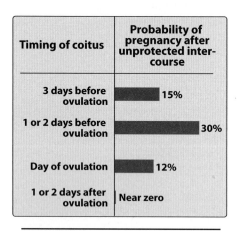

Timing of coitus	Probability of pregnancy after unprotected inter-course
3 days before ovulation	15%
1 or 2 days before ovulation	30%
Day of ovulation	12%
1 or 2 days after ovulation	Near zero

Figure 25.9
Risk of pregnancy after unprotected intercourse in young couples in their mid twenties.

B. Mechanism of action

The mechanism of action for these contraceptives is not completely understood. It is likely that the combination of estrogen and progestin administered over an approximately 3-week period inhibits ovulation. [Note: The estrogen provides a negative feedback on the release of LH and follicle-stimulating hormone (FSH) by the pituitary gland, thus preventing ovulation. The progestin also inhibits LH release and thickens the cervical mucus, thus hampering the transport of sperm. Withdrawal of the progestin stimulates menstrual bleeding during the placebo week].

C. Adverse effects

Most adverse effects are believed to be due to the estrogen component, but cardiovascular effects reflect the action of both estrogen and progestin. The incidence of adverse effects with oral contraceptives is relatively low and is determined by the specific compounds and combinations used.

1. **Major adverse effects:** The major adverse effects are breast fullness, depression, fluid retention, headache, nausea, and vomiting.

2. **Cardiovascular:** Although rare, the most serious adverse effect of oral contraceptives is cardiovascular disease, including thromboembolism, thrombophlebitis, hypertension, increased incidence of myocardial infarction, and cerebral and coronary thrombosis. These adverse effects are most common among women who smoke and who are older than 35 years, although they may affect women of any age.

3. **Carcinogenicity:** Oral contraceptives have been shown to decrease the incidence of endometrial and ovarian cancer. Their ability to induce other neoplasms is controversial. The production of benign tumors of the liver that may rupture and hemorrhage is rare.

4. **Metabolic:** Abnormal glucose tolerance (similar to the changes seen in pregnancy) is sometimes associated with oral contraceptives. Weight gain is common in women who are taking the *nortestosterone* derivatives.

5. **Serum lipids:** The combination pill causes a change in the serum lipoprotein profile: Estrogen causes an increase in HDL and a decrease in LDL (a desirable occurrence), whereas progestins may negate some of the beneficial effects of estrogen. [Note: The potent progestin *norgestrel* causes the greatest increase in the LDL:HDL ratio. Therefore, estrogen-dominant preparations are best for individuals with elevated serum cholesterol.]

6. **Contraindications:** Oral contraceptives are contraindicated in the presence of cerebrovascular and thromboembolic disease, estrogen-dependent neoplasms, liver disease, and pregnancy. Combination oral contraceptives should not be used in patients over the age of 35 who are heavy smokers.

VI. ANDROGENS

The androgens are a group of steroids that have anabolic and/or masculinizing effects in both males and females. *Testosterone* [tess-TOSS-te-rone], the most important androgen in humans, is synthesized by Leydig cells in the testes and, in smaller amounts, by cells in the ovary of the female and by the adrenal gland in both sexes. Other androgens secreted by the testes are *5α-dihydrotestosterone* (*DHT*), *androstenedione*, and *dehydroepiandrosterone* (DHEA) in small amounts. In adult males, *testosterone* secretion by Leydig cells is controlled by gonadotropin-releasing hormone from the hypothalamus, which stimulates the anterior pituitary gland to secrete FSH and LH. [Note: LH stimulates steroidogenesis in the Leydig cells, whereas FSH is necessary for spermatogenesis.] *Testosterone* or its active metabolite, *DHT*, inhibits production of these specific trophic hormones through a negative feedback loop and, thus, regulates *testosterone* production (Figure 25.10). The androgens are required for 1) normal maturation in the male, 2) sperm production, 3) increased synthesis of muscle proteins and hemoglobin, and 4) decreased bone resorption. Synthetic modifications of the androgen structure are designed to modify solubility and susceptibility to enzymatic breakdown (thus prolonging the half-life of the hormone) and to separate anabolic and androgenic effects.

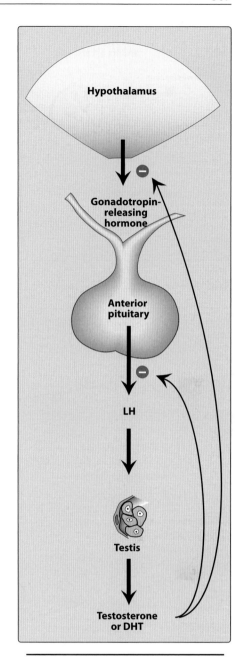

Figure 25.10
Regulation of secretion of testosterone. DHT = 5-α-dihydro testosterone; LH = luteinizing hormone.

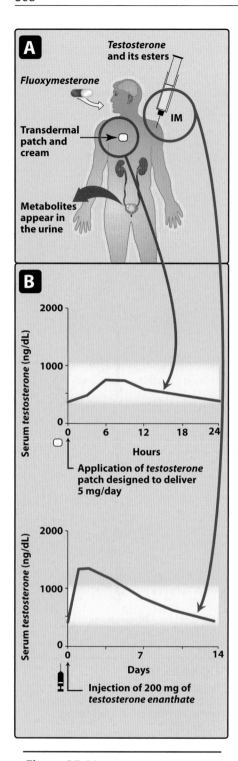

Figure 25.11
A. Administration and fate of androgens. B. Serum testosterone concentrations after administration by injection or transdermal patch to hypogonadal men. The yellow band indicates the upper and lower limits of normal range.

A. Mechanism of action

Like the estrogens and progestins, androgens bind to a specific nuclear receptor in a target cell. Although *testosterone* itself is the active ligand in muscle and liver, in other tissues it must be metabolized to derivatives, such as *DHT*. For example, after diffusing into the cells of the prostate, seminal vesicles, epididymis, and skin, *testosterone* is converted by 5α-reductase to *DHT*, which binds to the receptor. In the brain, liver, and adipose tissue, *testosterone* is biotransformed to *estradiol* by cytochrome P450 aromatase. The hormone-receptor complex binds to DNA and stimulates the synthesis of specific RNAs and proteins. [Note: *Testosterone* analogs that cannot be converted to DHT have less effect on the reproductive system than they do on the skeletal musculature.]

B. Therapeutic uses

1. **Androgenic effects:** Androgenic steroids are used for males with inadequate androgen secretion. [Note: Hypogonadism can be caused by testicular dysfunction (primary hypogonadism) or due to failure of the hypothalamus or pituitary (secondary hypogonadism). In each instance, androgen therapy is indicated.]

2. **Anabolic effects:** Anabolic steroids can be used to treat senile osteoporosis and chronic wasting associated with human immunodeficiency virus or cancer. They may also be used as adjunct therapy in severe burns and to speed recovery from surgery or chronic debilitating diseases.

3. **Endometriosis:** *Danazol* [DAH-nah-zole], a mild androgen, is used in the treatment of endometriosis (ectopic growth of the endometrium) and fibrocystic breast disease. It inhibits release of FSH and LH but has no effect on the aromatase. Weight gain, acne, decreased breast size, deepening voice, increased libido, and increased hair growth are among the adverse effects. *Danazol* has been reported occasionally to suppress adrenal function.

4. **Unapproved use:** Anabolic steroids are used to increase lean body mass, muscle strength, and endurance in athletes and body builders (see below). In some popular publications, *DHEA* (a precursor of *testosterone* and estrogen) has been touted as the anti-aging hormone as well as a "performance enhancer." With its ready availability in health food stores, the drug has been abused. There is no definitive evidence that it slows aging, however, or that it improves performance at normal therapeutic doses.

C. Pharmacokinetics

1. **Testosterone:** This agent is ineffective orally because of inactivation by first-pass metabolism. As with the other sex steroids, *testosterone* [tes-TOS-ter-own] is rapidly absorbed and is metabolized to relatively or completely inactive compounds that are excreted primarily in the urine. *Testosterone* and its C_{17}-esters (for example, *testosterone cypionate* or *enanthate*) are administered intramuscularly. [Note: The addition of the esterified lipid makes the hormone more lipid soluble, thereby increasing its duration of action.] Transdermal patches, topical gels, and buccal tablets of *testosterone* are also available. Figure 25.11 shows serum levels of testosterone achieved by injection and by a transdermal patch in hypogonadal men. *Testosterone* and its esters demonstrate a 1:1 relative ratio of androgenic to anabolic activity.

2. **Testosterone derivatives:** Alkylation of the 17α position of *testosterone* allows oral administration of the hormone. Agents such as *fluoxymesterone* [floo-ox-ee-MESS-teh-rone] have a longer half-life in the body than that of the naturally occurring androgen. *Fluoxymesterone* is effective when given orally, and it has a 1:2 androgenic to anabolic ratio. *Oxandrolone* [ox-AN-droe-lone] is another orally active testosterone derivative with anabolic activity 3 to 13 times that of *testosterone*. Hepatic adverse effects have been associated with the 17α-alkylated androgens.

D. Adverse effects

1. **In females:** Androgens can cause masculinization, with acne, growth of facial hair, deepening of the voice, male pattern baldness, and excessive muscle development. Menstrual irregularities may also occur. *Testosterone* should not be used by pregnant women because of possible virilization of the female fetus.

2. **In males:** Excess androgens can cause priapism, impotence, decreased spermatogenesis, and gynecomastia. Cosmetic changes such as those described for females may occur as well. Androgens can also stimulate growth of the prostate.

3. **In children:** Androgens can cause abnormal sexual maturation and growth disturbances resulting from premature closing of the epiphyseal plates.

4. **General effects:** Androgens increase serum LDL and lower serum HDL levels; therefore, they increase the LDL:HDL ratio and potentially increase the risk for premature coronary heart disease. Androgens can also cause fluid retention, leading to edema.

5. **In athletes:** Use of anabolic steroids, (for example, *DHEA* or *nandrolone* [NAN-dro-lone]) by athletes can cause premature closing of the epiphysis of the long bones, which stunts growth and interrupts development. The high doses taken by these young athletes may result in reduction of testicular size, hepatic abnormalities, increased aggression ("roid rage"), major mood disorders, and the other adverse effects described above.

E. Antiandrogens

Antiandrogens counter male hormonal action by interfering with the synthesis of androgens or by blocking their receptors. For example, at high doses, the antifungal drug *ketoconazole* inhibits several of the cytochrome P450 enzymes involved in steroid synthesis. *Finasteride* [fin-AS-ter-ide] and *dutasteride* [doo-TAS-ter-ride], agents used for the treatment of benign prostatic hypertrophy, inhibit 5α-reductase (Figure 25.12). The resulting decrease in formation of *DHT* in the prostate leads to a reduction in prostate size. Antiandrogens, such as *flutamide* [FLOO-tah-mide], act as competitive inhibitors of androgens at the target cell. *Flutamide* is used in the treatment of prostatic carcinoma in males. Two other potent antiandrogens, *bicalutamide* [bye-ka-LOO-ta-mide] and *nilutamide* [nye-LOO-tah-mide], are effective orally for the treatment of metastatic prostate cancer.

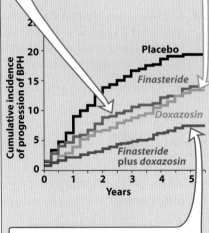

α₁-Adrenergic antagonists

- *Terazosin, doxazosin, tamsulosin,* and *alfuzosin* relieve outlet obstruction of the bladder by reducing the tension of prostatic smooth muscle in the prostate, prostate capsule, and bladder neck.

- The most important side effects are orthostatic hypotension and dizziness.

5 α-Reductase inhibitors

- *Finasteride* and *dutasteride* act by reducing the size of the prostate gland. Treatment for 6 to 12 months is generally needed before prostate size is sufficiently reduced to improve symptoms.

- The major side effects of the 5 α-reductase inhibitors are decreased libido and ejaculatory or erectile dysfunction.

Combination therapy

- Combination therapy with an α₁-adrenergic antagonist plus a 5 α-reductase inhibitor produces the greatest reduction in the symptoms of BPH, such as acute urinary retention, urinary incontinence, renal insufficiency, or recurrent urinary tract infections.

Figure 25.12
Therapy for benign prostatic hyperplasia (BPH).

Study Questions

Choose the ONE best answer.

25.1 Young athletes who abuse androgens should be made aware of the side effects of these drugs. Which one of the following is, however, not of concern?

    A. Increased muscle mass.
    B. Anemia due to bone marrow failure.
    C. Overly aggressive behavior.
    D. Decreased spermatogenesis.
    E. Stunted growth.

Correct answer = B. Anabolic steroids stimulate the bone marrow and have been used in the treatment of anemia. Erythropoietin has largely replaced them in this regard. All the other choices are possible problems stemming from androgen abuse.

25.2 A 70-year-old woman is being treated with raloxifene for osteoporosis. There is an increased risk of her developing:

    A. Breast cancer.
    B. Uterine cancer.
    C. Vein thrombosis.
    D. Atrophic vaginitis.
    E. Hypercholesterolemia.

Correct answer = C. Unlike estrogen and tamoxifen, raloxifene does not result in an increased incidence of breast or uterine cancer. It lowers cholesterol, and the incidence of vaginitis is essentially the same as that in patients taking a placebo.

25.3 A 23-year-old woman has failed to become pregnant after 2 years of unprotected intercourse. Which of the following would be effective in treating infertility due anovulatory cycles?

    A. A combination of an estrogen and progestin.
    B. Estrogen alone.
    C. Clomiphene.
    D. Raloxifene.

Correct answer = C. Clomiphene is a SERM that increases the secretion of gonadotropin-releasing hormone and gonadotropins by inhibiting the negative feedback caused by estrogens. The other treatments would have the opposite effect.

25.4 Which of the following is inappropriate for treating osteoporosis?

    A. Dehydroepiandrosterone.
    B. Estradiol.
    C. Tamoxifen.
    D. Norethindrone.
    E. Mestranol.

Correct answer = D. Norethindrone is a progestin and has no effect on bone resorption. Estradiol, tamoxifen, and mestranol (a synthetic estrogen) can decrease bone resorption, as can the synthetic androgen DHEA, which is converted to testosterone in the body.

25.5 Estrogen replacement therapy in menopausal women:

    A. Restores bone loss accompanying osteoporosis.
    B. May induce "hot flashes."
    C. May cause atrophic vaginitis.
    D. Is most effective if instituted at the first signs of menopause.
    E. Requires higher doses of estrogen than with oral contraceptive therapy.

Correct answer = D. Estrogens decrease, but do not restore, the age-related loss of bone. Vasomotor symptoms of menopause, such as hot flashes, are decreased with estrogen replacement therapy. Symptoms of menopause, such as atrophic vaginitis, are decreased with estrogen replacement therapy. Oral contraceptives contain higher doses of estrogen than are used with estrogen replacement therapy.

Adrenal Hormones

26

I. OVERVIEW

The adrenal gland consists of the cortex and the medulla. The latter secretes epinephrine, whereas the cortex, the subject of this chapter, synthesizes and secretes two major classes of steroid hormones—the adrenocorticosteroids (glucocorticoids and mineralocorticoids; Figure 26.1), and the adrenal androgens. The adrenal cortex is divided into three zones that synthesize various steroids from cholesterol and then secrete them (Figure 26.2). The outer zona glomerulosa produces mineralocorticoids (for example, aldosterone), which are responsible for regulating salt and water metabolism. Production of aldosterone is regulated primarily by the renin-angiotensin system (see p. 216). The middle zona fasciculata synthesizes glucocorticoids (for example, cortisol), which are involved with normal metabolism and resistance to stress. The inner zona reticularis secretes adrenal androgens (for example, *dehydroepiandrosterone*). Secretion by the two inner zones and, to some extent, the outer zone is controlled by pituitary *corticotropin adrenocorticotropic hormone [ACTH; also called corticotropin]*, which is released in response to the hypothalamic corticotropin-releasing hormone (CRH; also called corticotropin-releasing factor). Glucocorticoids serve as feedback inhibitors of *corticotropin* and CRH secretion. Hormones of the adrenal cortex are used in replacement therapy; in the treatment and management of asthma as well as other inflammatory diseases, such as rheumatoid arthritis; in the treatment of severe allergic reactions; and in the treatment of some cancers.

II. ADRENOCORTICOSTEROIDS

The adrenocorticoids bind to specific intracellular cytoplasmic receptors in target tissues. [Note: The glucocorticoid receptor is widely distributed throughout the body, whereas the mineralocorticoid receptor is confined mainly to excretory organs, such as the kidney, colon, and salivary and sweat glands.] After dimerizing, the receptor-hormone complex translocates into the nucleus, where it attaches to gene promoter elements, acting as a transcription factor to turn genes on or off, depending on the tissue (Figure 26.3)[1]. This mechanism requires time to produce an effect, but other glucocorticoid effects, such as their interaction with catecholamines to mediate relaxation of bronchial musculature or lipolysis, have effects that are immediate. Some normal actions and some selected mechanisms of adrenocorticoids are described in this section.

[1]See p. 449 in *Lippincott's Illustrated Reviews: Biochemistry* (4th ed.) for a discussion of the regulation of gene expression.

ADRENAL CORTICOSTEROIDS

CORTICOSTEROIDS

— *Beclomethasone*
— *Betamethasone*
— *Cortisone*
— *Desoxycorticosterone*
— *Dexamethasone*
— *Fludrocortisone*
— *Hydrocortisone*
— *Methylprednisolone*
— *Prednisolone*
— *Prednisone*
— *Triamcinolone*

INHIBITORS OF ADRENOCORTICOID BIOSYNTHESIS OR FUNCTION

— *Aminoglutethimide*
— *Eplerenone*
— *Ketoconazole*
— *Metyrapone*
— *Mifepristone*
— *Spironolactone*
— *Trilostane*

Figure 26.1
Summary of adrenal corticosteroids.

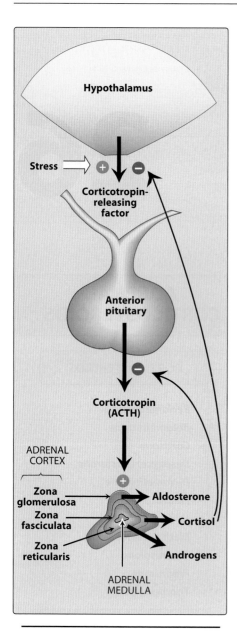

Figure 26.2
Regulation of corticosteroid secretion.

A. Glucocorticoids

Cortisol is the principal human glucocorticoid. Normally, its production is diurnal, with a peak early in the morning followed by a decline and then a secondary, smaller peak in the late afternoon. Factors such as stress and levels of the circulating steroid influence secretion. The effects of cortisol are many and diverse. In general, all glucocorticoids:

1. **Promote normal intermediary metabolism:** Glucocorticoids favor gluconeogenesis through increasing amino acid uptake by the liver and kidney and elevating activities of gluconeogenic enzymes. They stimulate protein catabolism (except in the liver) and lipolysis, thereby providing the building blocks and energy that are needed for glucose synthesis. [Note: Glucocorticoid insufficiency may result in hypoglycemia (for example, during stressful periods or fasting).] Lipolysis results as a consequence of the glucocorticoid augmenting the action of growth hormone on adipocytes, causing an increase in the activity of hormone-sensitive lipase.

2. **Increase resistance to stress:** By raising plasma glucose levels, glucocorticoids provide the body with the energy it requires to combat stress caused, for example, by trauma, fright, infection, bleeding, or debilitating disease. Glucocorticoids can cause a modest rise in blood pressure, apparently by enhancing the vasoconstrictor action of adrenergic stimuli on small vessels. [Note: Individuals with adrenal insufficiency may respond to severe stress by becoming hypotensive.]

3. **Alter blood cell levels in plasma:** Glucocorticoids cause a decrease in eosinophils, basophils, monocytes, and lymphocytes by redistributing them from the circulation to lymphoid tissue. In contrast to this effect, they increase the blood levels of hemoglobin, erythrocytes, platelets, and polymorphonuclear leukocytes. [Note: The decrease in circulating lymphocytes and macrophages compromises the body's ability to fight infections. However, this property is important in the treatment of leukemia (see p. 478).]

4. **Have anti-inflammatory action:** The most important therapeutic property of the glucocorticoids is their ability to dramatically reduce the inflammatory response and to suppress immunity. The exact mechanism is complex and incompletely understood. However, the lowering and inhibition of peripheral lymphocytes and macrophages is known to play a role. Also involved is the indirect inhibition of phospholipase A_2 (due to the steroid-mediated elevation of lipocortin), which blocks the release of arachidonic acid—the precursor of the prostaglandins and leukotrienes—from membrane-bound phospholipid. Cyclooxygenase-2 synthesis in inflammatory cells is further reduced, lowering the availability of prostaglandins. In addition, interference in mast cell degranulation results in decreased histamine and capillary permeability.

5. **Affect other components of the endocrine system:** Feedback inhibition of *corticotropin* production by elevated glucocorticoids causes inhibition of further glucocorticoid synthesis as well as further production of thyroid-stimulating hormone. In contrast, growth hormone production is increased.

6. **Can have effects on other systems:** Adequate cortisol levels are essential for normal glomerular filtration. However, the effects of corticosteroids on other systems are mostly associated with the adverse effects of the hormones. High doses of glucocorticoids stimulate gastric acid and pepsin production and may exacerbate ulcers. Effects on the central nervous system that influence mental status have been identified. Chronic glucocorticoid therapy can cause severe bone loss. Myopathy leads patients to complain of weakness.

B. Mineralocorticoids

Mineralocorticoids help to control the body's water volume and concentration of electrolytes, especially sodium and potassium. Aldosterone acts on kidney tubules and collecting ducts, causing a reabsorption of sodium, bicarbonate, and water. Conversely, aldosterone decreases reabsorption of potassium, which, with H+, is then lost in the urine. Enhancement of sodium reabsorption by aldosterone also occurs in gastrointestinal mucosa and in sweat and salivary glands. [Note: Elevated aldosterone levels may cause alkalosis and hypokalemia, whereas retention of sodium and water leads to an increase in blood volume and blood pressure. Hyperaldosteronism is treated with *spironolactone.*] Target cells for aldosterone action contain mineralocorticoid receptors that interact with the hormones in a manner analogous to that of the glucocorticoid receptor (see above).

C. Therapeutic uses of the adrenal corticosteroids

Several semisynthetic derivatives of the glucocorticoids have been developed that vary in their anti-inflammatory potency, degree to which they cause sodium retention, and duration of action. These are summarized in Figure 26.4.

1. **Replacement therapy for primary adrenocortical insufficiency (Addison's disease):** This disease is caused by adrenal cortex dysfunction (as diagnosed by the lack of patient response to *corticotropin* administration). *Hydrocortisone* [hye-droe-KOR-ti-sone], which is identical to natural cortisol, is given to correct the deficiency. Failure to do so results in death. The dosage of *hydrocortisone* is divided so that two-thirds of the normal daily dose is given in the morning and one-third is given in the afternoon. [Note: The goal of this regimen is to approximate the daily hormone levels resulting from the circadian rhythm exhibited by cortisol, which causes plasma levels to be maximal around 8 AM and then decrease throughout the day to their lowest level around 1 AM] Administration of *fludrocortisone* [floo-droe-KOR-tih-sone], a potent synthetic mineralocorticoid with some glucocorticoid activity, may also be necessary to raise the mineralocorticoid activity to normal levels.

2. **Replacement therapy for secondary or tertiary adrenocortical insufficiency:** These deficiencies are caused by a defect either in CRH production by the hypothalamus or in *corticotropin* production by the pituitary. [Note: Under these conditions, the synthesis of mineralocorticoids in the adrenal cortex is less impaired than that of glucocorticoids.] The adrenal cortex responds to *corticotropin* (*ACTH*) administration by synthesizing and releasing the adrenal corticosteroids. *Hydrocortisone* is also used for these deficiencies.

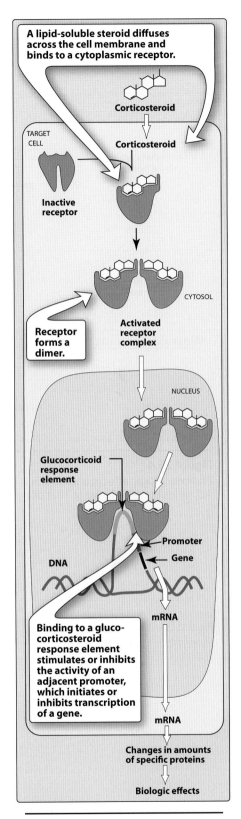

Figure 26.3
Gene regulation by glucocorticoids.

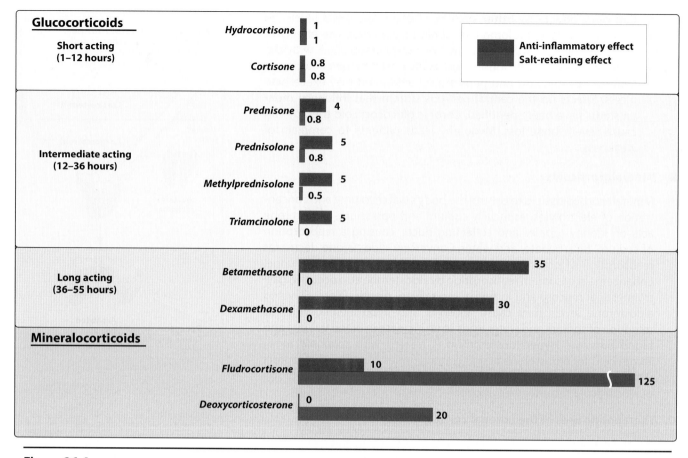

Figure 26.4
Pharmacologic effects and duration of action of some commonly used natural and synthetic corticosteroids. Activities are all relative to that of *hydrocortisone*, which is considered to be 1.

3. **Diagnosis of Cushing's syndrome:** Cushing's syndrome is caused by a hypersecretion of glucocorticoids that results either from excessive release of corticotropin by the anterior pituitary or an adrenal tumor. The *dexamethasone* [dex-a-METH-a-sone] suppression test is used to diagnose the cause of an individual's case of Cushing's syndrome. This synthetic glucocorticoid suppresses cortisol release in individuals with pituitary-dependent Cushing's syndrome, but it does not suppress glucocorticoid release from adrenal tumors. [Note: Chronic treatment with high doses of glucocorticoid is a frequent cause of iatrogenic Cushing's syndrome.]

4. **Replacement therapy for congenital adrenal hyperplasia:** This is a group of diseases resulting from an enzyme defect in the synthesis of one or more of the adrenal steroid hormones. This condition may lead to virilization in females due to overproduction of adrenal androgens (see below). Treatment of this condition requires administration of sufficient corticosteroids to normalize the patient's hormone levels by suppressing release of CRH and ACTH. This decreases production of adrenal androgens. The choice of replacement hormone depends on the specific enzyme defect.

5. **Relief of inflammatory symptoms:** Glucocorticoids dramatically reduce the manifestations of inflammations (for example, rheumatoid and osteoarthritic inflammations, as well as inflammatory conditions of the skin), including the redness, swelling, heat, and ten-

derness that are commonly present at the inflammatory site. The effect of glucocorticoids on the inflammatory process is the result of a number of actions, including the redistribution of leukocytes to other body compartments, thereby lowering their blood concentration (their function is also compromised). Other effects include an increase in the concentration of neutrophils; a decrease in the concentration of lymphocytes (T and B cells), basophils, eosinophils, and monocytes; and an inhibition of the ability of leukocytes and macrophages to respond to mitogens and antigens. The decreased production of prostaglandins and leukotrienes is believed to be central to the anti-inflammatory action. Glucocorticoids also influence the inflammatory response by their ability to reduce the amount of histamine that is released from basophils and mast cells, thus diminishing the activation of the kinin system [Note: The ability of glucocorticoids to inhibit the immune response is also a result of the other actions described above.]

6. **Treatment of allergies:** Glucocorticoids are beneficial in the treatment of the symptoms of bronchial asthma, allergic rhinitis, and drug, serum, and transfusion allergic reactions. These drugs are not, however, curative. [Note: *Beclomethasone dipropionate* [bek-loe-METH-ah-sone], *triamcinolone* [tri-am-SIN-o-lone], and others (see Figure 26.4) are applied topically to the respiratory tract through inhalation from a metered-dose dispenser. This minimizes systemic effects and allows the patient to significantly reduce or eliminate the use of oral steroids.]

7. **Acceleration of lung maturation:** Respiratory distress syndrome is a problem in premature infants. Fetal cortisol is a regulator of lung maturation. Consequently, a dose of *beclomethasone* is administered intramuscularly to the mother 48 hours prior to birth, followed by a second dose 24 hours before delivery.

D. Pharmacokinetics

1. **Absorption and fate:** Synthetic glucocorticoid preparations with unique pharmacokinetic characteristics are used therapeutically. Those that are administered orally are readily absorbed from the gastrointestinal tract. Selected compounds can also be administered intravenously, intramuscularly, intra-articularly (for example, into arthritic joints), topically, or as an aerosol for inhalation (Figure 26.5). Greater than 90 percent of the absorbed glucocorticoids are bound to plasma proteins—most to corticosteroid-binding globulin, and the remainder to albumin. Corticosteroids are metabolized by the liver microsomal oxidizing enzymes. The metabolites are conjugated to glucuronic acid or sulfate, and the products are excreted by the kidney. [Note: The half-life of adrenal steroids may increase dramatically in individuals with hepatic dysfunction.] The only glucocorticoid that has no effect on the fetus in pregnancy is *prednisone* [PRED-ni-sone]. It is a prodrug that is not converted to the active compound, *prednisolone* [pred-NIH-so-lene], in the fetal liver. Any *prednisolone* formed in the mother is biotransformed to *prednisone* by the fetus.

2. **Dosage:** In determining the dosage of adrenocortical steroids, many factors need to be considered, including glucocorticoid versus mineralocorticoid activity, duration of action, type of preparation, and

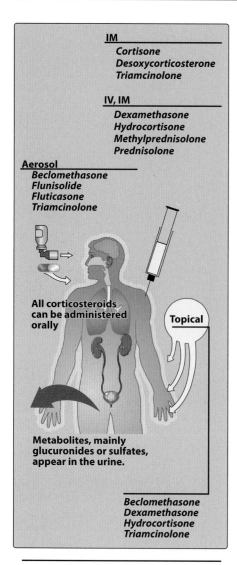

IM

Cortisone
Desoxycorticosterone
Triamcinolone

IV, IM

Dexamethasone
Hydrocortisone
Methylprednisolone
Prednisolone

Aerosol
Beclomethasone
Flunisolide
Fluticasone
Triamcinolone

All corticosteroids can be administered orally

Topical

Metabolites, mainly glucuronides or sulfates, appear in the urine.

Beclomethasone
Dexamethasone
Hydrocortisone
Triamcinolone

Figure 26.5
Routes of administration and elimination of corticosteroids.

time of day when the steroid is administered. For example, when large doses of the hormone are required over an extended period of time (more than 2 weeks), suppression of the hypothalamic-pituitary-adrenal (HPA) axis occurs. To prevent this adverse effect, a regimen of alternate-day administration of the adrenocortical steroid may be useful. This schedule allows the HPA axis to recover/function on the days the hormone is not taken.

E. Adverse effects

The common side effects of long-term corticosteroid therapy are summarized in Figure 26.6. Osteoporosis is the most common adverse effect due to the ability of glucocorticoids to suppress intestinal Ca^{2+} absorption, inhibit bone formation, and decrease sex hormone synthesis. Alternate-day dosing does not prevent osteoporosis. Patients are advised to take calcium and vitamin D supplements. Drugs that are effective in treating osteoporosis may also be beneficial. [Note: Increased appetite is not necessarily an adverse effect. In fact, it is one of the reasons for the use of *prednisone* in cancer chemotherapy.] The classic Cushing-like syndrome—redistribution of body fat, puffy face, increased body hair growth, acne, insomnia, and increased appetite—are observed when excess corticosteroids are present. Increased frequency of cataracts also occurs with long-term corticosteroid therapy. Hyperglycemia may develop and lead to diabetes mellitus. Diabetics should monitor their blood glucose and adjust their medications accordingly. Hypokalemia caused by corticosteroid therapy can be counteracted by potassium supplementation. Coadministration of medications that induce or inhibit the hepatic mixed-function oxidases may require adjustment of the glucocorticoid dose.

F. Withdrawal

Withdrawal from these drugs can be a serious problem, because if the patient has experienced HPA suppression, abrupt removal of the corticosteroids causes an acute adrenal insufficiency syndrome that can be lethal. This, coupled with the possibility of psychologic dependence on the drug and the fact that withdrawal might cause an exacerbation of the disease, means the dose must be tapered according to the individual, possibly through trial and error. The patient must be monitored carefully.

G. Inhibitors of adrenocorticoid biosynthesis

Several substances have proven to be useful as inhibitors of the synthesis of adrenal steroids: *metyrapone, aminoglutethimide, ketoconazole, trilostane, spironolactone,* and *eplerenone. Mifepristone* competes with glucocorticoids for the receptor.

1. **Metyrapone:** *Metyrapone* [me-TEER-ah-pone] is used for tests of adrenal function and can be used for the treatment of pregnant women with Cushing's syndrome. [Note: *Dexamethasone* suppression is now used more commonly for diagnosis.] *Metyrapone* interferes with corticosteroid synthesis by blocking the final step (11-hydroxylation) in glucocorticoid synthesis, leading to an increase in 11-deoxycortisol as well as adrenal androgens and the potent mineralocorticoid 11-deoxycorticosterone. The adverse effects encountered with *metyrapone* include salt and water retention, hirsutism, transient dizziness, and gastrointestinal disturbances.

2. **Aminoglutethimide:** This drug acts by inhibiting the conversion of cholesterol to pregnenolone. As a result, the synthesis of all hormonally active steroids is reduced. *Aminoglutethimide* [ah-mee-noe-glu-TETH-ih-mide] has been used therapeutically in the treatment of breast cancer to reduce or eliminate androgen and estrogen production. [Note: *Tamoxifen* has largely replaced *aminoglutethimide* in the treatment of breast cancer.] In these cases, it is used in conjunction with *dexamethasone*. However, it increases the clearance of *dexamethasone*. *Aminoglutethimide* may also be useful in the treatment of malignancies of the adrenal cortex to reduce the secretion of steroids. Recent studies indicate it is an aromatase inhibitor.

3. **Ketoconazole:** *Ketoconazole* [kee-toe-KON-ah-zole] is an antifungal agent that strongly inhibits all gonadal and adrenal steroid hormone synthesis. It is used in the treatment of patients with Cushing's syndrome.

4. **Trilostane:** *Trilostane* [TRYE-loe-stane] reversibly inhibits 3β-hydroxysteroid dehydrogenase and, thus, affects aldosterone, cortisol, and gonadal hormone synthesis. Its side effects are gastrointestinal.

5. **Mifepristone:** At high doses, *mifepristone* [mih-feh-PRIH-stone] is a potent glucocorticoid antagonist as well as an antiprogestin. It forms a complex with the glucocorticoid receptor, but the rapid dissociation of the drug from the receptor leads to a faulty translocation into the nucleus. Its use is presently limited to the treatment of inoperable patients with ectopic ACTH syndrome.

6. **Spironolactone:** This antihypertensive drug competes for the mineralocorticoid receptor and, thus, inhibits sodium reabsorption in the kidney. It can also antagonize aldosterone and testosterone synthesis. It is effective against hyperaldosteronism. *Spironolactone* [speer-oh-no-LAK-tone] is also useful in the treatment of hirsutism in women, probably due to interference at the androgen receptor of the hair follicle. Adverse effects include hyperkalemia, gynecomastia, menstrual irregularities, and skin rashes.

7. **Eplerenone:** *Eplerenone* [e-PLER-en-one] specifically binds to the mineralocorticoid receptor, where it acts as an aldosterone antagonist. This specificity avoids the side effect of gynecomastia that is associated with the use of *spironolactone*. It is approved as an antihypertensive.

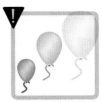

Decreased growth
in children

**Negative Calcium
Balance**

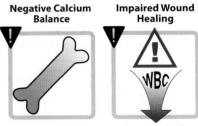

Osteoporosis

**Impaired Wound
Healing**

Increased risk
of infection

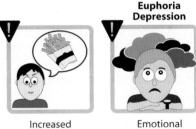

Increased
appetite

**Euphoria
Depression**

Emotional
disturbances

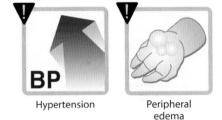

Hypertension

Peripheral
edema

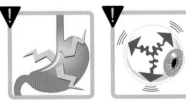

Peptic Ulcer

Glaucoma

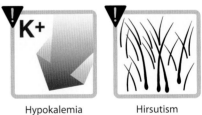

Hypokalemia

Hirsutism

Figure 26.6
Some commonly observed effects
of long-term corticosteroid therapy.

Study Questions

Choose the ONE best answer.

26.1 Measurements of cortisol precursors and plasma dehydroepiandrosterone sulfate confirm the diagnosis of congenital adrenal hyperplasia (CAH) in a child. This condition can be effectively treated by:

A. Suppressing the release of ACTH.
B. Administering an androgen antagonist.
C. Administering metapyrone to decrease cortisol synthesis.
D. Removing the adrenal gland surgically.

Correct answer = A. CAH is the most common disorder of infancy and childhood. Because cortisol synthesis is decreased, feedback inhibition of ACTH formation and release is also decreased, resulting in enhanced ACTH formation. This in turn leads to increased levels of adrenal androgens and/or mineralocorticoids. The treatment is to administer a glucocorticoid, such as hydrocortisone (in infants) or prednisone, which would restore the feedback inhibition. The other options are inappropriate.

26.2 Osteoporosis is a major adverse effect caused by the glucocorticoids. It is due to their ability to:

A. Increase the excretion of calcium.
B. Inhibit absorption of calcium.
C. Stimulate the HPA axis.
D. Decrease production of prostaglandins.

Correct answer = B. Glucocorticoid-induced osteoporosis is attributed to inhibition of calcium absorption as well as bone formation. Increased intake of calcium plus vitamin D or calcitonin, or of other drugs that are effective in this condition, is indicated. Glucocorticoids suppress rather than stimulate the HPA axis. The decreased production of prostaglandins does not play a role in bone formation.

26.3 A child with asthma is being treated effectively with an inhaled preparation of beclomethasone dipropionate. Which of the following adverse effects is of particular concern?

A. Hypoglycemia.
B. Hirsutism.
C. Growth suppression.
D. Cushing's syndrome.
E. Cataract formation.

Correct answer = C. Growth hormone may be decreased by this treatment. Chronic treatment with the medication therefore may lead to growth suppression, so linear growth should be monitored periodically. Hyperglycemia, not hypoglycemia, is a possible adverse effect. Hirsutism, Cushing's syndrome, and cataract formation are unlikely with the dose that the child would receive by inhalation.

Respiratory System

27

I. OVERVIEW

Asthma, chronic obstructive pulmonary disease (COPD), and allergic rhinitis are commonly encountered respiratory diseases. Each of these conditions may be associated with a troublesome cough, which may be the patient's only presenting complaint. Asthma is a chronic disease characterized by hyperresponsive airways, affecting 10 million patients (four to five percent of the U.S. population), and resulting annually in 2 million emergency room visits, 500,000 hospitalizations, and 5,000 deaths. COPD, also called emphysema or chronic bronchitis, affects approximately 30 million Americans and is currently the fourth most common cause of preventable deaths in the United States. Allergic rhinitis, characterized by itchy, watery eyes, runny nose, and a nonproductive cough, is an extremely common condition that significantly decreases patient-reported quality of life. Allergic rhinitis affects approximately 20 percent of the population, or over 61 million Americans. Coughing is an important defensive respiratory response to irritants and has been cited as the number-one reason why patients seek medical care. A troublesome cough may represent several etiologies, such as the common cold, sinusitis, and/or an underlying chronic respiratory disease.

Each of these respiratory conditions can be adequately controlled through a combined approach of appropriate lifestyle changes and medication management. Drugs used to treat respiratory conditions can be delivered topically to the nasal mucosa, inhaled into the lungs, or given orally or parenterally for systemic absorption. Topical delivery methods, such as nasal sprays or inhalers, are preferred so as to target affected tissues while minimizing systemic side effects. Clinically useful drugs mitigate the specific pathology, such as by relaxing bronchial smooth muscle or modulating the inflammatory response. Medications used to treat these commonly encountered respiratory disorders are summarized in Figure 27.1.

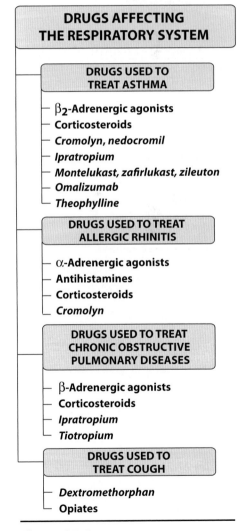

Figure 27.1
Summary of drugs affecting the respiratory system.

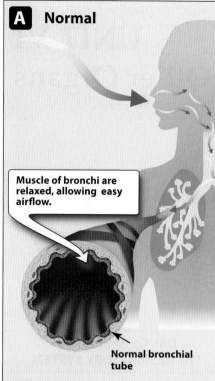

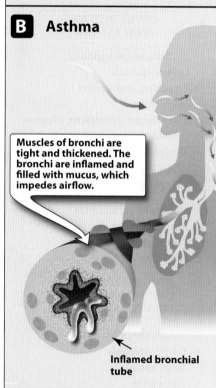

Figure 27.2
Comparison of bronchi of normal and asthmatic individuals.

II. FIRST-LINE DRUGS USED TO TREAT ASTHMA

Asthma is an inflammatory disease of the airways characterized by episodes of acute bronchoconstriction causing shortness of breath, cough, chest tightness, wheezing, and rapid respiration. These acute symptoms may resolve spontaneously, with nonpharmacologic relaxation exercises, or with use of "quick relief" medications, such as a short-acting β_2-adrenergic agonist (see p. 72). Unlike chronic bronchitis, cystic fibrosis, or bronchiectasis, asthma is usually not a progressive disease; that is, it does not inevitably lead to crippled airways. Asthma is a chronic disease with an underlying inflammatory pathophysiology that, if untreated, may incur airway remodeling, resulting in increased severity and incidence of exacerbations and/or death. Deaths due to asthma are relatively infrequent, but significant morbidity results in high outpatient costs, numerous hospitalizations, and decreased quality of life.

A. Goals of therapy

1. Reducing impairment:

  a. Prevent chronic and troublesome symptoms.

  b. Require infrequent use (≤2 days a week) of inhaled short-acting β_2 agonist for quick relief of symptoms.

  c. Maintain (near) "normal" pulmonary function.

  d. Maintain normal activity levels (including exercise and other physical activity and attendance at work or school).

  e. Meet patients' and family expectations of and satisfaction with asthma care.

2. Reducing risk:

  a. Prevent recurrent exacerbations of asthma, and minimize the need for emergency department visits or hospitalizations.

  b. Prevent progressive loss of lung function; for children, prevent reduced lung growth.

  c. Provide optimal pharmacotherapy with minimal or no adverse effects.

B. Role of inflammation in asthma

Airflow obstruction in asthma is due to bronchoconstriction that results from contraction of bronchial smooth muscle, inflammation of the bronchial wall, and increased mucous secretion (Figure 27.2). Asthmatic attacks may be related to recent exposure to allergens or inhaled irritants, leading to bronchial hyperactivity and inflammation of the airway mucosa. The symptoms of asthma may be effectively treated by several drugs, but no agent provides a cure for this obstructive lung disease.

C. Role of phenotype in asthma

Recent research demonstrates a link between β-receptor polymorphism (phenotype) and response to long-acting β_2 agonists for approximately 16 to 20 percent of the patient population affected by asthma. Three asthma phenotypes have been reported: homozygous glycine, heterozygous glycine/arginine, and homozygous arginine. Evidence from clinical trials and postmarketing analysis suggests patients with

CLASSIFICATION	BRONCHO-CONSTRICTIVE EPISODES	RESULTS OF PEAK FLOW OR SPIROMETRY	LONG-TERM CONTROL	QUICK RELIEF OF SYMPTOMS
Mild intermittent	Less than two per week	Near normal*	No daily medication	Short-acting β_2 agonist
Mild persistent	More than two per week	Near normal*	Low-dose inhaled corticosteroids	Short-acting β_2 agonist
Moderate persistent	Daily	60 to 80 percent of normal	Low- to medium-dose inhaled corticosteroids and a long-acting β_2 agonist	Short-acting β_2 agonist
Severe persistent	Continual	Less than 60 percent of normal	High-dose inhaled corticosteroids and a long-acting β_2 agonist	Short-acting β_2 agonist

Figure 27.3
Treatment of asthma. In all asthmatic patients, quick relief is provided by a short-acting β_2 agonist as needed for symptoms. *Eighty percent or more of predicted function.

the homozygous arginine polymorphism may be at risk for worsening symptoms with long-acting β_2 agonists therapy. Because population-based genotyping to determine β-receptor phenotype is not feasible at this time, clinicians prescribing any new long-acting β_2 agonists prescription should counsel patients to carefully monitor symptoms for any signs of worsening. If the patient reports worsening symptoms, the long-acting β_2 agonists therapy should be discontinued with a subsequent increase in corticosteroid dosing as clinically appropriate. Further research is underway examining the mechanism of the various asthma phenotypes and how to appropriately target therapy to each for improved control.

D. Adrenergic agonists

Inhaled adrenergic agonists with β_2 activity are the drugs of choice for mild asthma—that is, in patients showing only occasional, intermittent symptoms (Figure 27.3). Direct-acting β_2 agonists are potent bronchodilators that relax airway smooth muscle.

1. **Quick relief:** Most clinically useful β_2 agonists have a rapid onset of action (5–30 minutes) and provide relief for 4 to 6 hours. They are used for symptomatic treatment of bronchospasm, providing quick relief of acute bronchoconstriction. [Note: *Epinephrine* is the drug of choice for treatment of acute anaphylaxis.] β_2 Agonists have no anti-inflammatory effects, and they should never be used as the sole therapeutic agents for patients with persistent asthma. Monotherapy with short-acting β_2 agonists may be appropriate only for patients identified as having mild intermittent asthma, such as exercise-induced asthma. The direct-acting β_2-selective agonists, such as *pirbuterol* [peer-BYOO-ter-ole], *terbutaline* [ter-BYOO-ta-leen], and *albuterol* [al-BYOO-teh-rall], offer the advantage of providing maximally attainable bronchodilation with little of the undesired effect of α or β_1 stimulation. (See p. 69 for the receptor-specific actions of adrenergic agonists.) The β_2 agonists are not catecholamines and, thus, are not inactivated by catechol-*O*-methyltransferase. Adverse effects, such as tachycardia, hyperglycemia, hypokalemia, and hypomagnesemia are minimized with dosing via inhalation versus systemic routes. Although tolerance to the effects of β_2 agonists on nonairway tissues occurs, it is uncommon with normal dosages. All

patients with asthma should be prescribed a quick-relief inhaler and regularly assessed for appropriate inhaler technique.

2. **Long-term control:** *Salmeterol* [sal-ME-te-rol] *xinafoate* and *formoterol* [for-MOH-ter-ol] are long-acting β_2 agonists bronchodilators. They are chemical analogs of *albuterol* but differ by having a lipophilic side chain, increasing the affinity of the drug for the β_2-adrenoceptor. *Salmeterol* and *formoterol* have a long duration of action, providing bronchodilation for at least 12 hours. Both *salmeterol* and *formoterol* have slower onsets of action and should not be used for quick relief of an acute asthma attack. long-acting β_2 agonists should be prescribed for routine administration. Whereas inhaled corticosteroids remain the long-term control drugs of choice in asthma, long-acting β_2 agonists are considered to be useful adjunctive therapy for attaining asthma control. Adverse effects of the long-acting β_2 agonists are similar to quick-relief β_2 agonists. Appropriate inhaler technique with long-acting β_2 agonists is critical to the success of therapy, may differ from the patient's other inhalers (metered-dose inhaler versus dry powder inhaler), and should be reassessed regularly.

E. Corticosteroids

Inhaled corticosteroids (ICS) are the drugs of first choice in patients with any degree of persistent asthma (mild, moderate, or severe; see Figure 27.3). Severe persistent asthma may require the addition of a short course of oral glucocorticoid treatment. No other medications are as effective as ICS in the long-term control of asthma in children and adults. If appropriately prescribed and used, ICS therapy may reduce or eliminate the need for oral glucocorticoids in patients with severe asthma. To be effective in controlling inflammation, glucocorticoids must be taken continuously. (See p. 313 for a summary of the mechanism of action of corticosteroids.) Current guidelines recommend selecting ICS therapy for a newly diagnosed patient with asthma at dosing equivalent to the patient's asthma classification (National Heart, Lung, and Blood Institute [NHLBI] "Step Up" therapy). Patients achieving 3 to 6 consecutive months of improved asthma control may be considered for a reduction in ICS dosing (NHLBI "Step Down" therapy) as clinically indicated.

1. **Actions on lung:** ICS do not directly affect the airway smooth muscle. Instead, ICS therapy directly targets underlying airway inflammation by decreasing the inflammatory cascade (eosinophils, macrophages, and T lymphocytes), reversing mucosal edema, decreasing the permeability of capillaries, and inhibiting the release of leukotrienes. After several months of regular use, ICS reduce the hyperresponsiveness of the airway smooth muscle to a variety of bronchoconstrictor stimuli, such as allergens, irritants, cold air, and exercise.

2. **Route of administration**

   a. **Inhalation:** The development of ICS has markedly reduced the need for systemic corticosteroid treatment to achieve asthma control. Appropriate inhalation technique is critical to the success of therapy. Metered-dose inhalers have propellants that eject the active medication from the canister. Patients should be instructed to SLOWLY and DEEPLY inhale upon activation of these inhalers to avoid impaction of the medication onto the laryngeal mucosa rather than the bronchial smooth muscle. Improper use

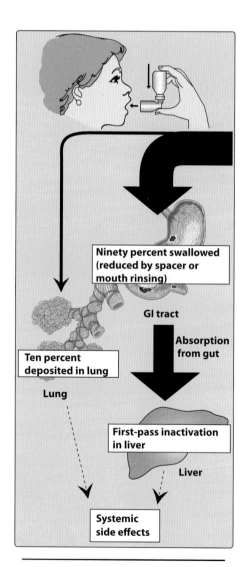

Figure 27.4
Pharmacokinetics of inhaled glucocorticoids.

of a metered-dose inhaler can result in a large fraction (typically 80–90 percent) of inhaled glucocorticoids to be deposited in the mouth, pharynx, and/or swallowed (Figure 27.4). The 10 to 20 percent of the metered dose of inhaled glucocorticoids that is not swallowed is deposited in the airway. If ICS are inappropriately inhaled, systemic absorption and adverse effects are much more likely. ICS delivered by dry powder inhalers require a different inhaler technique. Patients should be instructed to inhale QUICKLY and DEEPLY to optimize drug delivery to the lungs. Even properly administered, corticosteroid deposition on the oral and laryngeal mucosa can cause adverse effects such as oropharyngeal candidiasis and hoarseness. Patient counseling incorporating a rinsing of these tissues via the "swish and spit" method should avoid these adverse events.

b. **Oral/systemic:** Patients with severe exacerbation of asthma (status asthmaticus) may require intravenous administration of *methylprednisolone* or oral *prednisone*. Once the patient has improved, the dose of drug is gradually reduced, leading to discontinuance in 1 to 2 weeks. In most cases, suppression of the hypothalamic-pituitary axis will not occur during the short course of oral prednisone "burst" typically prescribed for an asthma exacerbation; therefore, dose reduction is not necessary.

c. **Spacers:** A spacer is a large-volume chamber attached to a metered-dose inhaler. Spacers decrease the deposition of drug in the mouth caused by improper inhaler technique (Figure 27.5). The chamber reduces the velocity of the injected aerosol before entering the mouth, allowing large drug particles to be deposited in the device. The smaller, higher-velocity drug particles are less likely to be deposited in the mouth and more likely to reach the target airway tissue. Spacers minimize the problem of adrenal suppression by reducing the amount of glucocorticoid deposited in the oropharynx. Spacers improve delivery of inhaled glucocorticoids and are advised for virtually all patients, especially children less than 5 years old and elderly patients who may have difficulty coordinating actuation with inhalation. Patients should be counseled about regular washing and/or rinsing of spacers to reduce the risk of bacterial, mold, or mildew growth inducing an asthma attack.

3. **Adverse effects:** Oral or parenteral glucocorticoids have a variety of potentially serious side effects (see p. 317); inhaled glucocorticoids, particularly if used with a spacer, have few systemic effects. Studies have demonstrated the effect of ICS on vertical bone growth in children to be negligible, whereas the retardation of vertical bone growth secondary to low oxygenated blood levels from uncontrolled asthma can occur in more severe cases.

III. ALTERNATIVE DRUGS USED TO TREAT ASTHMA

These drugs are useful for treatment of moderate to severe allergic asthma in patients who are poorly controlled by conventional therapy or experience adverse effects secondary to high-dose or prolonged corticosteroid treatment. These drugs should be used in conjunction with ICS therapy, not as sole therapies.

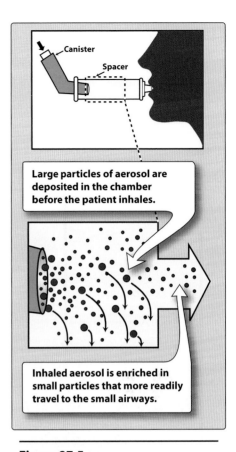

Figure 27.5
Effect of a spacer on the delivery of an inhaled aerosol.

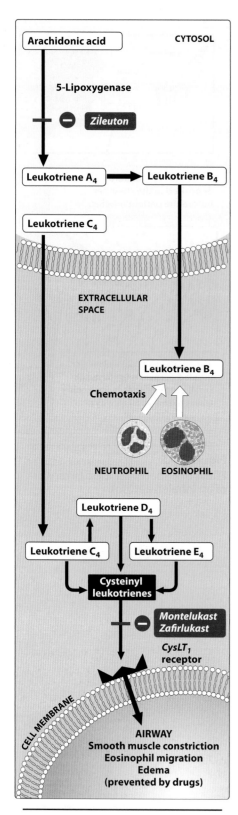

Figure 27.6
Sites of action of leukotriene-modifying drugs. $CysLT_1$ = cysteinyl leukotriene-1.

A. Leukotriene antagonists

Leukotriene (LT) B_4 and the cysteinyl leukotrienes, LTC_4, LTD_4, and LTE_4, are products of the 5-lipoxygenase pathway of arachidonic acid metabolism and part of the inflammatory cascade.[1] 5-Lipoxygenase is found in cells of myeloid origin, such as mast cells, basophils, eosinophils, and neutrophils. LTB_4 is a potent chemoattractant for neutrophils and eosinophils, whereas the cysteinyl leukotrienes constrict bronchiolar smooth muscle, increase endothelial permeability, and promote mucous secretion. *Zileuton* [zye-LOO-ton] is a selective and specific inhibitor of 5-lipoxygenase, preventing the formation of both LTB_4 and the cysteinyl leukotrienes. *Zafirlukast* [za-FIR-loo-kast] and *montelukast* [mon-tee-LOO-kast] are selective, reversible inhibitors of the cysteinyl leukotriene-1 receptor, thereby blocking the effects of cysteinyl leukotrienes (Figure 27.6). *Montelukast*, the market leader in this pharmacologic class, claims two primary advantages: dosing recommendations for children 1 year of age and older as well as being available in chewable tablets and granule formulations. All three drugs are approved for the prophylaxis of asthma but are not effective in situations where immediate bronchodilation is required. Modest reductions in the doses of β_2-adrenergic agonists and corticosteroids, as well as improved respiratory function, are among the therapeutic benefits.

1. **Pharmacokinetics:** All three drugs are orally active, although food impairs the absorption of *zafirlukast*. Greater than 90 percent of each drug is bound to plasma protein. The drugs are extensively metabolized. *Zileuton* and its metabolites are excreted in the urine, whereas *zafirlukast* and *montelukast* and their metabolites undergo biliary excretion.

2. **Adverse effects:** Elevations in serum hepatic enzymes have occurred with all three agents, requiring periodic monitoring and discontinuation when enzymes exceed three to five times the upper limit of normal. Although rare, eosinophilic vasculitis (Churg-Strauss syndrome) has been reported with all agents, particularly when the dose of concurrent glucocorticoids is reduced. Other effects include headache and dyspepsia. Both *zafirlukast* and *zileuton* are inhibitors of cytochrome P450. Both drugs can increase serum levels of *warfarin*. Figure 27.6 summarizes the drugs that modify the action of leukotrienes.

B. Cromolyn and nedocromil

Cromolyn [KROE-moe-lin] and *nedocromil* [ne-doe-KROE-mil] are effective prophylactic anti-inflammatory agents. However, they are not useful in managing an acute asthma attack, because they are not direct bronchodilators. These agents can block the initiation of immediate and delayed asthmatic reactions. For use in asthma, *cromolyn* is administered either by inhalation of a microfine powder or as an aerosolized solution. Because it is poorly absorbed, only minor adverse effects are associated with it. Pretreatment with *cromolyn* blocks allergen- and exercise-induced bronchoconstriction. *Cromolyn* is also useful in reducing the symptoms of allergic rhinitis. A 4 to 6-week trial is required to deter-

[1] See p. 213 in *Lippincott's Illustrated Reviews: Biochemistry* (4th ed.) for a discussion of leukotriene synthesis.

mine efficacy. Given its safety, an initial trial of *cromolyn* is often recommended, particularly in children and pregnant women. Toxic reactions are mild and include a bitter taste and irritation of the pharynx and larynx. Due to short duration of action, these agents require frequent daily dosing, which has been shown to affect adherence and, therefore, therapeutic efficacy. Neither *cromolyn* nor *nedocromil* should replace ICS or quick-relief β_2 agonists as the mainstay of asthma therapy.

C. Cholinergic antagonists

Anticholinergic agents are generally less effective than β_2-adrenergic agonists. They block the vagally mediated contraction of airway smooth muscle and mucus secretion. Inhaled *ipratropium* [i-pra-TROE-pee-um], a quaternary derivative of *atropine*, is useful in patients who are unable to tolerate adrenergic agonists. *Ipratropium* is slow in onset and nearly free of side effects. These agents are not traditionally effective for patients with asthma unless COPD is also present.

D. Theophylline

Theophylline [thee-OFF-i-lin] is a bronchodilator that relieves airflow obstruction in chronic asthma and decreases its symptoms. *Theophylline* is well absorbed by the gastrointestinal tract, and several sustained-release preparations are available. Previously the mainstay of asthma therapy, *theophylline* has been largely replaced with β_2 agonists and corticosteroids due to a narrow therapeutic window, high side-effect profile, and potential for drug interactions. Overdose may cause seizures or potentially fatal arrhythmias. *Theophylline* is metabolized in the liver, is a CYP1A2 and 3A4 substrate, and interacts adversely with many drugs.

E. Omalizumab

Omalizumab [oh-mah-lye-ZOO-mab] is a recombinant DNA–derived monoclonal antibody that selectively binds to human immunoglobulin E (IgE). This leads to decreased binding of IgE to the high-affinity IgE receptor on the surface of mast cells and basophils. Reduction in surface-bound IgE limits the degree of release of mediators of the allergic response. *Omalizumab* may be particularly useful for treatment of moderate to severe allergic asthma in patients who are poorly controlled with conventional therapy. Due to the high cost of the drug (approximately $600 for a 150-mg vial), limitations on dosage, and available clinical trial data, it is not presently used as first-line therapy.

IV. DRUGS USED TO TREAT CHRONIC OBSTRUCTIVE PULMONARY DISEASE

Chronic obstructive pulmonary disease is a chronic, irreversible obstruction of airflow. Smoking is the greatest risk factor for COPD and is directly linked to the progressive decline of lung function as demonstrated by forced expiratory volume (FEV). Smoking cessation and/or continued avoidance should be recommended regardless of stage/severity of COPD and age of patient. Inhaled bronchodilators, such as anticholinergic agents (*ipratropium* and *tiotropium*) and β_2-adrenergic agonists, are the foundation of therapy for COPD (Figure 27.7). These drugs increase airflow, alleviate symptoms, and decrease exacerbation of disease. Combinations of an anticholinergic plus a β_2 agonist may be helpful in patients for whom a single inhaled bronchodilator has failed to provide an adequate response. For example, the com-

STAGE	CHARACTERISTICS	LONG-TERM CONTROL
I: Mild COPD	FEV$_1$ greater than 80 percent predicted	Short-acting bronchodilator when needed
II: Moderate COPD	FEV$_1$ 50 to 80 percent predicted	Regular treatment with one or more bronchodilators Inhaled glucocorticosteroid
III: Severe COPD	FEV$_1$ less than 30 percent predicted	Regular treatment with one or more bronchodilators Inhaled glucocorticosteroid Antibiotics for acute exacerbations of COPD characterized by increased volume and purulence of secretions Long-term oxygen therapy

Figure 27.7
Treatment of stable chronic obstructive pulmonary disease (COPD). FEV$_1$ = forced expiratory volume in one second.

bination of *albuterol* and *ipratropium* provides greater bronchodilation than with either drug alone. Longer-acting drugs, such as *salmeterol* and *tiotropium* [tee-oh-TROE-pee-um], have the advantage of less frequent dosing. ICS should be restricted to patients with an FEV in 1 second (FEV$_1$) of less than 50 percent of predicted and three or more exacerbations in the last 3 years (Stage III or IV). Whereas the addition of ICS may provide symptomatic relief, the progressive decline in FEV$_1$ is not impacted. Addition of a long-acting β_2 agonists such as *salmeterol*, improves lung function compared to either a short-acting β_2 agonist or steroid alone.

V. DRUGS USED TO TREAT ALLERGIC RHINITIS

Rhinitis is an inflammation of the mucous membranes of the nose and is characterized by sneezing, itchy nose/eyes, watery rhinorrhea, and nasal congestion. An attack may be precipitated by inhalation of an allergen (such as dust, pollen, or animal dander). The foreign material interacts with mast cells coated with IgE generated in response to a previous allergen exposure (Figure 27.8). The mast cells release mediators, such as histamine, leukotrienes, and chemotactic factors, that promote bronchiolar spasm and mucosal thickening from edema and cellular infiltration. Combinations of oral antihistamines with decongestants are the first-line therapies for allergic rhinitis. Systemic effects associated with these oral preparations (sedation, insomnia, and, rarely, cardiac arrhythmias) have prompted interest in topical intranasal delivery of drugs.

A. Antihistamines (H$_1$-receptor blockers)

Antihistamines are the most frequently used agents in the treatment of sneezing and watery rhinorrhea associated with allergic rhinitis. H$_1$-histamine receptor blockers, such as *diphenhydramine, chlorpheniramine, loratadine,* and *fexofenadine*, are useful in treating the symptoms of allergic rhinitis caused by histamine release. Ocular and nasal antihistamine delivery devices are available over-the-counter for more targeted tissue delivery. Combinations of antihistamines with decongestants (see below) are effective when congestion is a feature of rhinitis. Antihistamines differ in their ability to cause sedation and in their duration of action. In general, anticholinergic side effects of the first-generation antihistamines (dry eyes/mouth, difficulty urinating and/or defecating) are transient and may resolve in 7 to 10 days. Constipation associated with chronic use of the first-generation antihistamines is not transient and may require treatment with a stool softener, especially in more susceptible patients.

B. α-Adrenergic agonists

Short-acting α-adrenergic agonists ("nasal decongestants"), such as *phenylephrine*, constrict dilated arterioles in the nasal mucosa and reduce airway resistance. Longer-acting *oxymetazoline* [ok-see-met-AZ-oh-leen] is also available. When administered as an aerosol, these drugs have a rapid onset of action and show few systemic effects. Oral administration results in longer duration of action but also increased systemic effects. Combinations of these agents with antihistamines are frequently used. The α-adrenergic agonists should be used no longer than several days due to the risk of rebound nasal congestion (rhinitis medicamentosa). α-Adrenergic agents have no place in the long-term treatment of allergic rhinitis.

C. Corticosteroids

Corticosteroids, such as *beclomethasone, budesonide, fluticasone, flunisolide,* and *triamcinolone*, are effective when administered as nasal sprays. [Note: Systemic absorption is minimal, and side effects of intranasal corticosteroid treatment are localized. These include nasal irritation, nosebleed, sore throat, and rarely, candidiasis.] To avoid systemic absorption, patient counseling should emphasize the importance of topical deposition of the drug (tell patients NOT to deeply inhale while administering these drugs because the target tissue is in the nose, not in the lungs or the throat). Topical steroids may be more effective than systemic antihistamines in relieving the nasal symptoms of both allergic and nonallergic rhinitis. The effects of long-term usage are unknown, but these agents are considered to be generally safe. Periodic assessment of the patient is advised. Treatment of chronic rhinitis may not result in improvement until 1 to 2 weeks after starting therapy.

D. Cromolyn

Intranasal *cromolyn* may be useful, particularly when administered before contact with an allergen. To optimize the therapeutic effect of cromolyn, dosing should occur at least 1 to 2 weeks prior to allergen exposure. Due to a short duration of action, *cromolyn* requires multiple daily dosing, which may deleteriously impact adherence and, therefore, therapeutic efficacy.

VI. DRUGS USED TO TREAT COUGH

Codeine [KOE-deen] is the gold-standard treatment for cough suppression due to its long history of availability and use. *Codeine* decreases the sensitivity of cough centers in the central nervous system to peripheral stimuli and decreases mucosal secretion. These therapeutic effects occur at doses lower than those required for analgesia but still incur common sides effects like constipation, dysphoria, and fatigue, in addition to its addictive potential. (See p. 159 for a more complete discussion of the opiates.) *Dextromethorphan* [dek-stroe-METH-or-fan] is a synthetic derivative of *morphine* that suppresses the response of the central cough center. It has no analgesic effects, has a low addictive profile, but may cause dysphoria at high doses, which may explain its status as a potential drug of abuse. *Dextromethorphan* has a significantly better side effect profile than *codeine* and has been demonstrated to be equally effective for cough suppression.

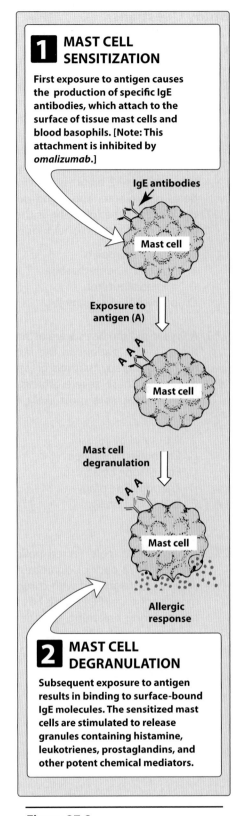

Figure 27.8
Hypersensitivity reactions mediated by immunoglobulin E (IgE) molecules can cause rhinitis.

Study Questions

Choose the ONE best answer.

27.1 A 12-year-old girl with a childhood history of asthma complained of cough, dyspnea, and wheezing after visiting a riding stable. Her symptoms became so severe that her parents brought her to the emergency room. Physical examination revealed diaphoresis, dyspnea, tachycardia, and tachypnea. Her respiratory rate was 42 breaths per minute, pulse rate 110 beats per minute, and blood pressure 132/65 mm Hg. Which of the following is the most appropriate drug to rapidly reverse her bronchoconstriction?

A. Inhaled cromolyn.
B. Inhaled beclomethasone.
C. Inhaled albuterol.
D. Intravenous propranolol.

Correct answer = C. Inhalation of a rapid-acting β_2 agonist, such as albuterol, usually provides immediate bronchodilation. An acute asthmatic crisis often requires intravenous corticosteroids, often methylprednisolone. Inhaled beclomethasone will not deliver enough steroid to fully combat airway inflammation. Propranolol is a β-blocker and would aggravate the patient's bronchoconstriction. Cromolyn can be used prophylactically to reduce the inflammatory response but is ineffective in relieving acute symptoms.

27.2 A 9-year-old girl has severe asthma, which required three hospitalizations in the last year. She is now receiving therapy that has greatly reduced the frequency of these severe attacks. Which of the following therapies is most likely responsible for this benefit?

A. Albuterol by aerosol.
B. Cromolyn by inhaler.
C. Fluticasone by aerosol.
D. Theophylline orally.
E. Zafirlukast orally.

Correct answer = C. Administration of a corticosteroid directly to the lung significantly reduces the frequency of severe asthma attacks. This benefit is accomplished with minimal risk of the severe systemic adverse effects of corticosteroid therapy. Albuterol is only used to treat acute asthmatic episodes. The other agents may reduce the severity of attacks but not to the same degree or consistency as fluticasone (or other corticosteroids).

27.3 A 68-year-old male retired police officer who has smoked a 1/2 pack of cigarettes a day for the past 40 years is diagnosed with chronic obstructive pulmonary disease (COPD). He has a difficulty in expiration during breathing, but the symptms are mild and intermittent. Which one of the following agents would most appropratate initial therapy.

A. Systemic corticosteroids
B. Albuterol
C. Salmeterol
D. Tiotropium plus salmeterol
E. Theophylline

Correct answer = B. All symptomatic patients with COPD should be prescribed a short-acting bronchodilator to be used on an as-needed basis. A regularly scheduled long-acting bronchodilator, such as salmeterol, could be added if symptoms are inadequately controlled with short-acting bronchodilator therapy. Systemic corticosteroids are used to treat exacerbations in patients with COPD. Tiotropium plus salmeterol are indicated in moderate to severe disease. Theophylline is an oral bronchodilator that is beneficial to some patients with stable COPD. Because of its toxic potential, it would not be considered for initial therapy.

Gastrointestinal and Antiemetic Drugs

28

I. OVERVIEW

This chapter describes drugs used to treat three common medical conditions involving the gastrointestinal tract: peptic ulcers and gastro-esophageal reflux disease (GERD), chemotherapy-induced emesis, and diarrhea and constipation. Many drugs described in other chapters also find application in the treatment of gastrointestinal disorders. For example, the *meperidine* derivative *diphenoxylate*, which decreases peristaltic activity of the gut, is useful in the treatment of severe diarrhea, and the corticosteroid *dexamethasone* has excellent antiemetic properties. Other drugs, (for example, H_2-receptor antagonists and proton-pump inhibitors (PPIs), are employed to heal peptic ulcers; the selective inhibitors of the serotonin receptors, such as *ondansetron* or *granisetron*, which prevent vomiting, are used almost exclusively to treat gastrointestinal tract disorders.

II. DRUGS USED TO TREAT PEPTIC ULCER DISEASE

Although the pathogenesis of peptic ulcer disease is not fully understood, several major causative factors are recognized: nonsteroidal anti-inflammatory drug (NSAID) use, infection with gram-negative <u>Helicobacter pylori</u>, increased hydrochloric acid secretion, and inadequate mucosal defense against gastric acid. Treatment approaches include 1) eradicating the <u>H</u>. <u>pylori</u> infection, 2) reducing secretion of gastric acid with the use of H_2-receptor antagonists or PPIs, and/or 3) providing agents that protect the gastric mucosa from damage, such as *misoprostol* and *sucralfate*. (Note: If patients are unable to tolerate the above therapies, neutralizing gastric acid with nonabsorbable antacids is an option). Figure 28.1 summarizes agents that are effective in treating peptic ulcer disease.

A. Antimicrobial agents

Optimal therapy for patients with peptic ulcer disease (both duodenal and gastric ulcers) who are infected with <u>H</u>. <u>pylori</u> requires antimicrobial treatment. To document infection with <u>H</u>. <u>pylori</u>, endoscopic biopsy of the gastric mucosa or various noninvasive methods are utilized, including serologic tests and urea breath tests. Figure 28.2 shows a biopsy sample in which <u>H</u>. <u>pylori</u> is closely associated with the gastric mucosa. Eradication of <u>H</u>. <u>pylori</u> results in rapid healing of active peptic ulcers and low recurrence rates (less than 15 percent compared with 60 to 100 percent per year for patients with initial ulcers healed by traditional antisecretory therapy). Successful eradication of <u>H</u>. <u>pylori</u> (80–90 percent) is possible with various combina-

---

DRUGS USED TO TREAT PEPTIC ULCER DISEASE

ANTIMICROBIAL AGENTS
- *Amoxicillin*
- **Bismuth compounds**
- *Clarithromycin*
- *Metronidazole*
- *Tetracycline*

H_2 - HISTAMINE RECEPTOR BLOCKERS
- *Cimetidine*
- *Famotidine*
- *Nizatidine*
- *Ranitidine*

INHIBITORS OF PROTON PUMP
- *Esomeprazole*
- *Lansoprazole*
- *Omeprazole*
- *Pantoprazole*
- *Rabeprazole*

PROSTAGLANDINS
- *Misoprostol*

Figure 28.1
Summary of drugs used to treat peptic ulcer disease.
(Figure continues on next page.)

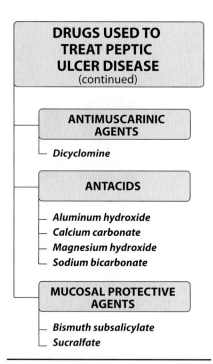

DRUGS USED TO TREAT PEPTIC ULCER DISEASE
(continued)

ANTIMUSCARINIC AGENTS

- *Dicyclomine*

ANTACIDS

- *Aluminum hydroxide*
- *Calcium carbonate*
- *Magnesium hydroxide*
- *Sodium bicarbonate*

MUCOSAL PROTECTIVE AGENTS

- *Bismuth subsalicylate*
- *Sucralfate*

Figure 28.1 (continued)
Summary of drugs used to treat peptic ulcer disease.

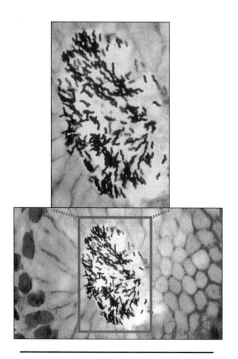

Figure 28.2
Helicobacter pylori in association with gastric mucosa.

tions of antimicrobial drugs. Currently, either triple therapy consisting of a PPI with either *metronidazole* or *amoxicillin* plus *clarithromycin*, or quadruple therapy of *bismuth subsalicylate* and *metronidazole* plus *tetracycline* plus a PPI, are administered for a 2-week course. This usually results in a 90 percent or greater eradication rate. Bismuth salts do not neutralize stomach acid, but they inhibit pepsin and increase the secretion of mucus, thus helping to form a barrier against the diffusion of acid in the ulcer. Treatment with a single antimicrobial drug is less effective (20 to 40 percent eradication rates), results in antimicrobial resistance and is absolutely not recommended; switching of antibiotics is also not recommended (that is, do not substitute *amoxicillin* for *ampicillin* or *erythromycin* for *clarithromycin* or *doxycycline* for *tetracycline*). [Note: GERD (that is, a heartburn-like sensation) is not associated with H. pylori infection and does not respond to treatment with antibiotics.]

B. Regulation of gastric acid secretion

Gastric acid secretion by parietal cells of the gastric mucosa is stimulated by acetylcholine, histamine, and gastrin (Figure 28.3). The receptor-mediated binding of acetylcholine, histamine, or gastrin results in the activation of protein kinases, which in turn stimulates the H^+/K^+–adenosine triphosphatase (ATPase) proton pump to secrete hydrogen ions in exchange for K^+ into the lumen of the stomach. A Cl^- channel couples chloride efflux to the release of H^+. In contrast, receptor binding of prostaglandin E_2 and somatostatin diminish gastric acid production. [Note: Histamine binding causes activation of adenylyl cyclase, whereas binding of prostaglandin E_2 inhibits this enzyme. Gastrin and acetylcholine act by inducing an increase in intracellular calcium levels.]

C. H₂-receptor antagonists

Although antagonists of the histamine H_2 receptor block the actions of histamine at all H_2 receptors, their chief clinical use is to inhibit gastric acid secretion, being particularly effective against nocturnal acid secretion. By competitively blocking the binding of histamine to H_2 receptors, these agents reduce the intracellular concentrations of cyclic adenosine monophosphate and, thereby, secretion of gastric acid. The four drugs used in the United States—*cimetidine* [si-MET-ih-deen], *ranitidine* [ra-NI-tih-deen], *famotidine* [fa-MOE-ti-deen], and *nizatidine* [nye-ZA-ti-deen]—potently inhibit (greater than 90 percent) basal, food-stimulated, and nocturnal secretion of gastric acid after a single dose. *Cimetidine* is the prototype histamine H_2-receptor antagonist; however, its utility is limited by its adverse effect profile and drug interactions.

1. **Actions:** The histamine H_2-receptor antagonists—*cimetidine*, *ranitidine*, *famotidine*, and *nizatidine*—act selectively on H_2 receptors in the stomach, blood vessels, and other sites, but they have no effect on H_1 receptors. They are competitive antagonists of histamine and are fully reversible. These agents completely inhibit gastric acid secretion induced by histamine or gastrin. However, they only partially inhibit gastric acid secretion induced by acetylcholine or *bethanechol*.

2. **Therapeutic uses:** The use of these agents has decreased with the advent of the PPIs.

   a. **Peptic ulcers:** All four agents are equally effective in promoting healing of duodenal and gastric ulcers. However, recurrence is common after treatment with H_2 antagonists is stopped (60–100

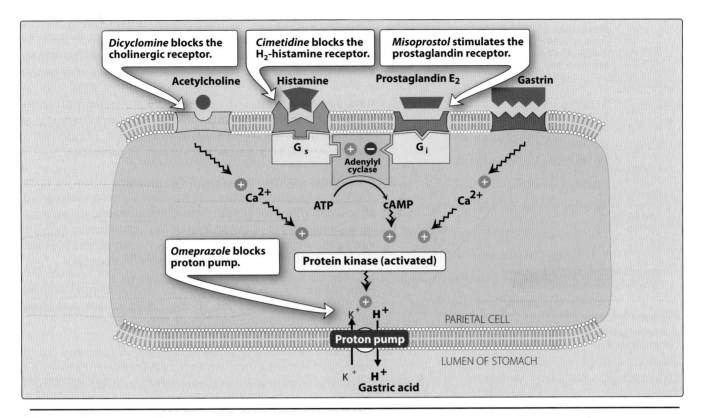

Figure 28.3
Effects of acetylcholine, histamine, prostaglandin E_2, and gastrin on gastric acid secretion by the parietal cells of stomach. G_s and G_i are membrane proteins that mediate the stimulatory or inhibitory effect of receptor coupling to adenylyl cyclase.

percent per year). Patients with NSAID-induced ulcers should be treated with PPIs, because these agents heal and prevent future ulcers better than H_2 antagonists.

b. **Acute stress ulcers:** These drugs are useful in managing acute stress ulcers associated with major physical trauma in high-risk patients in intensive care units. They are usually injected intravenously.

c. **Gastroesophageal reflux disease:** Low doses of H_2 antagonists, recently released for over-the-counter sale, appear to be effective for prevention and treatment of heartburn (gastroesophageal reflux). However, about 50 percent of patients do not find benefit, and PPIs are now used preferentially in the treatment of this disorder. Because H_2-receptor antagonists act by stopping acid secretion, they may not relieve symptoms for at least 45 minutes. Antacids more efficiently, but temporarily, neutralize secreted acid already in the stomach. Finally, tolerance to the effects of H_2 antagonists can be seen within 2 weeks of therapy.

3. **Pharmacokinetics:**

a. **Cimetidine:** *Cimetidine* and the other H_2 antagonists are given orally, distribute widely throughout the body (including into breast milk and across the placenta), and are excreted mainly in the urine (Figure 28.4). *Cimetidine* normally has a short serum half-life, which is increased in renal failure. Approximately 30 percent of a dose of *cimetidine* is slowly inactivated by the liver's

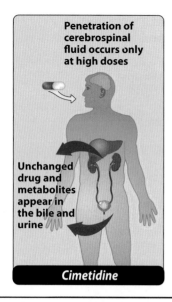

Figure 28.4
Administration and fate of *cimetidine*.

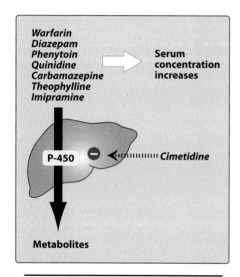

Figure 28.5
Drug interactions with *cimetidine*.

microsomal mixed-function oxygenase system (see p. 14) and can interfere in the metabolism of many other drugs; the other 70 percent is excreted unchanged in the urine. The dosage of all these drugs must be decreased in patients with hepatic or renal failure. *Cimetidine* inhibits cytochrome P450 and can slow metabolism (and, thus, potentiate the action) of several drugs (for example, *warfarin, diazepam, phenytoin, quinidine, carbamazepine, theophylline,* and *imipramine;* Figure 28.5), sometimes resulting in serious adverse clinical effects.

b. Ranitidine: Compared to *cimetidine, ranitidine* is longer acting and is five- to ten-fold more potent. *Ranitidine* has minimal side effects and does not produce the antiandrogenic or prolactin-stimulating effects of *cimetidine.* Unlike *cimetidine,* it does not inhibit the mixed-function oxygenase system in the liver and, thus, does not affect the concentrations of other drugs.

c. Famotidine: *Famotidine* is similar to *ranitidine* in its pharmacologic action, but it is 20 to 50 times more potent than *cimetidine,* and 3 to 20 times more potent than *ranitidine.*

d. Nizatidine: *Nizatidine* is similar to *ranitidine* in its pharmacologic action and potency. In contrast to *cimetidine, ranitidine,* and *famotidine,* which are metabolized by the liver, *nizatidine* is eliminated principally by the kidney. Because little first-pass metabolism occurs with *nizatidine,* its bioavailability is nearly 100 percent. No intravenous preparation is available.

4. **Adverse effects:** The adverse effects of *cimetidine* are usually minor and are associated mainly with the major pharmacologic activity of the drug—namely, reduced gastric acid production. Side effects occur only in a small number of patients and generally do not require discontinuation of the drug. The most common side effects are headache, dizziness, diarrhea, and muscular pain. Other central nervous system effects (confusion, hallucinations) occur primarily in elderly patients or after intravenous administration. *Cimetidine* can also have endocrine effects, because it acts as a nonsteroidal antiandrogen. These effects include gynecomastia, galactorrhea (continuous release/discharge of milk), and reduced sperm count. Except for *famotidine,* all these agents inhibit the gastric first-pass metabolism of ethanol. Drugs such as *ketoconazole,* which depend on an acidic medium for gastric absorption, may not be efficiently absorbed if taken with one of these antagonists.

D. Inhibitors of the H⁺/K⁺-ATPase proton pump

Omeprazole [oh-MEH-pra-zole] is the first of a class of drugs that bind to the H⁺/K⁺-ATPase enzyme system (proton pump) of the parietal cell, thereby suppressing secretion of hydrogen ions into the gastric lumen. The membrane-bound proton pump is the final step in the secretion of gastric acid (see Figure 28.3). Four additional PPIs are now available: *lansoprazole* [lan-SO-pra-zole], *rabeprazole* [rah-BEH-pra-zole], *pantoprazole* [pan-TOE-pra-zole], and *esomeprazole* [es-oh-MEH-pra-zole].

1. **Actions:** These agents are prodrugs with an acid-resistant enteric coating to protect them from premature degradation by gastric acid. The coating is removed in the alkaline duodenum, and the prodrug, a weak base, is absorbed and transported to the parietal cell canali-

culus. There, it is converted to the active form, which reacts with a cysteine residue of the H^+/K^+-ATPase, forming a stable covalent bond. It takes about 18 hours for the enzyme to be resynthesized. At standard doses, all PPIs inhibit both basal and stimulated gastric acid secretion by more than 90 percent. Acid suppression begins within 1 to 2 hours after the first dose of *lansoprazole* and slightly earlier with *omeprazole*. There is also an oral product containing *omeprazole* combined with *sodium bicarbonate* for faster absorption. It is available in powder to be dissolved in water and taken orally as well as in capsule form.

2. **Therapeutic uses:** The superiority of the PPIs over the H_2 antagonists for suppressing acid production and healing peptic ulcers has made them the preferred drugs for treating erosive esophagitis and active duodenal ulcer and for long-term treatment of pathologic hypersecretory conditions (for example, Zollinger-Ellison syndrome, in which a gastrin-producing tumor causes hypersecretion of HCl). They are approved for the treatment of GERD. Clinical studies have shown that PPIs reduce the risk of bleeding from an ulcer caused by *aspirin* and other NSAIDs. They are also successfully used with antimicrobial regimens to eradicate H. pylori. For maximum effect, PPIs should be taken 30 minutes before breakfast or the largest meal of the day. If an H_2-receptor antagonist is also needed, it should be taken well after the PPI for best effect. The H_2 antagonists will reduce the activity of the proton pump, and PPIs require active pumps to be effective. In patients with GERD in whom once-daily PPI is partially effective, increasing to a twice-daily regimen or keeping the PPI in the morning and adding an H_2 antagonist in the evening may improve symptom control.

3. **Pharmacokinetics:** All these agents are delayed-release formulations and are effective orally. [Note: Some are also available for intravenous injection.] Metabolites of these agents are excreted in urine and feces.

4. **Adverse effects:** The PPIs are generally well tolerated, but concerns about long-term safety have been raised due to the increased secretion of gastrin. In animal studies, the incidence of gastric carcinoid tumors increased, possibly related to the effects of prolonged hypochlorhydria and secondary hypergastrinemia. However, this has not been found in humans. Increased concentrations of viable bacteria in the stomach have been reported with continued use of these drugs. *Omeprazole* inhibits the metabolism of *warfarin, phenytoin, diazepam,* and *cyclosporine.* However, drug interactions are not a problem with the other PPIs. Prolonged therapy with agents that suppress gastric acid, such as the PPIs and H_2 antagonists, may result in low vitamin B_{12}, because acid is required for its absorption. Another problem with prolonged elevation of gastric pH is that calcium carbonate products require low gastric pH to be absorbed in the upper intestine. Increasing gastric pH increases the potential for incomplete absorption of calcium carbonate products. An effective option would be to use calcium citrate as a source of calcium by patients taking prolonged acid-suppressing medications. The absorption of the citrate salt is not affected by gastric pH. There are increased reports of diarrhea and Clostridium difficile colitis in community patients receiving PPIs; therefore, patients must be counseled to discontinue PPI therapy if they have diarrhea for several days and to contact their physicians for further follow-up.

E. Prostaglandins

Prostaglandin E_2, produced by the gastric mucosa, inhibits secretion of HCl and stimulates secretion of mucus and bicarbonate (cytoprotective effect). A deficiency of prostaglandins is thought to be involved in the pathogenesis of peptic ulcers. *Misoprostol* [mye-soe-PROST-ole], a stable analog of prostaglandin E_1, as well as some PPIs, are approved for prevention of gastric ulcers induced by NSAIDs (Figure 28.6). It is less effective than H_2 antagonists and the PPIs for acute treatment of peptic ulcers. Although *misoprostol* has cytoprotective actions, it is clinically effective only at higher doses that diminish gastric acid secretion. Routine prophylactic use of *misoprostol* may not be justified except in patients who are taking NSAIDs and are at high risk of NSAID-induced ulcers, such as the elderly or patients with ulcer complications. Like other prostaglandins, *misoprostol* produces uterine contractions and is contraindicated during pregnancy. Dose-related diarrhea and nausea are the most common adverse effects and limit the use of this agent.

F. Antimuscarinic agents (anticholinergic agents)

Muscarinic receptor stimulation increases gastrointestinal motility and secretory activity. A cholinergic antagonist, such as *dicyclomine* [dye-SYE-kloe-meen], can be used as an adjunct in the management of peptic ulcer disease and Zollinger-Ellison syndrome, particularly in patients who are refractory to standard therapies. However, its many side effects (for example, cardiac arrhythmias, dry mouth, constipation, and urinary retention) limit its use.

G. Antacids

Antacids are weak bases that react with gastric acid to form water and a salt, thereby diminishing gastric acidity. Because pepsin is inactive at a pH greater than 4, antacids also reduce pepsin activity.

1. **Chemistry of antacids:** Antacid products vary widely in their chemical composition, acid-neutralizing capacity, sodium content, palatability, and price. The acid-neutralizing ability of an antacid depends on its capacity to neutralize gastric HCl and on whether the stomach is full or empty (food delays stomach emptying, allowing more time for the antacid to react). Commonly used antacids are salts of aluminum and magnesium, such as *aluminum hydroxide* (usually a mixture of $Al(OH)_3$ and aluminum oxide hydrates) or *magnesium hydroxide* [$Mg(OH)_2$], either alone or in combination. *Calcium carbonate* [$CaCO_3$] reacts with HCl to form CO_2 and $CaCl_2$ and is a commonly used preparation. Systemic absorption of *sodium bicarbonate* [$NaHCO_3$] can produce transient metabolic alkalosis; therefore, this antacid is not recommended for long-term use.

2. **Therapeutic uses:** Aluminum- and magnesium-containing antacids are used for symptomatic relief of peptic ulcer disease and GERD; they may promote healing of duodenal ulcers, but the evidence for efficacy in the treatment of acute gastric ulcers is less compelling; therefore, these agents are used as last-line therapy. [Note: *Calcium carbonate* preparations are also used as calcium supplements for the treatment of osteoporosis.]

3. **Adverse effects:** *Aluminum hydroxide* tends to be constipating, and *magnesium hydroxide* tends to produce diarrhea. Preparations that combine these agents aid in normalizing bowel function. The

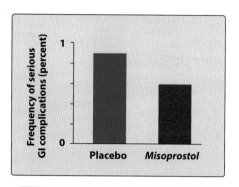

Figure 28.6
Misoprostol reduces serious gastrointestinal (GI) complications in patients with rheumatoid arthritis receiving nonsteroidal anti-inflammatory drugs.

binding of phosphate by aluminum-containing antacids can lead to hypophosphatemia. In addition to the potential for systemic alkalosis, *sodium bicarbonate* liberates CO_2, causing belching and flatulence. Absorption of the cations from antacids (Mg^{2+}, Al^{3+}, Ca^{2+}) is usually not a problem in patients with normal renal function, but the sodium content of antacids can be an important consideration in patients with hypertension or congestive heart failure. Adverse effects may also occur in patients with renal impairment, caused by accumulation of magnesium, calcium, sodium, and other electrolytes. Excessive intake of *calcium carbonate* along with calcium foods can result in hypercalcemia.

H. Mucosal protective agents

These compounds, known as cytoprotective compounds, have several actions that enhance mucosal protection mechanisms, thereby preventing mucosal injury, reducing inflammation, and healing existing ulcers.

1. **Sucralfate:** This complex of *aluminum hydroxide and sulfated sucrose* binds to positively charged groups in proteins of both normal and necrotic mucosa. By forming complex gels with epithelial cells, *sucralfate* [soo-KRAL-fate] creates a physical barrier that impairs diffusion of HCl and prevents degradation of mucus by pepsin and acid. It also stimulates prostaglandin release as well as mucus and bicarbonate output, and it inhibits peptic digestion. By these and other mechanisms, *sucralfate* effectively heals duodenal ulcers and is used in long-term maintenance therapy to prevent their recurrence. Because it requires an acidic pH for activation, *sucralfate* should not be administered with H_2 antagonists or antacids. Little of the drug is absorbed systemically. It is very well tolerated, but it can interfere with the absorption of other drugs by binding to them. This agent does not prevent NSAID-induced ulcers, nor does it heal gastric ulcers.

2. **Bismuth subsalicylate:** Preparations of this compound effectively heal peptic ulcers. In addition to their antimicrobial actions, they inhibit the activity of pepsin, increase secretion of mucus, and interact with glycoproteins in necrotic mucosal tissue to coat and protect the ulcer crater.

III. DRUGS USED TO CONTROL CHEMOTHERAPY- INDUCED EMESIS

Although nausea and vomiting may occur in a variety of conditions (for example, motion sickness, pregnancy, or hepatitis) and are always unpleasant for the patient, it is the nausea and vomiting produced by many chemotherapeutic agents that demand effective management. Nearly 70 to 80 percent of all patients who undergo chemotherapy experience nausea or vomiting. Several factors influence the incidence and severity of chemotherapy-induced emesis (Figure 28.7), including the specific chemotherapeutic drug, dose, route, schedule of administration, and patient variables. For example, the young and women are more susceptible than older patients and men, and 10 to 40 percent of patients experience nausea or vomiting in anticipation of their chemotherapy (anticipatory vomiting). Emesis not only affects the quality of life but can lead to rejection of potentially curative antineoplastic treatment. In addition, uncontrolled vomiting can produce dehydration, profound metabolic imbalances, and nutrient depletion.

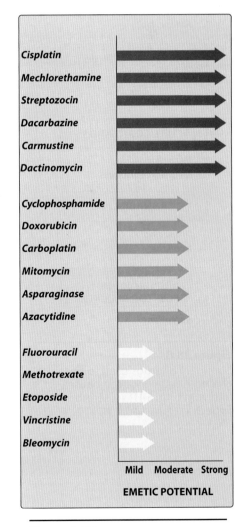

Figure 28.7
Comparison of emetic potential of anticancer drugs.

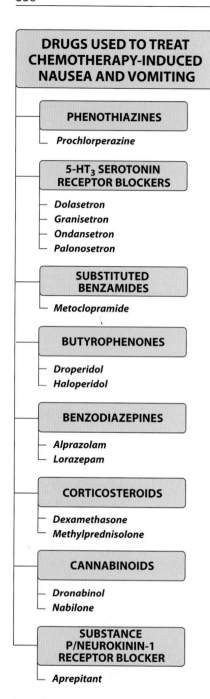

DRUGS USED TO TREAT CHEMOTHERAPY-INDUCED NAUSEA AND VOMITING

PHENOTHIAZINES
— *Prochlorperazine*

5-HT₃ SEROTONIN RECEPTOR BLOCKERS
— *Dolasetron*
— *Granisetron*
— *Ondansetron*
— *Palonosetron*

SUBSTITUTED BENZAMIDES
— *Metoclopramide*

BUTYROPHENONES
— *Droperidol*
— *Haloperidol*

BENZODIAZEPINES
— *Alprazolam*
— *Lorazepam*

CORTICOSTEROIDS
— *Dexamethasone*
— *Methylprednisolone*

CANNABINOIDS
— *Dronabinol*
— *Nabilone*

SUBSTANCE P/NEUROKININ-1 RECEPTOR BLOCKER
— *Aprepitant*

Figure 28.8
Summary of drugs used to treat chemotherapy-induced nausea and vomiting. 5-HT₃ = serotonin Type 3.

A. Mechanisms that trigger vomiting

Two brainstem sites have key roles in the vomiting reflex pathway. The chemoreceptor trigger zone, which is located in the area postrema (a circumventricular structure at the caudal end of the fourth ventricle) is outside the blood-brain barrier. Thus, it can respond directly to chemical stimuli in the blood or cerebrospinal fluid. The second important site, the vomiting center, which is located in the lateral reticular formation of the medulla, coordinates the motor mechanisms of vomiting. The vomiting center also responds to afferent input from the vestibular system, the periphery (pharynx and gastrointestinal tract), and higher brainstem and cortical structures. The vestibular system functions mainly in motion sickness.

B. Emetic actions of chemotherapeutic agents

Chemotherapeutic agents (or their metabolites) can directly activate the medullary chemoreceptor trigger zone or vomiting center; several neuroreceptors, including dopamine receptor Type 2 and serotonin Type 3 (5-HT₃), play critical roles. Often, the color or smell of chemotherapeutic drugs (and even stimuli associated with chemotherapy, such as cues in the treatment room or the physician or nurse who administers the therapy) can activate higher brain centers and trigger emesis. Chemotherapeutic drugs can also act peripherally by causing cell damage in the gastrointestinal tract and releasing serotonin from the enterochromaffin cells of the small intestinal mucosa. The released serotonin activates 5-HT₃ receptors on vagal and splanchnic afferent fibers, which then carry sensory signals to the medulla, leading to the emetic response.

C. Antiemetic drugs

Considering the complexity of the mechanisms involved in emesis, it is not surprising that antiemetics represent a variety of classes (Figure 28.8) and offer a range of efficacies (Figures 28.9). Anticholinergic drugs, especially the muscarinic receptor antagonist, *scopolamine*, and H₁-receptor antagonists, such as *dimenhydrinate, meclizine*, and *cyclizine*, are very useful in motion sickness but are ineffective against substances that act directly on the chemoreceptor trigger zone. The major categories of drugs used to control chemotherapy-induced nausea and vomiting include the following:

1. **Phenothiazines:** The first group of drugs shown to be effective antiemetic agents, phenothiazines, such as *prochlorperazine* [proe-klor-PER-ah-zeen], acts by blocking dopamine receptors. It is effective against low or moderately emetogenic chemotherapeutic agents (for example, *fluorouracil* and *doxorubicin*; see Figure 28.7). Although increasing the dose improves antiemetic activity, side effects, including hypotension and restlessness, are dose limiting. Other adverse reactions include extrapyramidal symptoms and sedation.

2. **5-HT₃ receptor blockers:** This class of agents commands an important place in treating emesis linked with chemotherapy. They have the advantage of a long duration of action. The specific antagonists of the 5-HT₃ receptor—*ondansetron* [on-DAN-seh-tron], *granisetron* [gra-NI-seh-tron], *palonosetron* [pa-low-NO-seh-tron] and *dolasetron* [dol-A-se-tron]—selectively block 5-HT₃ receptors in the periphery (visceral vagal afferent fibers) and in the brain (chemoreceptor trigger zone). These drugs can be administered as a single dose prior to chemotherapy (intravenously or orally) and are efficacious against

all grades of emetogenic therapy. One trial reported *ondansetron* and *granisetron* prevented emesis in 50 to 60 percent of *cisplatin*-treated patients. These agents are extensively metabolized by the liver, with hydroxydolasetron being an active metabolite of *dolasetron*. Thus, doses of these agents should be adjusted in patients with hepatic insufficiency. Elimination is through the urine. Headache is a common side effect. Electrocardiographic changes, such as prolongation of the QT interval, can occur with *dolasetron*; therefore, patients who may be at risk should receive this medication with caution. These drugs are costly.

3. **Substituted benzamides:** One of several substituted benzamides with antiemetic activity, *metoclopramide* [met-oh-kloe-PRAH-mide], is highly effective at high doses against the highly emetogenic *cisplatin*, preventing emesis in 30 to 40 percent of patients and reducing emesis in the majority. Antidopaminergic side effects, including sedation, diarrhea, and extrapyramidal symptoms, limit its high-dose use.

D2 antagonist

4. **Butyrophenones:** *Droperidol* [droe-PER-i-doll] and *haloperidol* [hal-oh-PER-i-doll] act by blocking dopamine receptors. The butyrophenones are moderately effective antiemetics. *Droperidol* had been used most often for sedation in endoscopy and surgery, usually in combination with opiates or benzodiazepines. However, it may prolong the QT interval, and current practice reserves it for patients whose response to other agents is inadequate. High-dose *haloperidol* was found to be nearly as effective as high-dose *metoclopramide* in preventing *cisplatin*-induced emesis.

5. **Benzodiazepines:** The antiemetic potency of *lorazepam* [lor-A-ze-pam] and *alprazolam* [al-PRAH-o-lam] is low. Their beneficial effects may be due to their sedative, anxiolytic, and amnesic properties. These same properties make benzodiazepines useful in treating anticipatory vomiting.

6. **Corticosteroids:** *Dexamethasone* [dex-a-MEH-tha-sone] and *methylprednisolone* [meth-ill-pred-NIH-so-lone], used alone, are effective against mildly to moderately emetogenic chemotherapy. Most frequently, however, they are used in combination with other agents. Their antiemetic mechanism is not known, but it may involve blockade of prostaglandins. These drugs can cause insomnia as well as hyperglycemia in patients with diabetes mellitus.

7. **Cannabinoids:** Marijuana derivatives, including *dronabinol* [droe-NAB-i-nol] and *nabilone* [NAB-il-own], are effective against moderately emetogenic chemotherapy. However, they are seldom first-line antiemetics because of their serious side effects, including dysphoria, hallucinations, sedation, vertigo, and disorientation. In spite of their psychotropic properties, the antiemetic action of cannabinoids may not involve the brain, because synthetic cannabinoids, which have no psychotropic activity, nevertheless are antiemetic.

8. **Substance P/neurokinin-1 receptor blocker:** *Aprepitant* [ah-PRE-pih-tant] belongs to a new family of antiemetic agents. It targets the neurokinin receptor in the brain and blocks the actions of the natural substance. *Aprepitant* is usually administered orally with *dexamethasone* and *palonosetron*. It undergoes extensive metabolism, primarily by CYP3A4. Thus, as would be expected, it can affect the metabolism of other drugs that are metabolized by this enzyme. *Aprepitant* can also induce this enzyme and, thus, affect responses

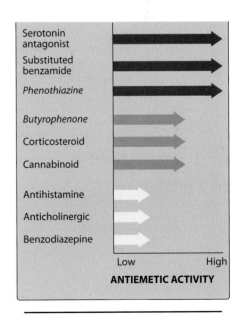

Figure 28.9
Potencies of antiemetic drugs.

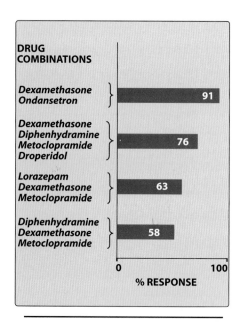

Figure 28.10
Effectiveness of antiemetic activity
of some drug combinations against
emetic episodes in the first 24 hours
after *cisplatin* chemotherapy.

to other agents; for example, concomitant use with *warfarin* can shorten the half-life of the anticoagulant. Constipation and fatigue appear to be the major side effects.

9. **Combination regimens:** Antiemetic drugs are often combined to increase antiemetic activity or decrease toxicity (Figure 28.10). Corticosteroids, most commonly *dexamethasone*, increase antiemetic activity when given with high-dose *metoclopramide*, a 5-HT$_3$ antagonist, *phenothiazine*, *butyrophenone*, a cannabinoid, or a benzodiazepine. Antihistamines, such as *diphenhydramine*, are often administered in combination with high-dose *metoclopramide* to reduce extrapyramidal reactions or with corticosteroids to counter *metoclopramide*-induced diarrhea.

IV. ANTIDIARRHEALS

Increased motility of the gastrointestinal tract and decreased absorption of fluid are major factors in diarrhea. Antidiarrheal drugs include antimotility agents, adsorbents, and drugs that modify fluid and electrolyte transport (Figure 28.11).

A. Antimotility agents

Two drugs that are widely used to control diarrhea are *diphenoxylate* [dye-fen-OX-see-late] and *loperamide* [loe-PER-ah-mide]. Both are analogs of *meperidine* and have opioid-like actions on the gut, activating presynaptic opioid receptors in the enteric nervous system to inhibit acetylcholine release and decrease peristalsis. At the usual doses, they lack analgesic effects. Side effects include drowsiness, abdominal cramps, and dizziness. Because these drugs can contribute to toxic megacolon, they should not be used in young children or in patients with severe colitis.

B. Adsorbents

Adsorbent agents, such as *bismuth subsalicylate*, *methylcellulose* [meth-ill-CELL-you-lowse], and *aluminum hydroxide* are used to control diarrhea. Presumably, these agents act by adsorbing intestinal toxins or microorganisms and/or by coating or protecting the intestinal mucosa. They are much less effective than antimotility agents. They can interfere with the absorption of other drugs.

C. Agents that modify fluid and electrolyte transport

Bismuth subsalicylate, used for traveler's diarrhea, decreases fluid secretion in the bowel. Its action may be due to its salicylate component as well as its coating action.

V. LAXATIVES

Laxatives are commonly used to accelerate the movement of food through the gastrointestinal tract. These drugs can be classified on the basis of their mechanism of action as irritants or stimulants of the gut, bulking agents, and stool softeners. They all have a risk of being habit-forming. Laxatives also increase the potential of loss of pharmacologic effect of poorly absorbed, delayed-acting, and extended-release oral preparations by accelerating their transit through the intestines. They may cause electrolyte imbalances when used chronically.

A. Irritants and stimulants

Senna is a widely used stimulant laxative. Its active ingredient is a group of sennosides, a natural complex of anthraquinone glycosides. Taken orally, it causes evacuation of the bowels within 8 to 10 hours. It also causes water and electrolyte secretion into the bowel. In combination products with a *docusate*-containing stool softener, it is useful in treating opioid-induced constipation. *Bisacodyl,* available as suppositories and enteric-coated tablets, is a potent stimulant of the colon. It acts directly on nerve fibers in the mucosa of the colon. Adverse effects include abdominal cramps and the potential for atonic colon with prolonged use. Antacids should not be taken at the same time as the enteric-coated tablets. The antacid would cause the enteric coating to dissolve prematurely in the stomach, resulting in stomach irritation and pain. The same adverse effects could be expected with milk, H_2-receptor antagonists, and PPIs. *Castor oil* is broken down in the small intestine to ricinoleic acid, which is very irritating to the gut, and promptly increases peristalsis. It should be avoided by pregnant patients, because it may stimulate uterine contractions.

B. Bulk laxatives

The bulk laxatives include hydrophilic colloids (from indigestible parts of fruits and vegetables). They form gels in the large intestine, causing water retention and intestinal distension, thereby increasing peristaltic activity. Similar actions are produced by *methylcellulose, psyllium seeds,* and *bran.* They should be used cautiously in patients who are bed-bound, due to the potential for intestinal obstruction.

C. Saline and osmotic laxatives

Saline cathartics, such as *magnesium citrate, magnesium sulfate, sodium phosphate*, and *magnesium hydroxide*, are nonabsorbable salts (anions and cations) that hold water in the intestine by osmosis and distend the bowel, increasing intestinal activity and producing defecation in a few hours. Electrolyte solutions containing *polyethylene glycol* (PEG) are used as colonic lavage solutions to prepare the gut for radiologic or endoscopic procedures. PEG powder for solution is available as a prescription and also an over-the-counter laxative. *Lactulose* is a semisynthetic disaccharide sugar that also acts as an osmotic laxative. It is a product that cannot be hydrolyzed by intestinal enzymes. Oral doses are degraded in the colon by colonic bacteria into lactic, formic, and acetic acids. This increases osmotic pressure, thereby accumulating fluid, distending the colon, creating a soft stool, and causing defecation.

D. Stool softeners (emollient laxatives or surfactants)

Surface-active agents that become emulsified with the stool produce softer feces and ease passage. These include *docusate sodium, docusate calcium*, and *docusate potassium*. They may take days to become effective. They should not be taken together with mineral oil because of the potential for absorption of the mineral oil.

E. Lubricant laxatives

Mineral oil and *glycerin suppositories* are considered to be lubricants. They facilitate the passage of hard stools. Mineral oil should be taken orally in an upright position to avoid its aspiration and potential for lipid or lipoid pneumonia.

DRUGS USED TO TREAT DIARRHEA AND CONSTIPATION

ANTIDIARRHEALS

- Aluminum hydroxide
- Bismuth subsalicylate
- Diphenoxylate
- Loperamide
- Methylcellulose

LAXATIVES

- Bisacodyl
- Bran
- Castor oil
- Docusate sodium
- Docusate calcium
- Glycerin suppositories
- Hydrophilic colloids
- Lactulose
- Magnesium citrate
- Magnesium hydroxide
- Magnesium sulfate
- Methylcellulose
- Mineral oil
- Polyethylene glycol
- Psyllium seeds
- Senna
- Sodium phosphate

Figure 28.11
Summary of drugs used to treat diarrhea and constipation.

Study Questions

Choose the ONE best answer.

28.1 A 68-year-old patient with cardiac failure is diagnosed with ovarian cancer. She is started on cisplatin but becomes nauseous and suffers from severe vomiting. Which of the following medications would be most effective to counteract the emesis in this patient without exacerbating her cardiac problem?

    A. Droperidol.
    B. Dolasetron.
    C. Prochlorperazine.
    D. Dronabinol.
    E. Ondansetron.

Correct answer = E. Ondansetron is a 5-HT$_3$ antagonist that is effective against drugs with high emetogenic activity, such as cisplatin. Although dolasetron is also in this category, its propensity to have effects on the heart makes it a poor choice for this patient. Droperidol also has effects on the heart and now is generally a second-line drug used in combination with opiates or benzodiazepines. The antiemetic effect of prochlorperazine, a phenothiazine, and dronabinol, a cannabinoid, are most beneficial against anticancer drugs with moderate to low emetogenic properties.

28.2 A 45-year-old woman is distressed by the dissolution of her marriage. She has been drinking heavily and overeating. She complains of persistent heartburn and an unpleasant, acid-like taste in her mouth. The clinician suspects gastrointestinal reflux disease and advises her to raise the head of her bed 6 to 8 inches, not to eat for several hours before retiring, to avoid alcohol, and to eat smaller meals. Two weeks later, she returns and says the symptoms have subsided slightly but still are a concern. The clinician prescribes:

    A. An antacid such as aluminum hydroxide.
    B. Dicyclomine.
    C. An antianxiety agent such as alprazolam.
    D. Esomeprazole.

Correct answer = D. It is appropriate to treat this patient with a PPI. Acid production would be reduced and healing promoted. An H$_2$-receptor antagonist might also be effective, but the PPIs are preferred. An antacid would decrease gastric acid, but its effects are short-lived compared to those of the PPIs and H$_2$-receptor inhibitors. Dicyclomine is an antimuscarinic drug and would decrease acid production, but it is not as effective as the PPIs or the H$_2$ receptor inhibitors. An antianxiety agent might have antiemetic action but would have no effect on the acid production.

28.3 Which of the following agents interferes with most of the cytochrome P450 enzymes and, thus, leads to many drug-drug interactions?

    A. Famotidine.
    B. Omeprazole.
    C. Cimetidine.
    D. Sucralfate.
    E. Ondansetron.

Correct answer = C. Cimetidine interferes in the metabolism of many drugs that are metabolized by the cytochrome P450 enzymes. These include warfarin, phenytoin, metoprolol, propranolol, calcium-channel blockers, and many others. Famotidine, another H$_2$-receptor antagonist, does not have this property, nor do the other drugs listed.

28.4 A couple celebrating their fortieth wedding anniversary is given a trip to Peru to visit Machu Picchu. Due to past experiences while traveling, they ask their doctor to prescribe an agent for diarrhea. Which of the following would be effective?

    A. Omeprazole.
    B. Loperamide.
    C. Famotidine.
    D. Lorazepam.

Correct answer = B. Loperamide is the only drug in this set that has antidiarrheal activity. Omeprazole is a PPI, famotidine antagonizes the H$_2$ receptor, and lorazepam is a benzodiazepine that is a sedative and anxiolytic agent.

Other Therapies

29

I. DRUGS USED TO TREAT ERECTILE DYSFUNCTION

Erectile dysfunction (ED)—that is, the inability to maintain penile erection for the successful performance of sexual activity—has many physical and psychological causes, including vascular disease, diabetes, medications, depression, and sequelae to prostatic surgery. ED is estimated to affect more than 30 million men in the United States. Previous therapies have included penile implants, intrapenile injections of *alprostadil*, and intraurethral suppositories of *alprostadil*. However, because of their efficacy, ease of use, and safety, oral phosphodiesterase (PDE) inhibitors are now considered to be first-line therapy for men with ED. Three PDE-5 inhibitors, *sildenafil* [sil-DEN-a-fil], *vardenafil* [var-DEN-na-fil], and *tadalafil* [ta-DAL-a-fil], are approved for the treatment of ED (Figure 29.1).

DRUGS FOR ERECTILE DYSFUNCTION

- ***Sildenafil***
- ***Tadalafil***
- ***Vardenafil***

DRUGS FOR OSTEOPOROSIS

- ***Alendronate***
- ***Calcitonin***
- ***Ibandronate***
- ***Risedronate***
- ***Raloxifene***
- ***Teriparatide***
- ***Zoledronic acid***

DRUGS FOR DISORDERS OF BONE REMODELING

- ***Etidronate***
- ***Pamidronate***
- ***Tiludronate***

DRUGS FOR OBESITY

- ***Diethylpropion***
- ***Orlistat***
- ***Phentermine***
- ***Sibutramine***

Figure 29.1
Summary of drugs used in the treatment of erectile dysfunction, osteoporosis, and obesity.

A. PDE-5 inhibitors

All three PDE-5 inhibitors are equally effective in treating ED, and the adverse effect profiles of the drugs are similar. However, the duration of action of PDE-5 inhibitors differ, as do the effects of food on the rates of drug absorption.

1. **Mechanism of penile erection:** Sexual stimulation results in smooth muscle relaxation of the corpus cavernosum, increasing the inflow of blood (Figure 29.2). The mediator of this response is nitric oxide (NO). NO activates guanylyl cyclase, which forms cyclic guanosine monophosphate (cGMP) from guanosine triphosphate. cGMP produces smooth muscle relaxation through a reduction in the intracellular Ca^{2+} concentration. The duration of action of cyclic nucleotides is controlled by the action of PDE. At least 11 isozymes of PDE have been characterized. *Sildenafil*, *vardenafil*, and *tadalafil* inhibit PDE-5, the isozyme responsible for degradation of cGMP in the corpus cavernosum. The action of PDE-5 inhibitors is to increase the flow of blood into the corpus cavernosum at any given level of sexual stimulation (Figure 29.3). At recommended doses, PDE-5 inhibitors have no effect in the absence of sexual stimulation. PDE-5 inhibitors are indicated for the treatment of ED due to organic or psychogenic causes.

2. **Pharmacokinetics:** *Sildenafil* and *vardenafil* have similar pharmacokinetic properties. Both drugs should be taken approximately 1 hour prior to anticipated sexual activity, with erectile enhancement observed up to 4 hours after administration. Thus, administration of *sildenafil* and *vardenafil* must be timed so that sexual activity occurs within 1 to 4 hours. The absorption of both drugs

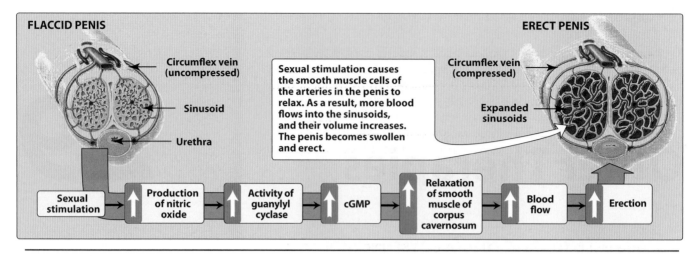

Figure 29.2
Mechanism of penile erection. cGMP = cyclic guanosine monophosphate.

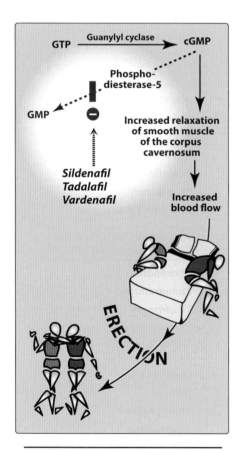

Figure 29.3
Effect of phosphodiesterase inhibitors on cyclic guanosine monophosphate (cGMP) levels in the smooth muscle of the corpus cavernosum. GTP = guanosine triphosphate.

is delayed by consumption of food, particularly high-fat meals. By contrast, *tadalafil* has a slower onset of action (Figure 29.4) but a significantly longer half-life of approximately 18 hours, resulting in enhanced erectile function for at least 36 hours. Furthermore, the absorption of *tadalafil* is not clinically influenced by food. The timing of sexual activity is less critical for *tadalafil* because of its prolonged duration of effect. All three PDE-5 inhibitors are metabolized by the cytochrome P450 3A4 (CYP3A4) enzyme. Dosage adjustments are recommended in patients with hepatic dysfunction.

3. **Adverse effects:** The most frequent adverse effects reported for PDE inhibitors are headache, flushing, dyspepsia, and nasal congestion. These effects are generally mild, and men with ED rarely discontinue treatment because of side effects. Disturbances in color vision (loss of blue/green discrimination) occur with *sildenafil*, probably because of inhibition of PDE-6 (a PDE found in the retina that is important in color vision). *Tadalafil* does not appear to disrupt PDE-6, and reports of changes in color vision have been rare with this medication. The incidence of these reactions appears to be dose dependent. Because there is an inherent cardiac risk associated with sexual activity, PDE-5 inhibitors should be used with caution in patients with a history of cardiovascular disease (CVD) or those with strong risk factors for CVD. PDE-5 inhibitors should not be used more than once per day.

4. **Drug interactions:** Because of the ability of PDE inhibitors to potentiate the activity of NO, administration of these agents in patients taking any form of organic nitrates is contraindicated. PDE-5 inhibitors may produce additive blood pressure–lowering effects when used in patients taking α-adrenergic antagonists (used to alleviate symptoms associated with benign prostatic hyperplasia). The combination of PDE-5 inhibitors and α-adrenergic antagonists should be used with caution. Patients should be on a stable dose of the α-adrenergic antagonist prior to the initiation of the PDE-5 inhibitor, and the PDE-5 inhibitor should be started at a low dose if this combination is to be used. Doses of PDE-5 inhibitors may need to be reduced in the presence of potent inhibitors of CYP3A4, such as protease inhibitors, *clarithromycin*, and *erythromycin*.

II. DRUGS USED TO TREAT OSTEOPOROSIS

Osteoporosis is a condition of skeletal fragility due to progressive loss of bone mass. It occurs in the elderly of both sexes but is most pronounced in postmenopausal women. Osteoporosis is characterized by frequent bone fractures, which are a major cause of disability among the elderly. Nondrug strategies to reduce bone loss in postmenopausal women include a diet adequate in calcium and vitamin D, weight-bearing exercise, and cessation of smoking. In addition, patients at risk for osteoporosis should avoid drugs that increase bone loss, such as glucocorticoids. Figure 29.5 shows the changes in bone morphology seen in osteoporosis.

A. Bisphosphonates

These analogs of pyrophosphate, including *etidronate* [e-TID-row-nate], *risedronate* [rih-SED-row-nate], *alendronate* [a-LEND-row-nate], *ibandronate* [eye-BAN-dro-nate], *pamidronate* [pah-MID-row-nate], *tiludronate* [till-UH-droe-nate], and *zoledronic* [zole-DROE-nick] *acid*, comprise an important drug group used for the treatment of disorders of bone remodeling, such as osteoporosis and Paget's disease, as well as for treatment of bone metastases and hypercalcemia of malignancy. In addition, *alendronate, risedronate,* and *ibandronate* have been approved for the prevention and treatment of osteoporosis. *Zoledronic acid* is also approved for the treatment of postmenopausal osteoporosis. The bisphosphonates decrease osteoclastic bone resorption via several mechanisms, including 1) inhibition of the osteoclastic proton pump necessary for dissolution of hydroxyapatite, 2) decrease in osteoclastic formation/activation, 3) increase in osteoclastic apoptosis (programmed cell death), and 4) inhibition of the cholesterol biosynthetic pathway important for osteoclast function. The relative importance of the mechanisms may differ among the individual bisphosphonates. The decrease in osteoclastic bone resorption results in a small but significant net gain in bone mass in osteoporotic patients, because the bone-forming osteoblasts are not inhibited. The beneficial effects of *alendronate* persist over several years of therapy (Figure 29.6), but discontinuation results in a gradual loss of its effects. Treatment with bisphosphonates decreases the risk of bone fracture in patients with osteoporosis. Bisphosphonates are preferred agents for the prevention and treatment of postmenopausal osteoporosis.

1. **Pharmacokinetics:** *Alendronate, risedronate,* and *ibandronate* are orally active agents for osteoporosis, although less than one percent of the administered dose is absorbed. *Alendronate* and *risedronate* may be dosed once daily or once weekly, whereas *ibandronate* is administered once monthly. Food significantly interferes with absorption. Bisphosphonates should be administered with 6 to 8 ounces of plain water at least 30 minutes (60 minutes for *ibandronate*) before eating breakfast or taking other medications. The bisphosphonates are rapidly cleared from the plasma, primarily because they avidly bind to the hydroxyapatite mineral of bone. Once bound to bone, they are cleared over a period of hours to years. Elimination from the body is primarily through renal clearance, and the bisphosphonates should not be given to individuals with severe renal impairment. For patients unable to tolerate oral bisphosphonates, intravenous *ibandronate* and *zoledronic acid* are alternative treatments for osteoporosis. Intravenous *ibandronate* is administered once every 3 months, and *zoledronic acid* is administered once yearly.

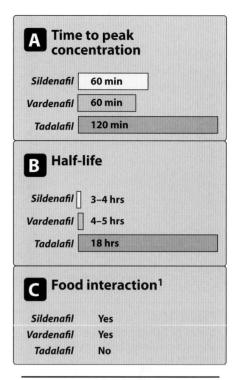

A Time to peak concentration

Sildenafil	60 min
Vardenafil	60 min
Tadalafil	120 min

B Half-life

Sildenafil	3–4 hrs
Vardenafil	4–5 hrs
Tadalafil	18 hrs

C Food interaction[1]

Sildenafil	Yes
Vardenafil	Yes
Tadalafil	No

Figure 29.4
Some properties of phosphodiesterase inhibitors. [1]Delay in time to reach peak drug concentration when taken with high-fat foods.

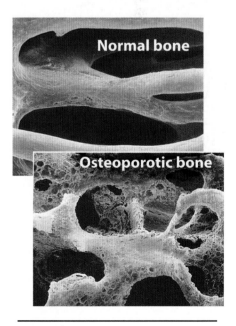

Normal bone

Osteoporotic bone

Figure 29.5
Changes in bone morphology seen in osteoporosis.

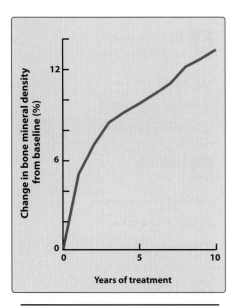

Figure 29.6
Effect of *alendronate* therapy on
the bone mineral density of the
lumbar spine.

Bisphosphonate	Antiresorptive activity
Etidronate	1
Pamidronate	100
Alendronate	1000
Risedronate	5,000
Ibandronate	10,000
Zoledronic acid	10,000

Figure 29.7
Antiresorptive activity of some
bisphosphonates.

2. **Adverse effects:** These include diarrhea, abdominal pain, and musculoskeletal pain. *Alendronate, risedronate, and ibandronate* are associated with esophagitis and esophageal ulcers. To minimize the risk of esophageal irritation, patients should remain upright for at least 30 minutes (60 minutes for *ibandronate*) after taking a bisphosphonate. Osteonecrosis of the jaw has been reported with bisphosphonates. *Etidronate* is the only member of the class that causes osteomalacia following long-term, continuous administration. Figure 29.7 shows the relative potencies of the bisphosphonates.

B. **Selective estrogen-receptor modulators**

Estrogen replacement is an effective therapy for the prevention of postmenopausal bone loss. When initiated in the immediate postmenopausal period, estrogen therapy prevents osteoporosis and reduces the risk of hip fracture. [Note: Estrogen-progestogen therapy is no longer the therapy of choice for the treatment of osteoporosis in postmenopausal women because of increased risk of breast cancer, stroke, venous thromboembolism, and coronary disease.] *Raloxifene* [rah-LOX-ih-feen] is a selective estrogen-receptor modulator approved for the prevention and treatment of osteoporosis. It increases bone density without increasing the risk of endometrial cancer. In addition, *raloxifene* may reduce the risk of invasive breast cancer. *Raloxifene* is a first-line alternative for postmenopausal osteoporosis in women who are intolerant to bisphosphonates. *Raloxifene* reduces serum total and low-density lipoprotein cholesterol concentrations. The risk of venous thromboembolism appears to be comparable to that with estrogen. Other adverse effects include hot flashes and leg cramps.

C. **Calcitonin**

Salmon *calcitonin* [cal-SIH-toe-nin], administered intranasally, is effective and well tolerated in the treatment of postmenopausal osteoporosis. The drug reduces bone resorption, but it is less effective than the bisphosphonates. A unique property of calcitonin is the relief of pain associated with osteoporotic fracture. Therefore, calcitonin may be beneficial in patients who have recently suffered a vertebral fracture. Common adverse effects of the intranasal formulation include rhinitis and other nasal symptoms. A parenteral formulation of *calcitonin* is available for intramuscular or subcutaneous injection, but it is infrequently used in the treatment of osteoporosis. Resistance to the effects of *calcitonin* has been observed with long-term use in patients with Paget's disease .

D. **Teriparatide**

Teriparatide [ter-ih-PAR-a-tide] is a recombinant segment of human parathyroid hormone that is administered subcutaneously for the treatment of osteoporosis. Parathyroid hormone given continuously leads to dissolution of bone, but when it is given subcutaneously once daily, bone formation is the predominant effect. It increases spinal bone density and decreases the risk of vertebral fracture. *Teriparatide* is the first approved treatment for osteoporosis that stimulates bone formation. Other drugs approved for this indication inhibit bone resorption. It is also effective in the treatment of glucocorticoid-induced osteoporosis. *Teriparatide* has been associated with an increased risk of osteosarcoma in rats. The safety and efficacy of this agent have not been evaluated beyond 24 months. *Teriparatide* should be reserved for patients at high risk of fractures or who cannot tolerate other osteoporosis therapies.

III. DRUGS USED TO TREAT OBESITY

Two classes of drugs are used in treating obesity: the anorexiants (appetite suppressants) *phentermine*, *diethylpropion*, and *sibutramine*, and a lipase inhibitor, *orlistat*. *Phentermine* and *diethylpropion* are indicated for short-term management of obesity. *Sibutramine* and *orlistat* have been approved for up to 2 and 4 years of use, respectively.

A. Phentermine, diethylpropion, and sibutramine

Phentermine [FEN-ter-meen] exerts its pharmacologic action by increasing release of norepinephrine and dopamine from the nerve terminals and by inhibiting reuptake of these neurotransmitters, thereby increasing levels of neurotransmitters in the brain. *Diethylpropion* [dye-eth-ill-PROE-pee-on] has similar effects on norepinephrine. *Sibutramine* [si-BYOO-tra-meen] inhibits central reuptake of serotonin, norepinephrine, and to a lesser extent, dopamine. Unlike the other agents, *sibutramine* does not cause the release of neurotransmitters. Figure 29.8 shows the effect of *sibutramine* treatment.

1. **Pharmacokinetics:** Limited information is available regarding the pharmacokinetics of *phentermine*. The duration of activity is dependent on the formulation, and the primary route of excretion is via the kidney. *Diethylpropion* is rapidly absorbed and undergoes extensive first-pass metabolism. Many of the metabolites are active. *Diethylpropion* and its metabolites are excreted mainly via the kidney. The half-life of the metabolites is 4 to 8 hours. *Sibutramine* undergoes first-pass demethylation to active metabolites, which are primarily responsible for its pharmacologic effects. The active metabolites are biotransformed further in the liver and excreted primarily in the urine. The half-life of the active metabolites is about 15 hours.

2. **Adverse effects and contraindications:** All of the appetite suppressants are Schedule IV controlled agents due to potential for dependence or abuse. Dry mouth, headache, insomnia, and constipation are common problems. Heart rate and blood pressure may be increased with these agents, and they should be avoided in patients with a history of hypertension, CVD, arrhythmias, congestive heart failure, or stroke. In addition, *phentermine* has been associated with heart valve disorders and pulmonary hypertension. Concomitant use of appetite suppressants and monoamine oxidase inhibitors should be avoided. *Sibutramine* should also be avoided in patients who are taking selective serotonin inhibitors such as *fluoxetine*, serotonin agonists for migraine such as *sumatriptan*, as well as *lithium*, *dextromethorphan*, or *pentazocine*. Drug interactions can occur when *sibutramine* is administered with drugs that inhibit CYP3A4, such as *ketoconazole*, *erythromycin*, and *cimetidine*. The clinical relevance of these interactions is not known.

B. Orlistat

Orlistat [OR-lih-stat] is the first drug in a class of antiobesity drugs known as lipase inhibitors. *Orlistat* is a pentanoic acid ester that inhibits gastric and pancreatic lipases, thus decreasing the breakdown of dietary fat into smaller molecules that can be absorbed. Fat absorption is decreased by about 30 percent. The loss of calories is the main cause of weight loss, but adverse gastrointestinal effects associated with the drug may also contribute to a decreased intake of food. *Orlistat* is administered

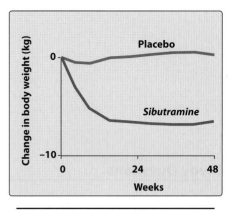

Figure 29.8
Effect of *sibutramine* treatment on body weight.

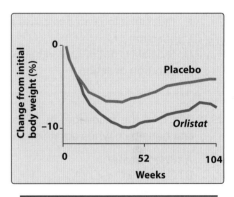

Figure 29.9
Effect of *orlistat* treatment on body weight.

three times daily with meals. Figure 29.9 shows the effects of *orlistat* treatment. The most common adverse effects associated with *orlistat* are gastrointestinal symptoms, such as oily spotting, flatulence with discharge, fecal urgency, and increased defecation. It interferes with the absorption of fat-soluble vitamins and β-carotene. Thus, patients should be advised to take a multivitamin supplement that contains vitamins A, D, E, and K and also β-carotene. The vitamin supplement should not be taken within 2 hours of orlistat. *Orlistat* is contraindicated in patients with chronic malabsorption syndrome or cholestasis.

Study Questions

Choose the ONE best answer.

29.1 A 66-year-old man complained of decreased libido and difficulty maintaining an erection. He is concerned about the use of drugs to restore sexual function, particularly about the need to time therapy with anticipated sexual activity. Which one of the following therapeutic options is indicated for this patient?

A. Sildenafil is indicated because of its long duration of action.
B. Vardenafil is indicated because its absorption is not affected by food.
C. Tadalafil is indicated because of its long duration of action
D. Tadalafil is not indicated because of its short duration of action.

> Correct answer = C. Tadalafil has a slow onset of action but a longer half-life of approximately 18 hours, resulting in enhanced erectile function for at least 36 hours. The timing of sexual activity is less critical for tadalafil because of its prolonged duration of effect.

29.2 Which of the following drugs causes osteomalacia and bone pain when administered chronically?

A. Risedronate.
B. Calcitonin.
C. Teriparatide.
D. Calcitriol.
E. Etidronate.

> Correct answer = E. The older bisphosphonates, such as etidronate, are not as potent inhibitors of osteoclast activity as the newer agents. Long-term therapy with etidronate also interferes with osteoblast activity, resulting in bone malformations and pain. The other drugs do not cause this problem.

29.3 A 58-year-old male has been effectively treated for Paget's disease for approximately 6 months. He is now beginning to experience renewed bone pain and radiologic evidence of advancing disease. Which of the following drugs is most likely to have resulted in this failure of therapy?

A. Alendronate.
B. Calcitonin.
C. Dihydrotachysterol.
D. Ergocalciferol.
E. Raloxifene.

> Correct answer = B. Paget's disease can be treated effectively with either a bisphosphonate or calcitonin. Calcitonin therapy is complicated by the fact that tolerance develops to the action of the hormone when administration is continuous over a long period of time. The other drugs are not effective in the treatment of Paget's disease.

Principles of Antimicrobial Therapy

30

I. OVERVIEW

Antimicrobial therapy takes advantage of the biochemical differences that exist between microorganisms and human beings. Antimicrobial drugs are effective in the treatment of infections because of their selective toxicity; that is, they have the ability to injure or kill an invading microorganism without harming the cells of the host. In most instances, the selective toxicity is relative rather than absolute, requiring that the concentration of the drug be carefully controlled to attack the microorganism while still being tolerated by the host.

II. SELECTION OF ANTIMICROBIAL AGENTS

Selection of the most appropriate antimicrobial agent requires knowledge of 1) the organism's identity, 2) the organism's susceptibility to a particular agent, 3) the site of the infection, 4) patient factors, 5) the safety of the agent, and 6) the cost of therapy. However, some critically ill patients require empiric therapy—that is, immediate administration of drug(s) prior to bacterial identification and susceptibility testing.

A. Identification of the infecting organism

Characterization of the organism is central to selection of the proper drug. A rapid assessment of the nature of the pathogen can sometimes be made on the basis of the Gram stain, which is particularly useful in identifying the presence and morphologic features of microorganisms in body fluids that are normally sterile (cerebrospinal fluid [CSF], pleural fluid, synovial fluid, peritoneal fluid, and urine). However, it is generally necessary to culture the infective organism to arrive at a conclusive diagnosis and to determine the susceptibility of the bacteria to antimicrobial agents. Thus, it is essential to obtain a sample culture of the organism prior to initiating treatment. Definitive identification of the infecting organism may require other laboratory techniques, such as detection of microbial antigens, microbial DNA

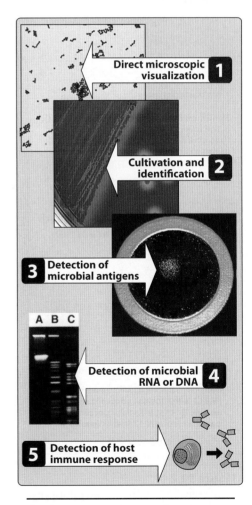

Figure 30.1
Some laboratory techniques that are useful in the diagnosis of microbia diseases.

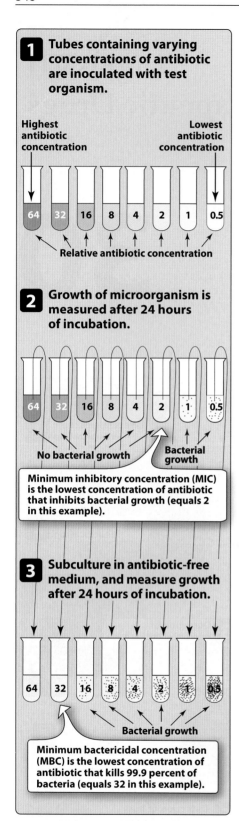

1 Tubes containing varying concentrations of antibiotic are inoculated with test organism.

Highest antibiotic concentration

Lowest antibiotic concentration

| 64 | 32 | 16 | 8 | 4 | 2 | 1 | 0.5 |

Relative antibiotic concentration

2 Growth of microorganism is measured after 24 hours of incubation.

| 64 | 32 | 16 | 8 | 4 | 2 | 1 | 0.5 |

No bacterial growth   Bacterial growth

Minimum inhibitory concentration (MIC) is the lowest concentration of antibiotic that inhibits bacterial growth (equals 2 in this example).

3 Subculture in antibiotic-free medium, and measure growth after 24 hours of incubation.

| 64 | 32 | 16 | 8 | 4 | 2 | 1 | 0.5 |

Bacterial growth

Minimum bactericidal concentration (MBC) is the lowest concentration of antibiotic that kills 99.9 percent of bacteria (equals 32 in this example).

Figure 30.2
Determination of minimum inhibitory concentration (MIC) and minimum bactericidal concentration (MBC) of an antibiotic.

or RNA, or detection of an inflammatory or host immune response to the microorganism (Figure 30.1).[1]

B. Empiric therapy prior to identification of the organism

Ideally, the antimicrobial agent used to treat an infection is selected after the organism has been identified and its drug susceptibility established. However, in the critically ill patient, such a delay could prove fatal, and immediate empiric therapy is indicated.

1. **Timing:** Acutely ill patients with infections of unknown origin—for example, a neutropenic patient (one who has a reduction in neutrophils, predisposing the patient to infections), or a patient with severe headache, a rigid neck, and sensitivity to bright lights (symptoms characteristic of meningitis)—require immediate treatment. Therapy is initiated after specimens for laboratory analysis have been obtained but before the results of the culture are available.

2. **Selecting a drug:** The choice of drug in the absence of susceptibility data is influenced by the site of infection and the patient's history (for example, whether the infection was hospital- or community-acquired, whether the patient is immunocompromised, as well as the patient's travel record and age). Broad-spectrum therapy may be needed initially for serious infections when the identity of the organism is unknown or the site makes a polymicrobial infection likely. The choice of agents may also be guided by known association of particular organisms with infection in a given clinical setting. For example, a gram-positive coccus in the spinal fluid of a newborn infant is unlikely to be Streptococcus pneumoniae (pneumococcus) and most likely to be Streptococcus agalactiae (Group B), which is sensitive to *penicillin G*. By contrast, a gram-positive coccus in the spinal fluid of a 40-year-old patient is most likely to be S. pneumoniae. This organism is frequently resistant to *penicillin G* and often requires treatment with a third-generation cephalosporin (such as *cefotaxime* or *ceftriaxone*) or *vancomycin*.

C. Determination of antimicrobial susceptibility of infective organisms

After a pathogen is cultured, its susceptibility to specific antibiotics serves as a guide in choosing antimicrobial therapy. Some pathogens, such as Streptococcus pyogenes and Neisseria meningitidis, usually have predictable susceptibility patterns to certain antibiotics. In contrast, most gram-negative bacilli, enterococci, and staphylococcal species often show unpredictable susceptibility patterns to various antibiotics and require susceptibility testing to determine appropriate antimicrobial therapy. The minimum inhibitory and bactericidal concentrations of a drug can be experimentally determined (Figure 30.2).

1. **Bacteriostatic vs. bactericidal drugs:** Antimicrobial drugs are classified as either bacteriostatic or bactericidal. Bacteriostatic drugs arrest the growth and replication of bacteria at serum levels achievable in the patient, thus limiting the spread of infection while the body's immune system attacks, immobilizes, and eliminates the pathogens. If the drug is removed before the immune system has

 [1] See Chapter 4 in ***Lippincott's Illustrated Reviews: Microbiology*** (2nd ed.) for a more detailed presentation of the techniques used in diagnostic microbiology.

scavenged the organisms, enough viable organisms may remain to begin a second cycle of infection. Bactericidal drugs kill bacteria at drug serum levels achievable in the patient. Because of their more aggressive antimicrobial action, these agents are often the drugs of choice in seriously ill patients. Figure 30.3 shows a laboratory experiment in which the growth of bacteria is arrested by the addition of a bacteriostatic agent. Note that viable organisms remain even in the presence of the bacteriostatic drug. By contrast, addition of a bactericidal agent kills bacteria, and the total number of viable organisms decreases. Although practical, this classification may be too simplistic, because it is possible for an antibiotic to be bacteriostatic for one organism and bactericidal for another. For example, *chloramphenicol* is bacteriostatic against gram-negative rods and is bactericidal against other organisms, such as <u>S. pneumoniae.</u>

2. **Minimum inhibitory concentration:** To determine the minimum inhibitory concentration (MIC), tubes containing serial dilutions of an antibiotic are inoculated with the organism whose susceptibility is to be tested (see Figure 30.2). The tubes are incubated and later observed to determine the MIC—that is, the lowest concentration of antibiotic that inhibits bacterial growth. To provide effective antimicrobial therapy, the clinically obtainable antibiotic concentration in body fluids should be greater than the MIC. [Note: This assay is now done automatically using microtiter plates.]

3. **Minimum bactericidal concentration:** This quantitative assay determines the minimum concentration of antibiotic that kills the bacteria under investigation. The tubes that show no growth in the MIC assay are subcultured into antibiotic-free media. The minimum bactericidal concentration is the lowest concentration of antimicrobial agent that results in a 99.9 percent decline in colony count after overnight broth dilution incubations (see Figure 30.2).

D. **Effect of the site of infection on therapy: The blood-brain barrier**

Adequate levels of an antibiotic must reach the site of infection for the invading microorganisms to be effectively eradicated. Capillaries with varying degrees of permeability carry drugs to the body tissues. For example, the endothelial cells comprising the walls of capillaries of many tissues have fenestrations (openings that act like windows) that allow most drugs not bound by plasma proteins to penetrate. However, natural barriers to drug delivery are created by the structures of the capillaries of some tissues, such as the prostate, the vitreous body of the eye, and the central nervous system (CNS). Of particular significance are the capillaries in the brain, which help to create and maintain the blood-brain barrier. This barrier is formed by the single layer of tile-like endothelial cells fused by tight junctions that impede entry from the blood to the brain of virtually all molecules, except those that are small and lipophilic (Figure 30.4). This barrier can be demonstrated by injecting dyes into laboratory animals. Dyes injected into the circulation stain all tissues except brain. However, the same dyes injected into the CSF stain only the cells of the CNS (Figure 30.5). The blood-brain barrier prevents the dye from escaping from the blood vessels in the brain, although they readily leak from the vessels throughout the rest of the body. The penetration and concentration of an antibacterial agent in the CSF is particularly influenced by the following:

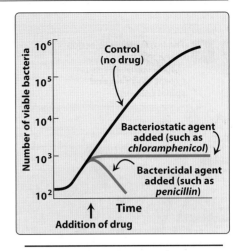

Figure 30.3
Effects of bactericidal and bacteriostatic drugs on the growth of bacteria in <u>vitro.</u>

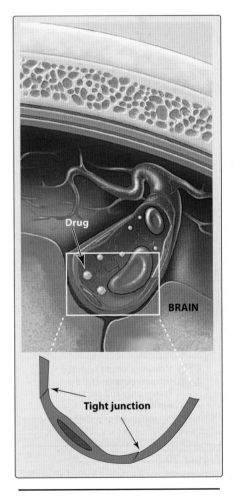

Figure 30.4
Essential features of the blood-brain barrier.

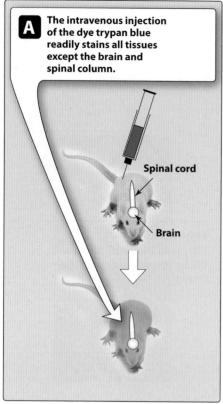

A The intravenous injection of the dye trypan blue readily stains all tissues except the brain and spinal column.

Spinal cord

Brain

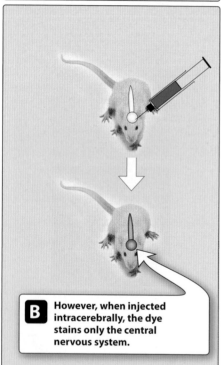

B However, when injected intracerebrally, the dye stains only the central nervous system.

Figure 30.5
Schematic representation of the blood-brain barrier.

1. **Lipid solubility of the drug:** All compounds without a specific transporter must pass intracellularly from the blood to the CSF (through two endothelial cell membranes; see Figure 30.5). The lipid solubility of a drug is therefore a major determinant of its ability to penetrate into the brain. For example, lipid-soluble drugs, such as the quinolones and *metronidazole*, have significant penetration into the CNS. In contrast, β-lactam antibiotics, such as *penicillin*, are ionized at physiologic pH and have low solubility in lipids. They therefore have limited penetration through the intact blood-brain barrier under normal circumstances. In infections such as meningitis, in which the brain becomes inflamed, the barrier does not function effectively, and local permeability is increased. Some β-lactam antibiotics can then enter the CSF in therapeutic amounts.

2. **Molecular weight of the drug:** A compound with a low molecular weight has an enhanced ability to cross the blood-brain barrier, whereas compounds with a high molecular weight (for example, *vancomycin*) penetrate poorly, even in the presence of meningeal inflammation.

3. **Protein binding of the drug:** A high degree of protein binding of a drug in the serum restricts its entry into the CSF. Therefore, the amount of free (unbound) drug in serum, rather than the total amount of drug present, is important for CSF penetration.

E. Patient factors

In selecting an antibiotic, attention must be paid to the condition of the patient. For example, the status of the patient's immune system, kidneys, liver, circulation, and age must be considered. In women, pregnancy or breast-feeding also affects selection of the antimicrobial agent.

1. **Immune system:** Elimination of infecting organisms from the body depends on an intact immune system. Antibacterial drugs decrease the microbial population (bactericidal) or inhibit further bacterial growth (bacteriostatic), but the host defense system must ultimately eliminate the invading organisms. Alcoholism, diabetes, infection with the human immunodeficiency virus, malnutrition, or advanced age can affect a patient's immunocompetence, as can therapy with immunosuppressive drugs. Higher-than-usual doses of bactericidal agents or longer courses of treatment are required to eliminate infective organisms in these individuals.

2. **Renal dysfunction:** Poor kidney function (10 percent or less of normal) causes accumulation in the body of antibiotics that ordinarily are eliminated by this route. This may lead to serious adverse effects unless drug accumulation is controlled by adjusting the dose or the dosage schedule of the antibiotic. Serum creatinine levels are frequently used as an index of renal function for adjustment of drug regimens.[2] However, direct monitoring of serum levels of some antibiotics (for example, aminoglycosides) is preferred to identify maximum and minimum values. Rising minimum values alert the physician to potential toxicity. [Note: The number of functioning nephrons

[2]See Chapter 287 in *Lippincott's Illustrated Reviews: Biochemitry* (4th ed.) for a discussion of creatinine.

decreases with age. Thus, elderly patients are particularly vulnerable to accumulation of drugs eliminated by the kidneys. Antibiotics that undergo extensive metabolism or are excreted via the biliary route may be favored in such patients.]

3. **Hepatic dysfunction:** Antibiotics that are concentrated or eliminated by the liver (for example, *erythromycin* and *tetracycline*) are contraindicated in treating patients with liver disease.

4. **Poor perfusion:** Decreased circulation to an anatomic area, such as the lower limbs of a diabetic, reduces the amount of antibiotic that reaches that area, making infections notoriously difficult to treat.

5. **Age:** Renal or hepatic elimination processes are often poorly developed in newborns, making neonates particularly vulnerable to the toxic effects of *chloramphenicol* and sulfonamides. Young children should not be treated with tetracyclines, which affect bone growth.

6. **Pregnancy:** All antibiotics cross the placenta. Adverse effects to the fetus are rare, except the for tooth dysplasia and inhibition of bone growth encountered with the tetracyclines. However, some anthelmintics are embryotoxic and teratogenic. Aminoglycosides should be avoided in pregnancy because of their ototoxic effect on the fetus. Figure 30.6 summarizes the U.S. Food and Drug Administration (FDA) categories of antibiotic use during pregnancy. The drug examples listed in Figure 30.6 are not all inclusive; they merely represent an example from each category. This current U.S. Food and Drug Administration category system can be difficult to apply to combination medications with many active ingredients and does not take into consideration the potential for any drug interactions. Of course, all drugs should be used only during pregnancy under the supervision of a patient's physician. Moreover, clinicians should reference the most current literature before prescribing medications for pregnant patients, to stay up-to-date for risk assessment reasons.

7. **Lactation:** Drugs administered to a lactating mother may enter the nursing infant via the breast milk. Although the concentration of an antibiotic in breast milk is usually low, the total dose to the infant may be enough to cause problems.

F. Safety of the agent

Many of the antibiotics, such as the penicillins, are among the least toxic of all drugs, because they interfere with a site unique to the growth of microorganisms. Other antimicrobial agents (for example, *chloramphenicol*) are less microorganism specific and are reserved for life-threatening infections because of the drug's potential for serious toxicity to the patient. [Note: As discussed above, safety is related not only to the inherent nature of the drug but also to patient factors that can predispose to toxicity.]

G. Cost of therapy

Often, several drugs may show similar efficacy in treating an infection but vary widely in cost. Figure 30.7 illustrates the cost of some antibacterial agents showing similar efficacy in eradicating the gram-negative bacillus <u>Helicobacter</u> <u>pylori</u> from the gastric mucosa. None of these agents shows a clear therapeutic superiority; thus, a combination of

CATE-GORY	DESCRIPTION	DRUG
A	No human fetal risk or remote possibility of fetal harm	
B	No controlled studies show human risk; animal studies suggest potential toxicity	β-Lactams β-Lactams with inhibitors Cephalosporins *Aztreonam Clindamycin Erythromycin Azithromycin Metronidazole Nitrofurantoin* Sulfonamides
C	Animal fetal toxicity demonstrated; human risk undefined	*Chloramphenicol Fluoroquinolones Clarithromycin Trimethoprim Vancomycin Gentamicin Trimethoprim-sulfa-methoxazole*
D	Human fetal risk present, but benefits outweigh risks	Tetracyclines Aminoglycosides (except *gentamicin*)
X	Human fetal risk present but does not outweigh benefits; contraindicated in pregnancy	

Figure 30.6
United States Food and Drug Administration categories of antimicrobials and fetal risk.

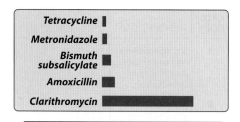

Figure 30.7
Relative cost of some drugs used for the treatment of peptic ulcers caused by <u>Helicobacter</u> <u>pylori</u>.

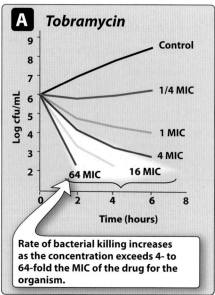

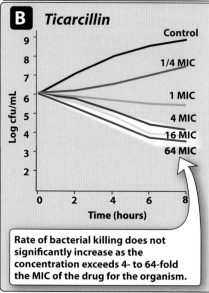

Figure 30.8
A. Significant dose-dependent killing effect shown by *tobramycin*. B. Nonsignificant dose-dependent killing effect shown by *ticarcillin*. cfu = colony forming units; MIC = minimum inhibitory concentration.

metronidazole with *bismuth subsalicylate* plus one other antibiotic is usually employed in the treatment of <u>H</u>. <u>pylori</u>–induced peptic ulcers. Selecting *clarithromycin* instead as the drug of choice would clearly make a considerable cost impact.

III. ROUTE OF ADMINISTRATION

The oral route of administration is chosen for infections that are mild and can be treated on an outpatient basis. In addition, economic pressures have prompted the use of oral antibiotic therapy in all but the most serious infectious diseases. In patients requiring a course of intravenous therapy initially, the switch to oral agents occurs as soon as possible. However, some antibiotics, such as *vancomycin*, the aminoglycosides, and *amphotericin B,* are so poorly absorbed from the gastrointestinal tract that adequate serum levels cannot be obtained by oral administration. Parenteral administration is used for drugs that are poorly absorbed from the gastrointestinal tract and for treatment of patients with serious infections, for whom it is necessary to maintain higher serum concentrations of antimicrobial agents than can be reliably obtained by the oral route.

IV. DETERMINANTS OF RATIONAL DOSING

Rational dosing of antimicrobial agents is based on their pharmacodynamics (the relationship of drug concentrations to antimicrobial effects) as well as their pharmacokinetic properties (the absorption, distribution, and elimination of the drug by the body). Three important properties that have a significant influence on the frequency of dosing are concentration-dependent killing, time-dependent killing, and postantibiotic effect. Utilizing these properties to optimize antibiotic dosing regimens will improve clinical outcomes and possibly decrease the development of resistance.

A. Concentration-dependent killing

Certain antimicrobial agents, including aminoglycosides, fluoroquinolones, and carbapenems show a significant increase in the rate of bacterial killing as the concentration of antibiotic increases from 4- to 64-fold the MIC of the drug for the infecting organism (Figure 30.8A). Giving drugs that exhibit this concentration-dependent killing by a once-a-day bolus infusion achieves high peak levels, favoring rapid killing of the infecting pathogen.

B. Time-dependent (concentration-independent) killing

By contrast, β-lactams, glycopeptides, macrolides, *clindamycin,* and *linezolid* do not exhibit this property; that is, increasing the concentration of antibiotic to higher multiples of the MIC does not significantly increase the rate of kill (Figure 30.8B). The clinical efficacy of antimicrobials that have a nonsignificant, dose-dependent killing effect is best predicted by the percentage of time that blood concentrations of a drug remain above the MIC. This effect is sometimes called concentration-independent or time-dependent killing. For example, for the penicillins and cephalosporins, dosing schedules that ensure blood levels greater than the MIC 60 to 70 percent of the time have been demonstrated to be clinically effective. Some experts therefore suggest that some severe infections are best treated by continuous infusion of these agents rather than by intermittent dosing.

C. Postantibiotic effect

The postantibiotic effect (PAE) is a persistent suppression of microbial growth that occurs after levels of antibiotic have fallen below the MIC. To measure the PAE of an antibiotic, a test culture is first incubated in antibiotic-containing medium and then transferred to antibiotic-free medium. The PAE is defined as the length of time it takes (after the transfer) for the culture to achieve log-phase growth.[3] Antimicrobial drugs exhibiting a long PAE (several hours) often require only one dose per day. For example, antimicrobials, such as aminoglycosides and fluoroquinolones, exhibit a long PAE, particularly against gram-negative bacteria.

V. AGENTS USED IN BACTERIAL INFECTIONS

In this book, the clinically useful antibacterial drugs are organized into six families—penicillins, cephalosporins, tetracyclines, aminoglycosides, macrolides, and fluoroquinolones—plus a seventh group labeled "Other" that is used to represent any drug not included in one of the other six drug families (Figure 30.9A). Here and throughout this book, these seven groups are graphically presented as a bar chart (as a "drug stack"). The drug(s) of choice within each family that is/are used for treating a specific bacterial infection are shown in bold print, as illustrated for <u>Staphylococcus</u> <u>aureus</u> in Figure 30.9B. A key to additional antibiotic symbols used in this book is shown in Figure 30.9C.

VI. CHEMOTHERAPEUTIC SPECTRA

In this book, the clinically important bacteria have been organized into eight groups based on Gram stain, morphology, and biochemical or other characteristics, and they are represented as wedges of a "pie chart" (Figure 30.10A). The ninth section of the bacterial pie chart is labeled "Other," and it is used to represent any organism not included in one of the other eight categories. In this chapter, the pie chart is used to illustrate the spectra of bacteria for which a particular class of antibiotics is therapeutically effective.

A. Narrow-spectrum antibiotics

Chemotherapeutic agents acting only on a single or a limited group of microorganisms are said to have a narrow spectrum. For example, *isoniazid* is active only against mycobacteria (Figure 30.10B).

B. Extended-spectrum antibiotics

Extended spectrum is the term applied to antibiotics that are effective against gram-positive organisms and also against a significant number of gram-negative bacteria. For example, *ampicillin* is considered to have an extended spectrum, because it acts against gram-positive and some gram-negative bacteria (Figure 30.10C).

C. Broad-spectrum antibiotics

Drugs such as *tetracycline* and *chloramphenicol* affect a wide variety of microbial species and are referred to as broad-spectrum antibiotics

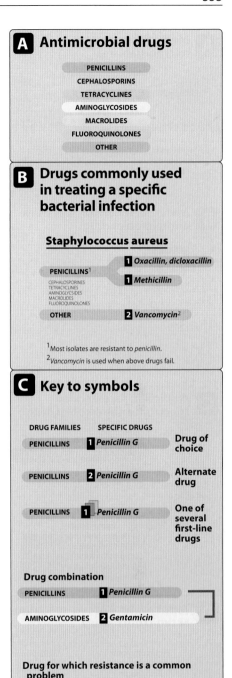

Figure 30.9
A. Bar chart showing the six most commonly used drug families.
B. An example of the bar chart with the drugs of choice for the treatment of <u>Staphylococcus</u> <u>aureus</u> shown in bold print. C. Key to symbols used in this book.

[3]See p. 54 in ***Lippincott's Illustrated Reviews: Microbiology*** (2nd ed.) for a discussion of the log phase of a bacterial growth curve.

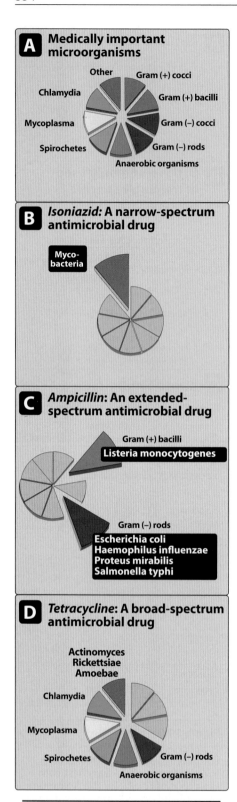

Figure 30.10
A. Color-coded representation of
medically important microorganisms.
B. *Isoniazid*, a narrow-spectrum
antimicrobial agent. C. *Ampicillin*,
an extended-spectrum antimicrobial
agent. D. *Tetracycline*, a broad-
spectrum antimicrobial agent.

(Figure 30.10D). Administration of broad-spectrum antibiotics can drasti-
cally alter the nature of the normal bacterial flora and precipitate a superinfection of an organism such as <u>Candida albicans</u>, the growth of which is
normally kept in check by the presence of other microorganisms.[4]

VII. COMBINATIONS OF ANTIMICROBIAL DRUGS

It is therapeutically advisable to treat patients with the single agent that is
most specific for the infecting organism. This strategy reduces the possibility of superinfection, decreases the emergence of resistant organisms (see
below), and minimizes toxicity. However, situations in which combinations
of drugs are employed do exist. For example, the treatment of tuberculosis
benefits from drug combinations.

A. Advantages of drug combinations

Certain combinations of antibiotics, such as β-lactams and aminoglycosides, show synergism; that is, the combination is more effective than
either of the drugs used separately. Because such synergism among
antimicrobial agents is rare, multiple drugs used in combination are
only indicated in special situations—for example, when an infection is
of unknown origin.

B. Disadvantages of drug combinations

A number of antibiotics act only when organisms are multiplying. Thus,
coadministration of an agent that causes bacteriostasis plus a second
agent that is bactericidal may result in the first drug interfering with the
action of the second. For example, bacteriostatic tetracycline drugs may
interfere with the bactericidal effect of penicillins and cephalosporins.

VIII. DRUG RESISTANCE

Bacteria are said to be resistant to an antibiotic if the maximal level of that
antibiotic that can be tolerated by the host does not halt their growth. Some
organisms are inherently resistant to an antibiotic. For example, gram-negative organisms are inherently resistant to *vancomycin*. However, microbial
species that are normally responsive to a particular drug may develop more
virulent, resistant strains through spontaneous mutation or acquired resistance and selection. Some of these strains may even become resistant to
more than one antibiotic.

A. Genetic alterations leading to drug resistance

Acquired antibiotic resistance requires the temporary or permanent
gain or alteration of bacterial genetic information. Resistance develops
due to the ability of DNA to undergo spontaneous mutation or to move
from one organism to another (Figure 30.11).

1. **Spontaneous mutations of DNA:** Chromosomal alteration may
    occur by insertion, deletion, or substitution of one or more nucle-
    otides within the genome.[5] The resulting mutation may persist, be
    corrected by the organism, or be lethal to the cell. If the cell survives,
    it can replicate and transmit its mutated properties to progeny cells.

[4]See p. 9 in ***Lippincott's Illustrated Reviews: Microbiology*** (2nd ed.) for a
discussion of the beneficial functions of normal flora.
[5]See p. 63 in ***Lippincott's Illustrated Reviews: Microbiology*** (2nd ed.) for a
discussion of DNA mutation.

Some spontaneous mutations have little or no effect on the susceptibility of the organism to antimicrobial agents. However, mutations that produce antibiotic-resistant strains can result in organisms that may proliferate under certain selective pressures. An example is the emergence of *rifampin*-resistant <u>Mycobacterium</u> <u>tuberculosis</u> when *rifampin* is used as a single antibiotic.

2. **DNA transfer of drug resistance:** Of particular clinical concern is resistance acquired due to DNA transfer from one bacterium to another. Resistance properties are usually encoded in extrachromosomal R factors (resistance plasmids). In fact, most resistance genes are plasmid mediated, although plasmid-mediated traits can become incorporated into host bacterial DNA. Plasmids may enter cells by processes such as transduction (phage mediated), transformation, or bacterial conjugation.[6]

B. **Altered expression of proteins in drug-resistant organisms**

Drug resistance may be mediated by a variety of mechanisms, such as a lack of or an alteration in an antibiotic target site, lowered penetrability of the drug due to decreased permeability, increased efflux of the drug, or presence of antibiotic-inactivating enzymes (see Figure 30.11).

[6]See p. 64 in ***Lippincott's Illustrated Reviews: Microbiology*** (2nd ed.) for a discussion of the integration of plasmid DNA into a host chromosome.

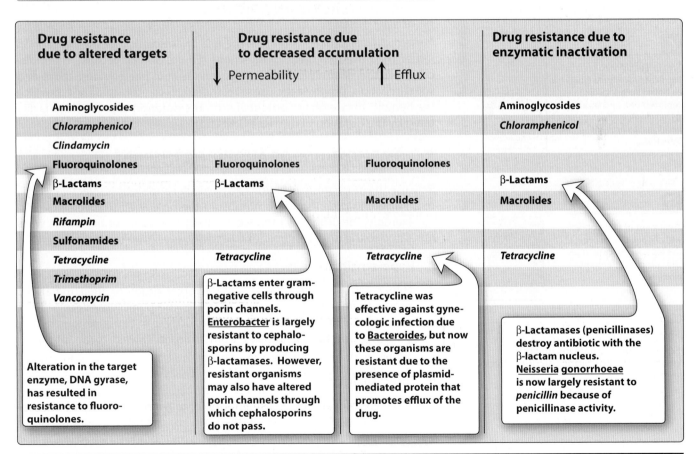

Drug resistance due to altered targets	Drug resistance due to decreased accumulation		Drug resistance due to enzymatic inactivation
	↓ Permeability	↑ Efflux	
Aminoglycosides			Aminoglycosides
Chloramphenicol			*Chloramphenicol*
Clindamycin			
Fluoroquinolones	Fluoroquinolones	Fluoroquinolones	
β-Lactams	β-Lactams		β-Lactams
Macrolides		Macrolides	Macrolides
Rifampin			
Sulfonamides			
Tetracycline	*Tetracycline*	*Tetracycline*	*Tetracycline*
Trimethoprim			
Vancomycin			

Alteration in the target enzyme, DNA gyrase, has resulted in resistance to fluoroquinolones.

β-Lactams enter gram-negative cells through porin channels. <u>Enterobacter</u> is largely resistant to cephalosporins by producing β-lactamases. However, resistant organisms may also have altered porin channels through which cephalosporins do not pass.

Tetracycline was effective against gynecologic infection due to <u>Bacteroides</u>, but now these organisms are resistant due to the presence of plasmid-mediated protein that promotes efflux of the drug.

β-Lactamases (penicillinases) destroy antibiotic with the β-lactam nucleus. <u>Neisseria gonorrhoeae</u> is now largely resistant to *penicillin* because of penicillinase activity.

Figure 30.11
Some mechanisms of resistance to antibiotics.

Prevention of strepto-coccal infections in patients with a history of rheumatic heart disease. Patients may require years of treatment.

Pretreatment of patients undergoing dental extractions who have implanted prosthetic devices, such as artificial heart valves, to prevent seeding of the prosthesis.

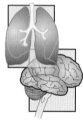

Prevention of tuber-culosis or meningitis among individuals who are in close contact with infected patients.

Treatment prior to certain surgical procedures (such as bowel surgery, joint replacement, and some gynecologic inter-ventions) to prevent infection.

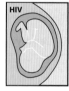

Treatment of the mother with *zidovudine* to protect the fetus in the case of an HIV-infected, pregnant woman.

Figure 30.12
Some clinical situations in which prophylactic antibiotics are indicated.

1. **Modification of target sites:** Alteration of an antibiotic's target site through mutation can confer organismal resistance to one or more related antibiotics. For example, S. pneumoniae resistance to β-lactam antibiotics involves alterations in one or more of the major bacterial *penicillin*-binding proteins, resulting in decreased binding of the antibiotic to its target.

2. **Decreased accumulation:** Decreased uptake or increased efflux of an antibiotic can confer resistance, because the drug is unable to attain access to the site of its action in sufficient concentrations to injure or kill the organism. For example, gram-negative organisms can limit the penetration of certain agents, including β-lactam anti-biotics, tetracyclines, and *chloramphenicol*, as a result of an altera-tion in the number and structure of porins (channels) in the outer membrane. Also, the presence of an efflux pump can limit levels of a drug in an organism.

3. **Enzymic inactivation:** The ability to destroy or inactivate the anti-microbial agent can also confer resistance on microorganisms. Examples of antibiotic-inactivating enzymes include 1) β-lactamases ("penicillinases") that hydrolytically inactivate the β-lactam ring of penicillins, cephalosporins, and related drugs; 2) acetyltransferases that transfer an acetyl group to the antibiotic, inactivating chloram-phenicol or aminoglycosides; and 3) esterases that hydrolyze the lactone ring of macrolides.

IX. PROPHYLACTIC ANTIBIOTICS

Certain clinical situations require the use of antibiotics for the prevention rather than the treatment of infections (Figure 30.12). Because the indis-criminate use of antimicrobial agents can result in bacterial resistance and superinfection, prophylactic use is restricted to clinical situations in which the benefits outweigh the potential risks. The duration of prophylaxis is dic-tated by the duration of the risk of infection.

X. COMPLICATIONS OF ANTIBIOTIC THERAPY

Because the mechanism of action of a particular antibiotic is selectively toxic to an invading organism does not insure the host against adverse effects. For example, the drug may produce an allergic response or be toxic in ways unrelated to the drug's antimicrobial activity.

A. Hypersensitivity

Hypersensitivity reactions to antimicrobial drugs or their metabolic products frequently occur. For example, the penicillins, despite their almost absolute selective microbial toxicity, can cause serious hyper-sensitivity problems, ranging from urticaria (hives) to anaphylactic shock.

B. Direct toxicity

High serum levels of certain antibiotics may cause toxicity by directly affecting cellular processes in the host. For example, aminoglycosides can cause ototoxicity by interfering with membrane function in the hair cells of the organ of Corti.

C. Superinfections

Drug therapy, particularly with broad-spectrum antimicrobials or combinations of agents, can lead to alterations of the normal microbial flora of the upper respiratory, intestinal, and genitourinary tracts, permitting the overgrowth of opportunistic organisms, especially fungi or resistant bacteria. These infections are often difficult to treat.

XI. SITES OF ANTIMICROBIAL ACTIONS

Antimicrobial drugs can be classified in a number of ways. These include 1) by their chemical structure (for example, β-lactams or aminoglycosides), 2) by their mechanism of action (for example, cell wall synthesis inhibitors), or 3) by their activity against particular types of organisms (for example, bacteria, fungi, or viruses). Chapters 31 through 33 are organized by the mechanisms of action of the drug, and Chapters 34 through 38 are organized according to the type of organisms affected by the drug (Figure 30.13).

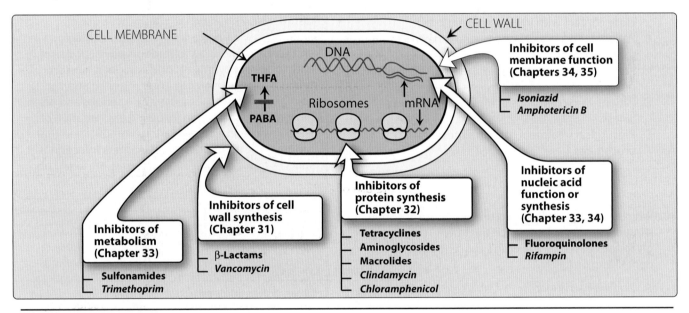

Figure 30.13
Classification of some antibacterial agents by their sites of action. (THFA = tetrahydrofolic acid; PABA = *p*-aminobenzoic acid)

Study Questions

Choose the ONE best answer.

30.1 Which one of the following patients is least likely to require antimicrobial treatment tailored to the individual's condition?

A. Patient undergoing cancer chemotherapy.
B. Patient with kidney disease.
C. Elderly patient.
D. Patient with hypertension.
E. Patient with liver disease.

Correct answer = D. Elevated blood pressure would not be expected to markedly influence the type of antimicrobial treatment employed. Anticancer drugs often suppress immune function, and these patients require additional antibiotics to eradicate infections. Impaired renal function may lead to accumulation of toxic levels of antimicrobial drugs. Renal and hepatic function are often decreased among the elderly. Impaired liver function may lead to the accumulation of toxic levels of antimicrobial drugs.

30.2 In which one of the following clinical situations is the prophylactic use of antibiotics not warranted?

A. Prevention of meningitis among individuals in close contact with infected patients.
B. Patient with a hip prosthesis who is having a tooth removed.
C. Presurgical treatment for implantation of a hip prosthesis.
D. Patient who complains of frequent respiratory illness.
E. Presurgical treatment in gastrointestinal procedures.

Correct answer = D. Respiratory illness may be of viral origin; furthermore, consequences of a chronic disorder may not warrant prophylactic use of antibiotics. Meningitis is a sufficiently contagious and serious disease to warrant prophylactic use of antibiotics. Following a tooth extraction, bacteria of the oral cavity can readily enter the circulation and colonize on a prosthesis, causing a serious and often fatal infection. Infection following implantation of a hip prosthesis is such a serious complication that prophylactic antibiotics are warranted. Infection is such a serious complication of gastrointestinal surgery that prophylactic antibiotics are warranted.

30.3 Which one of the following is the best route of administration/dosing schedule for treatment with aminoglycosides based on the drug's concentration-dependent killing property?

A. Oral every 8 hours.
B. Oral every 24 hours.
C. Parenterally by continuous intravenous infusion.
D. Parenterally every 8 hours.
E. Parenterally every 24 hours.

Correct answer = E. Giving a drug that exhibits concentration-dependent killing by once-a-day bolus infusion achieves high peak levels, favoring rapid killing of the infecting pathogen. The highly polar, polycationic structure of the aminoglycosides prevents adequate absorption after oral administration. Therefore, all aminoglycosides (except neomycin) must be given parenterally to achieve adequate serum levels.

Cell Wall Inhibitors

31

I. OVERVIEW

Some antimicrobial drugs selectively interfere with synthesis of the bacterial cell wall—a structure that mammalian cells do not possess. The cell wall is composed of a polymer called peptidoglycan that consists of glycan units joined to each other by peptide cross-links. To be maximally effective, inhibitors of cell wall synthesis require actively proliferating microorganisms; they have little or no effect on bacteria that are not growing and dividing. The most important members of this group of drugs are the β-lactam antibiotics (named after the β-lactam ring that is essential to their activity) and *vancomycin*. Figure 31.1 shows the classification of agents affecting cell wall synthesis.

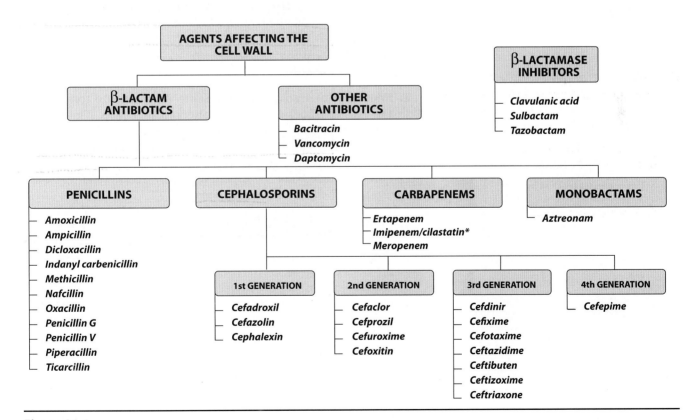

Figure 31.1
Summary of antimicrobial agents affecting cell wall synthesis. *Cilastatin* is not an antibiotic but a peptidase inhibitor that protects *imipenem* from degradation.

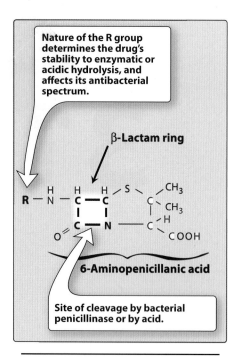

Figure 31.2
Structural features of β-lactam antibiotics.

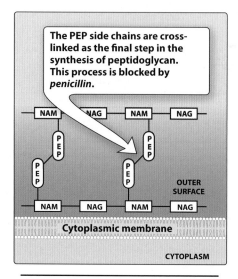

Figure 31.3
Bacterial cell wall of gram-positive bacteria. NAM = N-acetylmuramic acid; NAG = N-acetylglucosamine; PEP = cross-linking peptide.

II. PENICILLINS

The penicillins are among the most widely effective antibiotics and also the least toxic drugs known, but increased resistance has limited their use. Members of this family differ from one another in the R substituent attached to the 6-aminopenicillanic acid residue (Figure 31.2). The nature of this side chain affects the antimicrobial spectrum, stability to stomach acid, and susceptibility to bacterial degradative enzymes (β-lactamases).

A. Mechanism of action

The penicillins interfere with the last step of bacterial cell wall synthesis (transpeptidation or cross-linkage[1]), resulting in exposure of the osmotically less stable membrane. Cell lysis can then occur, either through osmotic pressure or through the activation of autolysins. These drugs are thus bactericidal. The success of a penicillin antibiotic in causing cell death is related to the antibiotic's size, charge, and hydrophobicity. Penicillins are only effective against rapidly growing organisms that synthesize a peptidoglycan cell wall. Consequently, they are inactive against organisms devoid of this structure, such as mycobacteria, protozoa, fungi, and viruses.

1. **Penicillin-binding proteins:** Penicillins inactivate numerous proteins on the bacterial cell membrane. These penicillin-binding proteins (PBPs) are bacterial enzymes involved in the synthesis of the cell wall and in the maintenance of the morphologic features of the bacterium. Exposure to these antibiotics can therefore not only prevent cell wall synthesis but also lead to morphologic changes or lysis of susceptible bacteria. The number of PBPs varies with the type of organism. Alterations in some of these target molecules provide the organism with resistance to the penicillins. [Note: *Methicillin*-resistant *Staphylococcus aureus* (MRSA) apparently arose because of such an alteration.]

2. **Inhibition of transpeptidase:** Some PBPs catalyze formation of the cross-linkages between peptidoglycan chains (Figure 31.3). Penicillins inhibit this transpeptidase-catalyzed reaction, thus hindering the formation of cross-links essential for cell wall integrity. As a result of this blockade of cell wall synthesis, the "Park nucleotide" (formerly called the "Park peptide"), UDP-acetylmuramyl-L-Ala-D-Gln-L-Lys-D-Ala-D-Ala, accumulates.

3. **Production of autolysins:** Many bacteria, particularly the gram-positive cocci, produce degradative enzymes (autolysins) that participate in the normal remodeling of the bacterial cell wall. In the presence of a penicillin, the degradative action of the autolysins proceeds in the absence of cell wall synthesis. [Note: The exact autolytic mechanism is unknown, but it may be due to a disinhibition of the autolysins.] Thus, the antibacterial effect of a penicillin is the result of both inhibition of cell wall synthesis and destruction of existing cell wall by autolysins.

[1]See p. 50 in *Lippincott's Illustrated Reviews: Microbiology* (2nd ed.) for a discussion of bacterial cell wall synthesis.

B. Antibacterial spectrum

The antibacterial spectrum of the various penicillins is determined, in part, by their ability to cross the bacterial peptidoglycan cell wall to reach the PBPs in the periplasmic space. Factors that determine the susceptibility of PBPs to these antibiotics include the size, charge, and hydrophobicity of the particular β-lactam antibiotic. In general, gram-positive microorganisms have cell walls that are easily traversed by penicillins and, therefore, in the absence of resistance are susceptible to these drugs. Gram-negative microorganisms have an outer lipopolysaccharide membrane (envelope) surrounding the cell wall that presents a barrier to the water-soluble penicillins. However, gram-negative bacteria have proteins inserted in the lipopolysaccharide layer that act as water-filled channels (called porins) to permit transmembrane entry. [Note: Pseudomonas aeruginosa lacks porins, making these organisms intrinsically resistant to many antimicrobial agents.]

1. **Natural penicillins:** These penicillins, which include those classified as antistaphylococcal, are obtained from fermentations of the mold Penicillium chrysogenum. Other penicillins, such as *ampicillin*, are called semisynthetic, because the different R groups are attached chemically to the 6-aminopenicillanic acid nucleus obtained from fermentation broths of the mold. *Penicillin* [pen-i-SILL-in] *G (benzylpenicillin)* is the cornerstone of therapy for infections caused by a number of gram-positive and gram-negative cocci, gram-positive bacilli, and spirochetes (Figure 31.4). *Penicillin G* is susceptible to inactivation by β-lactamases (penicillinases). *Penicillin V* has a spectrum similar to that of penicillin G, but it is not used for treatment of bacteremia because of its higher minimum bactericidal concentration (the minimum amount of the drug needed to eliminate the infection; see p. 343). *Penicillin V* is more acid-stable than *penicillin G*. It is often employed orally in the treatment of infections, where it is effective against some anaerobic organisms.

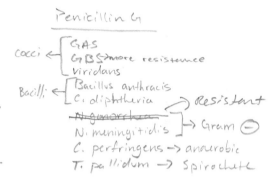

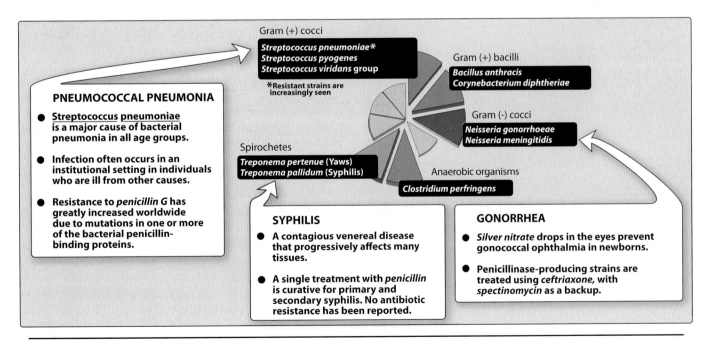

Figure 31.4
Typical therapeutic applications of *penicillin G*.

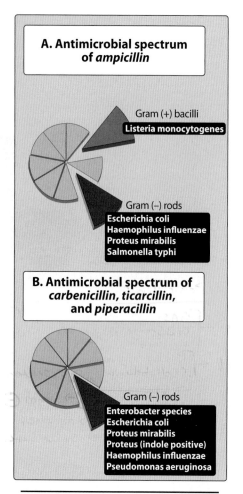

Figure 31.5
Typical therapeutic applications of *ampicillin* (A) and the antipseudomonal penicillins (B).

2. **Antistaphylococcal penicillins:** *Methicillin* [meth-i-SILL-in], *nafcillin* [naf-SILL-in], *oxacillin* [ox-a-SILL-in], and *dicloxacillin* [dye-klox-a-SILL-in] are penicillinase-resistant penicillins. Their use is restricted to the treatment of infections caused by penicillinase-producing staphylococci. [Note: Because of its toxicity, *methicillin* is not used clinically except to identify resistant strains of S. aureus]. Currently a serious source of nosocomial (hospital-acquired) infections, MRSA is usually susceptible to *vancomycin* and, rarely, to *ciprofloxacin* or *rifampin.*

3. **Extended-spectrum penicillins:** *Ampicillin* [am-pi-SILL-in] and *amoxicillin* [a-mox-i-SILL-in] have an antibacterial spectrum similar to that of *penicillin G* but are more effective against gram-negative bacilli. They are therefore referred to as extended-spectrum penicillins (Figure 31.5A). *Ampicillin* is the drug of choice for the gram-positive bacillus *Listeria monocytogenes*. These agents are also widely used in the treatment of respiratory infections, and *amoxicillin* is employed prophylactically by dentists for patients with abnormal heart valves who are to undergo extensive oral surgery. Resistance to these antibiotics is now a major clinical problem because of inactivation by plasmid-mediated penicillinase. [Note: *Escherichia coli* and *Haemophilus influenzae* are frequently resistant.] Formulation with a β-lactamase inhibitor, such as *clavulanic acid* or *sulbactam*, protects *amoxicillin* or *ampicillin*, respectively, from enzymatic hydrolysis and extends their antimicrobial spectrum.

4. **Antipseudomonal penicillins:** *Carbenicillin* [kar-ben-i-SILL-in], *ticarcillin* [tye-kar-SILL-in], and *piperacillin* [pip-er-a-SILL-in] are called antipseudomonal penicillins because of their activity against P. aeruginosa (Figure 31.5B). *Piperacillin* is the most potent of these antibiotics. They are effective against many gram-negative bacilli, but not against klebsiella, because of its constitutive penicillinase. Formulation of *ticarcillin* or *piperacillin* with *clavulanic acid* or *tazobactam*, respectively, extends the antimicrobial spectrum of these antibiotics to include penicillinase-producing organisms. (Figure 31.6 summarizes of the stability of the penicillins to acid or the action of penicillinase.)

5. **Penicillins and aminoglycosides:** The antibacterial effects of all the β-lactam antibiotics are synergistic with the aminoglycosides. Because cell wall synthesis inhibitors alter the permeability of bacterial cells, these drugs can facilitate the entry of other antibiotics (such as aminoglycosides) that might not ordinarily gain access to intracellular target sites. This can result in enhanced antimicrobial activity. [Note: Although the combination of a penicillin plus an aminoglycoside is used clinically, these drug types should never be placed in the same infusion fluid, because on prolonged contact, the positively charged aminoglycosides form an inactive complex with the negatively charged penicillins.]

C. **Resistance**

Natural resistance to the penicillins occurs in organisms that either lack a peptidoglycan cell wall (for example, mycoplasma) or have cell walls that are impermeable to the drugs. Acquired resistance to the penicillins by plasmid transfer has become a significant clinical problem, because an organism may become resistant to several antibiotics at the same time due to acquisition of a plasmid that encodes resistance to multiple agents. Multiplication of such an organism will lead to increased dissemination of the resistance genes. By obtaining a resistance plasmid, bacteria may acquire one or more of the following properties, thus allowing it to withstand β-lactam antibiotics.

1. **β-Lactamase activity:** This family of enzymes hydrolyzes the cyclic amide bond of the β-lactam ring, which results in loss of bactericidal activity (see Figure 31.2). They are the major cause of resistance to the penicillins and are an increasing problem. β-Lactamases are either constitutive or, more commonly, are acquired by the transfer of plasmids. Some of the β-lactam antibiotics are poor substrates for β-lactamases and resist cleavage, thus retaining their activity against β-lactamase producing organisms. [Note: Certain organisms may have chromosome-associated β-lactamases that are inducible by β-lactam antibiotics (for example, *cefoxitin*).] Gram-positive organisms secrete β-lactamases extracellularly, whereas gram-negative bacteria confine the enzymes in the periplasmic space between the inner and outer membranes.

2. **Decreased permeability to the drug:** Decreased penetration of the antibiotic through the outer cell membrane prevents the drug from reaching the target PBPs. The presence of an efflux pump can also reduce the amount of intracellular drug.

3. **Altered PBPs:** Modified PBPs have a lower affinity for β-lactam antibiotics, requiring clinically unattainable concentrations of the drug to effect inhibition of bacterial growth. This mechanism may explain MRSA, although it does not explain its resistance to non-β-lactam antibiotics like *erythromycin*, to which they are also refractory.

D. Pharmacokinetics

1. **Administration:** The route of administration of a β-lactam antibiotic is determined by the stability of the drug to gastric acid and by the severity of the infection.

   a. **Routes of administration:** *Ticarcillin, carbenicillin, piperacillin,* and the combinations of *ampicillin* with *sulbactam, ticarcillin* with *clavulanic acid,* and *piperacillin* with *tazobactam,* must be administered intravenously (IV) or intramuscularly (IM). *Penicillin V, amoxicillin, amoxicillin* combined with *clavulanic acid,* and the indanyl ester of *carbenicillin* (for treatment of urinary tract infections) are available only as oral preparations. Others are effective by the oral, IV, or IM routes (see Figure 31.6).

   b. **Depot forms:** *Procaine penicillin G* and *benzathine penicillin G* are administered IM and serve as depot forms. They are slowly absorbed into the circulation and persist at low levels over a long time period.

2. **Absorption:** Most of the penicillins are incompletely absorbed after oral administration, and they reach the intestine in sufficient amounts to affect the composition of the intestinal flora. However, *amoxicillin* is almost completely absorbed. Consequently, it is not appropriate therapy for the treatment of shigella- or salmonella-derived enteritis, because therapeutically effective levels do not

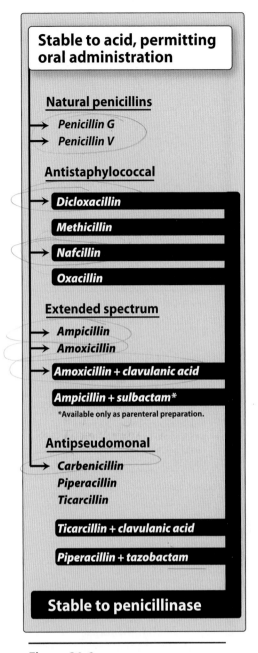

Figure 31.6
Stability of the penicillins to acid or the action of penicillinase.

Acid Stable Penicillins
Paid   Penicillin G
Pipers Penicillin V
Do   Dicloxacillin
Not   Nafcillin
Attempt Ampicillin
Any   Amoxicillin
Actual Amox + clav.
Crimes Carbenicillin

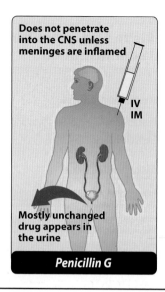

Figure 31.7
Administration and fate of
penicillin.

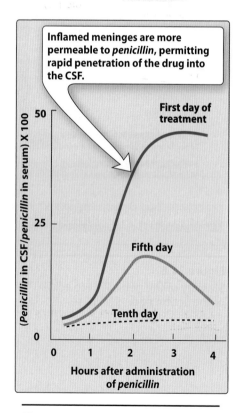

Figure 31.8
Enhanced penetration of *penicillin*
into the cerebral spinal fluid (CSF)
during inflammation.

reach the organisms in the intestinal crypts. Absorption of all the penicillinase-resistant penicillins is decreased by food in the stomach, because gastric emptying time is lengthened, and the drugs are destroyed in the acidic environment. Therefore, they must be administered 30 to 60 minutes before meals or 2 to 3 hours postprandially. Other penicillins are less affected by food.

3. **Distribution:** The β-lactam antibiotics distribute well throughout the body. All the penicillins cross the placental barrier, but none has been shown to be teratogenic. However, penetration into certain sites, such as bone or cerebrospinal fluid (CSF), is insufficient for therapy unless these sites are inflamed (Figures 31.7 and 31.8). [Note: During the acute phase of infection, the inflamed meninges are more permeable to the penicillins, resulting in an increased ratio of the amount of drug in the central nervous system compared to the amount in the serum. As the infection abates, inflammation subsides, and permeability barriers are reestablished.] *Penicillin* levels in the prostate are insufficient to be effective against infections.

4. **Metabolism:** Host metabolism of the β-lactam antibiotics is usually insignificant, but some metabolism of *penicillin G* has been shown to occur in patients with impaired renal function.

5. **Excretion:** The primary route of excretion is through the organic acid (tubular) secretory system of the kidney as well as by glomerular filtration. Patients with impaired renal function must have dosage regimens adjusted. Thus, the half-life of *penicillin G* can increase from a normal of between 30 minutes and 1 hour, to 10 hours in individuals with renal failure. *Probenecid* inhibits the secretion of penicillins by competing for active tubular secretion via the organic acid transporter and, thus, can increase blood levels. *Nafcillin* is eliminated primarily through the biliary route. [Note: This is also the preferential route for the acylureido penicillins in cases of renal failure.] The penicillins are also excreted into breast milk.

E. Adverse reactions

Penicillins are among the safest drugs, and blood levels are not monitored. However, the following adverse reactions may occur (Figure 31.9).

1. **Hypersensitivity:** This is the most important adverse effect of the penicillins. The major antigenic determinant of penicillin hypersensitivity is its metabolite, penicilloic acid, which reacts with proteins and serves as a hapten to cause an immune reaction. Approximately five percent of patients have some kind of reaction, ranging from maculopapular rash (the most common rash seen with *ampicillin* hypersensitivity) to angioedema (marked swelling of the lips, tongue, and periorbital area) and anaphylaxis. Among patients with mononucleosis who are treated with *ampicillin*, the incidence of maculopapular rash approaches 100 percent. Cross-allergic reactions occur among the β-lactam antibiotics.

2. **Diarrhea:** This effect, which is caused by a disruption of the normal balance of intestinal microorganisms, is a common problem. It occurs to a greater extent with those agents that are incompletely

absorbed and have an extended antibacterial spectrum. As with some other antibiotics, pseudomembranous colitis[2] may occur.

3. **Nephritis:** All penicillins, but particularly *methicillin*, have the potential to cause acute interstitial nephritis. [Note: *Methicillin* is therefore no longer available.]

4. **Neurotoxicity:** The penicillins are irritating to neuronal tissue, and they can provoke seizures if injected intrathecally or if very high blood levels are reached. Epileptic patients are particularly at risk.

5. **Hematologic toxicities:** Decreased coagulation may be observed with the antipseudomonal penicillins (*carbenicillin* and *ticarcillin*) and, to some extent, with *penicillin G*. It is generally a concern when treating patients who are predisposed to hemorrhage (for example, uremics) or those receiving anticoagulants. Additional toxicities include eosinophilia.

6. **Cation toxicity:** Penicillins are generally administered as the sodium or potassium salt. Toxicities may be caused by the large quantities of sodium or potassium that accompany the penicillin. Sodium excess may result in hypokalemia. This can be avoided by using the most potent antibiotic, which permits lower doses of drug and accompanying cations.

III. CEPHALOSPORINS

The cephalosporins are β-lactam antibiotics that are closely related both structurally and functionally to the penicillins. Most cephalosporins are produced semisynthetically by the chemical attachment of side chains to 7-aminocephalosporanic acid. Cephalosporins have the same mode of action as penicillins, and they are affected by the same resistance mechanisms. However, they tend to be more resistant than the penicillins to certain β-lactamases.

A. Antibacterial spectrum

Cephalosporins have been classified as first, second, third, or fourth generation, based largely on their bacterial susceptibility patterns and resistance to β-lactamases (Figure 31.10). [Note: Cephalosporins are ineffective against MRSA, L. monocytogenes, Clostridium difficile, and the enterococci.]

1. **First generation:** The first-generation cephalosporins act as *penicillin G* substitutes. They are resistant to the staphylococcal penicillinase and also have activity against Proteus mirabilis, E. coli, and Klebsiella pneumoniae (the acronym PEcK has been suggested).

2. **Second generation:** The second-generation cephalosporins display greater activity against three additional gram-negative organisms: H. influenzae, Enterobacter aerogenes, and some Neisseria species, whereas activity against gram-positive organisms is weaker (the acronym HENPEcK has been suggested with the second genera-

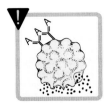

Hypersensitivity

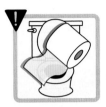

Diarrhea

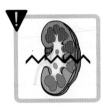

Nephritis

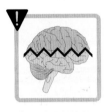

Neurotoxicity

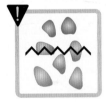

Hematologic toxicities

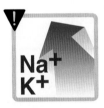

Cation toxicity

Figure 31.9
Summary of the adverse effects of *penicillin*.

1.) PEcK [+ Staph]
2) HENPEcK -Staph

[2]See p. 157 in *Lippincott's Illustrated Reviews: Microbiology* (2nd ed.) for a discussion of pseudomembranous colitis.

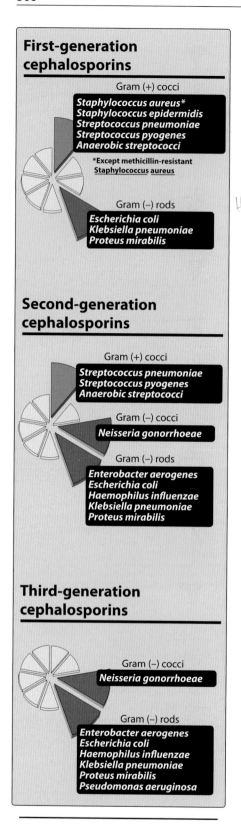

First-generation cephalosporins

Gram (+) cocci

*Staphylococcus aureus**
Staphylococcus epidermidis
Streptococcus pneumoniae
Streptococcus pyogenes
Anaerobic streptococci

*Except methicillin-resistant
Staphylococcus aureus

Gram (–) rods

Escherichia coli
Klebsiella pneumoniae
Proteus mirabilis

Second-generation cephalosporins

Gram (+) cocci

Streptococcus pneumoniae
Streptococcus pyogenes
Anaerobic streptococci

Gram (–) cocci

Neisseria gonorrhoeae

Gram (–) rods

Enterobacter aerogenes
Escherichia coli
Haemophilus influenzae
Klebsiella pneumoniae
Proteus mirabilis

Third-generation cephalosporins

Gram (–) cocci

Neisseria gonorrhoeae

Gram (–) rods

Enterobacter aerogenes
Escherichia coli
Haemophilus influenzae
Klebsiella pneumoniae
Proteus mirabilis
Pseudomonas aeruginosa

Figure 31.10
Summary of therapeutic applications of cephalosporins.

tion's increased coverage). [Note: The exception to this generalization is the structurally related cephamycin, *cefoxitin* [sef-OX-i-tin], which has little activity against H. influenzae yet is effective against the anaerobe Bacteroides fragilis [with some resistance occurring per 2007 antimicrobial guidelines.]

3. **Third generation:** These cephalosporins have assumed an important role in the treatment of infectious disease. Although inferior to first-generation cephalosporins in regard to their activity against gram-positive cocci, the third-generation cephalosporins have enhanced activity against gram-negative bacilli, including those mentioned above, as well as most other enteric organisms plus Serratia marcescens. *Ceftriaxone* [sef-trye-AKS-own] or *cefotaxime* [sef-oh-TAKS-eem] have become agents of choice in the treatment of meningitis. *Ceftazidime* [sef-TA-zi-deem] has activity against P. aeruginosa.

4. **Fourth generation:** *Cefepime* [SEF-eh-peem] is classified as a fourth-generation cephalosporin and must be administered parenterally. *Cefepime* has a wide antibacterial spectrum, being active against streptococci and staphylococci (but only those that are *methicillin*-susceptible). *Cefepime* is also effective against aerobic gram-negative organisms, such as enterobacter, E. coli, K. pneumoniae, P. mirabilis, and P. aeruginosa.

B. **Resistance**

Mechanisms of bacterial resistance to the cephalosporins are essentially the same as those described for the penicillins. [Note: Although they are not susceptible to hydrolysis by the staphylococcal penicillinase, cephalosporins may be susceptible to extended-spectrum β-lactamases.]

C. **Pharmacokinetics**

1. **Administration:** Many of the cephalosporins must be administered IV or IM (Figure 31.11) because of their poor oral absorption. Exceptions are noted in Figure 31.12.

2. **Distribution:** All cephalosporins distribute very well into body fluids. However, adequate therapeutic levels in the CSF, regardless of inflammation, are achieved only with the third-generation cephalosporins. For example, *ceftriaxone* or *cefotaxime* are effective in the treatment of neonatal and childhood meningitis caused by H. influenzae. *Cefazolin* [se-FA-zo-lin] finds application as a single prophylaxis dose prior to surgery because of its 1.8-hour half-life and its activity against penicillinase-producing S. aureus. However, additional intraoperative *cefazolin* doses may be required if the surgical procedure lasts longer than 3 hours. *Cefazolin* is effective for most surgical procedures, including orthopedic surgery because of its ability to penetrate bone. All cephalosporins cross the placenta.

3. **Fate:** Biotransformation of cephalosporins by the host is not clinically important. Elimination occurs through tubular secretion and/or glomerular filtration (see Figure 31.11). Therefore doses must be adjusted in cases of severe renal failure to guard against accumulation and toxicity. *Ceftriaxone* is excreted through the bile into the feces and, therefore, is frequently employed in patients with renal insufficiency.

D. Adverse effects

The cephalosporins produce a number of adverse affects, some of which are unique to particular members of the group.

1. Allergic manifestations: Patients who have had an anaphylactic response to penicillins should not receive cephalosporins. The cephalosporins should be avoided or used with caution in individuals who are allergic to penicillins (about 5–15 percent show cross-sensitivity). In contrast, the incidence of allergic reactions to cephalosporins is one to two percent in patients without a history of allergy to penicillins.

IV. OTHER β-LACTAM ANTIBIOTICS

A. Carbapenems

Carbapenems are synthetic β-lactam antibiotics that differ in structure from the penicillins in that the sulfur atom of the thiazolidine ring (see Figure 31.2) has been externalized and replaced by a carbon atom (Figure 31.13). *Imipenem* [i-mi-PEN-em], *meropenem* [mer-oh-PEN-em] and *ertapenem* [er-ta-PEN-em] are the only drugs of this group currently available. *Imipenem* is compounded with *cilastatin* to protect it from metabolism by renal dehydropeptidase.

1. Antibacterial spectrum: *Imipenem/cilastatin* and *meropenem* are the broadest-spectrum β-lactam antibiotic preparations currently available (Figure 31.14). *Imipenem* resists hydrolysis by most β-lactamases, but not the metallo-β-lactamases. The drug plays a role in empiric therapy because it is active against penicillinase-producing gram-positive and gram-negative organisms, anaerobes, and P. aeruginosa (although other pseudomonal strains are resistant, and resistant strains of P. aeruginosa have been reported to arise during therapy). *Meropenem* has antibacterial activity similar to that of *imipenem*. *Ertapenem* is not an alternative for P. aeruginosa coverage, because most strains exhibit resistance.

2. Pharmacokinetics: *Imipenem* and *meropenem* are administered IV and penetrate well into body tissues and fluids, including the CSF when the meninges are inflamed. They are excreted by glomerular filtration. *Imipenem* undergoes cleavage by a dehydropeptidase found in the brush border of the proximal renal tubule. This enzyme forms an inactive metabolite that is potentially nephrotoxic. Compounding the *imipenem* with *cilastatin* protects the parent drug and, thus, prevents the formation of the toxic metabolite. This allows the drug to be used in the treatment of urinary tract infections. *Meropenem* does not undergo metabolism. *Ertapenem* can be administered via IV or IM injection. [Note: Doses of these agents must be adjusted in patients with renal insufficiency.]

3. Adverse effects: *Imipenem/cilastatin* can cause nausea, vomiting, and diarrhea. Eosinophilia and neutropenia are less common than with other β-lactams. High levels of *imipenem* may provoke seizures, but *meropenem* is less likely to do so.

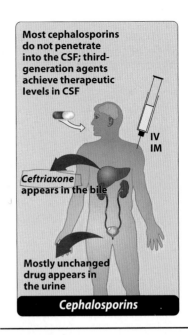

Most cephalosporins do not penetrate into the CSF; third-generation agents achieve therapeutic levels in CSF

IV IM

Ceftriaxone appears in the bile

Mostly unchanged drug appears in the urine

Cephalosporins

Figure 31.11
Administration and fate of the cephalosporins.

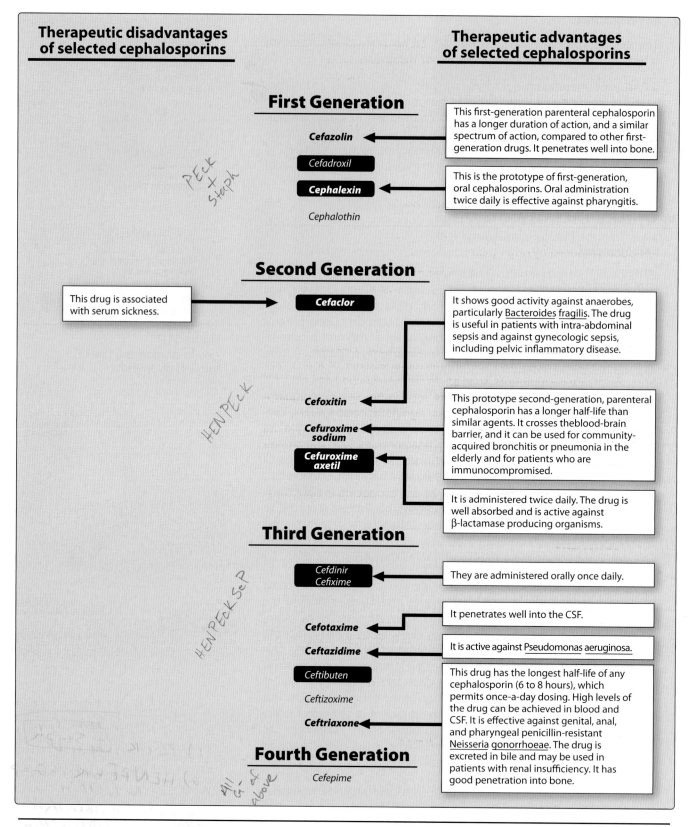

Figure 31.12
Characteristics of some clinically useful cephalosporins. [Note: Drugs that can be administered orally are shown in reverse type. More useful drugs shown in **bold**.] CSF = cerebrospinal fluid.

B. Monobactams

The monobactams, which also disrupt bacterial cell wall synthesis, are unique, because the β-lactam ring is not fused to another ring (see Figure 31.13). *Aztreonam* [az-TREE-oh-nam], which is the only commercially available monobactam, has antimicrobial activity directed primarily against the enterobacteriaceae, but it also acts against aerobic gram-negative rods, including P. aeruginosa. It lacks activity against gram-positive organisms and anaerobes. This narrow antimicrobial spectrum precludes its use alone in empiric therapy (see p. 342). *Aztreonam* is resistant to the action of β-lactamases. It is administered either IV or IM and is excreted in the urine. It can accumulate in patients with renal failure. *Aztreonam* is relatively nontoxic, but it may cause phlebitis, skin rash, and occasionally, abnormal liver function tests. This drug has a low immunogenic potential, and it shows little cross-reactivity with antibodies induced by other β-lactams. Thus, this drug may offer a safe alternative for treating patients who are allergic to penicillins and/or cephalosporins.

V. β-LACTAMASE INHIBITORS

Hydrolysis of the β-lactam ring, either by enzymatic cleavage with a β-lactamase or by acid, destroys the antimicrobial activity of a β-lactam antibiotic. β-Lactamase inhibitors, such as *clavulanic* [cla-vue-LAN-ick] *acid*, *sulbactam* [sul-BACK-tam], and *tazobactam* [ta-zoh-BACK-tam], contain a β-lactam ring but, by themselves, do not have significant antibacterial activity. Instead, they bind to and inactivate β-lactamases, thereby protecting the antibiotics that are normally substrates for these enzymes. The β-lactamase inhibitors are therefore formulated in combination with β-lactamase sensitive antibiotics. For example, Figure 31.15 shows the effect of *clavulanic acid* and *amoxicillin* on the growth of β-lactamase producing E. coli. [Note: *Clavulanic acid* alone is nearly devoid of antibacterial activity.]

VI. VANCOMYCIN

Vancomycin [van-koe-MYE-sin] is a tricyclic glycopeptide that has become increasingly important because of its effectiveness against multiple drug-resistant organisms, such as MRSA and enterococci. The medical community is presently concerned with emergence of *vancomycin* resistance in these organisms. [Note: *Bacitracin* [bass-i-TRAY-sin] is a mixture of polypeptides that also inhibits bacterial cell wall synthesis. It is active against a wide variety of gram-positive organisms. Its use is restricted to topical application because of its potential for nephrotoxicity with systemic use.]

A. Mode of action

Vancomycin inhibits synthesis of bacterial cell wall phospholipids as well as peptidoglycan polymerization by binding to the D-Ala-D-Ala side chain of the precursor pentapeptide. This prevents the transglycosylation step in peptidoglycan polymerization, thus weakening the cell wall and damaging the underlying cell membrane.

B. Antibacterial spectrum

Vancomycin is effective primarily against gram-positive organisms (Figure 31.16). It has been lifesaving in the treatment of MRSA and *methicillin*-resistant Staphylococcus epidermidis (MRSE) infections as well as enterococcal infections. With the emergence of resistant strains,

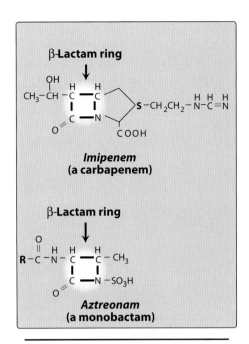

Figure 31.13
Structural features of *imipenem* and *aztreonam*.

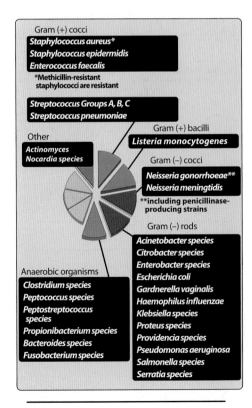

Figure 31.14
Antimicrobial spectrum of *imipenem*.

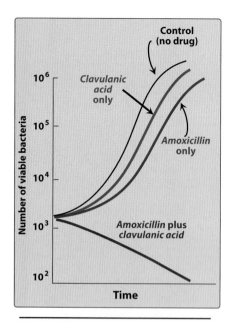

Figure 31.15
The in vitro growth of Escherichia coli in the presence of *amoxicillin*, with and without *clavulanic acid*.

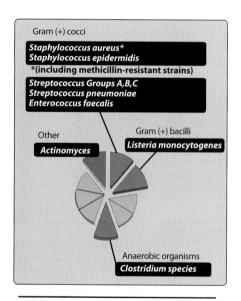

Figure 31.16
Antimicrobial spectrum of *vancomycin*.

it is important to curtail the increase in *vancomycin*-resistant bacteria (for example, Enterococcus faecium and Enterococcus faecalis) by restricting the use of *vancomycin* to the treatment of serious infections caused by β-lactam resistant, gram-positive microorganisms or for patients with gram-positive infections who have a serious allergy to the β-lactams. Oral *vancomycin* is limited to treatment for potentially life-threatening, antibiotic-associated colitis due to C. difficile or staphylococci. *Vancomycin* is used in individuals with prosthetic heart valves and in patients undergoing implantation with prosthetic devices. [Note: The latter is of particular concern in those hospitals where there is a problem with MRSA or MRSE. *Daptomycin*, a cyclic lipopeptide antibiotic, and two protein synthesis inhibitors—*quinopristin/dalfopristin* and *linezolid*—are currently available for the treatment of *vancomycin*-resistant organisms.] *Vancomycin* acts synergistically with the aminoglycosides, and this combination can be used in the treatment of enterococcal endocarditis.

C. Resistance

Vancomycin resistance can be caused by plasmid-mediated changes in permeability to the drug or by decreased binding of *vancomycin* to receptor molecules. [Note: An example of the latter is caused by the replacement of a D-Ala by D-lactate in resistant organisms.]

D. Pharmacokinetics

Slow IV infusion (60–90 minutes) is employed for treatment of systemic infections or for prophylaxis. Because *vancomycin* is not absorbed after oral administration, this route is employed only for the treatment of antibiotic-induced colitis due to C. difficile when *metronidazole* has proven to be ineffective. Inflammation allows penetration into the meninges. However, it is often necessary to combine *vancomycin* with other antibiotics, such as *ceftriaxone* for synergistic effects when treating menigits. Metabolism of the drug is minimal, and 90 to 100 percent is excreted by glomerular filtration (Figure 31.17). [Note: Dosage must be adjusted in renal failure, because the drug will accumulate. The normal half-life of *vancomycin* is 6 to 10 hours, compared to over 200 hours in end-stage renal disease.]

E. Adverse effects

Side effects are a serious problem with *vancomycin* and include fever, chills, and/or phlebitis at the infusion site. Flushing ("red man syndrome") and shock results from histamine release associated with a rapid infusion. If an infusion-related reaction occurs, slow the infusion rate to administer vancomycin over 2 hours, increase the dilution volume, or pretreat with an antihistamine 1 hour prior to administration. Additionally, reactions can be treated with antihistamines and steroids (Figure 31.18). Dose-related hearing loss has occurred in patients with renal failure who accumulate the drug. Ototoxicity and nephrotoxicity are more common when *vancomycin* is administered with another drug (for example, an aminoglycoside) that can also produce these effects.

VII. DAPTOMYCIN

Daptomycin [DAP-toe-mye-sin] is a cyclic lipopeptide antibiotic that is an alternative to other agents, such as *linezolid* and *quinupristin/dalfopristin*, for treating infections caused by resistant gram-positive organisms, including MRSA and vancomycin-resistant enterococci (VRE).

A. Mode of action

Upon binding to the bacterial cytoplasmic membrane, *daptomycin* induces rapid depolarization of the membrane, thus disrupting multiple aspects of membrane function and inhibiting intracellular synthesis of DNA, RNA, and protein. *Daptomycin* is bactericidal, and bacterial killing is concentration dependent.

B. Antibacterial spectrum

Daptomycin has a spectrum of activity limited to gram-positive organisms, which includes methicillin-susceptible and methicillin-resistant <u>S. aureus</u>, penicillin-resistant <u>Streptococcus pneumoniae</u>, <u>Streptococcus pyogenes</u>, <u>Corynebacterium jeikeium</u>, <u>E. faecalis</u>, and <u>E. faecium</u> (including VRE). *Daptomycin* is indicated for the treatment of complicated skin and skin structure infections and bacteremia caused by <u>S. aureus</u>, including those with right-sided infective endocarditis. Efficacy of treatment with *daptomycin* in left-sided endocarditis has not been demonstrated. Additionally, *daptomycin* is inactivated by pulmonary surfactants; thus, it is not indicated in the treatment of pneumonia.

C. Pharmacokinetics

Daptomycin is 90 to 95 percent protein bound and does not appear to undergo hepatic metabolism; however, the dosing interval needs to be adjusted in patients with renal impairment (creatinine clearance less than 30 mL/minute). In skin and soft tissue infections, *daptomycin* is administered at 4 mg/kg IV daily via a 30-minute infusion. Nevertheless, when treating bacteremia and endocarditis, dose should be increased to 6 mg/kg.

D. Adverse effects

The most common adverse effects reported in clinical trials included constipation, nausea, headache, and insomnia. Increased hepatic transaminases and also elevations in creatin phosphokinases occurred, suggesting weekly monitoring while the patient is receiving *daptomycin*. Although no clinically significant interactions have been identified, it is recommended to temporarily discontinue 3-hydroxy-3-methylglutary coenzyme A reductase inhibitors (statins) while receiving *daptomycin* due to the potential for additive muscle toxicity.

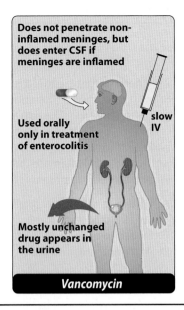

Figure 31.17
Administration and fate of *vancomycin*.

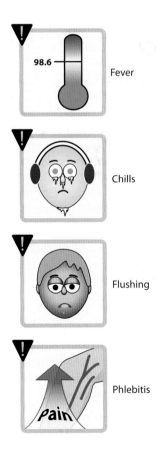

Figure 31.18
Some adverse effects of *vancomycin*.

Study Questions

Choose the ONE best answer

31.1 An elderly diabetic patient is admitted to the hospital with pneumonia. The sputum culture stains for a gram-negative rod. The patient is started on IV ampicillin. Two days later, the patient is not improving, and the microbiology laboratory reports the organism to be a β-lactamase producing H. influenzae. What course of treatment is indicated?

 A. Continue with the IV ampicillin.
 B. Switch to IV cefotaxime.
 C. Switch to oral vancomycin.
 D. Add gentamicin to the ampicillin therapy.

Correct answer = B. Cefotaxime, a third-generation cephalosporin, is not susceptible to hydrolysis by β-lactamase, is bactericidal, and has few adverse effects. To continue the ampicillin is not appropriate, because the organism is resistant to it. Vancomycin is used in the treatment of serious infections caused by β-lactamase resistant, gram-positive microorganisms (H. influenzae is gram-negative). Although gentamicin has some activity against H. influenzae, it also causes adverse effects, such as nephrotoxicity, which may harm the patient.

31.2 A 70-year-old alcoholic male with poor dental hygiene is to have his remaining teeth extracted for subsequent dentures. He has mitral valve stenosis with mild cardiac insufficiency and is being treated with captopril, digoxin, and furosemide. The dentist decides that his medical history warrants prophylactic antibiotic therapy prior to the procedure and prescribes which of the following drugs?

 A. Vancomycin.
 B. Amoxicillin.
 C. Tetracycline.
 D. Cotrimoxazole.
 E. Imipenem.

Correct answer = B. Multiple tooth extractions can lead to bacteremia, and the mitral valve stenosis and cardiac insufficiency place him at risk for developing endocarditis. The present American Heart Association guidelines indicate amoxicillin (2 g given 1 hour before procedure). Vancomycin is not an alternative medication currently listed as a prophylactic regimen for dental procedures. For penicillin-allergic patients, cephalexin, cefadroxil, clindamycin, clarithromycin or azithromycin are alternative medications listed as prophylactic regimens for dental procedures. Imipenem is also inappropriate, because its spectrum is too broad and only available IV.

31.3 A patient with degenerative joint disease is to undergo insertion of a hip prosthesis. To avoid complications due to postoperative infection, the surgeon will pretreat this patient with an antibiotic. This hospital has a significant problem with MRSA. Which of the following antibiotics should the surgeon select?

 A. Ampicillin.
 B. Imipenem/cilastatin.
 C. Gentamicin/piperacillin.
 D. Vancomycin.
 E. Cefazolin

Correct answer = D. The only antibiotic on the list that is effective against MRSA is vancomycin.

31.4 A 25-year-old male returns home from a holiday in the Far East and complains of 3 days of dysuria and a purulent urethral discharge. You diagnose this to be a case of gonorrhea. Which of the following is appropriate treatment?

 A. Ceftriaxone IM.
 B. Penicillin G IM.
 C. Gentamicin IM.
 D. Piperacillin/tazobactam IV.
 E. Vancomycin IV.

Correct answer = A. Most gonococcal infections are now resistant to penicillin, the previous drug of choice. The other antibiotics are inappropriate.

Protein Synthesis Inhibitors

32

I. OVERVIEW

A number of antibiotics exert their antimicrobial effects by targeting the bacterial ribosome, which has components that differ structurally from those of the mammalian cytoplasmic ribosome. In general, the bacterial ribosome is smaller (70S) than the mammalian ribosome (80S) and is composed of 50S and 30S subunits (as compared to 60S and 40S subunits). The mammalian mitochondrial ribosome, however, more closely resembles the bacterial ribosome. Thus, although drugs that interact with the bacterial target usually spare the host cells, high levels of drugs such as *chloramphenicol* or the tetracyclines may cause toxic effects as a result of interaction with the host mitochondrial ribosomes. Figure 32.1 lists the drugs discussed in this chapter.

II. TETRACYCLINES

The tetracyclines are a group of closely related compounds that, as the name implies, consist of four fused rings with a system of conjugated double bonds. Substitutions on these rings are responsible for variation in the drugs' individual pharmacokinetics, which cause small differences in their clinical efficacy.

A. Mechanism of action

Entry of these agents into susceptible organisms is mediated both by passive diffusion and by an energy-dependent transport protein mechanism unique to the bacterial inner cytoplasmic membrane. Nonresistant strains concentrate the tetracyclines intracellularly. The drug binds reversibly to the 30S subunit of the bacterial ribosome, thereby blocking access of the amino acyl-tRNA to the mRNA-ribosome complex at the acceptor site. By this mechanism, bacterial protein synthesis is inhibited (Figure 32.2).

B. Antibacterial spectrum

As broad-spectrum, bacteriostatic antibiotics, the tetracyclines are effective against gram-positive and gram-negative bacteria as well as against organisms other than bacteria. Tetracyclines are the drugs of choice for infections such as those shown in Figure 32.3.

C. Resistance

Widespread resistance to the tetracyclines limits their clinical use. The most commonly encountered, naturally occurring resistance

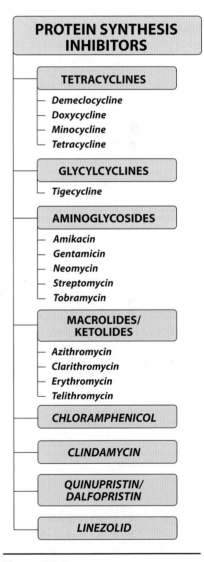

PROTEIN SYNTHESIS INHIBITORS

TETRACYCLINES
- *Demeclocycline*
- *Doxycycline*
- *Minocycline*
- *Tetracycline*

GLYCYLCYCLINES
- *Tigecycline*

AMINOGLYCOSIDES
- *Amikacin*
- *Gentamicin*
- *Neomycin*
- *Streptomycin*
- *Tobramycin*

MACROLIDES/ KETOLIDES
- *Azithromycin*
- *Clarithromycin*
- *Erythromycin*
- *Telithromycin*

CHLORAMPHENICOL

CLINDAMYCIN

QUINUPRISTIN/ DALFOPRISTIN

LINEZOLID

Figure 32.1
Summary of protein synthesis inhibitors.

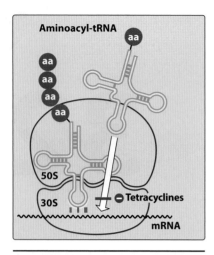

Figure 32.2
Tetracyclines binds to the 30S ribosomal subunit, thus preventing the binding of aminoacyl-tRNA to the ribosome. aa = amino acid.

("R") factor confers an inability of the organism to accumulate the drug, thus producing resistance. This is accomplished by Mg^{2+}-dependent, active efflux of the drug, mediated by the plasmid-encoded resistance protein, TetA. Other less important mechanisms of bacterial resistance to tetracyclines include enzymatic inactivation of the drug and production of bacterial proteins that prevent tetracyclines from binding to the ribosome. Any organism resistant to one tetracycline is resistant to all. The majority of penicillinase-producing staphylococci are now insensitive to tetracyclines.

D. Pharmacokinetics

1. **Absorption:** All tetracyclines are adequately but incompletely absorbed after oral ingestion (Figure 32.4). However, taking these drugs concomitantly with dairy foods in the diet decreases absorption due to the formation of nonabsorbable chelates of the tetracyclines with calcium ions. Nonabsorbable chelates are also formed with other divalent and trivalent cations (for example, those found in magnesium and aluminum antacids and in iron preparations). [Note: This presents a problem if a patient self-treats the epigastric upsets caused by tetracycline ingestion with antacids (Figure 32.5).] *Doxycycline* [dox-i-SYE-kleen] and *minocycline* [min-oh-SYE-kleen] are almost totally absorbed on oral administration. Currently, *doxycycline* is the preferred tetracycline for parenteral administration.

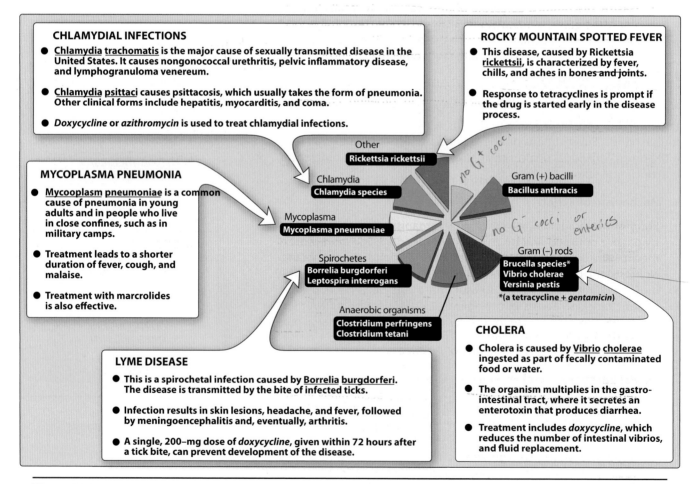

Figure 32.3
Typical therapeutic applications of tetracyclines.

2. **Distribution:** The tetracyclines concentrate in the liver, kidney, spleen, and skin, and they bind to tissues undergoing calcification (for example, teeth and bones) or to tumors that have a high calcium content (for example, gastric carcinoma). Penetration into most body fluids is adequate. Although all tetracyclines enter the cerebrospinal fluid (CSF), levels are insufficient for therapeutic efficacy, except for *minocycline*. *Minocycline* enters the brain in the absence of inflammation and also appears in tears and saliva. Although useful in eradicating the meningococcal carrier state, *minocycline* is not effective for central nervous system infections. All tetracyclines cross the placental barrier and concentrate in fetal bones and dentition.

3. **Fate:** All the tetracyclines concentrate in the liver, where they are, in part, metabolized and conjugated to form soluble glucuronides. The parent drug and/or its metabolites are secreted into the bile. Most tetracyclines are reabsorbed in the intestine via the enterohepatic circulation and enter the urine by glomerular filtration. Obstruction of the bile duct and hepatic or renal dysfunction can increase their half-lives. Unlike other tetracyclines, *doxycycline* can be employed for treating infections in renally compromised patients, because it is preferentially excreted via the bile into the feces. [Note: Tetracyclines are also excreted in breast milk.]

E. **Adverse effects**

1. **Gastric discomfort:** Epigastric distress commonly results from irritation of the gastric mucosa (Figure 32.6) and is often responsible for noncompliance in patients treated with these drugs. The discomfort can be controlled if the drug is taken with foods other than dairy products.

2. **Effects on calcified tissues:** Deposition in the bone and primary dentition occurs during calcification in growing children. This causes discoloration and hypoplasia of the teeth and a temporary stunting of growth.

3. **Fatal hepatotoxicity:** This side effect has been known to occur in pregnant women who received high doses of tetracyclines, especially if they were experiencing pyelonephritis.

4. **Phototoxicity:** Phototoxicity, such as severe sunburn, occurs when a patient receiving a tetracycline is exposed to sun or ultraviolet rays. This toxicity is encountered most frequently with *tetracycline* [tet-rah-SYE-kleen], *doxycycline*, and *demeclocycline* [dem-e-kloe-SYE-kleen].

5. **Vestibular problems:** These side effects (for example, dizziness, nausea, and vomiting) occur particularly with *minocycline*, which concentrates in the endolymph of the ear and affects function. *Doxycycline* may also cause vestibular effects.

6. **Pseudotumor cerebri:** Benign, intracranial hypertension characterized by headache and blurred vision may occur rarely in adults. Although discontinuation of the drug reverses this condition, it is not clear whether permanent sequelae may occur.

7. **Superinfections:** Overgrowths of Candida (for example, in the vagina) or of resistant staphylococci (in the intestine) may occur. Pseudomembranous colitis due to an overgrowth of Clostridium difficile has also been reported.

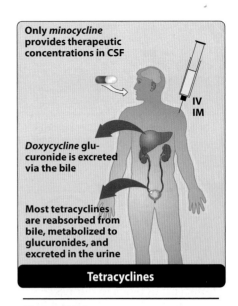

Figure 32.4
Administration and fate of tetracyclines.

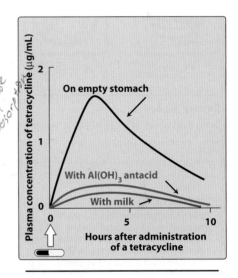

Figure 32.5
Effect of antacids and milk on the absorption of tetracyclines.

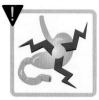

GI disturbance

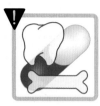

Deposition of
drug in bones
and teeth

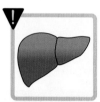

Liver failure

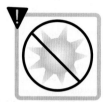

Photoxictiy

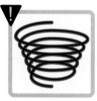

Vertigo

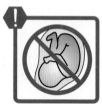

Avoid in pregnancy

Figure 32.6
Some adverse effects of *tetracycline*.

The aminoglycosides bind to the 30S
ribosomal subunit and distort its
structure, thus interfering with the
initiation of protein synthesis. They
also allow misreading of the mRNA,
causing mutations or premature chain
termination.

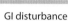

Figure 32.7
Mechanism of action of the aminoglycosides.

8. **Contraindications:** Renally impaired patients should not be treated with any of the tetracyclines except *doxycycline*. Accumulation of tetracyclines may aggravate preexisting azotemia (a higher-than-normal level of urea or other nitrogen-containing compounds in the blood) by interfering with protein synthesis, thus promoting amino acid degradation. The tetracyclines should not be employed in pregnant or breast-feeding women or in children less than 8 years of age.

III. GLYCYLCYCLINES

Tigecycline [tye-ge-SYE-kleen] is the first available member of a new class of antimicrobial agents called glycylcyclines. *Tigecycline*, a derivative of *minocycline*, is structurally similar to the tetracyclines and has a broad-spectrum activity against multidrug-resistant gram-positive pathogens, some gram-negative organisms, and anaerobic organisms. *Tigecycline* is indicated for treatment of complicated skin and soft tissue infections as well as complicated intra-abdominal infections.

A. Mechanism of action

Tigecycline exhibits bacteriostatic action by reversibly binding to the 30S ribosomal subunit and inhibiting protein translation.

B. Antibacterial spectrum — kills all but 3 Ps

Tigecycline exhibits expanded broad-spectrum activity that includes methicillin-resistant staphylococci, multidrug-resistant Streptococcus pneumoniae, and other susceptible strains of streptococcal species, *vancomycin*-resistant enterococci, extended-spectrum β-lactamase producing gram-negative bacteria, Acinetobacter baumannii, and many anaerobic organisms. However, *tigecycline* is not active against Proteus, Providencia, and Pseudomonas species.

C. Resistance

Tigecycline was developed to overcome the recent emergence of tetracycline class–resistant organisms that utilize efflux and ribosomal protection to infer resistance.

D. Pharmacokinetics

Following a 30- to 60-minute intravenous infusion every 12 hours, *tigecycline* is extensively distributed throughout plasma and body tissue. It does not undergo significant liver metabolism, but it is primarily eliminated via biliary/fecal excretion. No dose adjustment is necessary for patients who are renally impaired. However, dose adjustment is needed in severe hepatic dysfunction.

E. Adverse effects

Tigecycline is well tolerated, with the main adverse effects being similar to those of the tetracycline class. In clinical trials, the most commonly reported-class adverse effects were nausea and vomiting. Other similar tetracycline adverse effects that may occur with *tigecycline* include photosensitivity, pseudotumor cerebri, discoloration of permanent teeth when used during tooth development, and fetal harm when administered to a pregnant woman.

F. Drug interactions

The cytochrome P450 liver enzymes do not metabolize *tigecycline*; therefore, it will not be affected by medications that induce or inhibit these enzymes. Although *tigecycline* does not affect prothrombin time significantly, it has been found to inhibit the clearance of *warfarin*. Therefore, it is recommended that anticoagulation be monitored closely when *tigecycline* is coadministered with *warfarin*. No dose adjustment of *digoxin* is necessary with concomitant use of *tigecycline* even though *digoxin* C_{max} is increased. However, another method of contraception is suggested when *tigecycline* and oral contraceptives are coadministered, because the oral contraceptives may become less effective.

IV. AMINOGLYCOSIDES

Aminoglycoside antibiotics had been the mainstays for treatment of serious infections due to aerobic gram-negative bacilli. However, because their use is associated with serious toxicities, they have been replaced to some extent by safer antibiotics, such as the third- and fourth-generation cephalosporins, the fluoroquinolones, and the carbapenems. Aminoglycosides that are derived from Streptomyces have -mycin suffixes, whereas those derived from Micromonospora end in -micin. The terms "aminoglycoside" and "aminocyclitol" stem from their structure—two amino sugars joined by a glycosidic linkage to a central hexose (aminocyclitol) nucleus. Their polycationic nature precludes their easy passage across tissue membranes. All members of this family are believed to inhibit bacterial protein synthesis by the mechanism determined for *streptomycin* [strep-toe-MYE-sin] as described below.

A. Mechanism of action

Susceptible gram-negative organisms allow aminoglycosides to diffuse through porin channels in their outer membranes. These organisms also have an oxygen-dependent system that transports the drug across the cytoplasmic membrane. The antibiotic then binds to the 30S ribosomal subunit prior to ribosome formation (Figure 32.7). There, it interferes with assembly of the functional ribosomal apparatus and/or can cause the 30S subunit of the completed ribosome to misread the genetic code. Polysomes become depleted, because the aminoglycosides interrupt the process of polysome disaggregation and assembly. [Note: The aminoglycosides synergize with β-lactam antibiotics because of the latter's action on cell wall synthesis, which enhances diffusion of the aminoglycosides into the bacterium.]

B. Antibacterial spectrum

The aminoglycosides are effective in the empirical treatment of infections suspected of being due to aerobic gram-negative bacilli, including Pseudomonas aeruginosa. To achieve an additive or synergistic effect, aminoglycosides are often combined with a β-lactam antibiotic, or *vancomycin*, or a drug active against anaerobic bacteria. All aminoglycosides are bactericidal. The exact mechanism of their lethality is unknown because other antibiotics that affect protein synthesis are generally bacteriostatic. [Note: The aminoglycosides are effective only against aerobic organisms because strict anaerobes lack the oxygen-requiring drug transport system.] Some therapeutic applications of four commonly used aminoglycosides—*amikacin* [am-i KAY-sin], *gentamicin* [jen-ta-MYE-sin], *tobramycin* [toe-bra-MYE-sin], and *streptomycin*—are shown in Figure 32.8.

TULAREMIA

- Tularemia is commonly acquired during rabbit-hunting season by hunters skinning infected animals.

- Pneumonic tularemia results from infection by the respiratory route or by bacteremic seeding of lung.

- *Gentamicin* is effective in treating this rare lymphoid disease.

INFECTIONS DUE TO ENTEROCOCCI

- Enterococci are intrinsically resistant to most antibiotic classes and require two synergistic antibiotics for effective therapy.

- Recommended therapy is with *gentamicin* or *streptomycin* plus *vancomycin* or a β-lactam, such as *penicillin G*.

Gram (+) cocci

Enterococcus species
(*gentamicin + penicillin G*)
Streptococcus agalactiae
(*gentamicin + penicillin G*)

Gram (–) rods

Brucella species
(*gentamicin + doxycycline*)
Francisella tularensis
(*gentamicin*)
Klebsiella species
(*gentamicin + an antipseudomonal penicillin*)
Pseudomonas aeruginosa
(*tobramycin + an antipseudomonal penicillin*)
Yersinia pestis
(*streptomycin + doxycycline*)

INFECTIONS DUE TO PSEUDOMONAS AERUGINOSA

- Pseudomonas aeruginosa rarely attacks healthy individuals, but can cause infections under special circumstances, for example, in immunocompromised patients, and in burn victims.

- Treatment includes *tobramycin* alone or in combination with an antipseudomonal penicillin, such as *piperacillin* or *ticarcillin*.

Figure 32.8
Typical therapeutic applications of aminoglycosides.

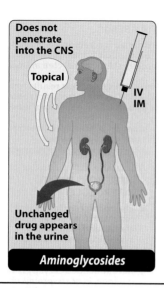

Figure 32.9
Administration and fate of aminoglycosides.

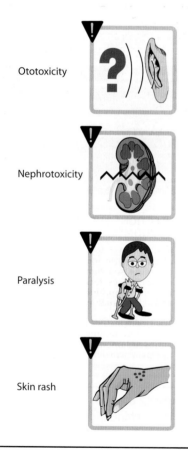

Figure 32.10
Some adverse effects of amino-glycosides.

C. Resistance

Resistance can be caused by 1) decreased uptake of drug when the oxygen-dependent transport system for aminoglycosides or porin channels are absent and 2) plasmid-associated synthesis of enzymes (for example, acetyl transferases, nucleotidyltransferases, and phospho-transferases) that modify and inactivate aminoglycoside antibiotics. Each of these enzymes has its own aminoglycoside specificity; therefore, cross-resistance is not an invariable rule. [Note: *Amikacin* is less vulnerable to these enzymes than are the other antibiotics of this group.]

D. Pharmacokinetics

1. **Administration:** The highly polar, polycationic structure of the amin-oglycosides prevents adequate absorption after oral administration (Figure 32.9). Therefore, all aminoglycosides (except *neomycin* [nee-oh-MYE-sin]) must be given parenterally to achieve adequate serum levels. [Note: The severe nephrotoxicity associated with *neomycin* precludes parenteral administration, and its current use is limited to topical application for skin infections or oral administration to prepare the bowel prior to surgery.] The bactericidal effect of aminoglycosides is concentration and time dependent; that is, the greater the concentration of drug, the greater the rate at which the organisms die. They also have a postantibiotic effect. Because of these properties, once-daily dosing with the aminoglycosides can be employed. This results in fewer toxicities and is less expensive to administer. The exceptions are pregnancy, neonatal infections, and bacterial endocarditis, in which these agents are administered in divided doses every 8 hours. [Note: The dose that is administered is calculated based on lean body mass, because these drugs do not distribute into fat.]

2. **Distribution:** All the aminoglycosides have similar pharmacokinetic properties. Levels achieved in most tissues are low, and penetration into most body fluids is variable. Concentrations in CSF are inadequate, even when the meninges are inflamed. Except for *neomycin*, the aminoglycosides may be administered intrathecally or intraven-tricularly. High concentrations accumulate in the renal cortex and in the endolymph and perilymph of the inner ear, which may account for their nephrotoxic and ototoxic potential. All aminoglycosides cross the placental barrier and may accumulate in fetal plasma and amniotic fluid.

3. **Fate:** Metabolism of the aminoglycosides does not occur in the host. All are rapidly excreted into the urine, predominantly by glomerular filtration (see Figure 32.9). Accumulation occurs in patients with renal failure and requires dose modification.

E. Adverse effects

It is important to monitor plasma levels of *gentamicin*, *tobramycin*, and *amikacin* to avoid concentrations that cause dose-related toxicities (Figure 32.10). [Note: When the drugs are administered two to three times daily, both peak and trough levels are measured. Peak levels are defined as those obtained 30 minutes to 1 hour after infusion. Trough levels are obtained immediately before the next dose. When once-daily dosing is employed, only the trough concentrations are monitored.] Patient factors, such as old age, previous exposure to aminoglycosides, and liver disease, tend to predispose patients to adverse reactions. The elderly are particularly susceptible to nephrotoxicity and ototoxicity.

1. **Ototoxicity:** Ototoxicity (vestibular and cochlear) is directly related to high peak plasma levels and the duration of treatment. The antibiotic accumulates in the endolymph and perilymph of the inner ear, and toxicity correlates with the number of destroyed hair cells in the organ of Corti. Deafness may be irreversible and has been known to affect fetuses in utero. Patients simultaneously receiving another ototoxic drug, such as *cisplatin* or the loop diuretics, *furosemide, bumetanide,* or *ethacrynic acid,* are particularly at risk. Vertigo and loss of balance (especially in patients receiving *streptomycin*) may also occur, because these drugs affect the vestibular apparatus.

2. **Nephrotoxicity:** Retention of the aminoglycosides by the proximal tubular cells disrupts calcium-mediated transport processes, and this results in kidney damage ranging from mild, reversible renal impairment to severe, acute tubular necrosis, which can be irreversible.

3. **Neuromuscular paralysis:** This side effect most often occurs after direct intraperitoneal or intrapleural application of large doses of aminoglycosides. The mechanism responsible is a decrease in both the release of acetylcholine from prejunctional nerve endings and the sensitivity of the postsynaptic site. Patients with myasthenia gravis are particularly at risk. Prompt administration of *calcium gluconate* or *neostigmine* can reverse the block.

4. **Allergic reactions:** Contact dermatitis is a common reaction to topically applied *neomycin.*

V. MACROLIDES

The macrolides are a group of antibiotics with a macrocyclic lactone structure to which one or more deoxy sugars are attached. *Erythromycin* [er-ith-roe-MYE-sin] was the first of these drugs to find clinical application, both as a drug of first choice and as an alternative to *penicillin* in individuals who are allergic to β-lactam antibiotics. The newer members of this family, *clarithromycin* [kla-rith-roe-MYE-sin] (a methylated form of *erythromycin*) and *azithromycin* [az-ith-roe-MYE-sin] (having a larger lactone ring), have some features in common with, and others that improve on, *erythromycin*. *Telithromycin* [tel-ith-roe-MYE-sin], a semisynthetic derivative of *erythromycin*, is the first "ketolide" antimicrobial agent that has been approved and is now in clinical use. Ketolides and macrolides have very similar antimicrobial coverage. However, the ketolides are active against many macrolide-resistant gram-positive strains.

A. Mechanism of action

The macrolides bind irreversibly to a site on the 50S subunit of the bacterial ribosome, thus inhibiting the translocation steps of protein synthesis (Figure 32.11). They may also interfere at other steps, such as transpeptidation. Generally considered to be bacteriostatic, they may be bactericidal at higher doses. Their binding site is either identical or in close proximity to that for *clindamycin* and *chloramphenicol*.

B. Antibacterial spectrum

1. **Erythromycin:** This drug is effective against many of the same organisms as *penicillin G* (Figure 32.12); therefore, it is used in patients who are allergic to the penicillins.

= Pen G

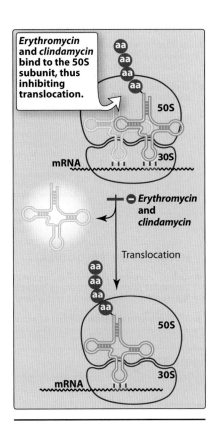

Figure 32.11
Mechanism of action of *erythromycin* and *clindamycin*.

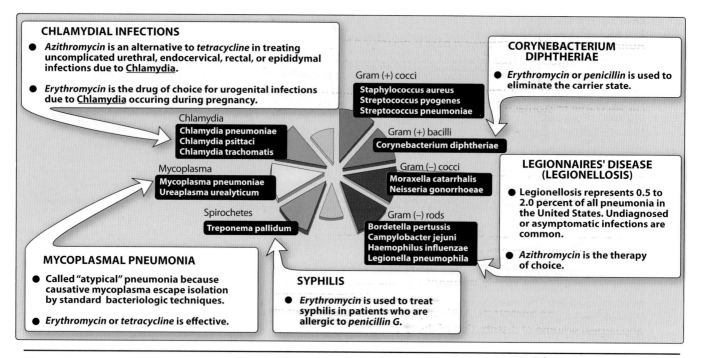

Figure 32.12
Typical therapeutic applications of macrolides.

Pen G + H. flu + intracellular pathogens

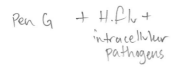

2. **Clarithromycin:** This antibiotic has a spectrum of antibacterial activity similar to that of *erythromycin*, but it is also effective against Haemophilus influenzae. Its activity against intracellular pathogens, such as Chlamydia, Legionella, Moraxella, and Ureaplasma species and Helicobacter pylori, is higher than that of *erythromycin*.

3. **Azithromycin:** Although less active against streptococci and staphylococci than *erythromycin*, *azithromycin* is far more active against respiratory infections due to H. influenzae and Moraxella catarrhalis. *Azithromycin* is now the preferred therapy for urethritis caused by Chlamydia trachomatis. It also has activity against Mycobacterium avium-intracellulare complex in patients with acquired immunodeficiency syndrome and disseminated infections.

Chlamydia + Respiratory infections

4. **Telithromycin:** This ketolide drug has an antibacterial spectrum similar to that of *azithromycin*. Moreover, the structural modification within ketolides neutralizes the most common resistance mechanisms (methylase-mediated and efflux-mediated) that make macrolides ineffective.

—Resistance

C. **Resistance**

Resistance to *erythromycin* is becoming a serious clinical problem. For example, most strains of staphylococci in hospital isolates are resistant to this drug. Several mechanisms have been identified: 1) the inability of the organism to take up the antibiotic or the presence of an efflux pump, both of which limit the amount of intracellular drug; 2) a decreased affinity of the 50S ribosomal subunit for the antibiotic, resulting from the methylation of an adenine in the 23S bacterial ribosomal RNA; and 3) the presence of a plasmid-associated *erythromycin* esterase. Both *clarithromycin* and *azithromycin* show cross-resistance with *erythromycin*, but *telithromycin* can be effective against macrolide-resistant organisms.

Figure 32.13
Administration and fate of the macrolide antibiotics.

D. Pharmacokinetics

1. **Administration:** The *erythromycin* base is destroyed by gastric acid. Thus, either enteric-coated tablets or esterified forms of the antibiotic are administered. All are adequately absorbed upon oral administration (Figure 32.13). *Clarithromycin, azithromycin,* and *telithromycin* are stable to stomach acid and are readily absorbed. Food interferes with the absorption of *erythromycin* and *azithromycin* but can increase that of *clarithromycin*. *Azithromycin* is available for intravenous infusion, but intravenous administration of *erythromycin* is associated with a high incidence of thrombophlebitis.

2. **Distribution:** *Erythromycin* distributes well to all body fluids except the CSF. It is one of the few antibiotics that diffuses into prostatic fluid, and it has the unique characteristic of accumulating in macrophages. All four drugs concentrate in the liver. Inflammation allows for greater tissue penetration. Similarly, *clarithromycin, azithromycin,* and *telithromycin* are widely distributed in the tissues. Serum levels of *azithromycin* are low; the drug is concentrated in neutrophils, macrophages, and fibroblasts. *Azithromycin* has the longest half-life and largest volume of distribution of the four drugs (Figure 32.14).

3. **Fate:** *Erythromycin* and *telithromycin* are extensively metabolized and are known to inhibit the oxidation of a number of drugs through their interaction with the cytochrome P450 system (see p. 14). Interference with the metabolism of drugs such as *theophylline* and *carbamazepine* has been reported for *clarithromycin* (see Figure 32.16). *Clarithromycin* is oxidized to the 14-hydroxy derivative, which retains antibiotic activity.

4. **Excretion:** *Erythromycin* and *azithromycin* are primarily concentrated and excreted in an active form in the bile (see Figure 32.13). Partial reabsorption occurs through the enterohepatic circulation. Inactive metabolites are excreted into the urine. In contrast, *clarithromycin* and its metabolites are eliminated by the kidney as well as the liver, and it is recommended that the dosage of this drug be adjusted in patients with compromised renal function.

E. Adverse effects

1. **Epigastric distress:** This side effect is common and can lead to poor patient compliance for *erythromycin*. *Clarithromycin* and *azithromycin* seem to be better tolerated by the patient, but gastrointestinal problems are their most common side effects (Figure 32.15).

2. **Cholestatic jaundice:** This side effect occurs especially with the estolate form of *erythromycin*, presumably as the result of a hypersensitivity reaction to the estolate form (the lauryl salt of the propionyl ester of *erythromycin*). It has also been reported for other forms of the drug.

3. **Ototoxicity:** Transient deafness has been associated with *erythromycin*, especially at high dosages.

4. **Contraindications:** Patients with hepatic dysfunction should be treated cautiously—if at all—with *erythromycin, telithromycin,* or *azithromycin*, because these drugs accumulate in the liver. Recent cases of severe hepatotoxicity with *telithromycin* use have empha-

	Erythromycin	Clarithromycin	Azithromycin	Telithromycin
Oral absorption	Yes	Yes	Yes	Yes
Half-life (hours)	2	3.5	>40	10
Conversion to an active metabolite	No	Yes	Yes	Yes
Percent excretion in urine	15	50	12	13

Figure 32.14
Some properties of the macrolide antibiotics.

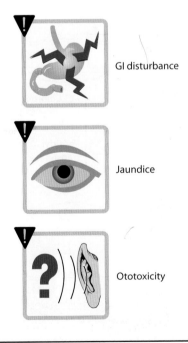

GI disturbance

Jaundice

Ototoxicity

Figure 32.15
Some adverse effects of macrolide antibiotics.

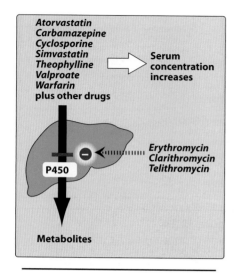

Figure 32.16
Inhibition of the cytochrome P450 system by *erythromycin, clarithromycin,* and *telithromycin*.

sized the caution needed when utilizing this agent. Additionally, *telithromycin* has the potential to prolongate the QTc interval in some patients. Therefore, it should be avoided in patients with congenital prolongation of the QTc interval and in those patients with proarrhythmic conditions. Similarly, patients who are renally compromised should be given *telithromycin* with caution. *Telithromycin* is contraindicated in patients with myasthenia gravis.

5. **Interactions:** *Erythromycin, telithromycin,* and *clarithromycin* inhibit the hepatic metabolism of a number of drugs, which can lead to toxic accumulations of these compounds (Figure 32.16). An interaction with *digoxin* may occur in some patients. In this case, the antibiotic eliminates a species of intestinal flora that ordinarily inactivates *digoxin,* thus leading to greater reabsorption of the drug from the enterohepatic circulation. No interactions have been reported for *azithromycin*.

VI. CHLORAMPHENICOL

Chloramphenicol [klor-am-FEN-i-kole] is active against a wide range of gram-positive and gram-negative organisms. However, because of its toxicity, its use is restricted to life-threatening infections for which no alternatives exist.

A. Mechanism of action

The drug binds to the bacterial 50S ribosomal subunit and inhibits protein synthesis at the peptidyl transferase reaction (Figure 32.17). Because of the similarity of mammalian mitochondrial ribosomes to those of bacteria, protein synthesis in these organelles may be inhibited at high circulating *chloramphenicol* levels, producing bone marrow toxicity.

B. Antimicrobial spectrum

Chloramphenicol, a broad-spectrum antibiotic, is active not only against bacteria but also against other microorganisms, such as rickettsiae. Pseudomonas aeruginosa is not affected, nor are the chlamydiae. *Chloramphenicol* has excellent activity against anaerobes. The drug is either bactericidal or (more commonly) bacteriostatic, depending on the organism.

C. Resistance

Resistance is conferred by the presence of an R factor that codes for an acetyl coenzyme A transferase. This enzyme inactivates *chloramphenicol.* Another mechanism for resistance is associated with an inability of the antibiotic to penetrate the organism. This change in permeability may be the basis of multidrug resistance.

D. Pharmacokinetics

Chloramphenicol may be administered either intravenously or orally (Figure 32.18). It is completely absorbed via the oral route because of its lipophilic nature, and is widely distributed throughout the body. It readily enters the normal CSF. The drug inhibits the hepatic mixed-function oxidases. Excretion of the drug depends on its conversion in the liver to a glucuronide, which is then secreted by the renal tubule. Only about 10 percent of the parent compound is excreted by glomerular filtration. *Chloramphenicol* is also secreted into breast milk.

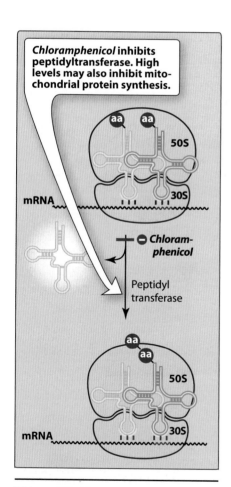

Figure 32.17
Mechanism of action of *chloramphenicol*.

E. Adverse effects

The clinical use of *chloramphenicol* is limited to life-threatening infections because of the serious adverse effects associated with its administration. In addition to gastrointestinal upsets, overgrowth of Candida albicans may appear on mucous membranes.

1. **Anemias:** Hemolytic anemia occurs in patients with low levels of glucose 6-phosphate dehydrogenase. Other types of anemia occurring as a side effect of *chloramphenicol* include reversible anemia, which is apparently dose-related and occurs concomitantly with therapy, and aplastic anemia, which although rare is idiosyncratic and usually fatal. [Note: Aplastic anemia is independent of dose and may occur after therapy has ceased.]

2. **Gray baby syndrome:** This adverse effect occurs in neonates if the dosage regimen of *chloramphenicol* is not properly adjusted. Neonates have a low capacity to glucuronylate the antibiotic, and they have underdeveloped renal function. Therefore, neonates have a decreased ability to excrete the drug, which accumulates to levels that interfere with the function of mitochondrial ribosomes. This leads to poor feeding, depressed breathing, cardiovascular collapse, cyanosis (hence the term "gray baby"), and death. Adults who have received very high doses of the drug can also exhibit this toxicity.

3. **Interactions:** *Chloramphenicol* is able to inhibit some of the hepatic mixed-function oxidases and, thus, blocks the metabolism of such drugs as *warfarin, phenytoin, tolbutamide,* and *chlorpropamide,* thereby elevating their concentrations and potentiating their effects (Figure 32.19).

VII. CLINDAMYCIN

Clindamycin [klin-da-MYE-sin] has a mechanism of action that is the same as that of *erythromycin. Clindamycin* is employed primarily in the treatment of infections caused by anaerobic bacteria, such as Bacteroides fragilis, which often causes abdominal infections associated with trauma. However, it is also significantly active against nonenterococcal, gram-positive cocci. Resistance mechanisms are the same as those for *erythromycin,* and cross-resistance has been described. [Note: Clostridium difficile is always resistant to *clindamycin.*] *Clindamycin* is well absorbed by the oral route. It distributes well into all body fluids except the CSF. Adequate levels of *clindamycin* are not achieved in the brain, even when meninges are inflamed. Penetration into bone occurs even in the absence of inflammation. *Clindamycin* undergoes extensive oxidative metabolism to inactive products. The drug is excreted into the bile or urine by glomerular filtration, but therapeutically effective levels of the parent drug are not achieved in the urine (Figure 32.20). Accumulation has been reported in patients with either severely compromised renal function or hepatic failure. In addition to skin rashes, the most serious adverse effect is potentially fatal pseudomembranous colitis caused by overgrowth of C. difficile, which elaborates necrotizing toxins. Oral administration of either *metronidazole* or *vancomycin* is usually effective in controlling this serious problem. [Note: *Vancomycin* should be reserved for a condition that does not respond to *metronidazole.*] Impaired liver function has also been reported.

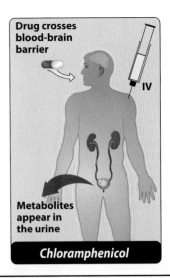

Figure 32.18
Administration and fate of *chloramphenicol.*

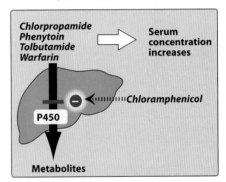

Figure 32.19
Inhibition of the cytochrome P450 system by *chloramphenicol.*

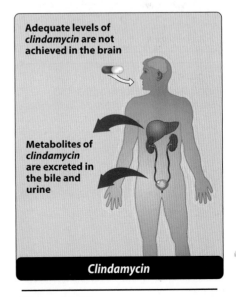

Figure 32.20
Administration and fate of *clindamycin.*

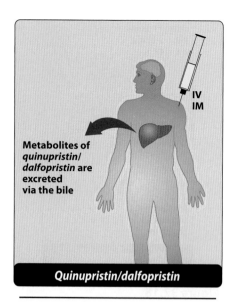

Figure 32.21
Administration and fate of
quinupristin/dalfopristin.

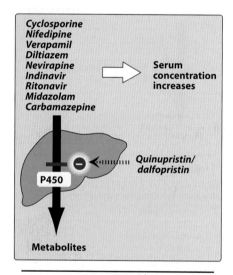

Figure 32.22
Inhibition of cytochrome P450
system by *quinupristin/dalfopristin*.

VIII. QUINUPRISTIN/DALFOPRISTIN

Quinupristin/dalfopristin [KWIN-yoo-pris-tin/DAL-foh-pris-tin] is a mixture of two streptogramins in a ratio of thirty to seventy, respectively. They are derived from a streptomycete and then chemically modified. The drug is normally reserved for the treatment of *vancomycin*-resistant Enterococcus faecium (VRE).

A. Mechanism of action

Each component of this combination drug binds to a separate site on the 50S bacterial ribosome, forming a stable ternary complex. Thus, they synergistically interrupt protein synthesis. The combination drug is bactericidal and has a long postantibiotic effect.

B. Resistance

Enzymatic processes commonly account for resistance to these agents. For example, the presence of a ribosomal enzyme that methylates the target bacterial 23S ribosomal RNA site can interfere in *quinupristin* binding. In some cases, the enzymatic modification can change the action from bactericidal to bacteriostatic. Plasmid-associated acetyltransferase inactivates *dalfopristin*. An active efflux pump can also decrease levels of the antibiotics in bacteria.

C. Antibacterial spectrum

The combination drug is active primarily against gram-positive cocci, including those resistant to other antibiotics (for example, *methicillin*-resistant staphylococci). Its primary use is in the treatment of E. faecium infections, including VRE strains. [Note: In the latter case, the effect is bacteriostatic rather than bactericidal.] The drug is not effective against Enterococcus faecalis.

D. Pharmacokinetics

Quinupristin/dalfopristin is injected intravenously in a 5 percent dextrose solution (the drug is incompatible with a saline medium). The combination drug penetrates macrophages and polymorphonucleocytes, a property that is important, because VRE are intracellular. Levels in the CSF are low. Both compounds undergo metabolism. The products are less active than the parent in the case of *quinupristin* and are equally active in the case of *dalfopristin*. Most of the parent drugs and metabolites are cleared through the liver and eliminated via the bile into the feces (Figure 32.21). Urinary excretion is secondary.

E. Adverse effects

1. **Venous irritation:** This commonly occurs when *quinupristin/dalfopristin* is administered through a peripheral rather than a central line.

2. **Arthralgia and myalgia:** These have been reported when higher levels of the drugs are employed.

3. **Hyperbilirubinemia:** Total bilirubin is elevated in about 25 percent of patients, resulting from a competition with the antibiotic for excretion.

4. **Interactions:** Because of the ability of *quinupristin/dalfopristin* to inhibit the cytochrome P450 (CYP3A4) isozyme, concomitant administration with drugs that are metabolized by this pathway may lead to toxicities (Figure 32.22). A drug interaction with *digoxin* appears to occur by the same mechanism as that caused by *erythromycin*.

IX. LINEZOLID

Linezolid [lih-NEH-zo-lid] was introduced recently to combat resistant gram-positive organisms, such as *methicillin*- and *vancomycin*-resistant Staphylococcus aureus, *vancomycin*-resistant E. faecium and E. faecalis, and *penicillin*-resistant streptococci. *Linezolid* is a totally synthetic oxazolidinone.

A. Mechanism of action

The drug inhibits bacterial protein synthesis by inhibiting the formation of the 70S initiation complex. *Linezolid* binds to a site on the 50S subunit near the interface with the 30S subunit (Figure 32.23).

B. Resistance

Decreased binding to the target site confers resistance on the organism. Cross-resistance with other antibiotics does not occur.

C. Antibacterial spectrum

The antibacterial action of *linezolid* is directed primarily against gram-positive organisms, such as staphylococci, streptococci, and enterococci, as well as Corynebacterium species and Listeria monocytogenes (Figure 32.24). It is also moderately active against Mycobacterium tuberculosis. However, its main clinical use is against the resistant organisms mentioned above. Like other agents that interfere with bacterial protein synthesis, *linezolid* is bacteriostatic. However, it is cidal against the streptococci and Clostridium perfringens.

D. Pharmacokinetics

Linezolid is completely absorbed on oral administration. An intravenous preparation is also available. The drug is widely distributed throughout the body, having a volume of distribution of 40 to 50 liters. Two metabolites that are oxidation products have been identified, one of which has antimicrobial activity. However, cytochrome P450 enzymes are not involved in their formation. The drug is excreted both by renal and non-renal routes. The metabolites rely on the kidney for elimination.

E. Adverse effects

Linezolid is well-tolerated, with some reports of gastrointestinal upset, nausea, and diarrhea, as well as headaches and rash. Thrombocytopenia was found to occur in about 2 percent of patients who were on the drug for longer than 2 weeks. Although no reports have appeared that *linezolid* inhibits monoamine oxidase activity, patients are cautioned not to consume large quantities of tyramine-containing foods. Early oxazolidinones had been shown to inhibit monoamine oxidase activity. The condition was reversible when the drug was suspended. Reversible enhancement of the pressor effects of *pseudoephedrine* was shown to occur.

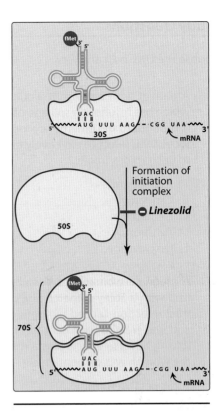

Figure 32.23
Mechanism of action of *linezolid*.

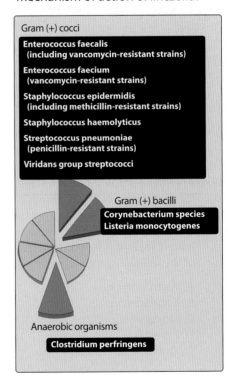

Figure 32.24
Antimicrobial spectrum of *linezolid*.

Study Questions

Choose the ONE best answer.

32.1 A patient with a gunshot wound to the abdomen, which has resulted in spillage of intestinal contents, is brought to the emergency room. Which antibiotic would you select to effectively treat an infection due to Bacteroides fragilis?

A. Aztreonam.
B. Clindamycin.
C. Gentamicin.
D. Azithromycin.
E. Doxycycline.

Correct answer = B. Bacteroides fragilis is an anaerobic organism. The only drug on the list that is effective against it is clindamycin.

32.2 A pregnant woman was hospitalized and catheterized with a Foley catheter. She developed a urinary tract infection caused by Pseudomonas aeruginosa and was treated with gentamicin. Which of the following adverse effects was a risk to the fetus when the woman was on gentamicin?

A. Skeletal deformity.
B. Hearing loss.
C. Teratogenesis.
D. Blindness.
E. Mental retardation.

Correct answer = B. Gentamicin can cross the placental barrier and cause hearing loss in the newborns of mothers who have received it.

32.3 Children younger than 8 years of age should not receive tetracyclines because these agents:

A. Cause rupture of tendons.
B. Do not cross into the CS.
C. Are not bactericidal.
D. Deposit in tissues undergoing calcification.
E. Can cause aplastic anemia.

Correct answer = D. It is true that tetracyclines are not bactericidal, but the reason they are contraindicated in this age group is that they are deposited in tissues undergoing calcification, such as teeth and bone, and therefore can stunt growth. Ciprofloxacin can interfere in cartilage formation and cause rupture of tendons, and it is also contraindicated in children. Tetracyclines can cross into the CSF but do not cause aplastic anemia—a property usually associated with chloramphenicol.

32.4 A 46-year-old woman is in the intensive care unit for treatment of a vancomycin-resistant strain of Enterococcus faecium–caused bacteremia. You want to limit the risk of drug interactions in this woman, who is receiving five other medications. Which one of the following antibiotics would you choose?

A. Azithromycin.
B. Clindamycin.
C. Doxycycline.
D. Linezolid.
E. Quinupristin/dalfopristin.

Correct answer = D. Azithromycin, clindamycin, and doxycycline do not have significant activity against this organism. Both linezolid and quinupristin/dalfopristin have activity against vancomycin-resistant Enterococcus faecium, but the latter antibiotic is a potent inhibitor of CYP3A4 isozymes. Linezolid is not an inhibitor of cytochrome P450 isozymes. Therefore, it would be less likely to have interactions with other drugs.

Quinolones, Folic Acid Antagonists, and Urinary Tract Antiseptics

33

I. FLUOROQUINOLONES

Introduction of the first fluorinated quinolone, *norfloxacin*, was rapidly followed by development of other members of this group, such as *ciprofloxacin*, which has had wide clinical application. Newer fluorinated quinolones offer greater potency, a broader spectrum of antimicrobial activity, greater in vitro efficacy against resistant organisms, and in some cases, a better safety profile than older quinolones and other antibiotics. Compared to *ciprofloxacin*, the new compounds are more active against gram-positive organisms, yet retain favorable activity against gram-negative microorganisms. It seems likely that the number of drugs in this class of antibiotics will increase due to its wide antibacterial spectrum, favorable pharmacokinetic properties, and relative lack of adverse reactions. Unfortunately, their overuse has already led to the emergence of resistant strains, resulting in limitations to their clinical usefulness. The fluoroquinolones and other antibiotics discussed in this chapter are listed in Figure 33.1.

A. Mechanism of action

The fluoroquinolones enter the bacterium by passive diffusion through water-filled protein channels (porins) in the outer membrane. Once inside the cell, they inhibit the replication of bacterial DNA by interfering with the action of DNA gyrase (topoisomerase II) and topoisomerase IV during bacterial growth and reproduction. [Note: Topoisomerases are enzymes that change the configuration or topology of DNA by a nicking, pass-through, and resealing mechanism. They do not change the DNA's primary sequence[1] (Figure 33.2).] Binding of the quinolone to both the enzyme and the DNA forms a ternary complex that inhibits the resealing step, and can cause cell death by inducing cleavage of the DNA. Because DNA gyrase is a bacteriospecific target for antimicrobial therapy, cross-resistance with other, more commonly used antimicrobial drugs is rare, but this is increasing in the case of multidrug-resistant organisms. The second site blocked by the fluoroquinolones—topoisomerase IV—is required by bacteria for cell division. It has been implicated in the process of segregating newly replicated DNA. In gram-negative organisms (for example, <u>Escherichia coli</u>), the inhibition of DNA gyrase is more significant than that of topoisomerase IV, whereas in gram-positive organisms (for example, the staphylococci), the opposite is true.

[1]See p. 401 in ***Lippincott's Illustrated Reviews: Biochemistry*** (4th ed.) for a discussion of topoisomerase activity.

QUINOLONES, FOLIC ACID ANTAGONISTS, AND URINARY TRACT ANTISEPTICS

FLUOROQUINOLONES

FIRST GENERATION
— *Nalidixic acid*
SECOND GENERATION
— *Ciprofloxacin*
— *Norfloxacin*
— *Ofloxacin*
THIRD GENERATION
— *Levofloxacin*
FOURTH GENERATION
— *Moxifloxacin*

INHIBITORS OF FOLATE SYNTHESIS

— *Mafenide*
— *Silver sulfadiazine*
— *Succinylsulfathiazole*
— *Sulfacetamide*
— *Sulfadiazine*
— *Sulfamethoxazole*
— *Sulfasalazine*
— *Sulfisoxazole*

Figure 33.1
Summary of drugs described in this chapter. (Figure continues on the next page.)

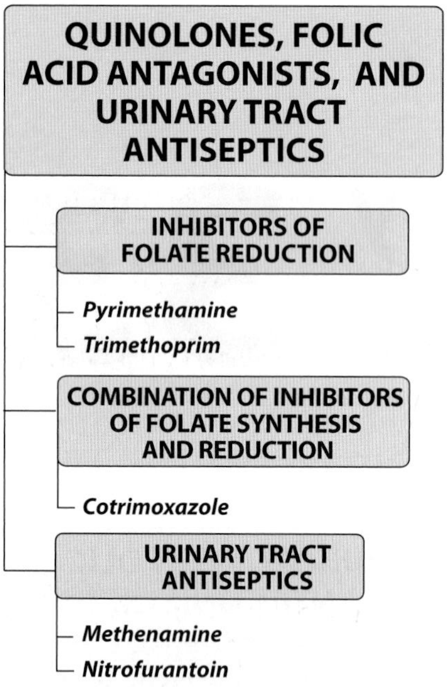

QUINOLONES, FOLIC ACID ANTAGONISTS, AND URINARY TRACT ANTISEPTICS

INHIBITORS OF FOLATE REDUCTION

— Pyrimethamine
— Trimethoprim

COMBINATION OF INHIBITORS OF FOLATE SYNTHESIS AND REDUCTION

— Cotrimoxazole

URINARY TRACT ANTISEPTICS

— Methenamine
— Nitrofurantoin

Figure 33.1 (continued)
Summary of drugs described in this chapter.

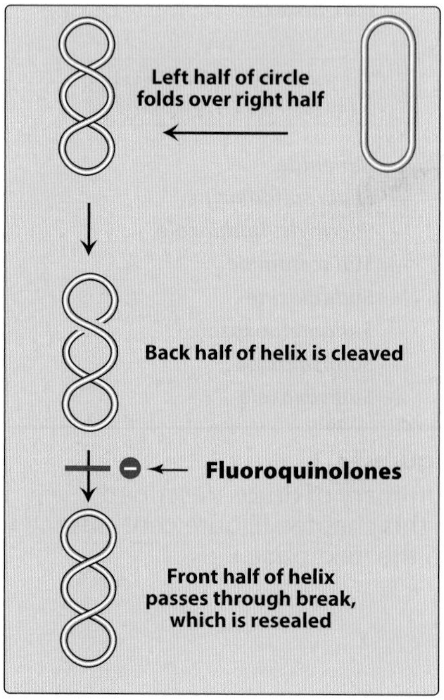

Figure 33.2
Action of Type II DNA topoisomerase.

Left half of circle folds over right half

Back half of helix is cleaved

Fluoroquinolones

Front half of helix passes through break, which is resealed

B. Antimicrobial spectrum

All the fluoroquinolones are bactericidal. Like aminoglycosides, the quinolones exhibit concentration-dependent bacterial killing. Bactericidal activity becomes more pronounced as the serum drug concentration increases to approximately 30-fold the minimum inhibitory concentration. In general, they are effective against gram-negative organisms such as the Enterobacteriaceae, Pseudomonas species, Haemophilus influenzae, Moraxella catarrhalis, Legionellaceae, chlamydia, and mycobacteria (except for Mycobacterium avium-intracellulare complex). They are effective in the treatment of gonorrhea but not syphilis. The newer agents (for example, *levofloxacin* and *moxifloxacin*) also have good activity against some gram-positive organisms, such as Streptococcus pneumoniae. *Moxifloxacin* has activity against many anaerobes. If used prophylactically before transurethral surgery, fluoroquinolones lower the incidence of postsurgical urinary tract infections (UTIs). It has become common practice to classify the fluoroquinolones into "generations," based on their antimicrobial targets (Figure 33.3). The nonfluorinated quinolone *nalidixic acid* is considered to be first generation, with a narrow spectrum of susceptible organisms usually confined to the urinary tract. *Ciprofloxacin* and *norfloxacin* are assigned to the second generation because of their activity against aerobic gram-negative and atypical bacteria. In addition, these fluoroquinolones exhibit significant intracellular penetration, allowing therapy for infections in which a bacterium spends part or all of its life cycle inside a host cell (for example, chlamydia, mycoplasma, and legionella). *Levofloxacin* is classified as third generation because of its increased activity against gram-positive bacteria. Lastly, the fourth generation includes only *moxifloxacin* because of its activity against anaerobic as well as gram-positive organisms.

C. Examples of clinically useful fluoroquinolones

1. **Ciprofloxacin:** This is the most frequently used fluoroquinolone in the United States (Figure 33.4). The serum levels of *ciprofloxacin* [sip-row-FLOX-a-sin] that are achieved are effective against many systemic infections, with the exception of serious infections caused by *methicillin*-resistant Staphylococcus aureus (MRSA), the enterococci, and pneumococci. *Ciprofloxacin* is also particularly useful in treating infections caused by many Enterobacteriaceae and other gram-negative bacilli. For example, traveler's diarrhea caused by E. coli can be effectively treated. *Ciprofloxacin* is also the drug of choice for prophylaxis and treatment of anthrax. It is the most potent of the fluoroquinolones for Pseudomonas aeruginosa infections and, therefore, is used in the treatment of pseudomonal infections associated with cystic fibrosis. The drug is also used as an alternative to more toxic drugs, such as the aminoglycosides. It may act synergistically with β-lactams and is also of benefit in treating resistant tuberculosis.

2. **Norfloxacin:** *Norfloxacin* (nor-FLOX-a-sin] is effective against both gram-negative (including P. aeruginosa) and gram-positive organisms in treating complicated and uncomplicated UTIs and prostatitis. It is not effective in systemic infections.

3. **Levofloxacin:** *Levofloxacin* [leave-oh-FLOX-a-sin] is an isomer of *ofloxacin* [oh-FLOX-a-sin] and has largely replaced it clinically. It can be used in the treatment of prostatitis due to E. coli and of sexually transmitted diseases, with the exception of syphilis. It may be used as alternative therapy in patients with gonorrhea. Additionally, due to its broad spectrum of activity, *levofloxacin* is utilized in a wide

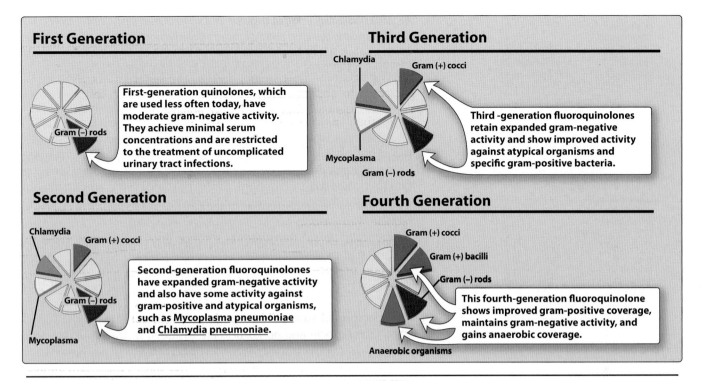

Figure 33.3
Summary of antimicrobial spectrum of quinolones. [Note: The antimicrobial spectrum of specific agents may differ from the generalizations shown in this figure.]

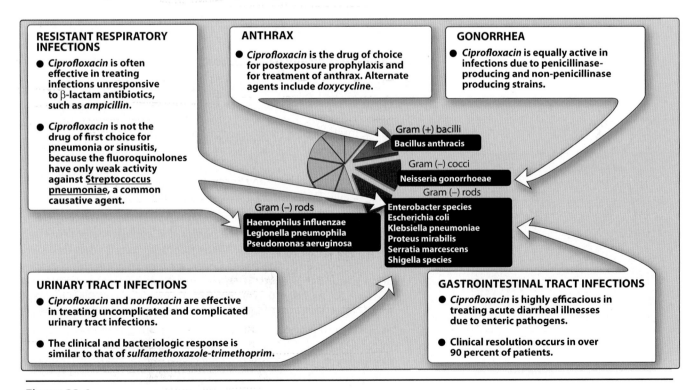

Figure 33.4
Typical therapeutic applications of *ciprofloxacin*.

range of infections, including skin infections, acute sinusitis, acute exacerbation of chronic bronchitis, community-acquired pneumonia, as well as nosocomial pneumonia. *Levofloxacin* has excellent activity against respiratory infections due to S. pneumoniae.

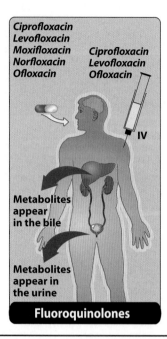

Figure 33.5
Administration and fate of the fluoroquinolones.

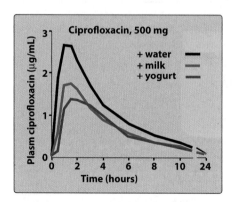

Figure 33.6
Effect of dietary calcium on the absorption of *ciprofloxacin*.

4. Moxifloxacin: *Moxifloxacin* [moxie-FLOX-a-sin] not only has enhanced activity against gram-positive organisms (for example, S. pneumoniae) but also has excellent activity against many anaerobes. It has very poor activity against P. aeruginosa.

D. Resistance

When the fluoroquinolones were first introduced, there was optimism that resistance would not develop. Although no plasmid-mediated resistance has been reported, resistant MRSA, pseudomonas, coagulase-negative staphylococci, and enterococci have unfortunately emerged due to chromosomal mutations. Cross-resistance exists among the quinolones. The mechanisms responsible for this resistance include the following.

1. **Altered target:** Mutations in the bacterial DNA gyrase have been associated with a decreased affinity for fluoroquinolones. Topoisomerase IV also undergoes mutations. Resistance is frequently associated with mutations in both gyrase and topoisomerase IV.

2. **Decreased accumulation:** Reduced intracellular concentration of the drugs in the bacterial cell is linked to two mechanisms. One involves a decreased number of porin proteins in the outer membrane of the resistant cell, thereby impairing access of the drugs to the intracellular topoisomerases. The other mechanism is associated with an energy-dependent efflux system in the cell membrane.

E. Pharmacokinetics

1. **Absorption:** Only 35 to 70 percent of orally administered *norfloxacin* is absorbed, compared with 85 to 95 percent of the other fluoroquinolones (Figure 33.5). Intravenous preparations of *ciprofloxacin*, *levofloxacin*, and *ofloxacin* are available. Ingestion of the fluoroquinolones with *sucralfate*, antacids containing aluminum or magnesium, or dietary supplements containing iron or zinc can interfere with the absorption of these antibacterial drugs. Calcium and other divalent cations have also been shown to interfere with the absorption of these agents (Figure 33.6). The fluoroquinolones with the longest half-lives (*levofloxacin* and *moxifloxacin*) permit once-daily dosing.

2. **Fate:** Binding to plasma proteins ranges from 10 to 40 percent. [Note: Achieved plasma levels of free *norfloxacin* are insufficient for treatment of systemic infections.] All the fluoroquinolones distribute well into all tissues and body fluids. Levels are high in bone, urine, kidney, and prostatic tissue (but not prostatic fluid), and concentrations in the lung exceed those in serum. Penetration into cerebrospinal fluid is low except for *ofloxacin*, for which concentrations can be as high as 90 percent of those in the serum. The fluoroquinolones also accumulate in macrophages and polymorphonuclear leukocytes, thus being effective against intracellular organisms such as Legionella pneumophila. They are excreted by the renal route.

F. Adverse reactions

In general, these agents are very well tolerated. Toxicities similar to those for *nalidixic acid* have been reported for the fluoroquinolones (Figure 33.7).

1. **Gastrointestinal:** The most common adverse effects of the fluoro-quinolones are nausea, vomiting, and diarrhea, which occur in three to six percent of patients.

2. **Central nervous system problems:** The most prominent central nervous system (CNS) effects of fluoroquinolone treatment are headache and dizziness or light-headedness. Thus, patients with CNS disorders, such as epilepsy, should be treated cautiously with these drugs. [Note: *Ciprofloxacin* interferes in the metabolism of *theophylline* and may evoke seizures.]

3. **Phototoxicity:** Patients taking fluoroquinolones are advised to avoid excessive sunlight and to apply sunscreens. However, the latter may not protect completely. Thus, it is advisable that the drug should be discontinued at the first sign of phototoxicity.

4. **Connective tissue problems:** Fluoroquinolones should be avoided in pregnancy, in nursing mothers, and in children under 18 years of age, because articular cartilage erosion (arthropathy) occurs in immature experimental animals. [Note: Children with cystic fibrosis who receive *ciprofloxacin* have had few problems, but careful monitoring is indicated.] In adults, fluoroquinolones can infrequently cause ruptured tendons.

5. **Contraindications:** *Moxifloxacin* may prolong the QTc interval and, thus, should not be used in patients who are predisposed to arrhythmias or are taking antiarrhythmic medications.

6. **Drug interactions:** The effect of antacids and cations on the absorption of these agents was considered above. *Ciprofloxacin* and *ofloxacin* can increase the serum levels of *theophylline* by inhibiting its metabolism (Figure 33.8). This is not the case with the third- and fourth-generation fluoroquinolones, which may raise the serum levels of *warfarin*, *caffeine*, and *cyclosporine*.

II. OVERVIEW OF THE FOLATE ANTAGONISTS

Enzymes requiring folate-derived cofactors are essential for the synthesis of purines and pyrimidines[2] (precursors of RNA and DNA) and other compounds necessary for cellular growth and replication. Therefore, in the absence of folate, cells cannot grow or divide. To synthesize the critical folate derivative, tetrahydrofolic acid, humans must first obtain preformed folate in the form of folic acid as a vitamin from the diet. In contrast, many bacteria are impermeable to folic acid and other folates and, therefore, must rely on their ability to synthesize folate de novo. The sulfonamides (sulfa drugs) are a family of antibiotics that inhibit this de novo synthesis of folate. A second type of folate antagonist—*trimethoprim*—prevents microorganisms from converting dihydrofolic acid to tetrahydrofolic acid, with minimal effect on a human cell's ability to make this conversion. Thus, both sulfonamides and *trimethoprim* interfere with the ability of an infecting bacterium to divide. Compounding the sulfonamide *sulfamethoxazole* with *trimethoprim* (the generic name for the combination is *cotrimoxazole*) provides a synergistic combination that is used as effective treatment of a variety of bacterial infections.

 [2]See p. 302 in ***Lippincott's Illustrated Reviews: Biochemistry*** (4th ed.) for a discussion of pyrimidine synthesis.

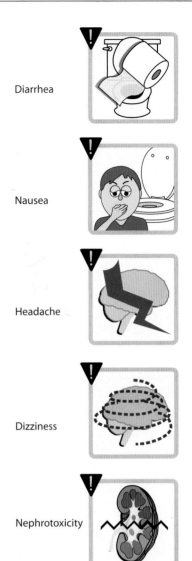

Diarrhea

Nausea

Headache

Dizziness

Nephrotoxicity

Figure 33.7
Some adverse reactions to fluoroquinolones.

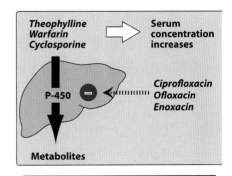

Figure 33.8
Drug interactions with fluoroquinolones.

III. SULFONAMIDES

The sulfa drugs are seldom prescribed alone except in developing countries, where they are still employed because of their low cost and their efficacy in certain bacterial infections, such as trachoma and those of the urinary tract. However, when *cotrimoxazole* was introduced in the mid-1970s, there was a renewed interest in the sulfonamides. Sulfa drugs differ from each other not only in their chemical and physical properties but also in their pharmacokinetics.

A. Mechanism of action

In many microorganisms, dihydrofolic acid is synthesized from *p*-amino-benzoic acid (PABA), pteridine, and glutamate (Figure 33.9). All the sulfonamides currently in clinical use are synthetic analogs of PABA.[3] Because of their structural similarity to PABA, the sulfonamides compete with this substrate for the bacterial enzyme, dihydropteroate synthetase. They thus inhibit the synthesis of bacterial dihydrofolic acid and, thereby, the formation of its essential cofactor forms.[4] The sulfa drugs, including *cotrimoxazole*, are bacteriostatic.

B. Antibacterial spectrum

Sulfa drugs are active against selected enterobacteria in the urinary tract and nocardia. In addition, *sulfadiazine* [sul-fa-DYE-a-zeen], in combination with the dihydrofolate reductase inhibitor *pyrimethamine* [pyri-METH-a-meen], is the preferred form of treatment for toxoplasmosis and chloroquine-resistant malaria.

C. Resistance

Only organisms that synthesize their folate requirements *de novo* are sensitive to the sulfonamides. Thus, humans, who synthesize critical folate cofactors from dietary folic acid, are not affected, and bacteria that can obtain folates from their environment are naturally resistant to these drugs. Acquired bacterial resistance to the sulfa drugs can arise

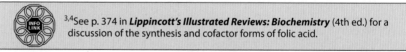

[3,4]See p. 374 in *Lippincott's Illustrated Reviews: Biochemistry* (4th ed.) for a discussion of the synthesis and cofactor forms of folic acid.

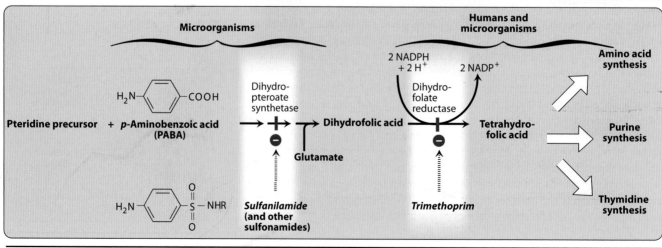

Figure 33.9
Inhibition of tetrahydrofolate synthesis by sulfonamides and *trimethoprim*.

from plasmid transfers or random mutations. [Note: Organisms resistant to one member of this drug family are resistant to all.] Resistance is generally irreversible and may be due to 1) an altered dihydropteroate synthetase, 2) decreased cellular permeability to sulfa drugs, or 3) enhanced production of the natural substrate, PABA.

D. Pharmacokinetics

1. **Administration:** After oral administration, most sulfa drugs are well absorbed via the small intestine (Figure 33.10). An exception is *sulfasalazine* [sul-fa-SAL-a-zeen]. It is not absorbed when administered orally or as a suppository and, therefore, is reserved for treatment of chronic inflammatory bowel disease (for example, Crohn's disease or ulcerative colitis). [Note: Local intestinal flora split *sulfasalazine* into sulfapyridine and 5-aminosalicylate, with the latter exerting the anti-inflammatory effect. Absorption of the *sulfapyridine* can lead to toxicity in patients who are slow acetylators (see below).] Intravenous sulfonamides are generally reserved for patients who are unable to take oral preparations. Because of the risk of sensitization, sulfas are not usually applied topically. However, in burn units, creams of *silver sulfadiazine* or *mafenide* [mah-FEN-ide] *acetate (α-amino-p-toluene-sulfonamide)* have been effective in reducing burn-associated sepsis, because they prevent colonization of bacteria. Superinfections with resistant bacteria or fungi may still occur. [Note: *Silver sulfadiazine* is preferred, because *mafenide* produces pain on application. Furthermore, *mafenide* can be absorbed in burn patients, causing an increased risk of acid-base imbalance.]

2. **Distribution:** Sulfa drugs are bound to serum albumin in the circulation, where the extent of binding depends on the particular agent's pK_a. In general, the lower the pK_a, the greater the binding. Sulfa drugs distribute throughout the body's water and penetrate well into cerebrospinal fluid—even in the absence of inflammation. They can also pass the placental barrier and enter fetal tissues.

3. **Metabolism:** The sulfa drugs are acetylated, primarily in the liver. The product is devoid of antimicrobial activity but retains the toxic potential to precipitate at neutral or acidic pH. This causes crystalluria ("stone formation"; see below) and, therefore, potential damage to the kidney.

4. **Excretion:** Sulfa drugs are eliminated by glomerular filtration. Therefore, depressed kidney function causes accumulation of both the parent compounds and their metabolites. The sulfonamides may also be eliminated in breast milk.

E. Adverse effects

1. **Crystalluria:** Nephrotoxicity develops as a result of crystalluria (Figure 33.11). Adequate hydration and alkalinization of urine prevent the problem by reducing the concentration of drug and promoting its ionization. Agents, such as *sulfisoxazole* [sul-fi-SOX-a-zole] and *sulfamethoxazole* [sul-fa-meth-OX-a-zole] are more soluble at urinary pH than are the older sulfonamides (for example, *sulfadiazine*) and are less liable to cause crystalluria .

2. **Hypersensitivity:** Hypersensitivity reactions, such as rashes, angioedema, and Stevens-Johnson syndrome, are fairly common. The latter occurs more frequently with the longer-acting agents.

exfoliative dermatitis

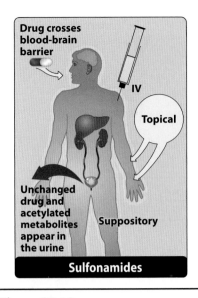

Figure 33.10
Administration and fate of the sulfonamides.

Disseminate to all compartments

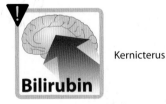

Figure 33.11
Some adverse reactions to sulfonamides.

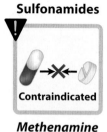

Figure 33.12
Contraindication for sulfonamide treatment.

3. **Hemopoietic disturbances:** Hemolytic anemia is encountered in patients with glucose 6-phosphate dehydrogenase deficiency. Granulocytopenia and thrombocytopenia can also occur.

4. **Kernicterus:** This disorder may occur in newborns, because sulfa drugs displace bilirubin from binding sites on serum albumin. The bilirubin is then free to pass into the CNS, because the baby's blood-brain barrier is not fully developed (see below).

5. **Drug potentiation:** Transient potentiation of the hypoglycemic effect of *tolbutamide* or the anticoagulant effect of *warfarin* results from their displacement from binding sites on serum albumin. Free *methotrexate* levels may also rise through displacement.

6. **Contraindications:** Due to the danger of kernicterus, sulfa drugs should be avoided in newborns and infants less than 2 months of age as well as in pregnant women at term. Because sulfonamides condense with formaldehyde, they should not be given to patients receiving *methenamine* for UTIs (Figure 33.12).

IV. TRIMETHOPRIM

Trimethoprim [trye METH-oh-prim], a potent inhibitor of bacterial dihydrofolate reductase, exhibits an antibacterial spectrum similar to that of the sulfonamides. *Trimethoprim* is most often compounded with *sulfamethoxazole*, producing the combination called *cotrimoxazole.*

A. Mechanism of action

The active form of folate is the tetrahydro-derivative that is formed through reduction of dihydrofolic acid by dihydrofolate reductase.[5] This enzymatic reaction (see Figure 33.9) is inhibited by *trimethoprim*, leading to a decreased availability of the tetrahydrofolate coenzymes required for purine, pyrimidine, and amino acid synthesis. The bacterial reductase has a much stronger affinity for *trimethoprim* than does the mammalian enzyme, which accounts for the drug's selective toxicity. [Note: Examples of other drugs that function as folate reductase inhibitors include *pyrimethamine,* which is used with sulfonamides in treating parasitic infections, and *methotrexate*, which is used in the treatment of cancer, rheumatoid arthritis, and psoriasis].

given w/ sulfadiazene

B. Antibacterial spectrum

The antibacterial spectrum of *trimethoprim* is similar to that of *sulfamethoxazole*. However, *trimethoprim* is 20- to 50-fold more potent than the sulfonamide. *Trimethoprim* may be used alone in the treatment of acute UTIs and in the treatment of bacterial prostatitis (although fluoroquinolones are preferred) and vaginitis.

Norfloxacin or Levafloxacin

C. Resistance

Resistance in gram-negative bacteria is due to the presence of an altered dihydrofolate reductase that has a lower affinity for *trimethoprim*. Overproduction of the enzyme may also lead to resistance, because this can decrease drug permeability.

 [5]See p. 374 in ***Lippincott's Illustrated Reviews: Biochemistry*** (4th ed.) for a discussion of the reaction catalyzed by dihydrofolate reductase.

D. Pharmacokinetics

The half-life of *trimethoprim* is similar to that of *sulfamethoxazole*. However, because the drug is a weak base, higher concentrations of *trimethoprim* are achieved in the relatively acidic prostatic and vaginal fluids. The drug also penetrates the cerebrospinal fluid. *Trimethoprim* undergoes some O-demethylation, but most of it is excreted unchanged through the kidney.

E. Adverse effects

Trimethoprim can produce the effects of folic acid deficiency.[6] These effects include megaloblastic anemia, leukopenia, and granulocytopenia, especially in pregnant patients and those having very poor diets. These blood disorders can be reversed by the simultaneous administration of *folinic acid*, which does not enter bacteria.

[handwritten: Mammals & bacteria share common pathway]

V. COTRIMOXAZOLE

The combination of *trimethoprim* with *sulfamethoxazole*, called *cotrimoxazole* [co-try-MOX-a-zole], shows greater antimicrobial activity than equivalent quantities of either drug used alone (see Figure 33.13). The combination was selected because of the similarity in the half-lives of the two drugs.

A. Mechanism of action

The synergistic antimicrobial activity of *cotrimoxazole* results from its inhibition of two sequential steps in the synthesis of tetrahydrofolic acid: *Sulfamethoxazole* inhibits the incorporation of PABA into dihydrofolic acid precursors, and *trimethoprim* prevents reduction of dihydrofolate to tetrahydrofolate (see Figure 33.9).

B. Antibacterial spectrum

Cotrimoxazole has a broader spectrum of antibacterial action than the sulfa drugs (Figure 33.14). It is effective in treating UTIs and respiratory tract infections as well as in Pneumocystis jiroveci pneumonia and *ampicillin-* or *chloramphenicol*-resistant systemic salmonella infections.

C. Resistance

Resistance to the *trimethoprim-sulfamethoxazole* combination is less frequently encountered than resistance to either of the drugs alone, because it would require that the bacterium have simultaneous resistance to both drugs. *[handwritten: → good]*

D. Pharmacokinetics

Trimethoprim is more lipid soluble than *sulfamethoxazole* and has a greater volume of distribution. Administration of one part *trimethoprim* to five parts of the sulfa drug produces a ratio of the drugs in the plasma of twenty parts *sulfamethoxazole* to one part *trimethoprim*. This ratio is optimal for the antibiotic effect. *Cotrimoxazole* is generally administered orally (Figure 33.15). An exception involves intravenous administration to patients with severe pneumonia caused by P. jiroveci or to patients who cannot take the drug by mouth. Both agents distribute throughout the body. *Trimethoprim* concentrates in the relatively acidic

[handwritten right margin: 1:5 Trim/sulfa yields   1:20 in plasma]

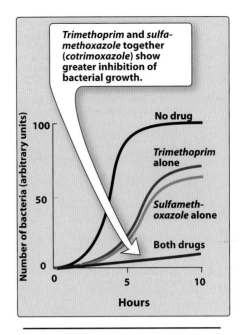

Figure 33.13
Synergism between *trimethoprim* and *sulfamethoxazole* on the inhibition of growth of Escherichia coli.

[6]See p. 375 in **Lippincott's Illustrated Reviews: Biochemistry** (4th ed.) for a discussion of folic acid deficiency.

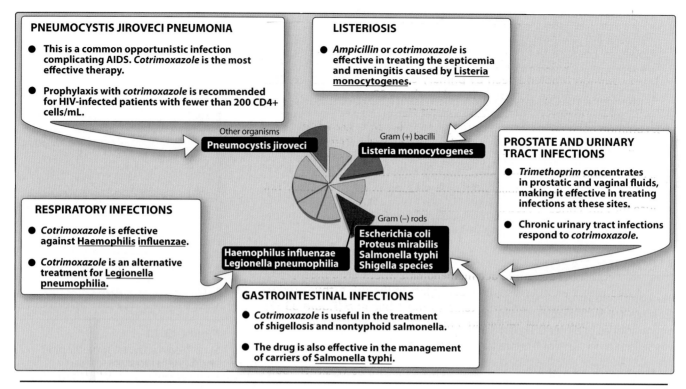

Figure 33.14
Typical therapeutic applications of *co-trimoxazole* (*sulfamethoxazole* plus *trimethoprim*).

milieu of prostatic and vaginal fluids, and it accounts for the use of the *trimethoprim-sulfamethoxazole* combination in infections at these sites. Both parent drugs and their metabolites are excreted in the urine.

E. Adverse effects

1. **Dermatologic:** Reactions involving the skin are very common and may be severe in the elderly (Figure 33.16).

2. **Gastrointestinal:** Nausea, vomiting, as well as glossitis and stomatitis are not unusual. → *Folate deficiency*

3. **Hematologic:** Megaloblastic anemia, leukopenia, and thrombocytopenia may occur. All these effects may be reversed by the concurrent administration of *folinic acid*, which protects the patient and does not enter the microorganism. Hemolytic anemia may occur in patients with glucose 6-phosphate dehydrogenase deficiency due to the *sulfamethoxazole*.

4. **Patients infected with human immunodeficiency virus:** Immunocompromised patients with P. jiroveci pneumonia frequently show drug-induced fever, rashes, diarrhea, and/or pancytopenia.

5. **Drug interactions:** Prolonged prothrombin times in patients receiving both *trimethoprim* and *warfarin* have been reported. The plasma half-life of *phenytoin* may be increased due to an inhibition of its metabolism. *Methotrexate* levels may rise due to displacement from albumin-binding sites by *sulfamethoxazole*.

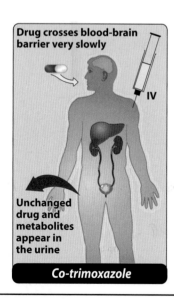

Figure 33.15
Administration and fate of the *cotrimoxazole*.

VI. URINARY TRACT ANTISEPTICS/ANTIMICROBIALS

Urinary tract infections (most commonly uncomplicated acute cystitis and pyelonephritis) in women of child-bearing age and in the elderly are one of the most common problems seen by primary care physicians. Escherichia coli is the most common pathogen, causing about 80 percent of uncomplicated upper and lower UTIs. Staphylococcus saprophyticus is the second most common bacterial pathogen causing UTIs, with other common causes including Klebsiella pneumoniae and Proteus mirabilis These infections may be treated with any one of a group of agents called urinary tract antiseptics, including *methenamine*, *nitrofurantoin*, and the quinolone *nalidixic acid*. These drugs do not achieve antibacterial levels in the circulation, but because they are concentrated in the urine, microorganisms at that site can be effectively eradicated.

A. Methenamine

1. **Mechanism of action:** To act, *methenamine* [meth-EN-a-meen] must decompose at an acidic pH of 5.5 or less in the urine, thus producing formaldehyde, which is toxic to most bacteria (Figure 33.17). The reaction is slow, requiring 3 hours to reach 90 percent decomposition. *Methenamine* should not be used in patients with indwelling catheters. Bacteria do not develop resistance to formaldehyde. [Note: *Methenamine* is frequently formulated with a weak acid, such as mandelic acid or hippuric acid.]

2. **Antibacterial spectrum:** *Methenamine* is primarily used for chronic suppressive therapy. Urea-splitting bacteria that alkalinize the urine, such as Proteus species, are usually resistant to the action of *methenamine*. *Methenamine* is used to treat lower UTIs but is not effective in upper UTIs.

3. **Pharmacokinetics:** *Methenamine* is administered orally. In addition to formaldehyde, ammonium ion is produced in the bladder. Because the liver rapidly metabolizes ammonia to form urea, *methenamine* is contraindicated in patients with hepatic insufficiency, in which elevated levels of circulating ammonium ions would be toxic to the CNS. *Methenamine* is distributed throughout the body fluids, but no decomposition of the drug occurs at pH 7.4. Thus, systemic toxicity does not occur. The drug is eliminated in the urine.

4. **Adverse effects:** The major side effect of *methenamine* treatment is gastrointestinal distress, although at higher doses, albuminuria, hematuria, and rashes may develop. *Methenamine mandelate* is contraindicated in patients with renal insufficiency, because mandelic acid may precipitate. [Note: Sulfonamides react with formaldehyde and must not be used concomitantly with *methenamine*.]

B. Nitrofurantoin

Nitrofurantoin [nye-troe-FYOOR-an-toyn] is less commonly employed for treating UTIs because of its narrow antimicrobial spectrum and its toxicity. Sensitive bacteria reduce the drug to an active agent that inhibits various enzymes and damages DNA. Antibiotic activity is greater in acidic urine. The drug is bacteriostatic. It is useful against E. coli, but other common urinary tract gram-negative bacteria may be resistant. Gram-positive cocci are susceptible. Adverse effects include gastrointestinal disturbances, acute pneumonitis, and neurologic problems.

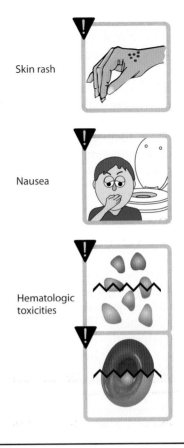

Skin rash

Nausea

Hematologic toxicities

Figure 33.16
Some adverse reactions to *cotrimoxazole*.

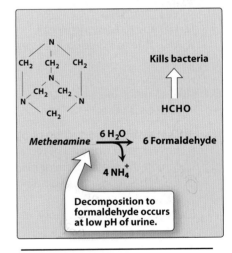

Figure 33.17
Formation of formaldehyde from *methenamine* at acid pH.

Study Questions

Choose the ONE best answer.

33.1 A 30-year-old male is diagnosed to be human immu-nodeficiency virus (HIV) positive. His CD4+ count is 200 cells/mm^3 and his viral load is 10,000 copies/mL. In addition to receiving antiviral therapy, which of the following is indicated to protect him against pneumonia due to <u>Pneumocystis</u> <u>jiroveci</u>?

    A. Trimethoprim.
    B. Ciprofloxacin.
    C. Cotrimoxazole.
    D. Clindamycin.

> Correct answer = C. Prophylaxis with cotrimoxazole is the standard treatment for HIV patients with CD4+ counts at 200 cells/mm^3 or lower. Trimethoprim is not effective as monotherapy. It can be used in combination with dapsone. Clindamycin is effective in pneumonia, which has already developed due to this organism, but is not employed for prophylaxis because of its adverse effect on the gastrointestinal tract. Ciprofloxacin lacks activity against this organism.

33.2 A 26-year-old young man presents with the symptoms of gonorrhea. Because this condition is often associated with an infection due to <u>Chlamydia trachomatis</u>, which of the following quinolones would be the best choice for treating him?

    A. Ciprofloxacin. → no activity against chlamydia
    B. Nalidixic acid.
    C. Norfloxacin.
    D. Levofloxacin. → all STDs but syphilis

> Correct answer = D. Levofloxacin has the best activity of all the quinolones against both gonorrheal and chlamydial infections. Nalidixic acid is without activity in these conditions.

33.3 In which one of the following infections is cipro-floxacin ineffective?

    A. Urinary tract infections due to a β-lactamase producing strain of Klebsiella.
    B. Pneumonia due to <u>Streptococcus</u> <u>pneumoniae</u>.
    C. Exacerbation of chronic bronchitis due to <u>Moraxella</u> <u>catarrhalis</u>.
    D. UTI due to <u>Escherichia</u> <u>coli</u>.
    E. UTIs due to Pseudomonas aeruginosa.

> Correct answer = B. Ciprofloxacin does not have sufficient activity against <u>S. pneumoniae</u> to be effective. Because it is not a β-lactam, ciprofloxacin is effective in treating UTIs caused by β-lactamase producing organisms. Ciprofloxacin is indicated for treatment of the other infections listed.

33.4 Sulfonamides increase the risk of neonatal kernicterus, because they:

    A. Diminish the production of plasma albumin.
    B. Increase the turnover of red blood cells.
    C. Inhibit the metabolism of bilirubin.
    D. Compete for bilirubin-binding sites on plasma albumin.
    E. Depress the bone marrow.

> Correct answer = D. Increased release of albumin-bound bilirubin increases the plasma concentration of free bilirubin, which can penetrate the CNS.

Antimycobacterials

34

I. OVERVIEW

Mycobacteria are slender, rod-shaped bacteria with lipid-rich cell walls that stain poorly with the Gram stain, but once stained, the walls cannot be easily decolorized by treatment with acidified organic solvents. Hence, they are termed "acid-fast." The most widely encountered mycobacterial infections is tuberculosis—the leading cause worldwide of death from infection. Members of the genus Mycobacterium also cause leprosy as well as several tuberculosis-like human infections. Mycobacterial infections are intracellular and, generally, result in the formation of slow-growing granulomatous lesions that are responsible for major tissue destruction.[1] There are four currently recommended first-line agents utilized for antituberculosis therapy (Figure 34.1). Second-line medications are either less effective, more toxic, or have not been studied as extensively. They are useful in patients who cannot tolerate the first-line drugs or who are infected with myobacteria that are resistant to the first-line agents.

II. CHEMOTHERAPY FOR TUBERCULOSIS

Mycobacterium tuberculosis, one of a number of mycobacteria, can lead to serious infections of the lungs, genitourinary tract, skeleton, and meninges. Treating tuberculosis as well as other mycobacterial infections presents therapeutic problems. The organism grows slowly; thus, the disease may have to be treated for 6 months to 2 years. Resistant organisms readily emerge, particularly in patients who have had prior therapy or who fail to adhere to the treatment protocol. It is currently estimated that about one-third of the world's population is infected with M. tuberculosis, with 30 million people having active disease. Worldwide, 8 million new cases occur, and approximately 2 million people die of the disease each year.

A. Strategies for addressing drug resistance

Strains of M. tuberculosis that are resistant to a particular agent emerge during treatment with a single drug. For example, Figure 34.2 shows that resistance rapidly develops in patients given only *streptomycin*. Therefore, multidrug therapy is employed when treating tuberculosis in an effort to delay or prevent the emergence of resistant strains. *Isoniazid, rifampin* (or *rifabutin* or *rifapentine*), *ethambutol*, and *pyrazin-*

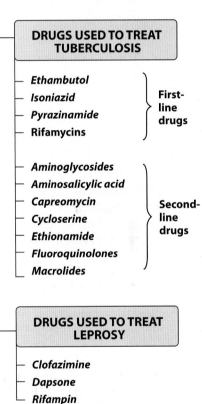

ANTIMYCOBACTERIAL AGENTS

DRUGS USED TO TREAT TUBERCULOSIS

— *Ethambutol*
— *Isoniazid*   First-line drugs
— *Pyrazinamide*
— *Rifamycins*

— *Aminoglycosides*
— *Aminosalicylic acid*
— *Capreomycin*
— *Cycloserine*   Second-line drugs
— *Ethionamide*
— *Fluoroquinolones*
— *Macrolides*

DRUGS USED TO TREAT LEPROSY

— *Clofazimine*
— *Dapsone*
— *Rifampin*

Figure 34.1
Summary of drugs used to treat mycobacterial infections.

[1]See p. 185 in **Lippincott's Illustrated Reviews: Microbiology** (2nd ed.) for a discussion of mycobacterial infections.

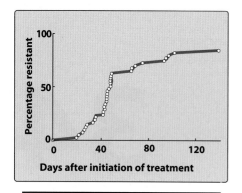

Figure 34.2
Cumulative percentage of strains of <u>Mycobacterium</u> <u>tuberculosis</u> showing resistance to *streptomycin*.

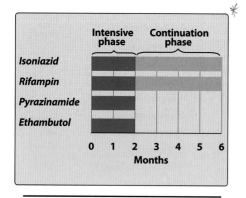

Figure 34.3
One of several recommended multi-drug schedules for the treatment of tuberculosis.

Targets for Isoniazid ← [*InhA*
                            kasA
↓
stops mycolic acid synthesis

amide are the principal or so-called "first-line" drugs because of their efficacy and acceptable degree of toxicity. Today, however, because of poor patient compliance and other factors, the number of multidrug-resistant organisms has risen. Some bacteria have been identified that are resistant to as many as seven antitubercular agents. Therefore, although treatment regimens vary in duration and in the agents employed, they always include a minimum of two drugs, preferably with both being bactericidal (see p. 348). The combination of drugs should prevent the emergence of resistant strains. The multidrug regimen is continued well beyond the disappearance of clinical disease to eradicate any persistent organisms. For example, the initial short-course chemotherapy for tuberculosis includes *isoniazid, rifampin, ethambutol,* and *pyrazinamide* for 2 months and then *isoniazid* and *rifampin* for the next 4 months (the "continuation phase"; Figure 34.3). Before susceptibility data are available, more drugs may be added to the first-line ones for patients who have previously had tuberculosis or those in whom multidrug-resistant tuberculosis is suspected. The added drugs normally include an aminoglycoside (*streptomycin, kanamycin,* or *amikacin*) or *capreomycin* (injectable agents), a fluoroquinolone, and perhaps a second-line antituberculosis agent such as *cycloserine, ethionamide,* or *para-aminosalicylic acid*. Once susceptibility data are available, the drug regimen can be individually tailored to the patient. Patient compliance is often low when multidrug schedules last for 6 months or longer. One successful strategy for achieving better treatment completion rates is "directly observed therapy," also known as DOT, in which patients take their medication while being supervised and observed. DOT have been shown to decrease drug resistance as well as relapse and mortality rates and to improve cure rates. Most local and state health departments offer DOT services.

B. Isoniazid

Isoniazid [eye-soe-NYE-a-zid], the hydrazide of isonicotinic acid, is a synthetic analog of pyridoxine. It is the most potent of the antitubercular drugs but is never given as a single agent in the treatment of active tuberculosis. Its introduction revolutionized the treatment of tuberculosis.

1. **Mechanism of action:** *Isoniazid*, often referred to as *INH*, is a prodrug that is activated by a mycobacterial catalase-peroxidase (KatG). Genetic and biochemical evidence has implicated at least two different target enzymes for *isoniazid* within the unique Type II fatty acid synthase system involved in the production of mycolic acids. [Note: Mycolic acid is a unique class of very-long-chain, β-hydroxylated fatty acids found in mycobacterial cell walls. Decreased mycolic acid synthesis corresponds with the loss of acid-fastness after exposure to *isoniazid*.] The targeted enzymes are enoyl acyl carrier protein reductase (InhA) and a β-ketoacyl-ACP synthase (KasA). The activated drug covalently binds to and inhibits these enzymes, which are essential for the synthesis of mycolic acid.

2. **Antibacterial spectrum:** For bacilli in the stationary phase, *isoniazid* is bacteriostatic, but for rapidly dividing organisms, it is bactericidal. It is effective against intracellular bacteria. *Isoniazid* is specific for treatment of <u>M</u>. tuberculosis, although <u>Mycobacterium</u> <u>kansasii</u> (an organism that causes three percent of the clinical illness known as tuberculosis) may be susceptible at higher drug levels. When it is used alone, resistant organisms rapidly emerge.

3. Resistance: This is associated with several different chromosomal mutations, each of which results in one of the following: mutation or deletion of KatG (producing mutants incapable of prodrug activation), varying mutations of the acyl carrier proteins, or overexpression of InhA. Cross-resistance does not occur between *isoniazid* and other antitubercular drugs.

4. Pharmacokinetics: Orally administered *isoniazid* is readily absorbed. Absorption is impaired if *isoniazid* is taken with food, particularly carbohydrates, or with aluminum-containing antacids. The drug diffuses into all body fluids, cells, and caseous material (necrotic tissue resembling cheese that is produced in tubercles). Drug levels in the cerebrospinal fluid (CSF) are about the same as those in the serum. The drug readily penetrates host cells and is effective against bacilli growing intracellularly. Infected tissue tends to retain the drug longer. *Isoniazid* undergoes N-acetylation and hydrolysis, resulting in inactive products. [Note: Acetylation is genetically regulated, with the fast acetylator trait being autosomally dominant. A bimodal distribution of fast and slow acetylators exists (Figure 34.4).] Chronic liver disease decreases metabolism, and doses must be reduced. Excretion is through glomerular filtration, predominantly as metabolites (Figure 34.5). Slow acetylators excrete more of the parent compound. Severely depressed renal function results in accumulation of the drug, primarily in slow acetylators.

5. Adverse effects: The incidence of adverse effects is fairly low. Except for hypersensitivity, adverse effects are related to the dosage and duration of administration.

a. Peripheral neuritis: Peripheral neuritis (manifesting as paresthesias of the hands and feet), which is the most common adverse effect, appears to be due to a relative pyridoxine deficiency. Most of the toxic reactions are corrected by supplementation of 25 to 50 mg per day of pyridoxine (vitamin B_6). [Note: *Isoniazid* can achieve levels in breast milk that are high enough to cause a pyridoxine deficiency in the infant unless the mother is supplemented with the vitamin.[2]]

b. Hepatitis and idiosyncratic hepatotoxicity: Potentially fatal hepatitis is the most severe side effect associated with *isoniazid*. It has been suggested that this is caused by a toxic metabolite of monoacetylhydrazine, formed during the metabolism of *isoniazid*. Its incidence increases among patients with increasing age, among patients who also take *rifampin*, or among those who drink alcohol daily.

c. Drug interactions: Because *isoniazid* inhibits metabolism of *phenytoin* (Figure 34.6), *isoniazid* can potentiate the adverse effects of that drug (for example, nystagmus and ataxia). Slow acetylators are particularly at risk .

d. Other adverse effects: Mental abnormalities, convulsions in patients prone to seizures, and optic neuritis have been observed. Hypersensitivity reactions include rashes and fever.

[2]See p. 378 in ***Lippincott's Illustrated Reviews: Biochemistry*** (4th ed.) for a discussion of pyridoxine.

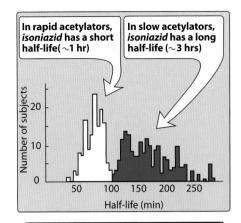

In rapid acetylators, *isoniazid* has a short half-life(~1 hr)

In slow acetylators, *isoniazid* has a long half-life (~3 hrs)

Figure 34 .4
Bimodal distribution of *isoniazid* half-lives caused by rapid and slow acetylation of the drug.

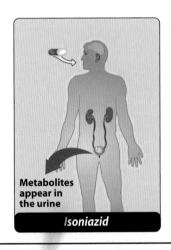

Metabolites appear in the urine

Isoniazid

Figure 34.5
Administration and fate of *isoniazid*.

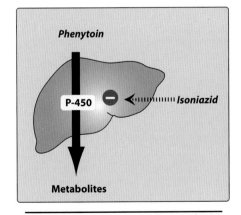

Phenytoin

P-450

Isoniazid

Metabolites

Figure 34.6
Isoniazid potentiates the adverse effects of *phenytoin*.

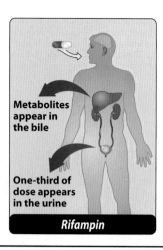

Figure 34.7
Administration and fate of *rifampin*. [Note: Patient should be warned that urine and tears may be orange-red in color.]

C. Rifamycins: Rifampin, rifabutin and rifapentine

Rifampin, rifabutin, and *rifapentine* are all considered to be rifamycins, a group of structurally similar macrocyclic antibiotics, which are first-line drugs for tuberculosis. Any of these rifamycins must always be used in conjunction with at least one other antituberculosis drug to which the isolate is susceptible.

1. **Rifampin:** *Rifampin* [rif-AM-pin], which is derived from the soil mold <u>Streptomyces</u>, has a broader antimicrobial activity than *isoniazid* and has found application in the treatment of a number of different bacterial infections. Because resistant strains rapidly emerge during therapy, it is never given as a single agent in the treatment of active tuberculosis.

   a. **Mechanism of action:** *Rifampin* blocks transcription by interacting with the β subunit of bacterial but not human DNA-dependent RNA polymerase. [Note: The drug is thus specific for prokaryotes.] *Rifampin* inhibits mRNA synthesis by suppressing the initiation step.

   b. **Antimicrobial spectrum:** *Rifampin* is bactericidal for both intracellular and extracellular mycobacteria, including <u>M. tuberculosis</u>, and atypical mycobacteria, such as <u>M. kansasii</u>. It is effective against many gram-positive and gram-negative organisms and is frequently used prophylactically for individuals exposed to meningitis caused by meningococci or <u>Haemophilus influenzae</u>. *Rifampin* is the most active antileprosy drug at present, but to delay the emergence of resistant strains, it is usually given in combination with other drugs. *Rifabutin*, an analog of *rifampin*, has some activity against <u>Mycobacterium avium-intracellulare</u> complex but is less active against tuberculosis.

   c. **Resistance:** Resistance to *rifampin* can be caused by a mutation in the affinity of the bacterial DNA-dependent RNA polymerase for the drug or by decreased permeability.

   d. **Pharmacokinetics:** Absorption is adequate after oral administration. Distribution of *rifampin* occurs to all body fluids and organs. Adequate levels are attained in the CSF even in the absence of inflammation. The drug is taken up by the liver and undergoes enterohepatic cycling. *Rifampin* itself can induce the hepatic mixed-function oxidases (see p. 14), leading to a shortened half-life. Elimination of metabolites and the parent drug is via the bile into the feces or via the urine (Figure 34.7). [Note: Urine and feces as well as other secretions have an orange-red color; patients should be forewarned. Tears may permanently stain soft contact lenses orange-red.]

   e. **Adverse effects:** Rifampin is generally well tolerated. The most common adverse reactions include nausea, vomiting, and rash. Hepatitis and death due to liver failure is rare; however, the drug should be used judiciously in patients who are alcoholic, elderly, or have chronic liver disease due to the increased incidence of severe hepatic dysfunction when *rifampin* is administered alone or concomitantly with *isoniazid*. Often, when *rifampin* is dosed intermittently, or in daily doses of 1.2 grams or greater, a flu-like syndrome is associated with fever, chills, and myalgias and sometimes is associated with acute renal failure, hemolytic anemia, and shock.

    f. Drug interactions: Because *rifampin* can induce a number of cytochrome P450 enzymes (see p. 14), it can decrease the half-lives of other drugs that are coadministered and metabolized by this system (Figure 34.8). This may lead to higher dosage requirements for these agents.

2. Rifabutin: *Rifabutin* [rif-a-BYOO-tin], a derivative of *rifampin*, is the preferred drug for use in tuberculosis-infected with the human immunodeficiency virus (HIV) patients who are concomitantly treated with protease inhibitors or nonnucleoside reverse transcriptase inhibitors, because it is a less potent inducer of cytochrome P450 enzymes. *Rifabutin* has adverse effects similar to those of *rifampin* but can also cause uveitis, skin hyperpigmentation, and neutropenia.

3. Rifapentine: *Rifapentine* [rih-fa-PEN-teen] has activity comparable to that of *rifampin* but has a longer half-life than *rifampin* and *rifabutin*, which permits weekly dosing. However, for the intensive phase (initial 2 months) of the short-course therapy for tuberculosis, *rifapentine* is given twice weekly. In the subsequent phase, *rifapentine* is dosed once per week for 4 months. To avoid resistance issues, *rifapentine* should not be used alone but, rather, be included in a three to four-drug regimen.

D. Pyrazinamide

Pyrazinamide [peer-a-ZIN-a-mide] is a synthetic, orally effective, bactericidal, antitubercular agent used in combination with *isoniazid*, *rifampin*, and *ethambutol*. It is bactericidal to actively dividing organisms, but the mechanism of its action is unknown. *Pyrazinamide* must be enzymatically hydrolyzed to pyrazinoic acid, which is the active form of the drug. Some resistant strains lack the pyrazinamidase. *Pyrazinamide* is active against tubercle bacilli in the acidic environment of lysosomes as well as in macrophages. *Pyrazinamide* distributes throughout the body, penetrating the CSF. It undergoes extensive metabolism. About one to five percent of patients taking *isoniazid*, *rifampin*, and *pyrazinamide* may experience liver dysfunction. Urate retention can also occur and may precipitate a gouty attack (Figure 34.9).

E. Ethambutol

Ethambutol [e-THAM-byoo-tole] is bacteriostatic and specific for most strains of M. tuberculosis and M. kansasii. *Ethambutol* inhibits arabinosyl transferase—an enzyme that is important for the synthesis of the mycobacterial arabinogalactan cell wall. Resistance is not a serious problem if the drug is employed with other antitubercular agents. *Ethambutol* can be used in combination with *pyrazinamide*, *isoniazid*, and *rifampin* to treat tuberculosis. Absorbed on oral administration, *ethambutol* is well distributed throughout the body. Penetration into the central nervous system (CNS) is therapeutically adequate in tuberculous meningitis. Both parent drug and metabolites are excreted by glomerular filtration and tubular secretion. The most important adverse effect is optic neuritis, which results in diminished visual acuity and loss of ability to discriminate between red and green. Visual acuity should be periodically examined. Discontinuation of the drug results in reversal of the optic symptoms. In addition, urate excretion is decreased by the drug; thus, gout may be exacerbated (see Figure 34.9). Figure 34.10 summa-

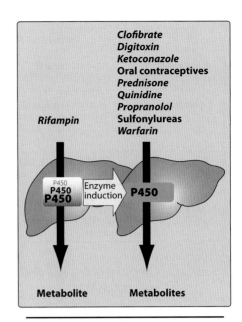

Figure 34.8
Rifampin induces cytochrome P450, which can decrease the half-lives of coadministered drugs that are metabolized by this system.

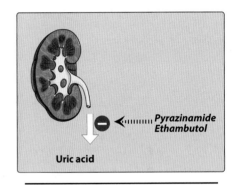

Figure 34.9
Pyrazinamide and *ethambutol* may cause urate retention and gouty attacks.

DRUG	ADVERSE EFFECTS	COMMENTS
Ethambutol	Optic neuritis with blurred vision, red-green color blindness	Establish baseline visual acuity and color vision; test monthly.
Isoniazid	Hepatic enzyme elevation, hepatitis, peripheral neuropathy	Take baseline hepatic enzyme measurements; repeat if abnormal or patient is at risk or symptomatic. Clinically significant interation with *phenytoin* and antifugal agents (azols).
Pyrazinamide	Nausea, hepatitis, hyperuricemia, rash, joint ache, gout (rare)	Take baseline hepatic enzymes and uric acid measurements; repeat if abnormal or patient is at risk or symptomatic.
Rifampin	Hepatitis, GI upset, rash, flu-like syndrome, significant interaction with several drugs	Take baseline hepatic enzyme measurements and CBC count; repeat if abnormal or patient is at risk or symptomatic. Warn patient that urine and tears may turn red-orange in color.

Figure 34.10
Some characteristics of first-line drugs used in treating tuberculosis. CBC = complete blood count.

rizes some of the characteristics of first-line drugs. [Note: As with any drug, antitubercular drugs have a therapeutic margin, which is the difference between the minimum drug concentration required to inhibit the growth of <u>M</u>. <u>tuberculosis</u> and the maximum concentration that can be given without provoking drug toxicity.]

F. Alternate second-line drugs

A number of drugs—*streptomycin*, [strep-toe-MY-sin], *para-aminosalicylic acid* [a-mee-noe-sal-i-SIL-ik], *ethionamide* [e-thye-ON-am-ide], *cycloserine* [sye-kloe-SER-een], *capreomycin* [kap-ree-oh-MYE sin], fluoroquinolones, and macrolides—are considered to be second-line drugs, either because they are no more effective than the first-line agents and their toxicities are often more serious or because they are particularly active against atypical strains of mycobacteria.

1. **Streptomycin:** This is the first antibiotic effective in the treatment of tuberculosis and is discussed with the aminoglycosides (see p. 377). Its action is directed against extracellular organisms. Infections due to *streptomycin*-resistant organisms may be treated with *kanamycin* or *amikacin*, to which these bacilli remain sensitive.

2. **Capreomycin:** This is a peptide that inhibits protein synthesis. It is administered parenterally. *Capreomycin* is primarily reserved for the treatment of multidrug-resistant tuberculosis. Careful monitoring of the patient is necessary to prevent its nephrotoxicity and ototoxicity.

3. **Cycloserine** is an orally effective, tuberculostatic agent that appears to antagonize the steps in bacterial cell wall synthesis involving D-alanine. It distributes well throughout body fluids, including the CSF. *Cycloserine* is metabolized, and both parent and metabolite are excreted in urine. Accumulation occurs with renal insufficiency. Adverse effects involve CNS disturbances, and epileptic seizure activity may be exacerbated. Peripheral neuropathies are also a problem, but they respond to pyridoxine.

4. **Ethionamide:** This is a structural analog of *isoniazid*, but it is not believed to act by the same mechanism. *Ethionamide* can inhibit acetylation of *isoniazid* (Figure 34.11). It is effective after oral administration and is widely distributed throughout the body, including the CSF. Metabolism is extensive, and the urine is the main route

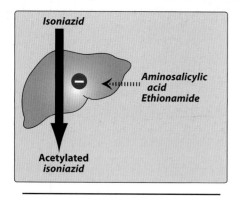

Figure 34.11
Aminosalicylic acid and *ethionamide* can inhibit the acetylation of *isoniazid*

of excretion. Adverse effects that limit its use include gastric irritation, hepatotoxicity, peripheral neuropathies, and optic neuritis. Supplementation with vitamin B$_6$ (pyridoxine) may lessen the severity of the neurologic side effects.

5. **Fluoroquinolones:** The fluoroquinolones, such as *moxifloxacin* and *levofloxacin,* have an important place in the treatment of multidrug-resistant tuberculosis. Some atypical strains of mycobacteria are also susceptible. These drugs are discussed in detail in Chapter 33.

6. **Macrolides:** The macrolides, such as *azithromycin* and *clarithromycin*, are part of the regimen that includes *ethambutol* and *rifabutin* used for the treatment of infections by M. avium-intracellulare complex. *Azithromycin* is preferred for HIV-infected patients because it is least likely to interfere with the metabolism of antiretroviral drugs. Details about the pharmacology of macrolides are found in Chapter 32.

III. CHEMOTHERAPY FOR LEPROSY

Leprosy (or, as it is specified by the U.S. Public Health Service, Hansen's disease) is rare in the United States, but a small number of cases, both imported and domestically acquired, are reported each year. Worldwide, it is a much larger problem (Figure 34.12). Approximately 70 percent of all cases in the world are located in India. Bacilli from skin lesions or nasal discharges of infected patients enter susceptible individuals via abraded skin or the respiratory tract. The World Health Organization recommends the triple-drug regimen of *dapsone, clofazimine,* and *rifampin* for 6 to 24 months. Figure 34.13 shows the effects of multi-drug therapy.

A. Dapsone

Dapsone [DAP-sone] is structurally related to the sulfonamides and similarly inhibits folate synthesis via dihydropteroate synthetase inhibiton. It is bacteriostatic for Mycobacterium leprae, but resistant strains are encountered. *Dapsone* is also employed in the treatment of pneumonia caused by Pneumocystis jiroveci in patients infected with the HIV. The drug is well absorbed from the gastrointestinal tract and is distributed throughout the body, with high levels concentrated in the skin. The parent drug enters the enterohepatic circulation and undergoes hepatic acetylation. Both parent drug and metabolites are eliminated through the urine. Adverse reactions include hemolysis, especially in patients with glucose 6-phosphate dehydrogenase deficiency, as well as methemoglobinemia, peripheral neuropathy, and the possibility of developing erythema nodosum leprosum (a serious and severe skin complication of leprosy). [Note: The latter is treated with corticosteroids or *thalidomide*.]

B. Clofazimine

Clofazimine [kloe-FA-zi-meen] is a phenazine dye that binds to DNA and prevents it from serving as a template for future DNA replication. Its redox properties may lead to the generation of cytotoxic oxygen radicals that are also toxic to the bacteria. *Clofazimine* is bactericidal to M. leprae and has some activity against M. avium-intracellulare complex. Following oral absorption, the drug accumulates in tissues, allowing intermittent therapy, but it does not enter the CNS. Patients may develop a red-brown discoloration of the skin. Eosinophilic enteritis has been reported as an adverse effect. The drug also has some anti-inflammatory activity; thus, erythema nodosum leprosum does not develop.

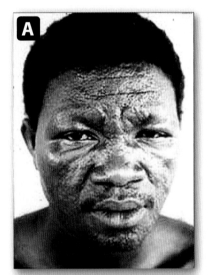

Figure 34.12
Reported prevalence of leprosy worldwide.

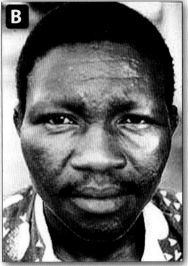

Figure 34.13
Leprosy patient. A. Before therapy. B. After 6 months of multidrug therapy.

Study Questions

Choose the ONE best answer.

34.1 A 31-year-old white intravenous drug user was admitted to the hospital with a 4-week history of cough and fever. A chest radiograph showed left upper lobe cavitary infiltrate. Cultures of sputum yielded <u>M. tuberculosis</u> susceptible to all antimycobacterial drugs. The patient received isoniazid, rifampin, and pyrazinamide. The patient's sputum remained culture-positive for the subsequent 4 months. Which one of the following is the most likely cause of treatment failure?

A. False-positive cultures.
B. Maladsorption of the medications.
C. Concomitant infection with HIV.
D. Noncompliance by the patient.
E. Drug resistance.

Correct answer = D. Although malabsorption of the drugs and the emergence of drug resistance are possibilities, the most common cause of treatment failure is nonadherence to the treatment protocol. Better treatment completion rates occur with "directly observed therapy." False-positive cultures is a possible but unlikely explanation.

34.2 A 40-year-old man has been on primary therapy for active pulmonary tuberculosis for the past 2 months. At his regular clinic visit, he complains of a "pins and needles" sensation in his feet. You suspect that he might be deficient in which one of the following vitamins?

A. Ascorbic acid.
B. Niacin.
C. Pyridoxine.
D. Calcitriol.
E. Folic acid.

Correct answer = C. Primary therapy for active pulmonary tuberculosis includes isoniazid. Isoniazid causes peripheral neuropathies with symptoms including paresthesias, such as "pins and needles" and numbness. This relative deficiency of pyridoxine appears to be due to the interference of isoniazid with its activation and enhancement of the excretion of pyridoxine. Concurrent administration of 100 mg of pyridoxine prevents the neuropathic actions of isoniazid.

34.3 A 35-year-old male, formerly a heroin abuser, has been on methadone maintenance for the last 13 months. Two weeks ago, he had a positive tuberculosis skin test (PPD test), and a chest radiograph showed evidence of right upper lobe infection. He was started on standard antimycobacterial therapy. He has come to the emergency department complaining of "withdrawal symptoms." Which of the following antimycobacterial drugs is likely to have caused this patient's acute withdrawal reaction?

A. Ethambutol.
B. Isoniazid.
C. Pyrazinamide.
D. Rifampin.
E. Streptomycin.

Correct answer = D. Rifampin is a potent inducer of cytochrome P450–dependent drug-metabolizing enzymes. The duration of action of methadone is dependent upon hepatic clearance, so enhanced drug metabolism will shorten the duration and increase the risk of withdrawal symptoms in individuals on methadone maintenance.

Antifungal Drugs

35

I. OVERVIEW

Infectious diseases caused by fungi are called mycoses, and they are often chronic in nature.[1] Many common mycotic infections are superficial and only involve the skin (cutaneous mycoses), but fungi may also penetrate the skin, causing subcutaneous infections. The fungal infections that are most difficult to treat are the systemic mycoses, which are often life-threatening. Unlike bacteria, fungi are eukaryotic. They have rigid cell walls composed largely of chitin—a polymer of N-acetylglucosamine—rather than peptidoglycan (a characteristic component of most bacterial cell walls). The fungal cell membrane contains ergosterol rather than the cholesterol found in mammalian membranes. These chemical characteristics are useful in targeting chemotherapeutic agents against fungal infections. Fungal infections are generally resistant to antibiotics used in the treatment of bacterial infections, and conversely, bacteria are resistant to the antifungal agents. The last two decades have seen a rise in the incidence of fungal infections so that candidemia is the fourth most common cause of septicemia. This increased incidence of fungal infections is associated with greater numbers of individuals who are on chronic immune suppression following organ transplant, undergoing chemotherapy for myelogenous and solid tumors, or infected with the human immunodeficiency virus (HIV). During this same period, there have been significant changes in the therapeutic options available to the clinician. For example, the ongoing development of new azole antifungal drugs offers effective therapy for all but the most serious mycotic infections. Clinically useful antifungal agents are listed in Figure 35.1.

II. DRUGS FOR SUBCUTANEOUS AND SYSTEMIC MYCOTIC INFECTIONS

The drugs used in the treatment of subcutaneous and systemic mycoses are listed in Figure 35.1. [Note: Additional azole drugs are effective in the topical treatment of candidiasis or dermatophytic infections.] The echinocandins are a new class of antifungal agents that exert their fungicidal activity by inhibiting 1,3-β-glucan synthesis for the fungal cell wall.

A. Amphotericin B

Amphotericin [am-foe-TER-i-sin] *B* is a naturally occurring, polyene macrolide antibiotic produced by <u>Streptomyces nodosus.</u> In spite of its toxic potential, *amphotericin B* is the drug of choice for the treat-

---

ANTIFUNGAL DRUGS

DRUGS FOR SUBCUTANEOUS AND SYSTEMIC MYCOSES

- *Amphotericin B*
- *Anidulafungin*
- *Caspofungin*
- *Fluconazole*
- *Flucytosine*
- *Itraconazole*
- *Ketoconazole*
- *Micafungin*
- *Posaconazole*
- *Voriconazole*

DRUGS FOR CUTANEOUS MYCOSES

- *Butoconazole*
- *Clotrimazole*
- *Econazole*
- *Griseofulvin*
- *Miconazole*
- *Nystatin*
- *Terbinafine*
- *Terconazole*

Figure 35.1
Summary of antifungal drugs.

---

[1]See Chapter 20 in ***Lippincott's Illustrated Reviews: Microbiology*** (2nd ed.) for a discussion of fungal infections.

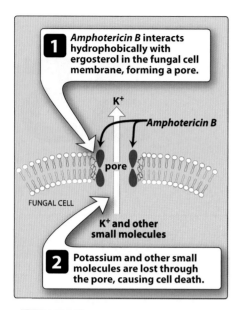

Figure 35.2
Model of a pore formed by
amphotericin B in the lipid bilayer
membrane.

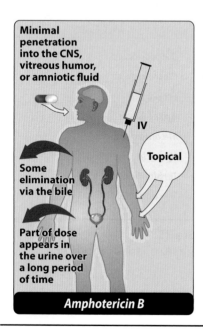

Figure 35.3
Administration and fate of
amphotericin B.

ment of life-threatening, systemic mycoses. [Note: Conventional *amphotericin* (*amphotericin B deoxycholate*, the nonlipid formulation) has undergone several formulation improvements to reduce the incidence of side effects, particularly nephrotoxicity.] The drug is also sometimes used in combination with *flucytosine* so that lower (less toxic) levels of *amphotericin B* are possible.

1. **Mechanism of action:** Several *amphotericin B* molecules bind to ergosterol in the plasma membranes of sensitive fungal cells. There, they form pores (channels) that require hydrophobic interactions between the lipophilic segment of the polyene antibiotic and the sterol (Figure 35.2). The pores disrupt membrane function, allowing electrolytes (particularly potassium) and small molecules to leak from the cell, resulting in cell death. [Note: Because the polyene antibiotics bind preferentially to ergosterol rather than to cholesterol—the sterol found in mammalian membranes—a relative (but not absolute) specificity is conferred.]

2. **Antifungal spectrum:** *Amphotericin B* is either fungicidal or fungistatic, depending on the organism and the concentration of the drug. It is effective against a wide range of fungi, including <u>Candida albicans</u>, <u>Histoplasma capsulatum</u>, <u>Cryptococcus neoformans</u>, <u>Coccidioides immitis</u>, <u>Blastomyces dermatitidis</u>, and many strains of aspergillus. [Note: *Amphotericin B* is also used in the treatment of the protozoal infection, leishmaniasis.]

3. **Resistance:** Fungal resistance, although infrequent, is associated with decreased ergosterol content of the fungal membrane.

4. **Pharmacokinetics:** *Amphotericin B* is administered by slow, intravenous infusion (Figure 35.3). *Amphotericin B* is insoluble in water, and injectable preparations require the addition of sodium deoxycholate, which produces a soluble colloidal dispersion. The more dangerous intrathecal route is sometimes chosen for the treatment of meningitis caused by fungi that are sensitive to the drug. *Amphotericin B* has also been formulated with a variety of artificial lipids that form liposomes. The three *amphotericin B* lipid formulations marketed in the United States are *Amphotec®*, *Abelcet®*, and *AmBisome®*. For example, the simplest and smallest of the liposome preparations, *AmBisome®*, is produced by the incorporation of *amphotericin B* into a single liposomal bilayer composed of phospholipids and cholesterol (Figure 35.4). These liposomal preparations have the primary advantage of reduced renal and infusion toxicity. However, because of their high cost, they are reserved mainly as salvage therapy for those individuals who cannot tolerate conventional *amphotericin B*. *Amphotericin B* is extensively bound to plasma proteins and is distributed throughout the body, becoming highly tissue bound. Inflammation favors penetration into various body fluids, but little of the drug is found in the cerebrospinal fluid (CSF), vitreous humor, or amniotic fluid. However, *amphotericin B* does cross the placenta. Low levels of the drug and its metabolites appear in the urine over a long period of time; some are also eliminated via the bile. Dosage adjustment is not required in patients with compromised hepatic function, but when renal dysfunction is due to the use of conventional *amphotericin B*, the total daily dose is decreased by 50% . Sodium loading with infusions of normal saline and the lipid-based *amphotericin B* products are alternatives utilized to minimize nephrotoxicity.

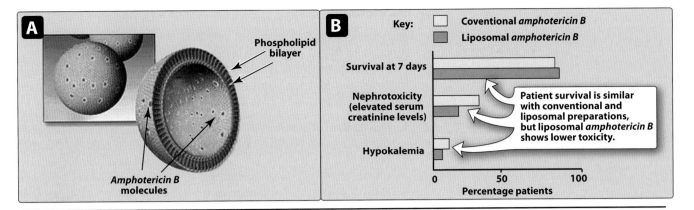

Figure 35.4
A. *Amphotericin B* intercalated between the phospholipids of a spherical liposome (AmBisome®). B. Outcomes of antifungal therapy in febrile, neutropenic cancer patients treated with conventional *amphotericin B* and liposomal *amphotericin B*.

5. **Adverse effects:** *Amphotericin B* has a low therapeutic index. A total adult daily dose should not exceed 1.5 mg/kg. Small test doses are usually administered to assess the degree of a patient's negative responses, such as anaphylaxis or convulsions. Other toxic manifestations include the following (Figure 35.5).

   a. **Fever and chills:** These occur most commonly 1 to 3 hours after starting the intravenous administration, but they usually subside with repeated administration of the drug. Premedication with a corticosteroid or an antipyretic helps to prevent this problem.

   b. **Renal impairment:** Despite the low levels of the drug excreted in the urine, patients may exhibit a decrease in glomerular filtration rate and renal tubular function. Creatinine clearance can drop, and potassium and magnesium are lost. [Note: Nephrotoxicity may be potentiated by sodium depletion; thus, a bolus infusion of normal saline before and after *amphotericin B* infusion may reduce the incidence of drug-induced nephrotoxicity.] Normal renal function usually returns on suspension of the drug, but residual damage is likely at high doses. Azotemia (elevated blood urea) is exacerbated by other nephrotoxic drugs, such as aminoglycosides, *cyclosporine*, or *pentamidine*, although adequate hydration can decrease its severity.

   c. **Hypotension:** A shock-like fall in blood pressure accompanied by hypokalemia may occur, requiring potassium supplementation. Care must be exercised in patients taking *digoxin*.

   d. **Anemia:** Normochromic, normocytic anemia caused by a reversible suppression of erythrocyte production may occur. This may be exacerbated in patients infected with HIV who are taking *zidovudine*.

   e. **Neurologic effects:** Intrathecal administration can cause a variety of serious neurologic problems.

   f. **Thrombophlebitis:** Adding *heparin* to the infusion can alleviate this problem.

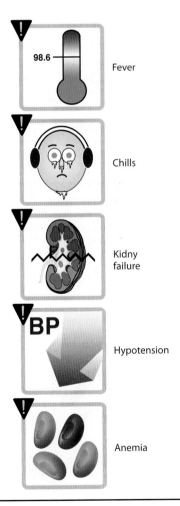

Figure 35.5
Adverse effects of *amphotericin B*.

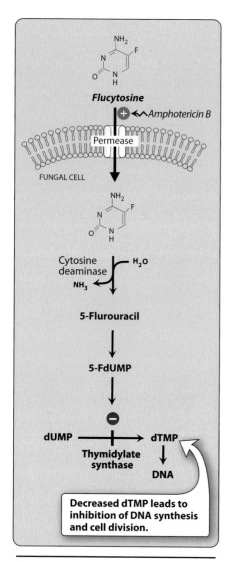

Figure 35.6
Mode of action of *flucytosine*.
5-FdUMP = 5-fluorodeoxyuridine
5'-monophosphate; dTMP = deoxythymidine 5'-monophosphate.

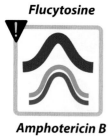

Figure 35.7
Synergism between *flucytosine*
and *amphotericin B*.

B. Flucytosine

Flucytosine [floo-SYE-toe-seen] (*5-FC*) is a synthetic pyrimidine anti-metabolite that is often used in combination with *amphotericin B*. This combination of drugs is administered for the treatment of systemic mycoses and for meningitis caused by Cryptococcus neoformans and Candida albicans.

1. **Mechanism of action:** *5-FC* enters fungal cells via a cytosine-specific permease—an enzyme not found in mammalian cells. *5-FC* is then converted by a series of steps to 5-fluorodeoxyuridine 5'-mono-phosphate. This false nucleotide inhibits thymidylate synthase, thus depriving the organism of thymidylic acid—an essential DNA component (Figure 35.6). The unnatural mononucleotide is further metabolized to a trinucleotide (5-fluorodeoxyuridine 5'-triphos-phate) and is incorporated into fungal RNA, thus disrupting nucleic acid and protein synthesis. [Note: *Amphotericin B* increases cell per-meability, allowing more *5-FC* to penetrate the cell. Thus, *5-FC* and *amphotericin B* are synergistic (Figure 35.7).]

2. **Antifungal spectrum:** *5-FC* is fungistatic. It is effective in combi-nation with *itraconazole* for treating chromoblastomycosis and in combination with *amphotericin B* for treating candidiasis or cryptococcosis.

3. **Resistance:** Resistance due to decreased levels of any of the enzymes in the conversion of *5-FC* to *5-fluorouracil* (*5-FU*) and beyond, or increased synthesis of cytosine, can develop during therapy. This is the primary reason that *5-FC* is not used as a single antimycotic drug. The rate of emergence of resistant fungal cells is lower with a combination of *5-FC* plus a second antifungal agent than it is with *5-FC* alone.

4. **Pharmacokinetics:** *5-FC* is well absorbed by the oral route. It distrib-utes throughout the body water and penetrates well into the CSF. *5-FU* is detectable in patients and is probably the result of metabo-lism of *5-FC* by intestinal bacteria. Excretion of both the parent drug and its metabolites is by glomerular filtration, and the dose must be adjusted in patients with compromised renal function.

5. **Adverse effects:** *5-FC* causes reversible neutropenia, thrombo-cytopenia, and dose-related bone marrow depression. Caution must be exercised in patients undergoing radiation or chemother-apy with drugs that depress bone marrow. Reversible hepatic dys-function with elevation of serum transaminases and alkaline phos-phatase may occur. Gastrointestinal disturbances, such as nausea, vomiting, and diarrhea, are common, and severe enterocolitis may occur. [Note: Some of these adverse effects may be related to *5-FU* formed by intestinal organisms from *5-FC*.]

C. Ketoconazole

Ketoconazole [kee-toe-KON-a-zole] was the first orally active azole avail-able for the treatment of systemic mycoses.

1. **Mechanism of action:** Azoles are predominantly fungistatic. They inhibit C-14 α-demethylase (a cytochrome P450 enzyme), thus blocking the demethylation of lanosterol to ergosterol—the princi-pal sterol of fungal membranes (Figure 35.8). This inhibition disrupts membrane structure and function and, thereby, inhibits fungal cell

growth. [Note: Unfortunately, as is often the case for the initial member of a class of drugs, the selectivity of *ketoconazole* toward its target is not as precise as those of later azoles. For example, in addition to blocking fungal ergosterol synthesis, the drug also inhibits human gonadal and adrenal steroid synthesis, leading to decreased testosterone and cortisol production. In addition, *ketoconazole* inhibits cytochrome P450–dependent hepatic drug-metabolizing enzymes.]

2. **Antifungal spectrum:** *Ketoconazole* is active against many fungi, including <u>Histoplasma</u>, <u>Blastomyces</u>, <u>Candida</u>, and <u>Coccidioides</u>, but not aspergillus species. Although *itraconazole* has largely replaced *ketoconazole* in the treatment of most mycoses because of its broader spectrum, greater potency, and fewer adverse effects, *ketoconazole*, as a second-line drug, is a less expensive alternative for the treatment of mucocutaneous candidiasis. Strains of several fungal species that are resistant to *ketoconazole* have been identified.

3. **Resistance:** This is becoming a significant clinical problem, particularly in the protracted therapy required for those with advanced HIV infection. Identified mechanisms of resistance include mutations in the C-14 α-demethylase gene, which cause decreased azole binding. Additionally, some strains of fungi have developed the ability to pump the azole out of the cell.

4. **Pharmacokinetics:** *Ketoconazole* is only administered orally (Figure 35.9). It requires gastric acid for dissolution and is absorbed through the gastric mucosa. Drugs that raise gastric pH, such as antacids, or that interfere with gastric acid secretion, such as H_2-histamine receptor blockers and proton-pump inhibitors, impair absorption. Administering acidifying agents, such as cola drinks, before taking the drug can improve absorption in patients with achlorhydria. *Ketoconazole* is extensively bound to plasma proteins. Although penetration into tissues is limited, it is effective in the treatment of histoplasmosis in lung, bone, skin, and soft tissues. The drug does not enter the CSF. Extensive metabolism occurs in the liver, and excretion is primarily through the bile. Levels of parent drug in the urine are too low to be effective against mycotic infections of the urinary tract.

5. **Adverse effects:** In addition to allergies, dose-dependent gastrointestinal disturbances, including nausea, anorexia, and vomiting, are the most common adverse effects of *ketoconazole* treatment. Endocrine effects, such as gynecomastia, decreased libido, impotence, and menstrual irregularities, result from the blocking of androgen and adrenal steroid synthesis by *ketoconazole*. Transient increases in serum transaminases are found in from 2 to 10 percent of patients. Frank hepatitis occurs rarely but requires immediate cessation of treatment. [Note: *Ketoconazole* may accumulate in patients with hepatic dysfunction. Plasma concentrations of the drug should be monitored in these individuals.]

6. **Drug interactions and contraindications:** By inhibiting cytochrome P450, *ketoconazole* can potentiate the toxicities of drugs such as *cyclosporine*, *phenytoin*, *tolbutamide*, and *warfarin*, among others (Figure 35.10). *Rifampin*, an inducer of the cytochrome P450 system, can shorten the duration of action of *ketoconazole* and the other azoles. Drugs that decrease gastric acidity, such as H_2-receptor

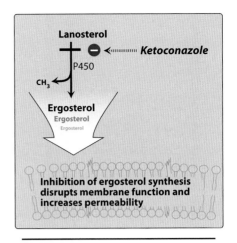

Figure 35.8
Mode of action of *ketoconazole*.

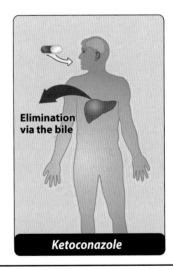

Figure 35.9
Administration and fate of *ketoconazole*.

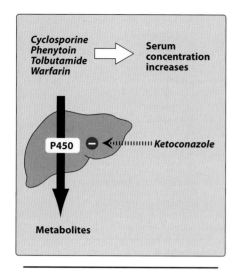

Figure 35.10
By inhibiting cytochrome P450, *ketoconazole* can potentiate the toxicities of other drugs.

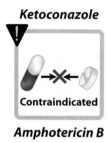

Figure 35.11
Ketoconazole and *amphotericin B* should not be used together.

blockers, antacids, proton-pump inhibitors, and *sucralfate*, can decrease absorption of *ketoconazole*. *Ketoconazole* and *amphotericin B* should not be used together, because the decrease in ergosterol in the fungal membrane reduces the fungicidal action of *amphotericin B* (Figure 35.11). Finally, *ketoconazole* is teratogenic in animals, and it should not be given during pregnancy.

D. Fluconazole

Fluconazole [floo-KON-a-zole] is clinically important because of its lack of the endocrine side effects of *ketoconazole* and its excellent penetrability into the CSF of both normal and inflamed meninges. *Fluconazole* is employed prophylactically, with some success, for reducing fungal infections in recipients of bone marrow transplants. It inhibits the synthesis of fungal membrane ergosterol in the same manner as *ketoconazole* and is the drug of choice for Cryptococcus neoformans, for candidemia, and for coccidioidomycosis. *Fluconazole* is effective against all forms of mucocutaneous candidiasis. [Note: Treatment failures due to resistance have been reported in some HIV-infected patients.] *Fluconazole* is administered orally or intravenously. Its absorption is excellent and, unlike that of *ketoconazole*, is not dependent on gastric acidity. Binding to plasma proteins is minimal. Unlike *ketoconazole*, *fluconazole* is poorly metabolized. The drug is excreted via the kidney, and doses must be reduced in patients with compromised renal function. The adverse effects caused by *fluconazole* treatment are less of a problem than those with *ketoconazole*. *Fluconazole* has no endocrinologic effects, because it does not inhibit the cytochrome P450 system responsible for the synthesis of androgens. However, it can inhibit the P450 cytochromes that metabolize other drugs listed in Figure 35.10. Nausea, vomiting, and rashes are a problem. Hepatitis is rare. *Fluconazole* is teratogenic, as are other azoles, and should not be used in pregnancy.

E. Itraconazole

Itraconazole [it-ra-KON-a-zole] is an azole antifungal agent with a broad antifungal spectrum. Like *fluconazole*, it is a synthetic triazole and also lacks the endocrinologic side effects of *ketoconazole*. Its mechanism of action is the same as that of the other azoles. *Itraconazole* is now the drug of choice for the treatment of blastomycosis, sporotrichosis, paracoccidioidomycosis, and histoplasmosis. Unlike *ketoconazole*, it is effective in acquired immunodeficiency syndrome–associated histoplasmosis. *Itraconazole* is well-absorbed orally, but it requires acid for dissolution. Food increases the bioavailability of some preparations. The drug is extensively bound to plasma proteins and distributes well throughout most tissues, including bone and adipose tissues. However, therapeutic concentrations are not attained in the CSF. Like *ketoconazole*, *itraconazole* is extensively metabolized by the liver, but it does not inhibit androgen synthesis. Its major metabolite, hydroxyitraconazole, is biologically active, with a similar antifungal spectrum. Little of the parent drug appears in the urine; thus, doses do not have to be reduced in renal failure. Adverse effects include nausea and vomiting, rash (especially in immunocompromised patients), hypokalemia, hypertension, edema, and headache. *Itraconazole* should be avoided in pregnancy. *Itraconazole* inhibits the metabolism of many drugs, including oral anticoagulants, statins, and *quinidine*. Inducers of the cytochrome P450 system increase the metabolism of *itraconazole*.

F. Voriconazole

Voriconazole [vor-i-KON-a-zole] has the advantage of being a broad-spectrum antifungal agent. It is available for intravenous administration and also for oral administration and is approximately 96% bioavailable. *Voriconazole* is approved for the treatment of invasive aspergillosis and seems to have replaced *amphotericin B* as the treatment of choice for this indication. *Voriconazole* is also approved for treatment of serious infections caused by <u>Scedosporium</u> <u>apiospermum</u> and <u>Fusarium</u> species. *Voriconazole* penetrates tissues well, including the CNS. Elimination is primarily by metabolism through the cytochrome P450 2C19, 2C9, and 3A4 enzymes. The significant number of drug interactions due to its metabolism through the various hepatic enzymes may limit its use. Side effects are similar to those of the other azoles. One unique problem is a transient visual disturbance that occurs within 30 minutes of dosing.

G. Posaconazole

Posaconazole [poe-sa-kon-a-zole] is a new oral, broad-spectrum antifungal agent with a chemical structure similar to that of *itraconazole*. It was approved in 2006 to prevent *Candida* and *Aspergillus* infections in severely immunocompromised patients and for the treatment of oropharyngeal candidiasis. Due to its spectrum of activity, *posaconazole* could possibly be used in the treatment of fungal infections caused by *Mucor* species and other zygomycetes. To date, *amphotericin B* formulations are the only other antifungal agents available for treatment of zygomycete infections. Overall, *posaconazole* is relatively well tolerated. The most common side effects observed were gastrointestinal issues (nausea, vomiting, diarrhea, and abdominal pain) and headaches. Like other azoles, *posaconazole* can cause an elevation of liver function tests aspartate aminotransferase and alanine aminotransferase. Additionally, in patients who are receiving concomitant *cyclosporine* or *tacrolimus* for management of transplant rejection, rare cases of hemolytic uremic syndrome, thrombotic thrombocytopenic purpura, and pulmonary embolus have been reported. Due to its inhibition of cytochrome P450 3A4 enzyme, *posaconazole* may increase the effect and toxicity of many drugs, including *cyclosporine*, *tacrolimus*, and *sirolumus*. Concomitant use of *posaconazole* with ergot alkaloids, *pimozide*, and *quinidine* is contraindicated. To be effective, *posaconazole* must be administered with a full meal or nutritional supplement. For treatment of oropharyngeal

	KETOCONAZOLE	FLUCONAZOLE	VORICONAZOLE	POSACONAZOLE
SPECTRUM	Narrow	Expanded	Expanded	Expanded
ROUTE(S) OF ADMINISTRATION	Oral	Oral, IV	Oral, IV	Oral
$t_{1/2}$ (HOURS)	6–9	30	6–24	20–66
CSF PENETRATION	No	Yes	Yes	Yes
RENAL EXCRETION	No	Yes	No	No
INTERACTION WITH OTHER DRUGS	Frequent	Occasional	Frequent	Frequent
INHIBITION OF MAMMALIAN STEROL SYNTHESIS	Dose-dependent inhibitory effect	No inhibition	No inhibition	No inhibition

Figure 35.12
Summary of some azole fungistatic drugs.

candidiasis, dosing is daily. However, for prophylaxis of *Candida* and *Aspergillus* infections, *posaconazole* must be dosed three times a day. Figure 35.12 summarizes the azole antifungal agents.

H. Echinocandins: Caspofungin, micafungin, and anidulafungin

1. **Caspofungin:** *Caspofungin* [kas-poh-FUN-jin] is the first approved member of the echinocandins class of antifungal drugs. Echinocandins interfere with the synthesis of the fungal cell wall by inhibiting the synthesis of $\beta(1,3)$-D-glucan, leading to lysis and cell death. This drug's spectrum is limited to <u>Aspergillus</u> and <u>Candida</u> species. *Caspofungin* is not active by the oral route. The drug is highly bound to serum proteins and has a half-life of 9 to 11 hours. It is slowly metabolized by hydrolysis and N-acetylation. Elimination is approximately equal between the urinary and fecal routes. Adverse effects include fever, rash, nausea, and phlebitis. Flushing occurs—probably due to the release of histamine from mast cells. *Caspofungin* should not be coadministered with *cyclosporine*. *Caspofungin* is a second-line antifungal for those who have failed or cannot tolerate *amphotericin B* or an azole.

2. **Micafungin and anidulafungin:** *Micafungin* (mi-ka-FUN-gin) and *anidulafungin* (ay-nid-yoo-la-FUN-jin) are the newer members of the echinocandins class of antifungal drugs. Like *caspofungin*, they are not orally active, are only available via intravenous infusion, and have histamine-mediated side effects. *Micafungin* and *anidulafungin* have similar efficacy against *Candida* species, but the efficacy for treatment of other fungal infections has not been established. Also, they are not substrates for cytochrome P450 enzymes and do not have any associated drug interactions.

III. DRUGS FOR CUTANEOUS MYCOTIC INFECTIONS

Fungi that cause superficial skin infections are called dermatophytes. Common dermatomycoses, such as tinea infections, are often referred to as "ringworm." This is a misnomer, because fungi rather than worms cause the disease.

A. Terbinafine

Terbinafine [TER-bin-a-feen] is the drug of choice for treating dermatophytoses and, especially, onychomycoses (fungal infections of nails). It is better tolerated, requires shorter duration of therapy, and is more effective than either *itraconazole* or *griseofulvin*.

1. **Mechanism of action:** *Terbinafine* inhibits fungal squalene epoxidase, thereby decreasing the synthesis of ergosterol (Figure 35.13). This plus the accumulation of toxic amounts of squalene result in the death of the fungal cell. [Note: Significantly higher concentrations of *terbinafine* are needed to inhibit human squalene epoxidase, an enzyme required for the cholesterol synthetic pathway.]

2. **Antifungal spectrum:** The drug is primarily fungicidal. Antifungal activity is limited to dermatophytes and <u>Candida albicans</u>. Therapy is prolonged—usually about 3 months—but considerably shorter than that with *griseofulvin*.

3. **Pharmacokinetics:** *Terbinafine* is orally active, although its bioavailability is only 40 percent due to first-pass metabolism. Absorption is not significantly enhanced by food. *Terbinafine* is greater than 99 percent bound to plasma proteins. It is deposited in the skin, nails, and

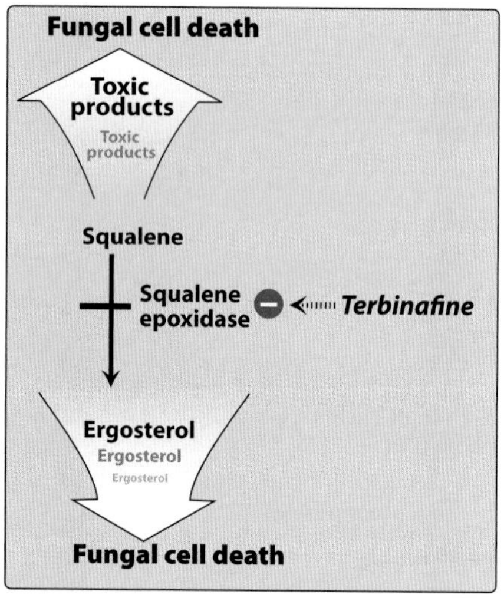

Figure 35.13
Mode of action of *terbinafine*.

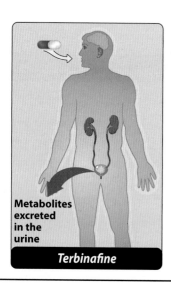

Figure 35.14
Administration and fate of *terbinafine*.

fat. *Terbinafine* accumulates in breast milk and, therefore, should not be given to nursing mothers. A prolonged terminal half-life of 200 to 400 hours may reflect the slow release from these tissues. *Terbinafine* is extensively metabolized prior to urinary excretion (Figure 35.14). Patients with either moderate renal impairment or hepatic cirrhosis have reduced clearance.

4. **Adverse effects:** The most common adverse effects due to *terbinafine* are gastrointestinal disturbances (diarrhea, dyspepsia, and nausea), headache, and rash. Taste and visual disturbances have been reported as well as transient elevations in serum liver enzyme levels. All adverse effects resolve upon drug discontinuation. Rarely, *terbinafine* may cause hepatotoxicity and neutropenia. Although *terbinafine* is extensively metabolized, there does not seem to be a significant risk of reduced clearance of other drugs. *Rifampin* decreases blood levels of *terbinafine*, whereas *cimetidine* increases blood levels of *terbinafine*.

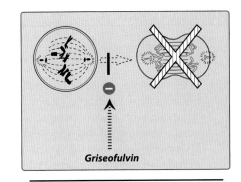

Figure 35.15
Inhibition of mitosis by *griseofulvin*.

B. Griseofulvin

Griseofulvin [gris-e-oh-FUL-vin] has been largely replaced by *terbinafine* for the treatment of dermatophytic infections of the nails. *Griseofulvin* requires treatment of 6 to 12 months in duration. It is only fungistatic, and it causes a number of significant drug interactions. *Griseofulvin* accumulates in newly synthesized, keratin-containing tissue, where it causes disruption of the mitotic spindle and inhibition of fungal mitosis (Figure 35.15). Duration of therapy is dependent on the rate of replacement of healthy skin or nails. Ultrafine crystalline preparations are absorbed adequately from the gastrointestinal tract; absorption is enhanced by high-fat meals. *Griseofulvin* induces hepatic cytochrome P450 activity (Figure 35.16). It also increases the rate of metabolism of a number of drugs, including anticoagulants. It may exacerbate intermittent porphyria. Patients should not drink alcoholic beverages during therapy, because griseofulvin potentiates the intoxicating effects of alcohol.

C. Nystatin

Nystatin [nye-STAT-in] is a polyene antibiotic, and its structure, chemistry, mechanism of action, and resistance resemble those of *amphotericin B*. Its use is restricted to topical treatment of <u>Candida</u> infections because of its systemic toxicity. The drug is negligibly absorbed from the gastrointestinal tract, and it is never used parenterally. It is administered as an oral agent ("swish and swallow" or "swish and spit") for the treatment of oral candidiasis. Excretion in the feces is nearly quantitative. Adverse effects are rare because of its lack of absorption, but nausea and vomiting occasionally occur.

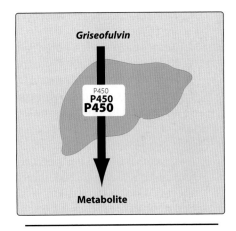

Figure 35.16
Induction of hepatic cytochrome P450 activity by *griseofulvin*.

D. Miconazole and other topical agents

Miconazole [my-KON-a-zole], *clotrimazole* [kloe-TRIM-a-zole], *butoconazole* [byoo-toe-KON-a-zole], and *terconazole* [ter-KON-a-zole] are topically active drugs that are only rarely administered parenterally because of their severe toxicity. Their mechanism of action and antifungal spectrum are the same as those of *ketoconazole*. Topical use is associated with contact dermatitis, vulvar irritation, and edema. *Miconazole* is a potent inhibitor of *warfarin* metabolism and has produced bleeding in warfarin-treated patients even when *miconazole* is applied topically. No significant difference in clinical outcomes is associated with any azole or *nystatin* in the treatment of vulvar candidiasis.

Study questions

Choose the ONE best answer.

35.1 A 25-year-old male patient with acquired immu-nodeficiency syndrome has a fever of 102°F and complains of severe headaches during the past week. Staining of his CSF with India ink reveals <u>Cryptococcus neoformans</u>. The patient is admitted to the hospital and is treated with:

A. Intravenous amphotericin B plus flucytosine.
B. Oral ketoconazole.
C. Intrathecal amphotericin B.
D. Oral fluconazole.
E. Intravenous amphotericin B plus ketoconazole.

Correct answer = C. Intrathecal administration of amphotericin B is indicated as the most effective way to treat cryptococcal meningitis. Although intravenous amphotericin B may be useful, the addition of flucytosine with its potential for bone marrow toxicity would not be appropriate therapy. Oral ketoconazole is also wrong because of its in-ability to cross into the CSF. Although fluconazole is very effective against <u>Cryptococcus neoformans</u> and does enter the CSF, the oral route is only used for chronic suppressive therapy and not as treatment for meningitis. The combination of amphotericin B and ketoconazole is a poor one, because ketocon-azole disrupts fungal membrane function and, thus, interferes with the action of amphotericin B.

35.2 A 30-year-old male has had a heart transplant and is being maintained on the immunosuppressant cyclosporine. He develops a Candida infection and is treated with ketoconazole. Why is this poor therapy?

A. Ketoconazole is not effective against <u>Candida</u> species.
B. Ketoconazole reacts with cyclosporine to inactivate it.
C. Ketoconazole has a potential for cardiotoxicity.
D. Ketoconazole inhibits cytochrome P450 enzymes that inactivate cyclosporine.
E. Ketoconazole causes gynecomastia and decreased libido in the male.

Correct answer = D. Ketoconazole is effective against Candida, but it does not react with cyclosporine species, and is not cardiotoxic. Ketoconazole inhibits the hepatic cytochrome P450 enzymes that inacti-vate cyclosporine. Thus, in this instance, the patient would be in danger of increased cyclosporine toxicity. Although ketoconazole does cause gyne-comastia and decreased libido, this would not be of primary concern.

35.3 A 22-year-old male has been treating his "athlete's foot" with an over-the-counter drug without much success. Upon examination, it is found that the nail bed of both great toes is infected. Which one of the following antifungal agents would be most appro-priate for this patient?

A. Caspofungin.
B. Fluconazole.
C. Griseofulvin.
D. Nystatin.
E. Terbinafine.

Correct answer = E. Terbinafine is the drug of choice for the treatment of dermatophytic infections. Be-cause it is fungicidal, it requires a shorter course of therapy than with griseofulvin. Drug interactions are also not a problem with terbinafine. Dermatophytes may respond to fluconazole, but this drug is re-served for more serious systemic infections. Nystatin and caspofungin are not useful in the treatment of dermatophytic infections.

Antiprotozoal Drugs

36

I. OVERVIEW

Protozoal infections are common among people in underdeveloped tropical and subtropical countries, where sanitary conditions, hygienic practices, and control of the vectors of transmission are inadequate. However, with increased world travel, protozoal diseases, such as malaria, amebiasis, leishmaniasis, trypanosomiasis, trichomoniasis, and giardiasis, are no longer confined to specific geographic locales. Because they are eukaryotes, the unicellular protozoal cells have metabolic processes closer to those of the human host than to prokaryotic bacterial pathogens. Protozoal diseases are thus less easily treated than bacterial infections, and many of the antiprotozoal drugs cause serious toxic effects in the host, particularly on cells showing high metabolic activity, such as neuronal, renal tubular, intestinal, and bone marrow stem cells. Most antiprotozoal agents have not proved to be safe for pregnant patients. Drugs used to treat protozoal infections are summarized in Figure 36.1.

II. CHEMOTHERAPY FOR AMEBIASIS

Amebiasis (also called amebic dysentery) is an infection of the intestinal tract caused by Entamoeba histolytica. The disease can be acute or chronic, with patients showing varying degrees of illness, from no symptoms to mild diarrhea to fulminating dysentery. The diagnosis is established by isolating E. histolytica from fresh feces. Therapy is aimed not only at the acutely ill patient but also at those who are asymptomatic carriers, because dormant E. histolytica may cause future infections in the carrier and be a potential source of infection for others.

A. Life cycle of Entamoeba histolytica

Entamoeba histolytica exists in two forms: cysts that can survive outside the body, and labile but invasive trophozoites that do not persist outside the body. Cysts, ingested through feces-contaminated food or water, pass into the lumen of the intestine, where the trophozoites are liberated. The trophozoites multiply, and they either invade and ulcerate the mucosa of the large intestine or simply feed on intestinal bacteria. [Note: One strategy for treating luminal amebiasis is to add antibiotics, such as *tetracycline*, to the treatment regimen, resulting in a reduction in intestinal flora—the ameba's major food source.] The trophozoites within the intestine are slowly carried toward the rectum, where they return to the cyst form and are excreted in feces.

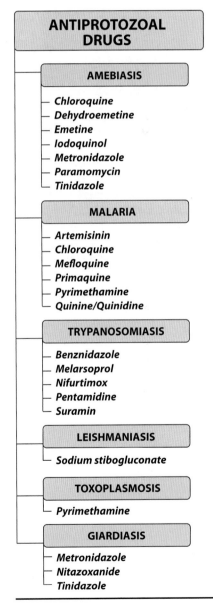

ANTIPROTOZOAL DRUGS

AMEBIASIS
- *Chloroquine*
- *Dehydroemetine*
- *Emetine*
- *Iodoquinol*
- *Metronidazole*
- *Paramomycin*
- *Tinidazole*

MALARIA
- *Artemisinin*
- *Chloroquine*
- *Mefloquine*
- *Primaquine*
- *Pyrimethamine*
- *Quinine/Quinidine*

TRYPANOSOMIASIS
- *Benznidazole*
- *Melarsoprol*
- *Nifurtimox*
- *Pentamidine*
- *Suramin*

LEISHMANIASIS
- *Sodium stibogluconate*

TOXOPLASMOSIS
- *Pyrimethamine*

GIARDIASIS
- *Metronidazole*
- *Nitazoxanide*
- *Tinidazole*

Figure 36.1
Summary of antiprotozoal agents.

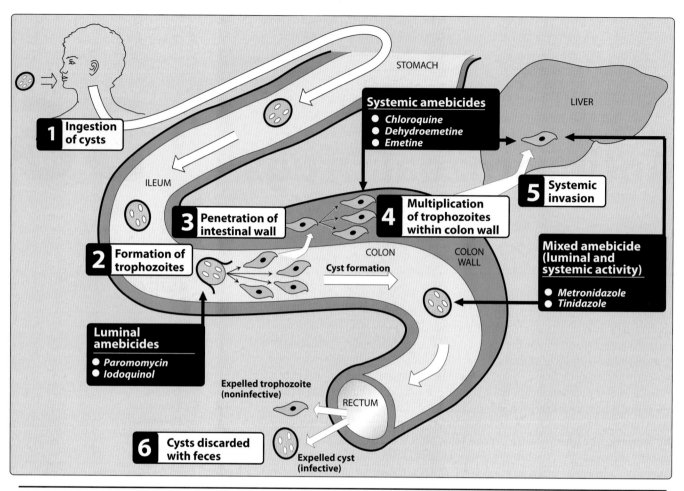

Figure 36.2
Life cycle of <u>Entamoeba</u> <u>histolytica</u>, showing the sites of action of amebicidal drugs.

Large numbers of trophozoites within the colon wall can also lead to systemic invasion. A summary of the life cycle of <u>E</u>. <u>histolytica</u> is presented in Figure 36.2.

B. Classification of amebicidal drugs

Therapeutic agents are classified as luminal, systemic, or mixed (luminal and systemic) amebicides according to the site where the drug is effective (see Figure 36.2). For example, luminal amebicides act on the parasite in the lumen of the bowel, whereas systemic amebicides are effective against amebas in the intestinal wall and liver. Mixed amebicides are effective against both the luminal and systemic forms of the disease, although luminal concentrations are too low for single-drug treatment.

C. Mixed amebicides (metronidazole and tinidazole)

1. **Metronidazole:** *Metronidazole* [me-troe-NYE-da-zole], a nitroimidazole, is the mixed amebicide of choice for treating amebic infections; it kills the <u>E. histolytica</u> trophozoites. [Note: *Metronidazole* also finds extensive use in the treatment of infections caused by <u>Giardia lamblia</u>, <u>Trichomonas vaginalis</u>, anaerobic cocci, and anaerobic gram-negative bacilli (for example, <u>Bacteroides</u> species). *Metronidazole* is the drug of choice for the treatment of pseudomembranous colitis

caused by the anaerobic, gram-positive bacillus <u>Clostridium difficile</u> and is also effective in the treatment of brain abscesses caused by these organisms.]

a. **Mechanism of action:** Some anaerobic protozoal parasites (including amebas) possess ferrodoxin-like, low-redox-potential, electron-transport proteins that participate in metabolic electron removal reactions. The nitro group of *metronidazole* is able to serve as an electron acceptor, forming reduced cytotoxic compounds that bind to proteins and DNA, resulting in cell death.

b. **Pharmacokinetics:** *Metronidazole* is completely and rapidly absorbed after oral administration (Figure 36.3). [Note: For the treatment of amebiasis, it is usually administered with a luminal amebicide, such as *iodoquinol* or *paromomycin*. This combination provides cure rates of greater than 90 percent.] *Metronidazole* distributes well throughout body tissues and fluids. Therapeutic levels can be found in vaginal and seminal fluids, saliva, breast milk, and cerebrospinal fluid (CSF). Metabolism of the drug depends on hepatic oxidation of the *metronidazole* side chain by mixed-function oxidase, followed by glucuronylation. Therefore, concomitant treatment with inducers of this enzymatic system, such as *phenobarbital*, enhances the rate of metabolism. Conversely, those drugs that inhibit this system, such as *cimetidine*, prolong the plasma half-life of *metronidazole*. The drug accumulates in patients with severe hepatic disease. The parent drug and its metabolites are excreted in the urine.

c. **Adverse effects:** The most common adverse effects are those associated with the gastrointestinal tract, including nausea, vomiting, epigastric distress, and abdominal cramps (Figure 36.4). An unpleasant, metallic taste is often experienced. Other effects include oral moniliasis (yeast infection of the mouth) and, rarely, neurotoxicologic problems, such as dizziness, vertigo, and numbness or paresthesias in the peripheral nervous system. [Note: The latter are reasons for discontinuing the drug.] If taken with alcohol, a *disulfiram*-like effect occurs (114).

d. **Resistance:** Resistance to *metronidazole* is not a therapeutic problem, although strains of trichomonads resistant to the drug have been reported.

2. **Tinidazole:** *Tinidazole* [tye-NI-da-zole] is a second-generation nitroimidazole that is similar to *metronidazole* in spectrum of activity, absorption, adverse effects and drug interactions. It was approved by the U.S. Food and Drug Administration in 2004 for treatment of amebiasis, amebic liver abcess, giardiasis, and trichomoniasis but was used outside the United States for decades prior to approval. *Tinidazole* is as effective as *metronidazole*, with a shorter course of treatment, yet is more expensive than generic *metronidazole*.

D. Luminal amebicides

After treatment of invasive intestinal or extraintestinal amebic disease is complete, a luminal agent, such as *iodoquinol*, *diloxanide furoate*, or *paromomycin*, should be administered for treatment of asymptomatic colonization state.

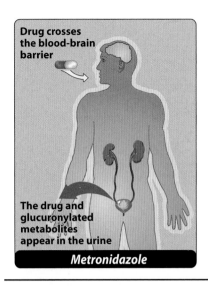

Figure 36.3
Administration and fate of *metronidazole*.

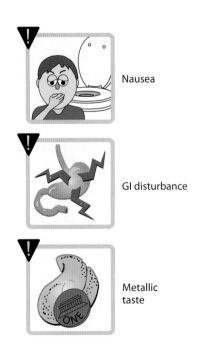

Figure 36.4
Adverse effects of *metronidazole*.

1. **Iodoquinol:** *Iodoquinol* [eye-oh-doe-QUIN-ole], a halogenated 8-hydroxy quinolone, is amebicidal against E. histolytica, and is effective against the luminal trophozoite and cyst forms. Side effects from *iodoquinol* include rash, diarrhea, and dose-related peripheral neuropathy, including a rare optic neuritis. Long-term use of this drug should be avoided.

2. **Paromomycin:** *Paromomycin* [par-oh-moe-MYE-sin], an aminoglycoside antibiotic, is only effective against the intestinal (luminal) forms of E. histolytica and tapeworm, because it is not significantly absorbed from the gastrointestinal tract. It is an alternative agent for cryptosporidiosis. Although directly amebicidal, *paromomycin* also exerts its antiamebic actions by reducing the population of intestinal flora. Its direct amebicidal action is probably due to the effects it has on cell membranes, causing leakage. Very little of the drug is absorbed on oral ingestion, but that which is absorbed is excreted in the urine. Gastrointestinal distress and diarrhea are the principal adverse effects.

E. Systemic amebicides

These drugs are useful for treating liver abscesses or intestinal wall infections caused by amebas.

1. **Chloroquine:** *Chloroquine* [KLOR-oh-kwin] is used in combination with *metronidazole* and *diloxanide furoate* to treat and prevent amebic liver abscesses. It eliminates trophozoites in liver abscesses, but it is not useful in treating luminal amebiasis. *Chloroquine* is also effective in the treatment of malaria.

2. **Emetine and dehydroemetine:** *Emetine* [EM-e-teen] and *dehydroemetine* [de-hye-dro-EM-e-teen] are alternative agents for the treatment of amebiasis. They inhibit protein synthesis by blocking chain elongation.[1] Intramuscular injection is the preferred route. *Emetine* is concentrated in the liver, where it persists for a month after a single dose. It is slowly metabolized and excreted, and it can accumulate. Its half-life in plasma is 5 days. The use of these ipecac alkaloids is limited by their toxicities (*dehydroemetine* is less toxic than *emetine*), and close clinical observation is necessary when these drugs are administered. They should not be taken for more than 5 days. *Dehydroemetine* is only available under a compassionate investigational new drug protocol through the Centers of Disease Control and Prevention. Among the untoward effects are pain at the site of injection, transient nausea, cardiotoxicity (for example, arrhythmias or congestive heart failure), neuromuscular weakness, dizziness, and rashes. A summary of the treatment of amebiasis is shown in Figure 36.5.

CLINICAL SYNDROME	DRUG
Asymptomatic cyst carriers	*Iodoquinol* or *Paromycin*
Diarrhea/dysentery Extraintestinal	*Metronidazole* plus *Iodoquinol* or *Paromycin*
Amebic liver absess	*Chloroquine* plus *Metronidazole* or *Emetine*

Figure 36.5
Some commonly used therapeutic options for the treatment of amebiasis.

III. CHEMOTHERAPY FOR MALARIA

Malaria is an acute infectious disease caused by four species of the protozoal genus Plasmodium. The parasite is transmitted to humans through the bite of a female Anopheles mosquito, which thrives in humid, swampy areas. Plasmodium falciparum is the most dangerous species, causing an

[1]See p. 431 in *Lippincott's Illustrated Reviews: Biochemistry* (4th ed.) for a more detailed discussion of protein synthesis.

acute, rapidly fulminating disease that is characterized by persistent high fever, orthostatic hypotension, and massive erythrocytosis (an abnormal elevation in the number of red blood cells accompanied by swollen and reddish condition of the limbs). P. falciparum infection can lead to capillary obstruction and death if treatment is not instituted promptly. Plasmodium vivax causes a milder form of the disease. Plasmodium malariae is common to many tropical regions, but Plasmodium ovale is rarely encountered. Resistance acquired by the mosquito to insecticides, and by the parasite to drugs, has led to new therapeutic challenges, particularly in the treatment of P. falciparum.

A. Life cycle of the malarial parasite

When an infected mosquito bites, it injects Plasmodium sporozoites into the bloodstream (Figure 36.6). The sporozoites migrate through the blood to the liver, where they form cyst-like structures containing thousands of merozoites. [Note: Diagnosis depends on laboratory identification of the parasites in red blood cells of peripheral blood smears.] Upon release, each merozoite invades a red blood cell, becoming a trophozoite and using hemoglobin as a nutrient. The trophozoites multiply and become merozoites. Eventually, the infected cell ruptures, releasing heme and merozoites that can enter other erythrocytes. [Note: Alternatively, released merozoites can become gametocytes,

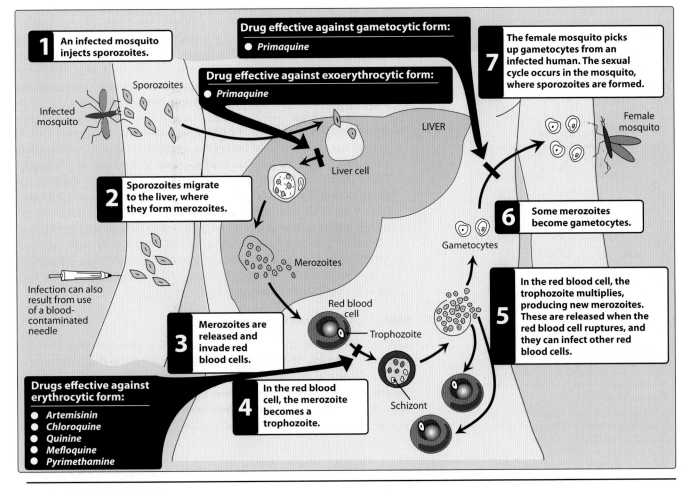

Figure 36.6
Life cycle of the malarial parasite, Plasmodium falciparum, showing the sites of action of antimalarial drugs.

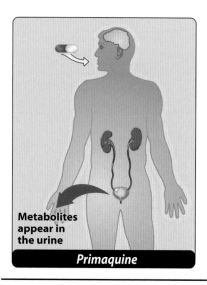

Figure 36.7
Administration and fate of *primaquine*.

Figure 36.8
Mechanism of *primaquine*-induced hemolytic anemia. GSH = reduced glutathione; GSSG = oxidized glutathione; NADP+ = nicotinamide adenine dinucleotide phosphate; NADPH = reduced nicotinamide adenine dinucleotide phosphate.

which are picked up by mosquitoes from the blood they ingest. The cycle thus begins again, with the gametocytes becoming sporozoites in the insect.] The effectiveness of a drug treatment is related to the particular species of infecting plasmodium and the stage of its life cycle that is targeted. A summary of the life cycle of the parasite and the sites of therapeutic interventions are presented in Figure 36.6.

B. Tissue schizonticide: Primaquine

Primaquine [PRIM-a-kwin] is an 8-aminoquinoline that eradicates primary exoerythrocytic forms of P. falciparum and P. vivax and the secondary exoerythrocytic forms of recurring malarias (P. vivax and P. ovale). [Note: *Primaquine* is the only agent that can lead to radical cures of the P. vivax and P. ovale malarias, which may remain in the liver in the exoerythrocytic form after the erythrocytic form of the disease is eliminated.] The sexual (gametocytic) forms of all four plasmodia are destroyed in the plasma or are prevented from maturing later in the mosquito, thus interrupting the transmission of the disease. [Note: *Primaquine* is not effective against the erythrocytic stage of malaria and, therefore, is often used in conjunction with a blood schizonticide, such as *chloroquine*, *quinine*, *mefloquine*, or *pyrimethamine*.]

1. **Mechanism of action:** This is not completely understood. Metabolites of *primaquine* are believed to act as oxidants that are responsible for the schizonticidal action as well as for the hemolysis and methemoglobinemia encountered as toxicities.

2. **Pharmacokinetics:** *Primaquine* is well absorbed on oral administration and is not concentrated in tissues. It is rapidly oxidized to many compounds, the major one being the deaminated drug. It has not been established which compound possesses the schizontocidal activity. Metabolites appear in the urine (Figure 36.7).

3. **Adverse effects:** *Primaquine* has a low incidence of adverse effects, except for drug-induced hemolytic anemia in patients with genetically low levels of glucose-6-phosphate dehydrogenase[2] (Figure 36.8). Other toxic manifestations observed after large doses of the drug include abdominal discomfort, especially when administered in combination with *chloroquine* (which may affect patient compliance), and occasional methemoglobinemia. Granulocytopenia and agranulocytosis are rarely seen, except in patients with lupus or arthritis (both conditions are aggravated by the drug). *Primaquine* is contraindicated during pregnancy. All Plasmodium species may develop resistance to *primaquine*.

C. Blood schizonticide: Chloroquine

Chloroquine [KLOR-oh-kwin] is a synthetic 4-aminoquinoline that has been the mainstay of antimalarial therapy, and it is the drug of choice in the treatment of erythrocytic P. falciparum malaria, except in resistant strains. *Chloroquine* is less effective against P. vivax malaria. It is highly specific for the asexual form of plasmodia. *Chloroquine* is also effective in the treatment of extraintestinal amebiasis. [Note: The anti-inflam-

---

[2]See p. 152 in ***Lippincott's Illustrated Reviews: Biochemistry*** (4th ed.) for a discussion of glucose-6-phosphate dehydrogenase deficiency.

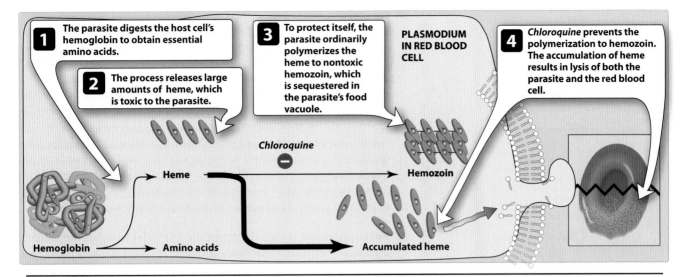

Figure 36.9
Action of *chloroquine* on the formation of hemozoin by <u>Plasmodium</u> species.

matory action of *chloroquine* explains its occasional use in rheumatoid arthritis and discoid lupus erythematosus.]

1. **Mechanism of action:** Although a detailed explanation of the mechanisms by which *chloroquine* kills plasmodial parasites is still incomplete, the following processes are essential for the drug's lethal action (Figure 36.9). After traversing the erythrocytic and plasmodial membranes, *chloroquine* (a diprotic weak base) is concentrated in the organism's acidic food vacuole, primarily by ion trapping. It is in the food vacuole that the parasite digests the host cell's hemoglobin to obtain essential amino acids. However, this process also releases large amounts of soluble heme (ferriprotoporphyrin IX), which is toxic to the parasite. To protect itself, the parasite ordinarily polymerizes the heme to hemozoin (a pigment), which is sequestered in the parasite's food vacuole. *Chloroquine* specifically binds to heme, preventing its polymerization to hemozoin. The increased pH and the accumulation of heme result in oxidative damage to the membranes, leading to lysis of both the parasite and the red blood cell. The binding to heme and prevention of its polymerization appear to be a crucial step in the drug's antiplasmodial activity, and this may represent a unifying mechanism for such diverse compounds as *chloroquine*, *quinidine*, and *mefloquine*.

2. **Pharmacokinetics:** *Chloroquine* is rapidly and completely absorbed following oral administration. Usually, 4 days of therapy suffice to cure the disease. The drug concentrates in erythrocytes, liver, spleen, kidney, lung, melanin-containing tissues, and leukocytes. Thus, it has a very large volume of distribution. It persists in erythrocytes (see "Mechanism of action" above). The drug also penetrates into the central nervous system (CNS) and traverses the placenta. *Chloroquine* is dealkylated by the hepatic mixed-function oxidase system, but some metabolic products retain antimalarial activity. Both parent drug and metabolites are excreted predominantly in the urine (Figure 36.10). The excretion rate is enhanced as urine is acidified.

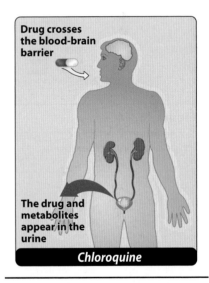

Figure 36.10
Administration and fate of *chloroquine*.

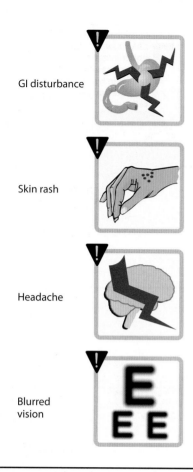

GI disturbance

Skin rash

Headache

Blurred
vision

Figure 36. 11
Some adverse effects commonly
associated with *chloroquine*.

3. **Adverse effects:** Side effects are minimal at the low doses used in the chemosuppression of malaria. At higher doses, many more toxic effects occur, such as gastrointestinal upset, pruritus, headaches, and blurring of vision (Figure 36.11). [Note: An ophthalmologic examination should be routinely performed.] Discoloration of the nail beds and mucous membranes may be seen on chronic administration. *Chloroquine* should be used cautiously in patients with hepatic dysfunction or severe gastrointestinal problems or in patients with neurologic or blood disorders. *Chloroquine* can cause electrocardiographic changes, because it has a *quinidine*-like effect. It may also exacerbate dermatitis produced by *gold* or *phenylbutazone* therapy. [Note: Patients with psoriasis or porphyria should not be treated with *chloroquine*, because an acute attack may be provoked.]

4. **Resistance:** Resistance of plasmodia to available drugs has become a serious medical problem throughout Africa, Asia, and most areas of Central and South America. *Chloroquine*-resistant P. falciparum exhibit multigenic alterations that confer a high level of resistance. [Note: When a *chloroquine*-resistant organism is encountered, therapy usually consists of an orally administered combination of *quinine*, *pyrimethamine*, and a sulfonamide, such as *sulfadoxine*.]

D. Blood schizonticide: Mefloquine

Mefloquine [MEF-lo-kween] appears to be promising as an effective single agent for suppressing and curing infections caused by multidrug-resistant forms of P. falciparum. Its exact mechanism of action remains to be determined, but like *quinine*, it can apparently damage the parasite's membrane. Resistant strains have been identified. *Mefloquine* is absorbed well after oral administration and concentrates in the liver and lung. It has a long half-life (17 days) because of its concentration in various tissues and its continuous circulation through the enterohepatic and enterogastric systems. The drug undergoes extensive metabolism. Its major excretory route is the feces. Adverse reactions at high doses range from nausea, vomiting, and dizziness to disorientation, hallucinations, and depression. Electrocardiographic abnormalities and cardiac arrest are possible if *mefloquine* is taken concurrently with *quinine* or *quinidine*.

E. Blood schizonticides: Quinine and quinidine

Quinine [KWYE-nine] and its stereoisomer, *quinidine* [KWIH-ni-deen], interfere with heme polymerization, resulting in death of the erythrocytic form of the plasmodial parasite. These drugs are reserved for severe infestations and for malarial strains that are resistant to other agents, such as *chloroquine*. Taken orally, *quinine* is well distributed throughout the body and can reach the fetus. Alkalinization of the urine decreases its excretion. The major adverse effect of *quinine* is cinchonism—a syndrome causing nausea, vomiting, tinnitus, and vertigo. These effects are reversible and are not considered to be reasons for suspending therapy. However, *quinine* treatment should be suspended if a positive Coombs' test for hemolytic anemia occurs. Drug interactions include potentiation of neuromuscular-blocking agents and elevation of *digoxin* levels if taken concurrently with *quinine*. *Quinine* absorption is retarded when the drug is taken with aluminum-containing antacids. *Quinine* is fetotoxic.

F. Blood schizonticide: Artemisinin

Artemisinin [ar-te-MIS-in-in] is derived from the qinghaosu plant, which has been used in Chinese medicine for more than two millennia in the treatment of fevers and malaria. *Artemisinin* (or one of its derivatives) is available for the treatment of severe, multidrug-resistant P. falciparum malaria. Its antimalarial action involves the production of free radicals within the plasmodium food vacuole, following cleavage of the drug's endoperoxide bridge by heme iron in parasitized erythrocytes. It is also believed to covalently bind to and damage specific malarial proteins. Oral, rectal, and intravenous preparations are available, but the short half-lives preclude their use in chemoprophylaxis. They are metabolized in the liver and are excreted primarily in the bile. Adverse effects include nausea, vomiting, and diarrhea, but overall, *artemisinin* is remarkably safe. Extremely high doses may cause neurotoxicity and prolongation of the QT interval.

G. Blood schizonticide and sporontocide: Pyrimethamine

The antifolate agent *pyrimethamine* [peer-i-METH-a-meen] is frequently employed to effect a radical cure as a blood schizonticide. It also acts as a strong sporonticide in the mosquito's gut when the mosquito ingests it with the blood of the human host. *Pyrimethamine* inhibits plasmodial dihydrofolate reductase[3] at much lower concentrations than those needed to inhibit the mammalian enzyme. The inhibition deprives the protozoan of tetrahydrofolate—a cofactor required in the de novo biosynthesis of purines and pyrimidines and in the interconversions of certain amino acids. *Pyrimethamine* alone is effective against P. falciparum. In combination with a sulfonamide, it is also used against P. malariae and Toxoplasma gondii. If megaloblastic anemia occurs with *pyrimethamine* treatment, it may be reversed with *leucovorin*. Figure 36.12 shows some therapeutic options in the treatment of malaria.

IV. CHEMOTHERAPY FOR TRYPANOSOMIASIS

Trypanosomiasis refers to two chronic and, eventually, fatal diseases caused by species of Trypanosoma: African sleeping sickness, and American sleeping sickness (Figure 36.13). In African sleeping sickness, the causative organisms, Trypanosoma brucei gambiense and Trypanosoma brucei rhodiense, initially live and grow in the blood. The parasite invades the CNS, causing an inflammation of the brain and spinal cord that produces the characteristic lethargy and, eventually, continuous sleep. Chagas' disease (American sleeping sickness) is caused by Trypanosoma cruzi and occurs in South America.

A. Melarsoprol

Melarsoprol [mel-AR-so-prol] is a derivative of mersalyl oxide, a trivalent arsenical. Its use is limited to the treatment of trypanosomal infections—usually in the late stage with CNS involvement—and it is lethal to these parasites.

1. **Mechanism of action:** The drug reacts with sulfhydryl groups of various substances, including enzymes in both the organism and host.

[3]See p. 374 in ***Lippincott's Illustrated Reviews: Biochemistry*** (4th ed.) for a discussion of dihydrofolate reductase.

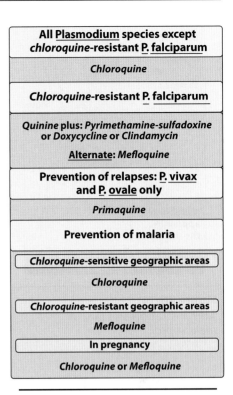

Figure 36.12
Treatment and prevention of malaria.

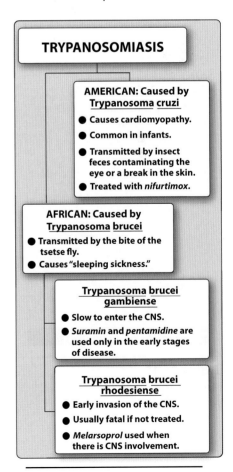

Figure 36.13
Summary of trypanosomiasis.

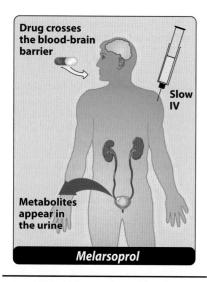

Figure 36.14
Administration and fate of
melarsoprol.

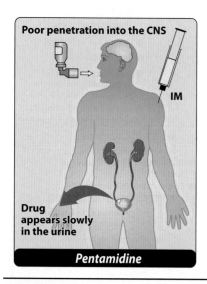

Figure 36.15
Administration and fate of
pentamidine.

The parasite's enzymes may be more sensitive than those of the host. There is evidence that mammalian cells may be less permeable to the drug and, thus, are protected from its toxic effects. Trypanosomal resistance may also be due to decreased permeability of the drug.

2. **Pharmacokinetics:** *Melarsoprol* usually is slowly administered intravenously through a fine needle, even though it is absorbed from the gastrointestinal tract. Because it is very irritating, care should be taken not to infiltrate surrounding tissue. Adequate trypanocidal concentrations appear in the CSF, in contrast to nonpenetration of the CSF by *pentamidine*. *Melarsoprol* is therefore the agent of choice in the treatment of T. brucei rhodesiense, which rapidly invades the CNS, as well as for meningoencephalitis caused by T. brucei gambiense. The host readily oxidizes *melarsoprol* to a relatively nontoxic, pentavalent arsenic compound. The drug has a very short half-life and is rapidly excreted into the urine (Figure 36.14).

3. **Adverse effects:** CNS toxicities are the most serious side effects of *melarsoprol* treatment. Encephalopathy may appear soon after the first course of treatment but usually subsides. It may, however, be fatal. Hypersensitivity reactions may also occur, and fever may follow injection. Gastrointestinal disturbances, such as severe vomiting and abdominal pain, can be minimized if the patient is in the fasting state during drug administration and for several hours thereafter. *Melarsoprol* is contraindicated in patients with influenza. Hemolytic anemia has been seen in patients with glucose 6-phosphate dehydrogenase deficiency.

B. Pentamidine isethionate

Pentamidine [pen-TAM-i-deen] is active against a variety of protozoal infections, including many trypanosomes, such as T. brucei gambiense, for which *pentamidine* is used to treat and prevent the organism's hematologic stage. However, some trypanosomes, including T. cruzi, are resistant. *Pentamidine* is also effective in the treatment of systemic blastomycosis (caused by the fungus Blastomyces dermatitidis) and in treating infections caused by Pneumocystis jiroveci (formerly called Pneumocystis carinii—a name now used to refer to the organism in animals). [Note: It is now considered to be a fungus, but it is not susceptible to antifungal drugs. *Trimethoprim-sulfamethoxazole* is preferred in the treatment of P. jiroveci infections. However, *pentamidine* is the drug of choice in treating patients with pneumonia caused by P. jiroveci who have failed to respond to *trimethoprim-sulfamethoxazole*. The drug is also used in treating P. jiroveci–infected individuals who are allergic to sulfonamides. Because of the increased incidence of pneumonia caused by this organism in immunocompromised patients, such as those infected with human immunodeficiency virus, *pentamidine* has assumed an important place in chemotherapy.] *Pentamidine* is also an alternative drug to *stibogluconate* in the treatment of leishmaniasis.

1. **Mechanism of action:** Trypanosoma brucei concentrates *pentamidine* by an energy-dependent, high-affinity uptake system. [Note: Resistance is associated with an inability of the trypanosome to concentrate the drug.] Although its mechanism of action has not been defined, evidence exists that the drug binds to the parasite's DNA and interferes with the synthesis of RNA, DNA, phospholipid, and protein by the parasite.

2. **Pharmacokinetics:** Fresh solutions of *pentamidine* are administered intramuscularly or as an aerosol (Figure 36.15). [Note: The intravenous route is avoided because of severe adverse reactions, such as a sharp fall in blood pressure and tachycardia.] The drug is concentrated and stored in the liver and kidney for a long period of time. Because it does not enter the CSF, it is ineffective against the meningoencephalitic stage of trypanosomiasis. The drug is not metabolized, and it is excreted very slowly into the urine. Its half-life in the plasma is about 5 days.

3. **Adverse effects:** Serious renal dysfunction may occur, which reverses on discontinuation of the drug. Other adverse reactions are hypotension, dizziness, rash, and toxicity to β cells of the pancreas.

C. Nifurtimox

Nifurtimox [nye-FER-tim-oks] has found use only in the treatment of acute T. cruzi infections (Chagas' disease), although treatment of the chronic stage of such infections has led to variable results. [Note: *Nifurtimox* is suppressive, not curative.] Being a nitroaromatic compound, *nifurtimox* undergoes reduction and, eventually, generates intracellular oxygen radicals, such as superoxide radicals and hydrogen peroxide[4] (Figure 36.16). These highly reactive radicals are toxic to T. cruzi, which lacks catalase.[5] [Note: Mammalian cells are partially protected from such substances by the presence of enzymes such as catalase, glutathione peroxidase, and superoxide dismutase.] *Nifurtimox* is administered orally, and it is rapidly absorbed and metabolized to unidentified products that are excreted in the urine. Adverse effects are common following chronic administration, particularly among the elderly. Major toxicities include immediate hypersensitivity reactions such as anaphylaxis, delayed hypersensitivity reactions such as dermatitis and icterus, and gastrointestinal problems that may be severe enough to cause weight loss. Peripheral neuropathy is relatively common, and disturbances in the CNS may also occur. In addition, cell-mediated immune reactions may be suppressed.

D. Suramin

Suramin [SOO-ra-min] is used primarily in the early treatment and, especially, the prophylaxis of African trypanosomiasis. It is very reactive and inhibits many enzymes, among them those involved in energy metabolism (for example, glycerol phosphate dehydrogenase[6]), which appears to be the mechanism most closely correlated with trypanocidal activity. The drug must be injected intravenously. It binds to plasma proteins and remains in the plasma for a long time, accumulating in the liver and in the proximal tubular cells of the kidney. The severity of the adverse reactions demands that the patient be carefully followed, especially if he or she is debilitated. Although infrequent, adverse reactions include nausea and vomiting (which cause further debilitation of the patient), shock and loss of consciousness, acute urticaria, and neurologic problems, including paresthesia, photophobia, palpebral edema (edema

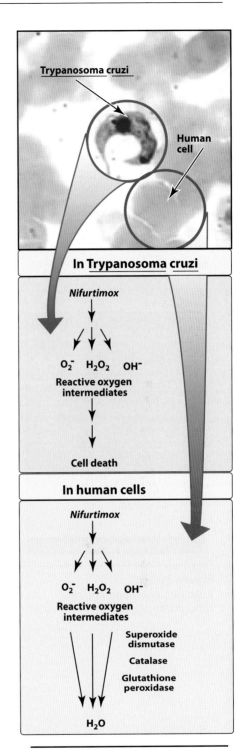

Figure 36.16
Generation of toxic intermediates by *nifurtimox*.

[4]See p. 148 in ***Lippincott's Illustrated Reviews: Biochemistry*** (4th ed.) for a discussion of reactive oxygen intermediates.
[5]See p. 148 in ***Lippincott's Illustrated Reviews: Biochemistry*** (4th ed.) for a discussion of catalase.
[6]See p. 189 in ***Lippincott's Illustrated Reviews: Biochemistry*** (4th ed.) for a discussion of glycerol phosphate dehydrogenase.

of the eyelids), and hyperesthesia of the hands and feet. Albuminuria tends to be common, but when cylindruria (the presence of renal casts in the urine) and hematuria occur, treatment should cease.

E. Benznidazole

Benznidazole [benz-NI-da-zole] is a nitroimidazole derivative that inhibits protein synthesis and ribonucleic acid synthesis in the <u>T. cruzi</u> cells. It is an alternative choice for treatment of acute and indeterminate phases of Chagas' disease, but therapy with *benznidazole* does not offer any significant efficacy or toxicity advantages over that with *nifurtimox*. However, *benznidazole* is recommended as prophylaxis for preventing infections caused by <u>T. cruzi</u> among hematopoietic stem cell transplant, recipients because treatment in potential donors is not always effective.

V. CHEMOTHERAPY FOR LEISHMANIASIS

There are three types of leishmaniasis: cutaneous, mucocutaneous, and visceral. [Note: In the visceral type (liver and spleen), the parasite is in the bloodstream and can cause very serious problems.] Leishmaniasis is transmitted from animals to humans (and between humans) by the bite of infected sandflies. The diagnosis is established by demonstrating the parasite in biopsy material and skin lesions. The treatments of leishmaniasis and trypanosomiasis are difficult, because the effective drugs are limited by their toxicities and failure rates. Pentavalent antimonials, such as *sodium stibogluconate*, are the conventional therapy used in the treatment of leishmaniasis, with *pentamidine* and *amphotericin B* as backup agents. *Allopurinol* has also been reported to be effective (it is converted to a toxic metabolite by the amastigote form[7] of the organism).

A. Life cycle of the causative organism: <u>Leishmania</u> species

The sandfly transfers the flagellated promastigote form of the protozoa, which is rapidly phagocytized by macrophages. In the macrophage, the promastigotes rapidly change to nonflagellated amastigotes and multiply, killing the cell. The newly released amastigotes are again phagocytized, and the cycle continues.

B. Sodium stibogluconate

Sodium stibogluconate [stib-o-GLOO-koe-nate] is not effective <u>in vitro</u>. Therefore, it has been proposed that reduction to the trivalent antimonial compound is essential for activity. The exact mechanism of action has not been determined. Evidence for inhibition of glycolysis in the parasite at the phosphofructokinase reaction[8] has been found. Because it is not absorbed on oral administration, *sodium stibogluconate* must be administered parenterally, and it is distributed in the extravascular compartment. Metabolism is minimal, and the drug is excreted in the urine (Figure 36.17). Adverse effects include pain at the injection site, gastrointestinal upsets, and cardiac arrhythmias. Renal and hepatic function should be monitored periodically.

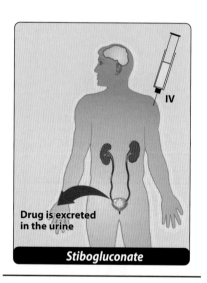

Figure 36.17
Administration and fate of *stibogluconate*.

[7]See p. 224 in ***Lippincott's Illustrated Reviews: Microbiology*** (2nd ed.) for a discussion of leishmaniasis.
[8]See p. 99 in ***Lippincott's Illustrated Reviews: Biochemistry*** (4th ed.) for a discussion of phosphofructokinase reaction.

VI. CHEMOTHERAPY FOR TOXOPLASMOSIS

One of the most common infections in humans is caused by the protozoan <u>Toxoplasma</u> <u>gondii</u>, which is transmitted to humans when they consume raw or inadequately cooked, infected meat.[9] An infected pregnant woman can transmit the organism to her fetus. Cats are the only animals that shed oocysts, which can infect other animals as well as humans. The treatment of choice for this condition is the antifolate drug *pyrimethamine*. A combination of *sulfadiazine* and *pyrimethamine* is also efficacious. *Leucovorin* is often administered to protect against folate deficiency. Other inhibitors of folate biosynthesis, such as *trimethoprim* and *sulfamethoxazole*, are without therapeutic efficacy in toxoplasmosis. [Note: At the first appearance of a rash, *pyrimethamine* should be discontinued, because hypersensitivity to this drug can be severe.]

VII. CHEMOTHERAPY FOR GIARDIASIS

<u>Giardia lamblia</u> is the most commonly diagnosed intestinal parasite in the United States.[10] It has only two life-cycle stages: the binucleate trophozoite with four flagellae, and the drug-resistant, four-nucleate cyst (Figure 36.18). Ingestion, usually from contaminated drinking water, leads to infection. The trophozoites exist in the small intestine and divide by binary fission. Occasionally, cysts are formed that pass out in the stool. Although some infections are asymptomatic, severe diarrhea can occur, which can be very serious in immune-suppressed patients. The treatment of choice is *metronidazole* for 5 days. One alternative agent is *tinidazole*, which is equally effective as *metronidazole* in treatment of giardiasis but with a much shorter course of treatment (2 g given once). *Nitazoxanide* [nye-ta-ZOX-a-nide], a nitrothiazole derivative structurally similar to *aspirin*, was recently approved for treatment of giardiasis. *Nitazoxanide* is also equally efficacious as *metronidazole* and, in comparison, has a 2 day shorter course of therapy.

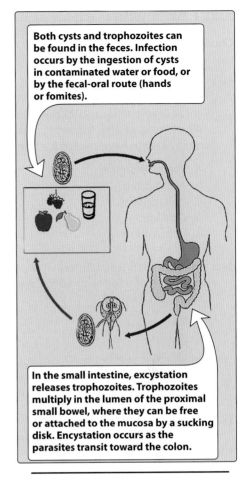

Both cysts and trophozoites can be found in the feces. Infection occurs by the ingestion of cysts in contaminated water or food, or by the fecal-oral route (hands or fomites).

In the small intestine, excystation releases trophozoites. Trophozoites multiply in the lumen of the proximal small bowel, where they can be free or attached to the mucosa by a sucking disk. Encystation occurs as the parasites transit toward the colon.

Figure 36.18
Life cycle of <u>Giardia</u> <u>lamblia</u>.

[9]See p. 223 in ***Lippincott's Illustrated Reviews: Microbiology*** (2nd ed.) for a discussion of toxoplasmosis.
[10]See p. 219 in ***Lippincott's Illustrated Reviews: Microbiology*** (2nd ed.) for a discussion of giardiasis.

Study Questions

Choose the ONE best answer.

36.1 A 36-year-old male of Lebanese ancestry is being treated for <u>Plasmodium</u> <u>vivax</u> malaria. He experiences severe fatigue, back pain, and darkened urine. Which one of the following antimalarial drugs is most likely to have caused his symptoms?

    A. Pyrimethamine.
    B. Artemisinin.
    C. Chloroquine.
    D. Quinine.
    E. Primaquine.

Correct answer = E. The symptoms presented by the patient are consistent with hemolytic anemia. The patient is male and from the Mediterranean basin, both of which are factors associated with glucose 6-phosphate dehydrogenase deficiency. Primaquine is most likely to cause hemolytic anemia in such individuals.

36.2 Tinnitus, dizziness, blurred vision, and headache are indicative of toxicity to which one of the following antimalarial drugs?

    A. Primaquine.
    B. Quinine.
    C. Pyrimethamine.
    D. Chloroquine.
    E. Sulfadoxine.

Correct answer = B. The symptoms are characteristic of cinchonism, which is characteristic of quinine or quinidine.

37.3 Which of the following drugs is recommended for the treatment of severe, multidrug-resistant <u>Plasmodium</u> <u>falciparum</u> malaria?

    A. Artemisinin.
    B. Chloroquine.
    C. Quinine.
    D. Sodium stibogluconate.
    E. Primaquine.

Correct answer = A. Artemisinin is the antimalarial drug recommended for life-threatening, multidrug-resistant <u>Plasmodium</u> <u>falciparum</u> malaria. The parasite is resistant to chloroquine and quinine and would not be affected by primaquine or stibogluconate.

37.4 A 22-year-old man, who frequently backpacks, complains of diarrhea and fatigue. Examination of stool specimens shows binucleate organisms with four flagellae. Which one of the following drugs would be effective in treating this patient's infestation?

    A. Metronidazole.
    B. Quinidine.
    C. Pentamidine.
    D. Sulfadoxine.
    E. Stibogluconate.

Correct answer = A. The patient has giardiasis, and metronidazole is the drug of choice for this intestinal protozoal infection. He probably was infected by drinking contaminated water from a stream. The other drugs are not effective against giardia.

Anthelmintic Drugs

37

I. OVERVIEW

Three major groups of helminths (worms)—the nematodes, trematod, and cestodes—infect humans. As in all antibiotic regimens, the anthelmintic drugs (Figure 37.1) are aimed at metabolic targets that are present in the parasite but are either absent from or have different characteristics than those of the host. Figure 37.2 illustrates the high incidence of helmintic infections.

II. DRUGS FOR THE TREATMENT OF NEMATODES

Nematodes are elongated roundworms that possess a complete digestive system, including both a mouth and an anus. They cause infections of the intestine as well as the blood and tissues.

A. Mebendazole

Mebendazole [me-BEN-da-zole], a synthetic benzimidazole compound, is effective against a wide spectrum of nematodes. It is a drug of choice in the treatment of infections by whipworm (<u>Trichuris trichiura</u>), pinworm (<u>Enterobius vermicularis</u>), hookworms (<u>Necator americanus</u> and <u>Ancylostoma duodenale</u>), and roundworm (<u>Ascariasis lumbricoides</u>). *Mebendazole* acts by binding to and interfering with the assembly of the parasites' microtubules and also by decreasing glucose uptake. Affected parasites are expelled with the feces. *Mebendazole* is nearly insoluble in aqueous solution. Little of an oral dose (that is chewed) is absorbed by the body, unless it is taken with a high-fat meal. It undergoes first-pass metabolism to inactive compounds. *Mebendazole* is relatively free of toxic effects, although patients may complain of abdominal pain and diarrhea. It is, however, contraindicated in pregnant women (Figure 37.3), because it has been shown to be embryotoxic and teratogenic in experimental animals.

B. Pyrantel pamoate

Pyrantel pamoate [pi-RAN-tel PAM-oh-ate], along with *mebendazole*, is effective in the treatment of infections caused by roundworms, pinworms, and hookworms (Figure 37.4). *Pyrantel pamoate* is poorly absorbed orally and exerts its effects in the intestinal tract. It acts as a depolarizing, neuromuscular-blocking agent, causing persistent activation of the parasite's nicotinic receptors. The paralyzed worm is then expelled from the host's intestinal tract. Adverse effects are mild and include nausea, vomiting, and diarrhea.

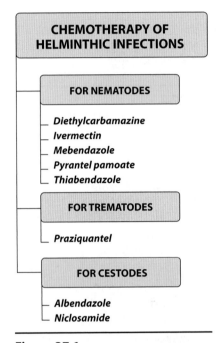

Figure 37.1
Summary of anthelmintic agents.

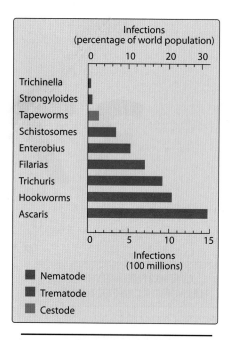

Figure 37.2
Relative incidence of helminth infections worldwide.

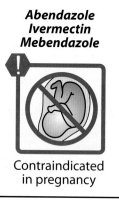

Contraindicated in pregnancy

Figure 37.3
Albendazole, ivermectin, and *mebendazole* are contraindicated in pregnancy.

C. Thiabendazole

Thiabendazole [thye-a-BEN-da-zole], another synthetic benzimidazole, is effective against strongyloidiasis caused by Strongyloides stercoralis (threadworm), cutaneous larva migrans, and early stages of trichinosis (caused by Trichinella spiralis; see Figure 37.4). *Thiabendazole,* like the other benzimidazoles, affects microtubular aggregation. Although nearly insoluble in water, the drug is readily absorbed on oral administration. It is hydroxylated in the liver and excreted in the urine. The adverse effects most often encountered are dizziness, anorexia, nausea, and vomiting. There have been reports of central nervous system (CNS) symptomatology. Among the cases of erythema multiforme and Stevens-Johnson syndrome reportedly caused by *thiabendazole,* there have been a number of fatalities. Its use is contraindicated during pregnancy.

D. Ivermectin

Ivermectin [eye-ver-MEK-tin] is the drug of choice for the treatment of onchocerciasis (river blindness) caused by Onchocerca volvulus and is a drug of first choice for cutaneous larva migrans and strongyloides. *Ivermectin* targets the parasite's glutamate-gated Cl⁻ channel receptors. Chloride influx is enhanced, and hyperpolarization occurs, resulting in paralysis of the worm. The drug is given orally. It does not cross the blood-brain barrier and, thus, has no pharmacologic effects in the CNS. However, it is contraindicated in patients with meningitis, because their blood-brain barrier is more permeable and CNS effects might be expected. *Ivermectin* is also contraindicated in pregnancy (see Figure 37.3). The killing of the microfilaria can result in a Mazotti-like reaction (fever, headache, dizziness, somnolence, and hypotension).

E. Diethylcarbamazine

Diethylcarbamazine [dye-eth-il-kar-BAM-a-zeen] is used in the treatment of filariasis because of its ability to immobilize microfilariae and render them susceptible to host defense mechanisms. Combined with *albendazole, diethylcarbamazine* is effective in the treatment of Wucheria bancrofti and Brugia malayi infections. It is rapidly absorbed following oral administration with meals and is excreted primarily in the urine. Urinary alkalosis or renal impairment may require dosage reduction. Adverse effects are primarily caused by host reactions to the killed organisms. The severity of symptoms is related to the parasite load and include fever, malaise, rash, myalgias, arthralgias, and headache. Most patients have leukocytosis. Antihistamines or steroids may be given to ameliorate many of the symptoms. Figure 37.4 summarizes the major infections caused by nematodes and the common therapies for them.

III. DRUGS FOR THE TREATMENT OF TREMATODES

The trematodes (flukes) are leaf-shaped flatworms that are generally characterized by the tissues they infect. For example, they may be categorized as liver, lung, intestinal, or blood flukes (Figure 37.5).

A. Praziquantel

Trematode infections are generally treated with *praziquantel* [pray-zi-KWON-tel]. This drug is an agent of choice for the treatment of all forms of schistosomiasis and other trematode infections and for cestode infections like cysticercosis. Permeability of the cell membrane to calcium is increased, causing contracture and paralysis of the parasite.

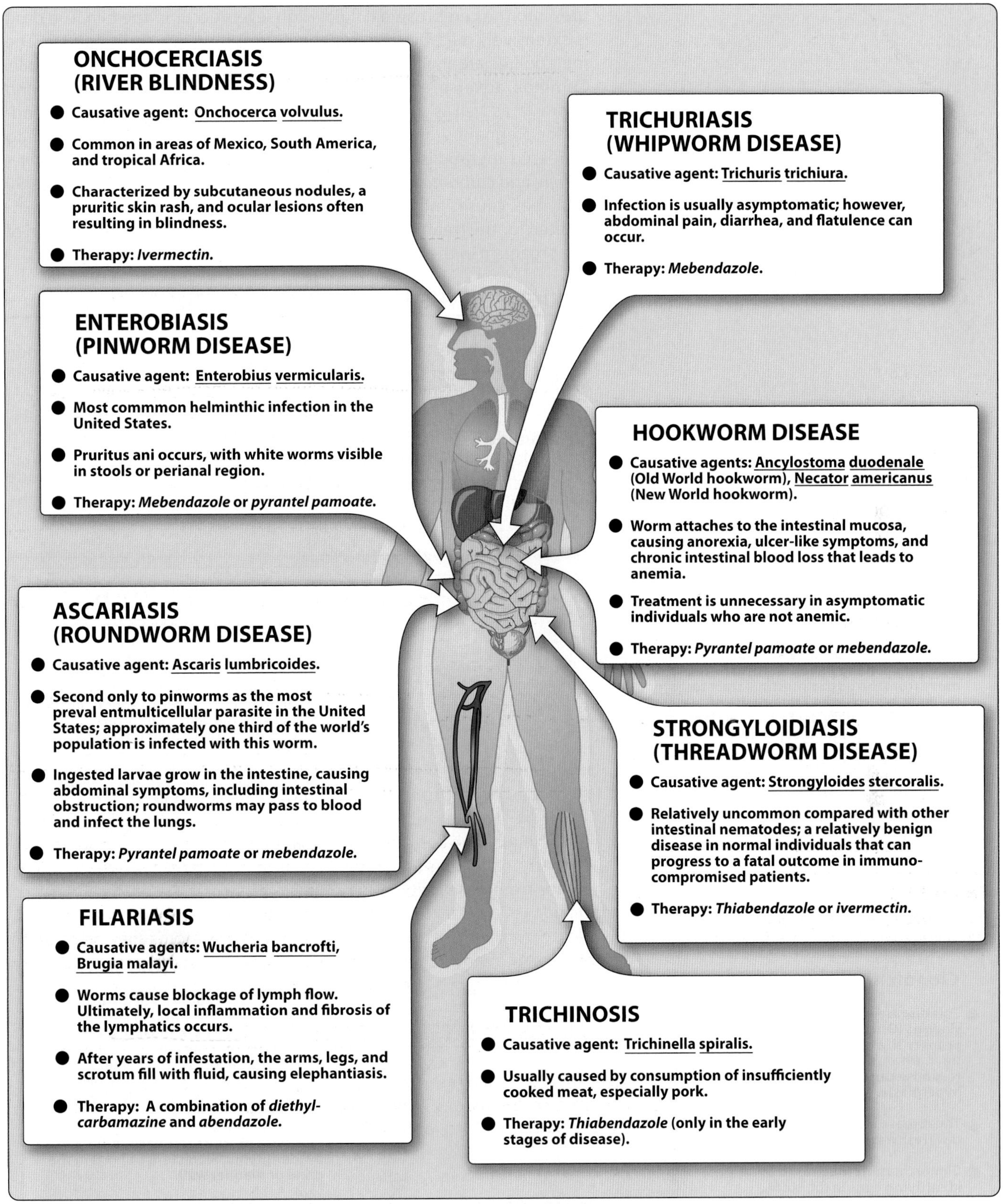

ONCHOCERCIASIS (RIVER BLINDNESS)

- Causative agent: <u>Onchocerca</u> <u>volvulus</u>.
- Common in areas of Mexico, South America, and tropical Africa.
- Characterized by subcutaneous nodules, a pruritic skin rash, and ocular lesions often resulting in blindness.
- Therapy: *Ivermectin*.

TRICHURIASIS (WHIPWORM DISEASE)

- Causative agent: <u>Trichuris</u> <u>trichiura</u>.
- Infection is usually asymptomatic; however, abdominal pain, diarrhea, and flatulence can occur.
- Therapy: *Mebendazole*.

ENTEROBIASIS (PINWORM DISEASE)

- Causative agent: <u>Enterobius</u> <u>vermicularis</u>.
- Most commmon helminthic infection in the United States.
- Pruritus ani occurs, with white worms visible in stools or perianal region.
- Therapy: *Mebendazole or pyrantel pamoate*.

HOOKWORM DISEASE

- Causative agents: <u>Ancylostoma</u> <u>duodenale</u> (Old World hookworm), <u>Necator</u> <u>americanus</u> (New World hookworm).
- Worm attaches to the intestinal mucosa, causing anorexia, ulcer-like symptoms, and chronic intestinal blood loss that leads to anemia.
- Treatment is unnecessary in asymptomatic individuals who are not anemic.
- Therapy: *Pyrantel pamoate or mebendazole*.

ASCARIASIS (ROUNDWORM DISEASE)

- Causative agent: <u>Ascaris</u> <u>lumbricoides</u>.
- Second only to pinworms as the most preval entmulticellular parasite in the United States; approximately one third of the world's population is infected with this worm.
- Ingested larvae grow in the intestine, causing abdominal symptoms, including intestinal obstruction; roundworms may pass to blood and infect the lungs.
- Therapy: *Pyrantel pamoate or mebendazole*.

STRONGYLOIDIASIS (THREADWORM DISEASE)

- Causative agent: <u>Strongyloides</u> <u>stercoralis</u>.
- Relatively uncommon compared with other intestinal nematodes; a relatively benign disease in normal individuals that can progress to a fatal outcome in immuno-compromised patients.
- Therapy: *Thiabendazole or ivermectin*.

FILARIASIS

- Causative agents: <u>Wucheria</u> <u>bancrofti</u>, <u>Brugia</u> <u>malayi</u>.
- Worms cause blockage of lymph flow. Ultimately, local inflammation and fibrosis of the lymphatics occurs.
- After years of infestation, the arms, legs, and scrotum fill with fluid, causing elephantiasis.
- Therapy: A combination of *diethyl-carbamazine* and *abendazole*.

TRICHINOSIS

- Causative agent: <u>Trichinella</u> <u>spiralis</u>.
- Usually caused by consumption of insufficiently cooked meat, especially pork.
- Therapy: *Thiabendazole* (only in the early stages of disease).

Figure 37.4
Characteristics of and therapy for commonly encountered nematode infections.

Praziquantel is rapidly absorbed after oral administration and distributes into the cerebrospinal fluid. High levels occur in the bile. The drug is extensively metabolized oxidatively, resulting in a short half-life. The metabolites are inactive and are excreted through the urine and bile. Common adverse effects include drowsiness, dizziness, malaise, and anorexia, as well as gastrointestinal upsets. The drug is not recommended for pregnant women or nursing mothers. Drug interactions due to increased metabolism have been reported with *dexamethasone*, *phenytoin*, and *carbamazepine*. *Cimetidine*, which inhibits cytochrome P450 isozymes, causes increased *praziquantel* levels. *Praziquantel* is contraindicated for the treatment of ocular cysticercosis, because destruction of the organism in the eye may damage the organ.

IV. DRUGS FOR THE TREATMENT OF CESTODES

The cestodes, or "true tapeworms," typically have a flat, segmented body and attach to the host's intestine (Figure 37.6). Like the trematodes, the tapeworms lack a mouth and a digestive tract throughout their life cycle.

A. Niclosamide

Niclosamide [ni-KLOE-sa-mide] is the drug of choice for most cestode (tapeworm) infections. Its action has been ascribed to inhibition of the

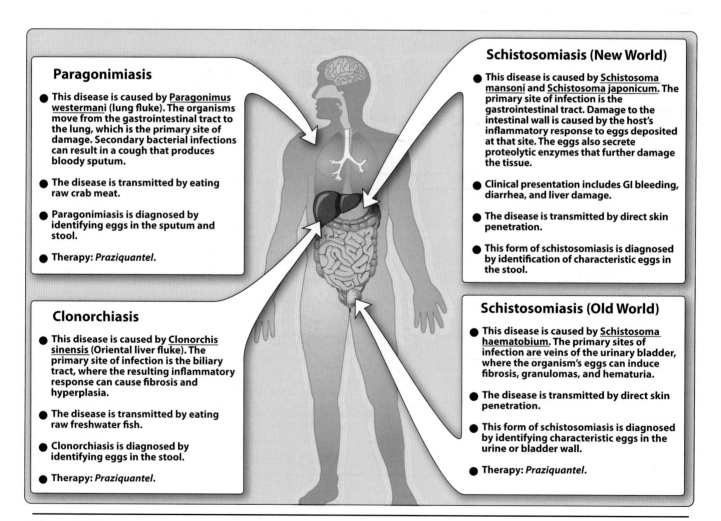

Paragonimiasis

- This disease is caused by <u>Paragonimus westermani</u> (lung fluke). The organisms move from the gastrointestinal tract to the lung, which is the primary site of damage. Secondary bacterial infections can result in a cough that produces bloody sputum.

- The disease is transmitted by eating raw crab meat.

- Paragonimiasis is diagnosed by identifying eggs in the sputum and stool.

- Therapy: *Praziquantel*.

Clonorchiasis

- This disease is caused by <u>Clonorchis sinensis</u> (Oriental liver fluke). The primary site of infection is the biliary tract, where the resulting inflammatory response can cause fibrosis and hyperplasia.

- The disease is transmitted by eating raw freshwater fish.

- Clonorchiasis is diagnosed by identifying eggs in the stool.

- Therapy: *Praziquantel*.

Schistosomiasis (New World)

- This disease is caused by <u>Schistosoma mansoni</u> and <u>Schistosoma japonicum</u>. The primary site of infection is the gastrointestinal tract. Damage to the intestinal wall is caused by the host's inflammatory response to eggs deposited at that site. The eggs also secrete proteolytic enzymes that further damage the tissue.

- Clinical presentation includes GI bleeding, diarrhea, and liver damage.

- The disease is transmitted by direct skin penetration.

- This form of schistosomiasis is diagnosed by identification of characteristic eggs in the stool.

Schistosomiasis (Old World)

- This disease is caused by <u>Schistosoma haematobium</u>. The primary sites of infection are veins of the urinary bladder, where the organism's eggs can induce fibrosis, granulomas, and hematuria.

- The disease is transmitted by direct skin penetration.

- This form of schistosomiasis is diagnosed by identifying characteristic eggs in the urine or bladder wall.

- Therapy: *Praziquantel*.

Figure 37.5
Characteristics of and therapy for commonly encountered trematode infections.

parasite's mitochondrial phosphorylation of adenosine diphospate, which produces usable energy in the form of adenosine triphospate. Anaerobic metabolism may also be inhibited. The drug is lethal for the cestode's scolex and segments of cestodes but not for the ova. A laxative is administered prior to oral administration of *niclosamide*. This is done to purge the bowel of all dead segments and so preclude digestion and liberation of the ova, which may lead to cysticercosis. Alcohol should be avoided within 1 day of *niclosamide*.

B. Albendazole

Albendazole [al-BEN-da-zole] is a benzimidazole that, like the others, inhibits microtubule synthesis and glucose uptake in nematodes. Its primary therapeutic application, however, is in the treatment of cestodal infestations, such as cysticercosis (caused by <u>Taenia solium</u> larvae) and hydatid disease (caused by <u>Echinococcus granulosis</u>). *Albendazole* is erratically absorbed after oral administration, but absorption is enhanced by a high-fat meal. It undergoes extensive first-pass metabolism, including formation of the sulfoxide, which is also active. *Albendazole* and its metabolites are primarily excreted in the urine. When used in short-

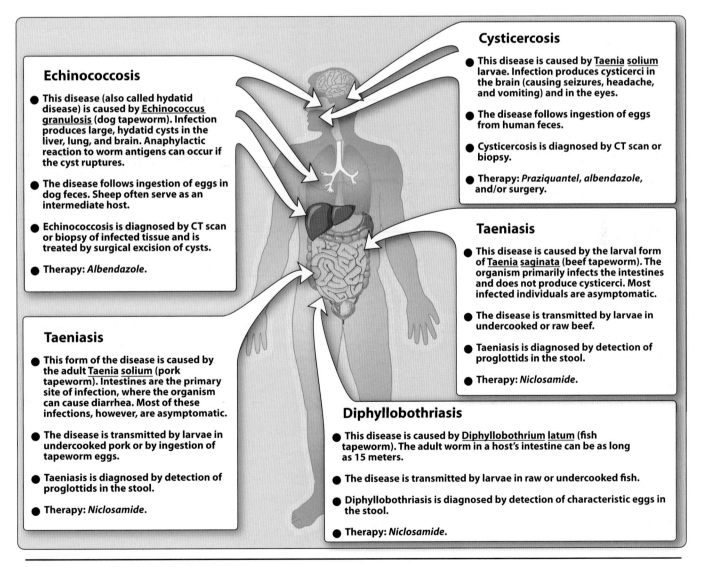

Cysticercosis

- This disease is caused by <u>Taenia solium</u> larvae. Infection produces cysticerci in the brain (causing seizures, headache, and vomiting) and in the eyes.
- The disease follows ingestion of eggs from human feces.
- Cysticercosis is diagnosed by CT scan or biopsy.
- Therapy: *Praziquantel, albendazole, and/or surgery.*

Echinococcosis

- This disease (also called hydatid disease) is caused by <u>Echinococcus granulosis</u> (dog tapeworm). Infection produces large, hydatid cysts in the liver, lung, and brain. Anaphylactic reaction to worm antigens can occur if the cyst ruptures.
- The disease follows ingestion of eggs in dog feces. Sheep often serve as an intermediate host.
- Echinococcosis is diagnosed by CT scan or biopsy of infected tissue and is treated by surgical excision of cysts.
- Therapy: *Albendazole.*

Taeniasis

- This disease is caused by the larval form of <u>Taenia saginata</u> (beef tapeworm). The organism primarily infects the intestines and does not produce cysticerci. Most infected individuals are asymptomatic.
- The disease is transmitted by larvae in undercooked or raw beef.
- Taeniasis is diagnosed by detection of proglottids in the stool.
- Therapy: *Niclosamide.*

Taeniasis

- This form of the disease is caused by the adult <u>Taenia solium</u> (pork tapeworm). Intestines are the primary site of infection, where the organism can cause diarrhea. Most of these infections, however, are asymptomatic.
- The disease is transmitted by larvae in undercooked pork or by ingestion of tapeworm eggs.
- Taeniasis is diagnosed by detection of proglottids in the stool.
- Therapy: *Niclosamide.*

Diphyllobothriasis

- This disease is caused by <u>Diphyllobothrium latum</u> (fish tapeworm). The adult worm in a host's intestine can be as long as 15 meters.
- The disease is transmitted by larvae in raw or undercooked fish.
- Diphyllobothriasis is diagnosed by detection of characteristic eggs in the stool.
- Therapy: *Niclosamide.*

Figure 37.6
Characteristics of and therapy for commonly encountered cestode infections.

course therapy (1–3 days) for nematodal infestations, adverse effects are mild and transient and include headache and nausea. Treatment of hydatid disease (3 months) has a risk of hepatotoxicity and, rarely, agranulocytosis or pancytopenia. Medical treatment of neurocysticercosis is associated with inflammatory responses to dying parasites in the CNS, including headache, vomiting, hyperthermia, convulsions, and mental changes. The drug should not be given during pregnancy (see Figure 37.3) or to children under 2 years of age.

Study Questions

Choose the ONE best answer.

37.1 A 48-year-old immigrant from Mexico presents with seizures and other neurologic symptoms. Eggs of Taenia solium are found upon examination of a stool specimen. A magnetic resonance image of the brain shows many cysts, some of which are calcified. Which one of the following drugs would be of benefit to this individual?

A. Ivermectin.
B. Pyrantel pamoate.
C. Albendazole.
D. Diethylcarbamazine.
E. Niclosamide.

Correct answer = C. The symptoms and other findings for this patient are consistent with neurocysticercosis. Albendazole is the drug of choice for the treatment of this infestation. The other drugs are not effective against the larval forms of tapeworms.

37.2 A 56-year-old man from South America is found to be parasitized by both schistosomes and Taenia solium—the pork tapeworm. Which of the following anthelmintic drugs would be effective for both infestations?

A. Albendazole.
B. Ivermectin.
C. Mebendazole.
D. Niclosamide.
E. Praziquantel.

Correct answer = E. Praziquantel is a primary drug for the treatment of trematode and cestode infestations. Although albendazole is effective in cysticercosis, it is not active against flukes, and this patient has no evidence of cysticercosis. Niclosamide is also active against tapeworms but has no activity against blood flukes.

Antiviral Drugs

38

I. OVERVIEW

Viruses are obligate intracellular parasites. They lack both a cell wall and a cell membrane, and they do not carry out metabolic processes. Viral reproduction uses much of the host's metabolic machinery, and few drugs are selective enough to prevent viral replication without injury to the host. Therapy for viral diseases is further complicated by the fact that the clinical symptoms appear late in the course of the disease, at a time when most of the virus particles have replicated. [Note: This contrasts with bacterial diseases, in which the clinical symptoms are usually coincident with bacterial proliferation.] At this late, symptomatic stage of the viral infection, administration of drugs that block viral replication has limited effectiveness. However, some antiviral agents are useful as prophylactic agents. Only a few virus groups, including those that cause the viral infections discussed in this chapter, respond to available antiviral drugs. To assist in the review of these drugs, they are grouped according to the organisms that are affected (Figure 38.1).

II. TREATMENT OF RESPIRATORY VIRUS INFECTIONS

Viral respiratory tract infections for which treatments exist include those of influenza A and B and respiratory syncytial virus (RSV). [Note: Immunization against influenza A is the preferred approach. However, antiviral agents are employed when patients are allergic to the vaccine, when the outbreak is due to an immunologic variant of the virus not covered by vaccines, or when outbreaks occur among unvaccinated individuals who are at risk and in closed settings (for example, in nursing homes).]

A. Neuraminidase inhibitors

Orthomyxoviruses that cause influenza contain the enzyme neuraminidase, which is essential to the life cycle of the virus. Viral neuraminidase can be selectively inhibited by the sialic acid analogs, oseltamivir [os-el-TAM-i-veer] and zanamivir [za-NA-mi-veer]. These drugs prevent the release of new virions and their spread from cell to cell. Unlike the adamantine analogs discussed below, oseltamivir and zanamivir are effective against both Type A and Type B influenza viruses. They do not interfere with the immune response to influenza A vaccine. Administered prior to exposure, neuraminidase inhibitors prevent infection, and when administered within the first 24 to 48 hours after the onset of infection, they have a modest effect on the intensity and duration of symptoms.

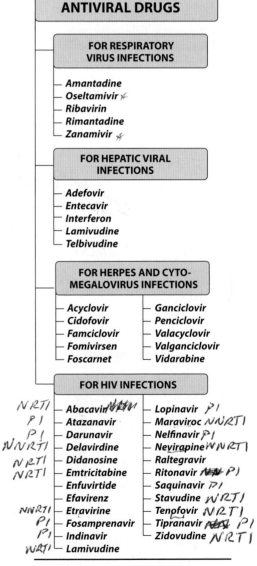

Figure 38.1
Summary of antiviral drugs. HIV = human immunodeficiency virus.

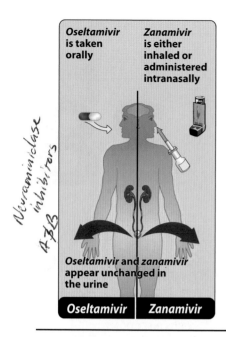

(handwritten, left margin: Neuraminidase inhibitors AZB)

Figure 38.2
Administration and metabolism of *oseltamivir* and *zanamivir*.

(handwritten: Amantadine takes off his coat)

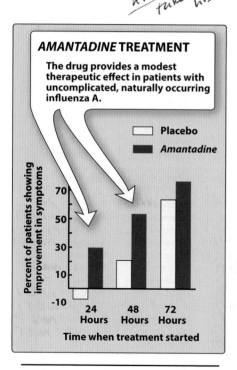

Figure 38.3
Improvement in symptoms of individuals with naturally occurring influenza infections treated with *amantadine*.

1. **Mode of action:** Influenza viruses employ a specific neuraminidase that is inserted into the host cell membrane for the purpose of releasing newly formed virions. *Oseltamivir* and *zanamivir* are transition-state analogs of the sialic acid substrate and serve as inhibitors of the enzyme activity. Virions accumulate at the internal infected cell surface.

2. **Pharmacokinetics:** *Oseltamivir* is an orally active prodrug that is rapidly hydrolyzed by the liver to its active form. *Zanamivir*, on the other hand, is not active orally and is either inhaled or administered intranasally. Both drugs are eliminated unchanged in the urine (Figure 38.2).

3. **Adverse effects:** The most common side effects of *oseltamivir* are gastrointestinal discomfort and nausea, which can be alleviated by taking the drug with food. *Zanamivir* is not associated with gastrointestinal disturbance, because it is administered directly to the airways. Irritation of the respiratory tract does occur, however. *Zanamivir* should be avoided in individuals with severe reactive asthma or chronic obstructive respiratory disease, because bronchospasm may occur with the risk of fatality. Neither drug has been reported to have clinically significant drug interactions.

4. **Resistance:** Mutations of the neuraminidase have been identified in adults treated with either of the neuraminidase inhibitors. These mutants, however, are often less infective and virulent than the wild type.

(handwritten: Oseltamivir & Zanamivir)

B. Inhibitors of viral uncoating

The therapeutic spectrum of the *adamantine* derivatives, *amantadine* [a-MAN-ta-deen] and *rimantadine* [ri-MAN-ta-deen], is limited to influenza A infections, for which the drugs have been shown to be equally effective in both treatment and prevention. For example, these drugs are 70 to 90 percent effective in preventing infection if treatment is begun at the time of—or prior to—exposure to the virus. Also, both drugs reduce the duration and severity of systemic symptoms if started within the first 48 hours after exposure to the virus (Figure 38.3). Neither impairs the immune response to influenza A vaccine, and either can be administered as a supplement to vaccination, thus providing protection until antibody response occurs (usually 2 weeks in healthy adults). Treatment is particularly useful in high-risk patients who have not been vaccinated and during epidemics. [Note: *Amantadine* is also effective in the treatment of some cases of Parkinson's disease (see p. 101).]

1. **Mode of action:** The primary antiviral mechanism of *amantadine* and *rimantadine* is to block the viral membrane matrix protein, M2, which functions as a channel for hydrogen ion. This channel is required for the fusion of the viral membrane with the cell membrane that ultimately forms the endosome (created when the virus is internalized by endocytosis). [Note: The acidic environment of the endosome is required for viral uncoating.] These drugs may also interfere with the release of new virions.

2. **Pharmacokinetics:** Both drugs are well absorbed orally. *Amantadine* distributes throughout the body and readily penetrates into the central nervous system (CNS), whereas *rimantadine* does not cross the blood-brain barrier to the same extent. *Amantadine* is not extensively metabolized. It is excreted into the urine and may accumulate

(handwritten: RIMANtadine REMAINs in the periphery)

to toxic levels in patients with renal failure. On the other hand, *rimantadine* is extensively metabolized by the liver, and both the metabolites and the parent drug are eliminated by the kidney (Figure 38.4).

3. **Adverse effects:** The side effects of *amantadine* are mainly associated with the CNS. Minor neurologic symptoms include insomnia, dizziness, and ataxia. More serious side effects have been reported (for example, hallucinations and seizures). The drug should be employed cautiously in patients with psychiatric problems, cerebral atherosclerosis, renal impairment, or epilepsy. *Rimantadine* causes fewer CNS reactions, because it does not efficiently cross the blood-brain barrier. Both drugs cause gastrointestinal intolerance. *Amantadine* and *rimantadine* should be used with caution in pregnant and nursing mothers, because they have been found to be embryotoxic and teratogenic in rats.

4. **Resistance:** Resistance can develop rapidly in up to 50 percent of treated individuals, and resistant strains can be readily transmitted to close contacts. Resistance has been shown to result from a change in one amino acid of the M2 matrix protein. Cross-resistance occurs between the two drugs.

Amantadine & Rimantadine

C. Ribavirin

Ribavirin [rye-ba-VYE-rin] is a synthetic guanosine analog. It is effective against a broad spectrum of RNA and DNA viruses. For example, *ribavirin* is used in treating infants and young children with severe RSV infections. [Note: It is not indicated for use in adults.] *Ribavirin* is also effective in chronic hepatitis C infections when used in combination with *interferon-a-2b*. *Ribavirin* may reduce the mortality and viremia of Lassa fever.

"avir" → nucleoside analogue

1. **Mode of action:** The mode of action of *ribavirin* has been studied only for the influenza viruses. The drug is first converted to the 5'-phosphate derivatives, the major product being the compound ribavirin-triphosphate, which exerts its antiviral action by inhibiting guanosine triphosphate formation, preventing viral mRNA capping,[1] and blocking RNA-dependent RNA polymerase. [Note: Rhinoviruses and enteroviruses, which contain preformed mRNA and do not need to synthesize mRNA in the host cell to initiate an infection, are relatively resistant to the action of *ribavirin*.]

2. **Pharmacokinetics:** *Ribavirin* is effective orally and intravenously. Absorption is increased if the drug is taken with a fatty meal. An aerosol is used in certain respiratory viral conditions, such as the treatment of RSV infection. Studies of drug distribution in primates have shown retention in all tissues, except brain. The drug and its metabolites are eliminated in the urine (Figure 38.5).

Bone marrow suppression

3. **Adverse effects:** Side effects reported for oral or parenteral use of *ribavirin* have included dose-dependent transient anemia. Elevated bilirubin has been reported. The aerosol may be safer, although respiratory function in infants can deteriorate quickly after initiation of aerosol treatment. Therefore, monitoring is essential. Because of teratogenic effects in experimental animals, *ribavirin* is contraindicated in pregnancy (Figure 38.6).

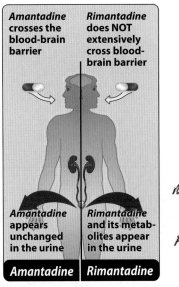

Figure 38.4
Administration and metabolism of *amantadine* and *rimantadine*.

*M2 protein blockers
A only*

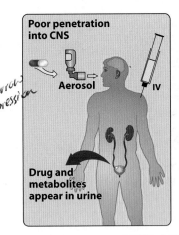

Figure 38.5
Administration and metabolism of *ribavirin*.

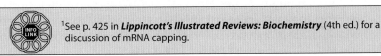
[1] See p. 425 in ***Lippincott's Illustrated Reviews: Biochemistry*** (4th ed.) for a discussion of mRNA capping.

Ribavirin

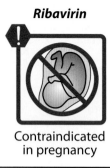

Contraindicated
in pregnancy

Figure 38.6
Ribavirin causes teratogenic
effects.

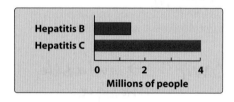

Figure 38.7
The prevalence of chronic hepatitis
B and C in the United States.

Interferon-α	Interferon-β	Interferon-γ
Chronic hepatitis B and C	Relapsing-remitting multiple sclerosis	Chronic granulo-matous disease
Genital warts caused by papilloma-virus		
Leukemia, hairy-cell		
Leukemia, chronic myelogenous		
Kaposi's sarcoma		

Figure 38.8
Some approved indications
for *interferon*.

III. TREATMENT OF HEPATIC VIRAL INFECTIONS

The hepatitis viruses thus far identified—A, B, C, D, and E—each have a pathogenesis specifically involving replication in and destruction of hepatocytes. Of this group, hepatitis B and hepatitis C are the most common causes of chronic hepatitis, cirrhosis, and hepatocellular carcinoma (Figure 38.7) and are the only hepatic viral infections for which therapy is currently available. [Note: Hepatitis A is a commonly encountered infection, but it is not a chronic disease.] Chronic hepatitis B is usually treated with *peginterferon-α-2a*, which is injected subcutaneously once weekly. [Note: *Interferon-α-2b* injected intramuscularly or subcutaneously three times weekly is also useful in the treatment of hepatitis B, but *pegintererfon-α-2a* has similar or slightly better efficacy.] Oral therapy includes *lamivudine, adefovir, enetecavir*, or *telbivudine*. Combination therapy of an *interferon* plus *lamivudine* is no more effective than monotherapy with *lamivudine*. Patients with acquired immunodeficiency syndrome (AIDS) who are coinfected with hepatitis B are usually poor responders to *interferon* therapy. In the treatment of chronic hepatitis C, the preferred treatment is the combination of *peginterferon-α-2a* or *peginterferon-α-2b* plus *ribavirin*, which is more effective than the combination of standard interferons and ribavirin.

A. Interferon

Interferon [in-ter-FEER-on] is a family of naturally occurring, inducible glycoproteins that interfere with the ability of viruses to infect cells. Although *interferon* inhibits the growth of many viruses in vitro, its activity in vivo against viruses has been disappointing. The interferons are synthesized by recombinant DNA technology. At least three types of *interferon* exist, α, β, and γ (Figure 38.8). One of the 15 *interferon-α glycoproteins—interferon-α-2b*—has been approved for treatment of hepatitis B and C, condylomata acuminata, and cancers such as hairy-cell leukemia and Kaposi's sarcoma. *Interferon-β* has some effectiveness in the treatment of multiple sclerosis. In so-called "pegylated" formulations, bis-monomethoxy polyethylene glycol has been covalently attached to either *interferon-α-2a* or *-α-2b* to increase the size of the molecule. The larger molecular size delays absorption from the injection site, lengthening the duration of action of the drug, and also decreases its clearance.

1. **Mode of action:** The antiviral mechanism is incompletely understood. It appears to involve the induction of host cell enzymes that inhibit viral RNA translation, ultimately leading to the degradation of viral mRNA and tRNA.

2. **Pharmacokinetics:** *Interferon* is not active orally, but it may be administered intralesionally, subcutaneously, or intravenously. Very little active compound is found in the plasma, and its presence is not correlated with clinical responses. Cellular uptake and metabolism by the liver and kidney account for the disappearance of *interferon* from the plasma. Negligible renal elimination occurs.

3. **Adverse effects:** Adverse effects include flu-like symptoms on injection, such as fever, chills, myalgias, arthralgias, and gastrointestinal disturbances. Fatigue and mental depression are common. These symptoms subside with subsequent administrations. The principal dose-limiting toxicities are bone marrow suppression including granulocytopenia, neurotoxicity characterized by somnolence and behavioral disturbances, severe fatigue and weight loss, autoim-

mune disorders such as thyroiditis, and rarely, cardiovascular problems such as congestive heart failure. Acute hypersensitivity reactions and hepatic failure are rare.

4. **Drug interactions:** *Interferon* interferes with hepatic drug metabolism, and toxic accumulations of *theophylline* have been reported. *Interferon* may also potentiate the myelosuppression caused by other bone marrow–depressing agents, such as *zidovudine*.

B. Lamivudine

This cytosine analog is an inhibitor of both hepatitis B virus (HBV) DNA polymerase and human immunodeficiency virus (HIV) reverse transcriptase. *Lamivudine* [la-MI-vyoo-deen] must be phosphorylated by host cellular enzymes to the triphosphate (active) form. This compound competitively inhibits HBV DNA polymerase at concentrations that have negligible effects on host DNA polymerase. As with many nucleotide analogs, the intracellular half-life of the triphosphate is many hours longer than its plasma half-life, which permits infrequent dosing. Chronic treatment is associated with decreased plasma HBV DNA levels, improved biochemical markers, and reduced hepatic inflammation. *Lamivudine* is well absorbed orally and is widely distributed. Its plasma half-life is about 9 hours. Seventy percent is excreted unchanged in the urine. Dose reductions are necessary when there is moderate renal insufficiency (creatinine clearance less than 50 mL/min). *Lamivudine* is well tolerated, with rare occurrences of headache and dizziness.

[handwritten note: → used in HAART as well]

C. Adefovir

Adefovir dipivoxil [ah-DEH-for-veer-die-pih-VOCKS-ill] is a nucleotide analog that is phosphorylated to adefovir diphosphate, which is then incorporated into viral DNA. This leads to termination of further DNA synthesis and prevents viral replication. *Adefovir* is administered once a day and is excreted in the urine, with 45 percent as the active compound. Clearance is influenced by renal function. Both decreased viral load and improved liver function have occurred in patients treated with *adefovir*. As with other agents, discontinuation of *adefovir* results in severe exacerbation of hepatitis in about 25 percent of patients. *Adefovir* does not seem to have significant drug interactions. The drug should be used cautiously in patients with existing renal dysfunction.

[handwritten note: HBV NRTIs — L - amivudine, A - defovir, T - elbivudine, E - ntecavir]

D. Entecavir

Entecavir [en-TECK-ah-veer] is a guanosine analog approved for the treatment of HBV infections. Following intracellular phosphorylation to the triphosphate, it competes with the natural substrate, deoxyguanosine triphosphate, for viral reverse transcriptase. *Entecavir* has been shown to be effective against *lamivudine*-resistant strains of HBV. Liver inflammation and scarring are improved. *Entecavir* need only be given once a day. *Entecavir* undergoes both glomerular filtration and tubular secretion. Very little, if any, drug is metabolized. Renal function must be assessed periodically, and drugs that have renal toxicity should be avoided. Patients should be monitored closely for several months after discontinuation of therapy because of the possibility of severe hepatitis.

E. Telbivudine

Telbivudine [tel-BIV-yoo-dine] is a thymidine analog that can be used in the treatment of HBV. Unlike *lamivudine* and *adefovir*, *telbivudine* is not effective against HIV or other viruses. The drug is phosphorylated intra-

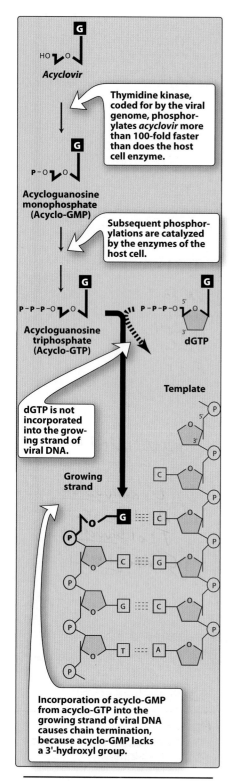

Figure 38.9
Incorporation of *acyclovir* into replicating viral DNA, causing chain termination. dGTP = deoxyguanosine triphosphate

cellularly to the triphosphate, which can either compete with endogenous thymidine triphosphate for incorporation into DNA or else be incorporated into viral DNA, where it serves to terminate further elongation of the DNA chain. The drug is administered orally, once a day, with or without food. *Telbivudine* is eliminated by glomerular filtration as the unchanged drug, and no metabolites have been detected. The dose must be adjusted in renal failure. Combination of *telbivudine* with *lamivudine* has been no more effective than *telbivudine* alone.

IV. TREATMENT OF HERPESVIRUS INFECTIONS

Herpesviruses are associated with a broad spectrum of diseases—for example, cold sores, viral encephalitis, and genital infections (the latter being a hazard to the newborn during parturition). The drugs that are effective against these viruses exert their actions during the acute phase of viral infections and are without effect during the latent phase. Except for *foscarnet* and *fomivirsen*, all are purine or pyrimidine analogs that inhibit viral DNA synthesis.

A. Acyclovir

Acyclovir [ay-SYE-kloe-ver] (acycloguanosine) is the prototypic antiherpetic therapeutic agent. It has a greater specificity than *vidarabine* against herpesviruses. Herpes simplex virus (HSV) Types 1 and 2, varicella-zoster virus (VZV), and some Epstein-Barr virus–mediated infections are sensitive to *acyclovir*. It is the treatment of choice in HSV encephalitis, and is more efficacious than *vidarabine* at increasing the rate of survival. The most common use of *acyclovir* is in therapy for genital herpes infections. It is also given prophylactically to seropositive patients before bone marrow and after heart transplants to protect such individuals during posttransplant immunosuppressive treatments.

1. **Mode of action:** *Acyclovir*, a guanosine analog that lacks a true sugar moiety, is monophosphorylated in the cell by the herpes virus–encoded enzyme, thymidine kinase (Figure 38.9). Therefore, virus-infected cells are most susceptible. The monophosphate analog is converted to the di- and triphosphate forms by the host cells. Acyclovir triphosphate competes with deoxyguanosine triphosphate as a substrate for viral DNA polymerase and is itself incorporated into the viral DNA, causing premature DNA-chain termination (see Figure 38.9). Irreversible binding of the *acyclovir*-containing template primer to viral DNA polymerase inactivates the enzyme. The drug is less effective against the host enzyme.

2. **Pharmacokinetics:** Administration of *acyclovir* can be by an intravenous, oral, or topical route. [Note: The efficacy of topical applications is doubtful.] The drug distributes well throughout the body, including the cerebrospinal fluid (CSF). *Acyclovir* is partially metabolized to an inactive product. Excretion into the urine occurs both by glomerular filtration and by tubular secretion (Figure 38.10). *Acyclovir* accumulates in patients with renal failure. The valyl ester, *valacyclovir* [val-a-SYE-kloe-veer], has greater oral bioavailability than *acyclovir*. This ester is rapidly hydrolyzed to *acyclovir* and achieves levels of the latter comparable to those from intravenous *acyclovir* administration.

3. **Adverse effects:** Side effects of *acyclovir* treatment depend on the route of administration. For example, local irritation may occur from topical application; headache, diarrhea, nausea, and vomiting may result after oral administration. Transient renal dysfunction may

occur at high doses or in a dehydrated patient receiving the drug intravenously. High-dose *valacyclovir* can cause gastrointestinal problems and thrombotic thrombocytopenia purpura in patients with AIDS.

4. **Resistance:** Altered or deficient thymidine kinase and DNA polymerases have been found in some resistant viral strains and are most commonly isolated from immunocompromised patients. Cross-resistance to the other cyclovirs occurs. [Note: Cytomegalovirus (CMV) is resistant, because it lacks a specific viral thymidine kinase.]

B. Cidofovir

Cidofovir [si-DOE-foe-veer] is approved for treatment of CMV-induced retinitis in patients with AIDS. *Cidofovir* is a nucleotide analog of cytosine, the phosphorylation of which is not dependent on viral enzymes. It inhibits viral DNA synthesis. Slow elimination of the active intracellular metabolite permits prolonged dosage intervals and eliminates the permanent venous access used for *ganciclovir* therapy. *Cidofovir* is available for intravenous, intravitreal (injection into the eye's vitreous humor between the lens and the retina), and topical administration. *Cidofovir* produces significant toxicity to the kidney (Figure 38.11), and it is contraindicated in patients with preexisting renal impairment or in those who are taking concurrent nephrotoxic drugs, including nonsteroidal anti-inflammatory drugs. Neutropenia, metabolic acidosis, and ocular hypotony also occur. *Probenecid* must be coadministered with *cidofovir* to reduce the risk of nephrotoxicity, but *probenecid* itself causes rash, headache, fever, and nausea. Since the introduction of HAART (highly active antiretroviral therapy), the prevalence of CMV infections in immunocompromised hosts has markedly declined, and the importance of *cidofovir* in the treatment of these patients has also diminished.

C. Fomivirsen

Fomivirsen [foe-MI-veer-sen] is an antisense oligonucleotide directed against CMV mRNA. Its use is limited to those who cannot tolerate—or have failed—other therapies for CMV retinitis. A 2- to 4-week hiatus after discontinuing *cidofovir* is desirable to reduce toxicity. The drug is administered intravitreally. The common adverse effects include iritis, vitritis, and changes in vision.

D. Foscarnet

Unlike most of the antiviral agents, *foscarnet* [fos-KAR-net] is not a purine or pyrimidine analog. Instead, it is phosphonoformate—a pyrophosphate derivative—and does not require activation by viral (or human) kinases. *Foscarnet* has broad in vitro antiviral activity. It is approved for CMV retinitis in immunocompromised hosts and for *acyclovir*-resistant HSV and herpes zoster infections. *Foscarnet* works by reversibly inhibiting viral DNA and RNA polymerases, thereby interfering with viral DNA and RNA synthesis. Mutation of the polymerase structure is responsible for resistant viruses. [Note: Cross-resistance between *foscarnet* and *ganciclovir* or *acyclovir* is uncommon.] *Foscarnet* is poorly absorbed orally and must be injected intravenously. It must also be given frequently to avoid relapse when plasma levels fall. It is dispersed throughout the body, and greater than 10 percent enters the bone matrix, from which it slowly leaves. The parent drug is eliminated by glomerular filtration and tubular secretion into the urine (Figure 38.12). Adverse effects include nephrotoxicity, anemia, nausea, and fever. Due to chelation with diva-

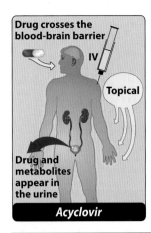

Figure 38.10
Administration and metabolism of *acyclovir*.

A – G
C – C
F – P

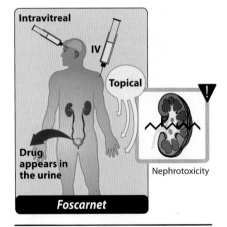

Figure 38.11
Administration, metabolism, and toxicity of *cidofovir*.

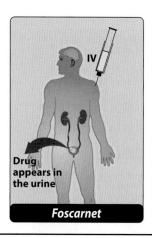

Figure 38.12
Administration and metabolism of *foscarnet*.

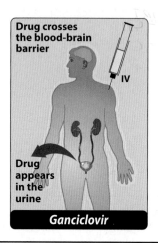

Figure 38.13
Administration and metabolism of *ganciclovir*.

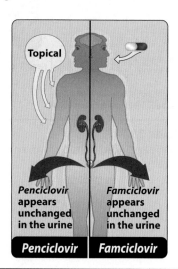

Figure 38.14
Administration and metabolism of *penciclovir* and *famciclovir*.

lent cations, hypocalcemia and hypomagnesemia are also seen. In addition, hypokalemia, hypo- and hyperphosphatemia, seizures, and arrhythmias have been reported.

E. Ganciclovir

Ganciclovir [gan-SYE-kloe-veer] is an analog of *acyclovir* that has 8- to 20-times greater activity against CMV—the only viral infection for which it is approved. It is currently available for treatment of CMV retinitis in immunocompromised patients and for CMV prophylaxis in transplant patients.

1. **Mode of action:** Like *acyclovir*, *ganciclovir* is activated through conversion to the nucleoside triphosphate by viral and cellular enzymes, with the actual pathway depending on the virus. CMV is deficient in thymidine kinase and, therefore, forms the triphosphate by another route. The nucleotide competitively inhibits viral DNA polymerase and can be incorporated into the DNA, thereby decreasing the rate of chain elongation.

2. **Pharmacokinetics:** *Ganciclovir* is administered intravenously and distributes throughout the body, including the CSF. Excretion into the urine occurs through glomerular filtration and tubular secretion (Figure 38.13). Like *acyclovir*, *ganciclovir* accumulates in patients with renal failure. *Valganciclovir* [val-gan-SYE-kloe-veer] is the valyl ester of *ganciclovir*. Like *valacyclovir*, *valganciclovir* has high oral bioavailability, because rapid hydrolysis in the intestine and liver after oral administration leads to high levels of *ganciclovir*.

3. **Adverse effects:** Adverse effects include severe, dose-dependent neutropenia. [Note: Combined treatment with *zidovudine, azathioprine,* or *mycophenolate mofetil* can result in additive neutropenia.] *Ganciclovir* is carcinogenic as well as embryotoxic and teratogenic in experimental animals.

4. **Resistance:** Resistant CMV strains have been detected that have lower levels of ganciclovir triphosphate.

F. Penciclovir and famciclovir

Penciclovir [pen-SYE-kloe-veer] is an acyclic guanosine nucleoside derivative that is active against HSV-I, HSV-2, and VZV. *Penciclovir* is only administered topically (Figure 38.14). It is monophosphorylated by viral thymidine kinase, and cellular enzymes form the nucleoside triphosphate, which inhibits HSV DNA polymerase. Penciclovir triphosphate has an intracellular half-life 20- to 30-fold longer than does acyclovir triphosphate. *Penciclovir* is negligibly absorbed upon topical application and is well tolerated. Both pain and healing are shortened approximately one-half day in duration compared to placebo-treated subjects. *Famciclovir* [fam-SYE-kloe-veer], another acyclic analog of 2'-deoxyguanosine, is a prodrug that is metabolized to the active *penciclovir*. The antiviral spectrum is similar to that of *ganciclovir*, but it is presently approved only for treatment of acute herpes zoster. The drug is effective orally (see Figure 38.14). Adverse effects include headaches and nausea. Studies in experimental animals have shown an increased incidence of mammary adenocarcinomas and testicular toxicity.

G. Vidarabine (ara-A)

Vidarabine [vye-DARE-a-been] (*arabinofuranosyl adenine, ara-A, adenine arabinoside*) is one of the most effective of the nucleoside analogs. However, it has been supplanted clinically by *acyclovir*, which is more efficacious and safe. Although *vidarabine* is active against HSV-1, HSV-2, and VZV, its use is limited to treatment of immunocompromised patients with herpetic and vaccinial keratitis and in HSV keratoconjunctivitis. [Note: *Vidarabine* is only available as an ophthalmic ointment.] *Vidarabine*, an adenosine analog, is converted in the cell to its 5′-triphosphate analog (ara-ATP), which is postulated to inhibit viral DNA synthesis. Some resistant HSV mutants have been detected that have altered polymerase.

H. Trifluridine

Trifluridine [trye-FLURE-i-deen] is a fluorinated pyrimidine nucleoside analog. It is structurally very similar to thymidine, the only difference being the replacement of a methyl group on the pyrimidine ring of thymidine with a trifluoromethyl group. Once converted to the triphosphate, the agent is believed to competitively inhibit the incorporation of thymidine triphosphate into viral DNA and, to a lesser extent, to be

Antiviral drug	Mechanism of action	Viruses or diseases affected	
Acyclovir	Metabolized to acyclovir triphosphate, which inhibits viral DNA polymerase	Herpes simplex, varicella-zoster, cytomegalovirus	Guanosine
Amantadine	Blockage of the M2 protein ion channel and its ability to modulate intracellular pH	Influenza A	M2-blocker
Cidofovir	Inhibition of viral DNA polymerase	Cytomegalovirus; indicated only for virus-induced retinitis	cytosine
Famciclovir	Same as penciclovir	Herpes simplex, varicella-zoster	guanosine
Foscarnet	Inhibition of viral DNA polymerase and reverse transcriptase at the pyrophosphate-binding site	Cytomegalovirus, acyclovir-resistant herpes simplex, acyclovir-resistant varicella-zoster	Pyrophosphate
Ganciclovir	Inhibits viral DNA polmerase	Cytomegalovirus	guanosine
Interferon-α	Induction of cellular enzymes that interfere with viral protein synthesis	Hepatitis B and C, human herpesvirus 8, papilloma virus, Kaposi's sarcoma, hairy-cell leukemia, chronic myelogenous leukemia	
Lamivudine	Inhibition of viral DNA polymerase and reverse transcriptase	Hepatitis B (chronic cases), human immunodeficiency virus type 1	cytosine
Oseltamivir	Inhibition of viral neuramidase	Influenza A	neuraminidase
Penciclovir	Metabolized to penciclovir triphosphate, which inhibits viral DNA polymerase	Herpes simplex	guanosine
Ribavirin	Interference with viral messenger RNA	Lassa fever, hantavirus (hemorrhagic fever renal syndrome), hepatitis C (in chronic cases in combination with *interferon-α* RSV in children and infants	guanosine
Rimantadine	Blockage of the M2 protein ion channel and its ability to modulate intracellular pH	Influenza A	M2-blocker
Valacyclovir	Same as acyclovir	Herpes simplex, varicella-zoster, cytomegalovirus	guanosine
Vidarabine	inhibits viral DNA synthesis	HSV-1, HSV-2, and VZV; its use is limited to treatment of immunocompromised patients with HSV keratitis	Adenine
Zanamivir	Inhibition of viral neuramidase	Influenza A	neuraminidase

Figure 38.15
Summary of selected antiviral agents.

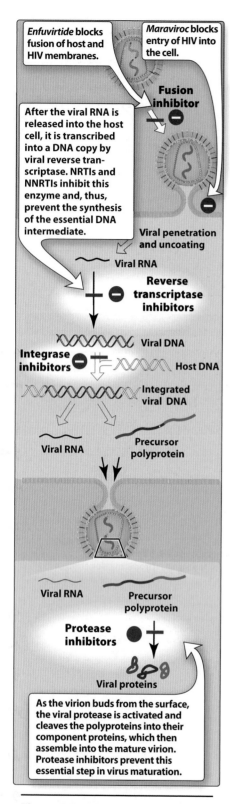

Figure 38.16
Drugs used to prevent HIV from replicating. [NRTI = nucleoside and nucleotide reverse transcriptase inhibitor; NNRTI = nonnucleoside reverse transcriptase inhibitor.

incorporated into viral DNA, leading to the synthesis of a defective DNA that renders the virus unable to reproduce. Trifluridine monophosphate is an irreversible inhibitor of viral thymidine synthase. *Trifluridine* is active against HSV-1, HSV-2, and vaccina virus. It is generally considered to be the drug of choice for treatment of HSV keratoconconjunctivitis and recurrent epithelial keratitis. Because the triphosphate form of trifluridine can also incorporate to some degree into cellular DNA, the drug is considered to be too toxic for systemic use; therefore, the use of *trifluridine* is restricted to topical application as a solution to the eye. A short half-life of approximately 12 minutes necessitates that the drug be applied frequently. Side effects include a transient irritation of the eye and palpebral (eyelid) edema.

Figure 38.15 summarizes selected antiviral agents.

V. OVERVIEW OF THE TREATMENT FOR HIV INFECTION

Prior to approval of *zidovudine* in 1987, treatment of HIV infections focused on decreasing the occurrence of opportunistic infections that caused a high degree of morbidity and mortality in AIDS patients rather than on inhibiting HIV itself. Today, the viral life cycle is understood (Figure 38.16), and a highly active regimen is employed that uses combinations of drugs to suppress replication of HIV and restore the number of CD4+ cells and immunocompetency to the host.[2] This multi drug regimen is commonly referred to as "highly active antiretroviral therapy," or HAART (Figure 38.17). There are five classes of antiretroviral drugs, each of which targets one of four viral processes. These classes of drugs are nucleoside and nucleotide reverse transcriptase inhibitors (NRTIs), non-nucleoside reverse transcriptase inhibitors (NNRTIs), protease inhibitors, entry inhibitors and the integrase inhibitors. The current recommendation for primary therapy is to administer two NRTIs with either a protease inhibitor or an NNRTI. Selection of the appropriate combination is based on 1) avoiding the use of two agents of the same nucleoside analog, 2) avoiding overlapping toxicities and genotypic and phenotypic characteristics of the virus, 3) patient factors such as disease symptoms and concurrent illnesses, 4) impact of drug interactions, and 5) ease of adherence to a frequently complex administration regimen. The goals of therapy are to maximally and durably suppress viral load replication, to restore and preserve immunologic function, to reduce HIV-related morbidity and mortality, and to improve quality of life.

VI. NRTIs USED TO TREAT HIV INFECTION

A. Overview of NRTIs

1. **Mechanism of action:** Nucleoside and nucleotide reverse transcriptase inhibitors (NRTIs) are analogs of native ribosides (nucleosides or nucleotides containing ribose), which all lack a 3'-hydroxyl group. Once they enter cells, they are phosphorylated by a variety of cellular enzymes to the corresponding triphosphate analog, which is preferentially incorporated into the viral DNA by virus reverse transcriptase. Because the 3'-hydroxyl group is not present, a 3'-5'-phosphodiester bond between an incoming nucleoside triphosphate and the growing DNA chain cannot be formed, and DNA chain elon-

 [2]See p. 293 in ***Lippincott's Illustrated Reviews: Microbiology*** (2nd ed.) for a discussion of retroviruses and AIDS.

gation is terminated. Affinities of the drugs for many host cell DNA polymerases are lower than they are for HIV reverse transcriptase, although mitochondrial DNA polymerase γ appears to be susceptible at therapeutic concentrations.

2. **Pharmacokinetics:** The NRTIs are primarily renally excreted, and all require dosage adjustment in renal insufficiency except *abacavir,* which is metabolized by alcohol dehydrogenase and glucuronyl transferase. Dosage adjustment is required when the creatinine clearance drops below 50 mL/min.

3. **Adverse effects**: Many of the toxicities of the NRTIs are believed to be due to inhibition of the mitochondrial DNA polymerase in certain tissues. As a general rule, the dideoxynucleosides, such as *zalcitabine*, *didanosine*, and *stavudine,* have a greater affinity for the mitochondrial DNA polymerase, leading to such toxicities as peripheral neuropathy, pancreatitis, and lipoatrophy. When more than one NRTI is given, care is taken not to have overlapping toxicities. All the NRTIs have been associated with a potentially fatal liver toxicity characterized by lactic acidosis and hepatomegaly with steatosis.

4. **Drug interactions:** Due to the renal excretion of the NRTIs, there are not many drug interactions encountered with these agents except for *zidovudine* and *tenofovir* (see below).

5. **Resistance:** NRTI resistance is well characterized, and the most common mutation is the mutation at viral codon 184, which confers a high degree of resistance to *lamivudine* but, more importantly, restores sensitivity to *zidovudine* and *tenofovir*. Cross-resistance and antagonism occur between agents of the same analog class (thymidine, cytosine, guanosine and adenosine) so concomitant use of agents in the same class is contraindicated (for example, *zidovudine* plus *stavudine*).

B. Zidovudine (AZT)

Approved in 1987, the first agent available for treatment of HIV infection is the pyrimidine analog, *3′-azido-3′-deoxythymidine (AZT)*. *AZT* has the generic name of *zidovudine* [zye-DOE-vyoo-deen]. *AZT* is approved for use in children and adults and to prevent prenatal infection in pregnancy. It is also recommended for prophylaxis in individuals exposed to HIV infection. The drug is well absorbed after oral administration. If taken with food, peak levels may be lower, but the total amount of drug absorbed is not affected. Penetration across the blood-brain barrier is excellent, and the drug has a half-life of 1 hour. The intracellular half-life, however, is approximately 3 hours. Most of the *AZT* is glucuronylated by the liver and then excreted in the urine (Figure 38.18). In spite of its seeming specificity, *AZT* is toxic to bone marrow. Headaches are also common. The toxicity of *AZT* is potentiated if glucuronylation is decreased by coadministration of drugs like *probenecid*, *acetaminophen*, *lorazepam*, *indomethacin*, and *cimetidine*. They should be avoided or used with caution in patients receiving *AZT*. Both *stavudine* and *ribavirin* are activated by the same intracellular pathways and should not be given with *AZT*.

C. Stavudine (d4T)

Stavudine [STAV-yoo-deen] is an analog of thymidine, in which a double bond joins the 2′ and 3′ carbons of the sugar. *Stavudine* is a strong inhibitor of cellular enzymes such as the β and γ DNA polymerases, thus

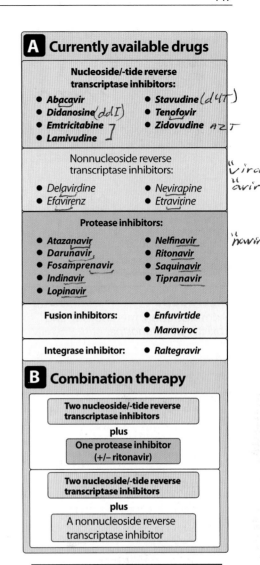

A **Currently available drugs**

Nucleoside/-tide reverse transcriptase inhibitors:

- *Abacavir*
- *Didanosine* (ddI)
- *Emtricitabine*
- *Lamivudine*
- *Stavudine* (d4T)
- *Tenofovir*
- *Zidovudine* AZT

Nonnucleoside reverse transcriptase inhibitors:

- *Delavirdine*
- *Efavirenz*
- *Nevirapine*
- *Etravirine*

"vira" "avir"

Protease inhibitors:

- *Atazanavir*
- *Darunavir*,
- *Fosamprenavir*
- *Indinavir*
- *Lopinavir*
- *Nelfinavir*
- *Ritonavir*
- *Saquinavir*
- *Tipranavir*

"navir"

Fusion inhibitors:
- *Enfuvirtide*
- *Maraviroc*

Integrase inhibitor:
- *Raltegravir*

B **Combination therapy**

Two nucleoside/-tide reverse transcriptase inhibitors

plus

One protease inhibitor (+/− ritonavir)

Two nucleoside/-tide reverse transcriptase inhibitors

plus

A nonnucleoside reverse transcriptase inhibitor

Figure 38.17

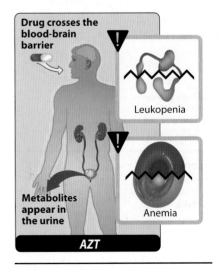

Figure 38.18
Administration, metabolism, and toxicity of *zidovudine (AZT)*.

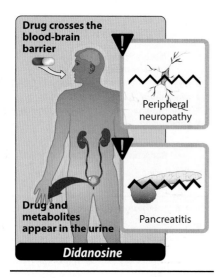

Figure 38.19
Administration, metabolism, and toxicity of *didanosine*.

reducing mitochondrial DNA synthesis, resulting in toxicity. The drug is almost completely absorbed on oral ingestion and is not affected by food. *Stavudine* penetrates the blood-brain barrier. About half of the parent drug can be accounted for in the urine. Renal impairment interferes with clearance. The major and most common clinical toxicity is peripheral neuropathy along with lipoatrophy and hyperlipidemia.

D. Didanosine (ddl)

The second drug approved to treat HIV-1 infection was *didanosine* [dye-DAN-oh-seen] (*dideoxyinosine, ddl*), which is missing both the 2'- and 3'-hydroxyl groups. Upon entry into the host cell, *ddl* is biotransformed into dideoxyadenosine triphosphate (ddATP) through a series of reactions that involve phosphorylation of the *ddl*, amination to dideoxyadenosine monophosphate, and further phosphorylation. Like *AZT*, the resulting ddATP is incorporated into the DNA chain, causing termination of chain elongation. Due to its acid lability, absorption is best if *ddl* is taken in the fasting state. The drug penetrates into the CSF, but to a lesser extent than does *AZT*. About 55 percent of the parent drug appears in the urine (Figure 38.19). Pancreatitis, which may be fatal, is a major toxicity of *ddl* treatment and requires monitoring of serum amylase. The dose-limiting toxicity of *ddl* is peripheral neuropathy. Because of its similar adverse effect profile, concurrent use of *stavudine* is not recommended.

E. Tenofovir (TDF)

Tenofovir [te-NOE-fo-veer] is the first approved drug that is a nucleotide analog—namely, an acyclic nucleoside phosphonate analog of adenosine 5'-monophosphate. It is converted by cellular enzymes to the diphosphate, which is the inhibitor of HIV reverse transcriptase. Cross-resistance with other NRTIs may occur, but some *AZT*-resistant strains retain susceptibility to *tenofovir*. *Tenofovir* should be taken with a meal to increase bioavailability. *Tenofovir* has a long half-life, allowing once-daily dosing. Most of the drug is recovered unchanged in the urine, and elimination is by filtration and active secretion. Serum creatinine must be monitored and doses adjusted in renal insufficiency. Gastrointestinal complaints are frequent and include nausea, diarrhea, and vomiting. (Figure 38.20). *Tenofovir* is the only NRTI with significant drug interactions. *Tenofovir* increases the concentrations of *ddl* to the point that *ddl* dosage reductions are required if the two are given together; however, these two agents are no longer recommended for combined use. *Tenofovir* decreases the concentrations of *atazanavir* such that *atazanavir* must be boosted with *ritonavir* (see p. 452) if given with *tenofovir* to maintain effective *atazanavir* concentrations.

F. Lamivudine (3TC)

Lamivudine [la-MI-vyoo-deen] (*2'-deoxy-3'-thiacytidine, 3TC*) is approved for treatment of HIV in combination with *AZT*, but it should not be used with other cytosine analogs due to antagonism. *Lamivudine* terminates the synthesis of the proviral DNA chain, and it inhibits the reverse transcriptase of both HIV and HBV. However, it does not affect mitochondrial DNA synthesis or bone marrow precursor cells. It has good bioavailability on oral administration, depends on the kidney for excretion, and is well tolerated.

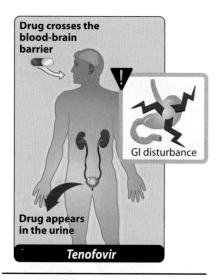

Figure 38.20
Administration, metabolism, and toxicity of *tenofovir*.

G. Emtricitabine (FTC)

Emtricitabine [em-tri-SIGH-ta-been], a fluoro-derivative of *lamivudine*, inhibits both HIV and HBV reverse transcriptase. In a small clinical trial, it was shown to be at least as effective as *lamivudine* in the treatment of HIV-infected individuals. *Emtricitabine* is orally active, with a mean bioavailability of 93 percent. Plasma half-life is about 10 hours, whereas it has a long intracellular half-life of 39 hours. *Emtricitabine* is eliminated essentially unchanged in the urine. It does not affect cytochrome P450 isozymes, and has no significant interactions with other drugs. Headache, diarrhea, nausea, and rash are its most common adverse effects. *Emtricitabine* causes hyperpigmentation of the soles and palms, and it has been associated with lactic acidosis, fatty liver, and hepatomegaly. Withdrawal of *emtricitabine* in HBV-infected patients may result in worsening of the hepatitis.

H. Zalcitabine (ddC)

Zacitabine [zal-SIGH-ta-been], was the first cytosine analog developed; however, due to severe toxicity, it was removed from the market.

I. Abacavir (ABC)

Abacavir [a-BA-ka-veer] is a guanosine analog. There may be some cross-resistance with strains resistant to *AZT* and *lamivudine*. *Abacavir* is well absorbed orally, and metabolites appear in the urine (Figure 38.21). Most of the drug is metabolized by non-cytochrome P450–dependent reactions. A carboxylic acid derivative and a glucuronylated form have been identified. Common side effects include gastrointestinal disturbances, headache, and dizziness. Approximately 5 percent of patients exhibit the "hypersensitivity reaction," which is characterized by drug fever, plus one or more of the following symptoms of rash, gastrointestinal symptoms, malaise, and respiratory distress (Figure. 38.22). Sensitized individuals should NEVER be rechallenged because of rapidly appearing, severe reactions that lead to death. There is a newly approved HLA genetic test available to screen patients for the potential of this reaction. Figure 38.23 show some adverse reactions commonly seen with nucleoside analogs.

VII. NNRTIs USED TO TREAT AIDS

Nonnucleoside reverse transcriptase inhibitors (NNRTIs) are highly selective, noncompetitive inhibitors of HIV-1 reverse transcriptase. They bind to HIV reverse transcriptase at a site adjacent to the active site, inducing a conformational change that results in enzyme inhibition. They do not require activation by cellular enzymes. Their major advantage is their lack of effect on the host blood-forming elements and their lack of cross-resistance with NRTIs. These drugs, however, do have common characteristics that include cross-resistance within the NNRTI class, drug interactions, and a high incidence of hypersensitivity reactions, including rash.

A. Nevirapine (NVP)

Nevirapine [ne-VYE-ra-peen] is used in combination with other antiretroviral drugs for the treatment of HIV-1 infections in adults and children. Due to potential severe hepatotoxicity, *nevirapine* should not be initiated in women with CD4+ T-cell counts of greater than 250 cells/mm^3 or in men with CD4+ T cell counts greater than 400 cells/mm^3. *Nevirapine* is well absorbed orally, and its absorption is not affected by food and antacids. The lipophilic nature of *nevirapine* accounts for its entrance into the fetus and mother's milk and for its wide tissue distribution, including the CNS. *Nevirapine* is dependent upon metabolism for elimination; most of the drug is excreted in the urine as the

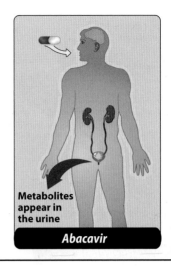

Figure 38.21
Administration and fate of the *abacavir*.

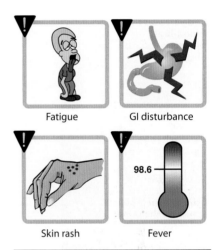

Fatigue GI disturbance

Skin rash Fever

Figure 38.22
Hypersensitivity reactions to *abacavir*.

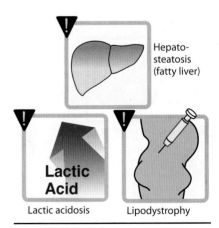

Hepato-steatosis (fatty liver)

Lactic Acid

Lactic acidosis Lipodystrophy

Figure 38.23
Some adverse reactions of nucleoside analogs.

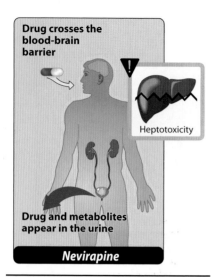

Figure 38.24
Administration, metabolism, and toxicity of *nevirapine*.

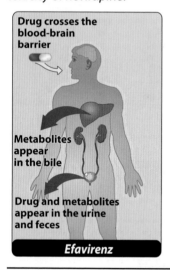

Figure 38.25
Administration and metabolism of *efavirenz*.

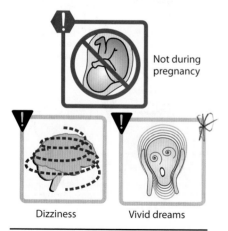

Figure 38.26
Adverse reactions of *efavirenz*.

glucuronides of hydroxylated metabolites (Figure 38.24). *Nevirapine* is an inducer of the CYP3A4 family of cytochrome P450 drug-metabolizing enzymes. *Nevirapine* does increase the metabolism of protease inhibitors, but most combinations do not require dosage adjustment. *Nevirapine* increases the metabolism of a number of drugs, such as oral contraceptives, *ketoconazole*, *methadone*, *metronidazole*, *quinidine*, *theophylline*, and *warfarin*. The most frequently observed side effects are rash, fever, headache, and elevated serum transaminases and fatal hepatotoxicity. Severe dermatologic effects have been encountered, including Stevens-Johnson syndrome and toxic epidermal necrolysis. A 14-day titration period at half the dose is mandatory to reduce the risk of serious epidermal reactions.

B. Delavirdine (DLV)

Delavirdine [de-LA-vir-deen] has not undergone clinical trials as extensive as those of *nevirapine* and is not recommended as a preferred or alternate agent in the U.S. Department of Health and Human Services (DHHS) guidelines for initial therapy. *Delavirdine* is rapidly absorbed after oral administration and is unaffected by the presence of food. *Delavirdine* is extensively metabolized, and very little is excreted as the parent compound. Fecal and urinary excretion each account for approximately half the elimination. *Delavirdine* is an inhibitor of cytochrome P450–mediated drug metabolism, including that of protease inhibitors. *Fluoxetine* and *ketoconazole* increase plasma levels of *delavirdine*, whereas *phenytoin*, *phenobarbital*, and *carbamazepine* result in substantial decreases in plasma levels of *delavirdine*. Rash is the most common side effect of *delavirdine*.

C. Efavirenz (EFV)

Efavirenz [e-FA-veer-enz] treatment results in increases in CD4+ cell counts and a decrease in viral load comparable to that achieved by protease inhibitors when used in combination with NRTIs; and therefore, it is the preferred NNRTI on the DHHS guidelines. Following oral administration, *efavirenz* is well distributed, including to the CNS (Figure 38.25). Bioavailability is enhanced when taken with a high-fat meal. Most of the drug is bound to plasma albumin (99 percent) at therapeutic doses. A half-life of more than 40 hours accounts for its recommended once-a-day dosing. *Efavirenz* is extensively metabolized to inactive products. *Efavirenz* is a potent inducer of cytochrome P450 enzymes; therefore, it may reduce the concentrations of drugs that are substrates of the cytochrome P450. Most adverse effects are tolerable and are associated with the CNS, including dizziness, headache, vivid dreams, and loss of concentration (Figure 38.26). Nearly half of the patients experience these complaints, which usually resolve within a few weeks. Rash is the other most common side effect, with an incidence of approximately 25 percent. Severe, life-threatening reactions are rare. *Efavirenz* should be avoided in pregnant women.

See p. 455 for a discussion of the second-generation NNRTI *entravirine*.

VIII. HIV PROTEASE INHIBITORS

Inhibitors of HIV protease have significantly altered the course of this devastating viral disease. Within a year of their introduction in 1995, the number of deaths in the United States due to AIDS declined, although the trend appears to be leveling off (Figure 38.27).

A. Overview

These potent agents have several common features that characterize their pharmacology.

1. **Mechanism of action:** All the drugs in this group are reversible inhibitors of the HIV aspartyl protease—the viral enzyme responsible for cleavage of the viral polyprotein into a number of essential enzymes (reverse transcriptase, protease, and integrase) and several structural proteins. The protease inhibitors exhibit at least a thousandfold greater affinity for HIV-1 and HIV-2 enzymes than they have for comparable human proteases, such as renin and cathepsin D/E. This accounts for their selective toxicity. The inhibition prevents maturation of the viral particles and results in the production of noninfectious virions. Treatment of antiretrovirally naïve patients (that is, patients who have never had HIV therapy) with a protease inhibitor and two NRTIs as recommended by the DHHS guidelines, results in a decrease in the plasma viral load to undetectable levels in 60 to 95 percent of patients. Treatment failures under these conditions are most likely due to a lack of patient adherence.

2. **Pharmacokinetics:** Most protease inhibitors have poor oral bioavailability. High-fat meals substantially increase the bioavailability of some, such as *nelfinavir* and *saquinavir*, whereas the bioavailability of *indinavir* is decreased and others are essentially unaffected. All are substrates for the CYP3A4 isozyme of cytochrome P450, and individual protease inhibitors are also metabolized by other P450 isozymes. Metabolism is extensive, and very little of the protease inhibitors are excreted unchanged in the urine. Dosage adjustments are unnecessary in renal impairment. Distribution into some tissues may be affected by the fact that the protease inhibitors are substrates for the P-glycoprotein multidrug efflux pump. The presence of this pump in endothelial cells of capillaries in the brain may limit protease inhibitor access to the CNS. The HIV protease inhibitors are all substantially bound to plasma proteins, specifically α_1-acid glycoprotein. This may be clinically important, because the concentration of α_1-acid glycoprotein increases in response to trauma and surgery.

3. **Adverse effects:** Protease inhibitors commonly cause parathesias, nausea, vomiting, and diarrhea (Figure 38.28). Disturbances in glucose and lipid metabolism also occur, including diabetes, hypertriglyceridemia, and hypercholesterolemia. Chronic administration results in fat redistribution, including loss of fat from the extremities and its accumulation in the abdomen and the base of the neck ("buffalo hump"; Figure 38.29), and breast enlargement. These physical changes may indicate to others that an individual is HIV positive.

4. **Drug interactions:** Drug interactions are a common problem for all protease inhibitors, because they are not only substrates but also potent inhibitors of CYP isozymes. The inhibitory potency of the compounds lies between that of *ritonavir*, the most potent, and that of *saquinavir*, the least potent inhibitor of CYP isozymes. Drug interactions are therefore quite common. Drugs that rely on metabolism for their termination of action may accumulate to toxic levels. Examples of potentially dangerous interactions from drugs that are contraindicated with protease inhibitors include rhabdomyolysis from *simvastatin* or *lovastatin*, excessive sedation from *midazolam*

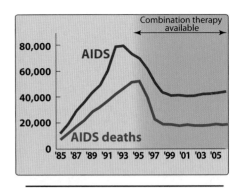

Figure 38.27
Estimated number of AIDS cases and deaths due to AIDS in the United States. Green background indicates years in which combination antiretroviral therapy came into common usage.

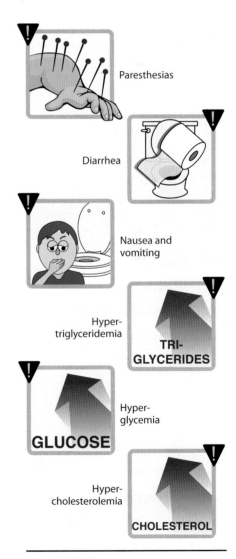

Figure 38.28
Some adverse effects of the HIV protease inhibitors.

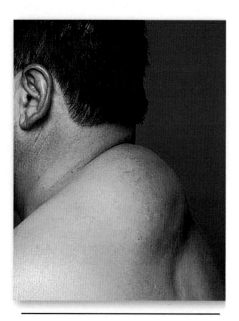

Figure 38.29
Accumulation of fat at the base of the neck in a patient receiving a protease inhibitor.

DRUG CLASS	EXAMPLE
ANTIARRHYTMICS	*Quinidine*
ERGOT DERIVATIVES	*Ergotamine*
ANTIMYCOBACTERIAL DRUGS	*Rifampin*
BENZODIAZEPINES	*Triazolam*
INHALED STEROIDS	*Fluticasone*
HERBAL SUPPLEMENTS	St. John's wart
HMG CoA REDUCTASE INHIBITORS	*Lovastatin* *Simvastatin*
NARCOTICS	*Fentanyl*

Contraindicated

PROTEASE INHIBITORS

Figure 38.30
Drugs that should not be coadministered with any protease inhibitor.

or *triazolam*, and respiratory depression from *fentanyl* (Figure 38.30). Other drug interactions that require dosage modification and cautious use include *warfarin*, *sildenafil* and *phenytoin* (Figure 38.31). In addition, inducers of CYP isozymes may result in the lowering of protease plasma concentrations to suboptimal levels, contributing to treatment failures. Thus, drugs such as *rifampin* and St. John's wort are also contraindicated with protease inhibitors. Meticulous attention must be paid to all these detrimental interactions.

5. **Resistance:** Resistance occurs as an accumulation of stepwise mutations of the protease gene. Initial mutations result in decreased ability of the virus to replicate, but as the mutations accumulate, virions with high levels of resistance to the protease emerge. Suboptimal concentrations result in the more rapid appearance of resistant strains.

B. Ritonavir (RTV)

Ritonavir [ri-TOE-na-veer] is no longer used as a single protease inhibitor but, instead, is used as a "pharmacokinetic enhancer or booster" of other protease inhibitors. *Ritonavir* is a potent inhibitor of CYP3A, and concomitant *ritonavir* administration (at low doses) increases the bioavailability of the second protease inhibitor and often allows for longer dosing intervals. The resulting higher Cmin levels of the "boosted protease inhibitors" also help to prevent the development of resistance. Therefore, the "boosted protease inhibitors" are the preferred agents in the DHHS treatment guidelines. Metabolism and biliary excretion are the primary methods of elimination. *Ritonavir* has a half-life of 3 to 5 hours. Because it is primarily an inhibitor of cytochrome P450 isozymes, numerous drug interactions have been identified. *Ritonavir* is also a self-inducer of its own metabolism as well as that of some substrates. Nausea, vomiting, diarrhea, headache, and circumoral parethesias are among the more common adverse effects.

C. Saquinavir (SQV)

To maximize bioavailability, *saquinavir* [sa-KWIH-na-veer] is given along with a low dose of *ritonavir*. High-fat meals also enhance absorption. Elimination of *saquinavir* is primarily by metabolism, followed by biliary excretion. Its half-life is 7 to 12 hours, requiring multiple daily doses. Drugs that enhance the metabolism of *saquinavir*, such as *rifampin*, *rifabutin*, *nevirapine*, *efavirenz*, and other enzyme inducers, should be avoided if possible. The most common adverse effects of *saquinavir* treatment include headache, fatigue, diarrhea, nausea, and other gastrointestinal disturbances. Increased levels of hepatic aminotransferases have been noted, particularly in patients with concurrent viral hepatitis B or C infections.

D. Indinavir (IDV)   "*in it goes*"

Indinavir [in-DIH-na-veer] is well absorbed orally and, of all the protease inhibitors, is the least protein-bound, at 60 percent. Acidic gastric conditions are necessary for absorption. Absorption is decreased when administered with meals, although a light, low-fat snack is permissible. *Ritonavir* overcomes this problem and also permits twice-a-day dosing. Metabolism and hepatic clearance account for elimination of *indinavir*. The dosage should therefore be reduced in the presence of hepatic insufficiency. *Indinavir* has the shortest half-life of the protease inhibitors, at 1.8 hours. It is well tolerated, with the usual gastrointestinal symptoms and headache predominating. *Indinavir* characteristically causes nephrolithiasis and hyperbilirubinemia. Adequate hydration is important to reduce the incidence of kidney stone formation, and patients should drink at least 1.5 L of water per day. Fat redistribution is particularly troublesome with this drug.

E. Nelfinavir (NFV)

Nelfinavir [nel-FIN-a-veer] is a non-peptide protease inhibitor. It is well absorbed and does not require strict food or fluid conditions; however, it is usually given with food. *Nelfinavir* undergoes metabolism by several CYP isozymes. The major metabolite of *nelfinavir* produced by isozyme CYP2C19 has an antiviral activity equal to that of the parent compound, but it achieves plasma concentrations only 40 percent of those of the parent compound. *Nelfinavir* is the only protease inhibitor that cannot be boosted by *ritonavir*, because it is not extensively metabolized by CYP3A. The half-life of *nelfinavir* is 5 hours. Diarrhea is the most common side effect and can be controlled by *loperamide*. Like other members of the class, *nelfinavir* can inhibit the metabolism of other drugs, resulting in required alterations of drug dosage or the prohibition of combined use.

F. Fosamprenavir (fAPV)

Fosamprenavir [fos-am-PREN-a-veer] is a prodrug that is metabolized to *amprenavir* following oral absorption. Its long plasma half-life permits twice-a-day dosing, and coadministration of *ritonavir* increases the plasma levels of *amprenavir* and lowers the total daily dose. *Fosamprenavir* boosted with *ritonavir* is one of the preferred protease inhibitors according to the DHHS treatment guidelines. Nausea, vomiting, diarrhea, fatigue, paresthesias, and headache are common adverse effects. Like other members of the class, *fosamprenavir* can inhibit the metabolism of other drugs, resulting in required alterations of drug dosage or the prohibition of combined use.

G. Lopinavir (LPVr)

Lopinavir [loe-PIN-a-veer] is a peptidomimetic protease inhibitor. It is one of the preferred protease inhibitors according to the DHHS treatment guidelines. *Lopinavir* has very poor intrinsic bioavailability, which is substantially enhanced by including a low dose of *ritonavir* in the formulation. [Note: Only the coformulation known as *lopinavir* is available in the United States.] Gastrointestinal adverse effects and hypertriglyceridemia are the most common side effects for lopinavir, in addition to the other protease inhibitor class side effects. Like other members of the class, *lopinavir* can inhibit the metabolism of other drugs, resulting in required alterations of drug dosage or the prohibition of combined use. Enzyme inducers as well as St. John's wort should be avoided, because they lower the plasma concentrations of *lopinavir*. The oral solution contains alcohol; thus, *disulfiram* or *metronidazole* administration can cause unpleasant reactions.

H. Atazanavir (ATV)

Atazanavir [ah-ta-ZA-na-veer] inhibits HIV protease and is structurally unrelated to other HIV protease inhibitors. *Atazanavir* in combination with *ritonavir* are the only once-daily preferred protease inhibitors. *Atazanavir* is well absorbed orally. Food increases absorption and bioavailability. The drug is highly protein bound (86 percent) and undergoes extensive CYP3A4-catalyzed biotransformation. It is excreted primarily in the bile. Its half-life is about 7 hours, but it only needs to be administered once a day. *Atazanavir* is a competitive inhibitor of

DRUG CLASS	EXAMPLE
ANTICOAGULANTS	*Warfarin*
ANTICONVULSANTS	*Phenytoin*
ANTIFUNGALS	*Voriconazole*
ANTIMYCOBACTERIALS	*Ribabutin*
ERECTILE DYSFUNCTION AGENTS	*Sildenafil* *Tadalafil* *Vardenafil*
LIPID-LOWERING AGENTS	*Atorvastatin*
NARCOTICS	*Methadone*

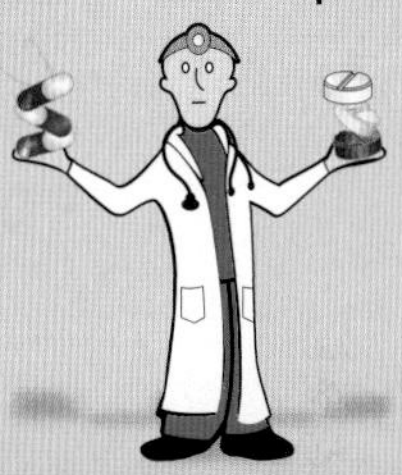

PROTEASE INHIBITORS

Figure 38.31
Drugs that require dose modifications or cautious use with any protease inhibitor.

glucuronyl transferase, and benign hyperbilirubinemia and jaundice are known side effects. In the heart, *atazanavir* prolongs the PR interval and slows the heart rate. *Atazanavir* exhibits a decreased risk of hyperlipidemia, but it is not known if *atazanavir* is less likely to cause insulin resistance and lipodystrophy, as seen with other protease inhibitors. Like the other protease inhibitors, *atazanavir* is a potent inhibitor of CYP3A4 and has the potential for many drug interactions. *Atazanavir* is contraindicated with use of prescription doeses of proton-pump inhibitors, and administration must be spaced 12 hours apart from H_2-blockers and antacids.

I. Tipranavir (TPV)

Tipranavir [ti-PRA-na-veer] inhibits HIV protease in viruses that are resistant to the other protease inhibitors. *Tipranavir* is well absorbed when taken with food. The half-life is 6 hours, and it must be administered twice daily in combination with *ritonavir*. *Tipranvir* has a unique action as a *cytochrome P450* inducer in addition to a substrate that is different from the other protease inhibitors. Side effects are similar to those of the other protease inhibitors with the exception of two "black box" warnings for severe and fatal hepatitis and rare cases of fatal and nonfatal intracranial hemorrhages. Most patients had underlying comorbidities. *Tipranavir* is useful in "salvage" regimens in patients with multidrug resistance.

J. Darunavir (DRV)

Darunavir [da-RU-na-veer] is the most recently approved protease inhibitor and is also active against HIV protease that is resistant to other protease inhibitors. *Darunavir* is well absorbed when given with food, and the terminal elimination half-life is 15 hours when combined with *ritonavir*. *Darunavir* is extensively metabolized by the CYP3A enzymes and is an inhibitor as well. The side effects are similar to those of the other protease inhibitors with the addition of possible rash. Early reports demonstrate a decreased risk of hyperlipidemia, but it is not known if *darunavir* is less likely to cause insulin resistance and lipodystrophy, as seen with other protease inhibitors. *Darunavir* is useful in "salvage" regimens in patients with multidrug resistance, and studies are underway in naïve patients.

A summary of protease inhibitors is presented in Figure 38.32

IX. ENTRY INHIBITORS

A. Enfuvirtide

Enfuvirtide [en-FU-veer-tide] is the first of new class of antiretroviral drugs known as entry inhibitors. *Enfuvirtide* is a fusion inhibitor. For HIV to gain entry into the host cell, it must fuse its membrane with that of the host cell. This is accomplished by changes in the conformation of the viral transmembrane glycoprotein gp41, which occurs when HIV binds to the host cell surface. *Enfuvirtide* is a 36-amino-acid peptide that binds to gp41, preventing the conformational change. *Enfuvirtide*, in combination with other antiretrovirals, is approved for therapy of treatment-experienced patients with evidence of viral replication despite ongoing antiretroviral drug therapy. As a peptide, it must be given subcutaneously. Most of the adverse effects are related to the injection, including pain, erythema, induration, and nodules, which occur in almost all patients. However, only 3 percent discontinue treatment because of them. *Enfuvirtide* must be reconstituted prior to administration. It is an expensive medication.

B. Maraviroc

Maraviroc [ma-RA-vi-roc] is the second entry inhibitor. Because it is well absorbed orally, it is formulated as an oral tablet. *Maraviroc* blocks the CCR5 coreceptor that works together with gp41 to facilitate HIV entry through the membrane into the cell. HIV may express either the CCR5 coreceptor or the CXCR4 coreceptor, or both. A test to determine tropism is required to distinguish the CCR5 from the CXCR4 coreceptor as well as mixed and dual tropic virus. Only the CCR5-expressing virus can be treated with *maraviroc*. *Maraviroc* is metabolized by cytochromeP450 liver enzymes, and the dose must be reduced when given with the protease inhibitors. *Maraviroc* is generally well tolerated.

X. INTEGRASE INHIBITORS

A. Raltegravir (RAL)

Raltegravir [ral TEG ra veer] is the first of new class of antiretroviral drugs known as integrase inhibitors. *Ragtegravir* specifically inhibits the final step in integration of stand transfer of the viral DNA into our own host cell DNA. *Raltegravir* has a half-life of approximately 9 hours and is therefore dosed twice daily. The route of metabolism is UGT1A1-mediated glucuronidation, therefore drug interactions with CYP450 inducers, inhibitors or substrates do not occur. *Raltegravir* is well-tolerated with nausea, headache and diarrhea as the most common side effects. *Raltegravir*, in combination with other antiretrovirals, is approved for therapy of treatment-experienced patients with evidence of viral replication despite ongoing antiretroviral drug therapy.

Note added in proof: *Etravirine* [et-ra-VYE-rine] is the first second generation NNRTI. It is active against many of the strains of HIV that are resistant to the first generation NNRTI. HIV strains with the commonn K103N resistance mutation to the first generation of NNRTI's are fully susceptible to *entravirine*. Following oral administration, *etravirine* is well distributed and bioavailability is enhance when taken with a high-fat meal. Although it has a half-life of approximately 40 hours, it is indicated for twice daily dosing. *Etravirine* is extensively metabolized to inactive products. *Etravirine* is a potent inducer of cytochrome P450; therefore, the doses of cytochrome P450 substrates may need to be increased when given with *etravirine*. Rash is the most common side effect. *Etravirine* is otherwsie well tolerated and does not have the CNS side effects that are seen with *efavirenz* and *etravirine* is pregnany category B. *Etravirine* is indicaated for HIV treatment-experienced, multi-drug resistant adult patients who have evidence of ongoing viral replication.

DRUGS	MAJOR TOXICITIES AND CONCERNS
Atazanavir	Nausea, abdominal discomfort, headache, skin rash
Darunavir	Nausea, abdominal discomfort, headache, skin rash
Fosamprenavir	Nausea, diarrhea, vomiting, oral and perioral paresthesia, and rash
Indinavir	Benign hyperbilirubinemia, nephrolithiasis; take 1 hour before or 2 hours after food; may take with skim milk or a low-fat meal; drink >1.5 L of liquid daily
Lopinavir	Gastrointestinal, hyperlipidemia, insulin resistance
Nelfinavir	Diarrhea, nausea, flatulence, rash
Ritonavir	Diarrhea, nausea, taste perversion, vomiting, anemia, increased hepatic enzymes, increased triglycerides. Requires refrigeration; take with meals; chocolate milk improves the taste
Saquinavir	Diarrhea, nausea, abdominal discomfort, elevated transaminase levels. Take with high-fat meal or within 2 hours of a full meal
Tipranavir	Nausea, vomiting, diarrhea, rash, severe hepatotoxicity, intracranial hemorrhage

Figure 38.32
Summary of protease inhibitors. [Note: *Lopinavir* is co formulated with *ritonavir*; *ritonavir* inhibits the metabolism of *lopinavir*, thereby increasing its level in the plasma.]

Study Questions

Choose the ONE best answer.

38.1 A 30-year-old male patient with an HIV infection is being treated with a HAART regimen. Four weeks after initiating therapy, he comes to the emergency department complaining of fever, rash, and gras- tointestinal upset. Which one of the following drugs is most likely the cause of his symptoms?

   A. Zidovudine.
   B. Nelfinavir.
   C. Abacavir.
   D. Efavirenz.
   E. Darunavir.

> Correct answer = C. The abacavir hypersensitivity reaction is characterized by fever, rash, or gastrointestinal uspet. The patient must stop therapy and not be rechallenged.

38.2 Chills, fever, and muscle aches are common reactions to which one of the following antiviral drugs?

   A. Acyclovir.
   B. Ganciclovir.
   C. Oseltamivir.
   D. Interferon.
   E. Ribavirin

> Correct answer = D. Interferon causes flu-like symptoms, including chills, fever, and myalgias, upon injection. Pretreatment with acetaminophen decreases the reaction. The other drugs do not cause this particular adverse effect.

38.3 An HIV-positive woman is diagnosed with CMV retinitis. She has been on a HAART regimen containing zidovudine. Which of the following anti-CMV drugs is likely to cause additive myelosuppression with zidovudine?

   A. Acyclovir.
   B. Ganciclovir.
   C. Amantadine.
   D. Foscarnet.
   E. Ribavirin.

> Correct answer = B. Ganciclovir is myelosuppressive in and of itself and will add to the myelosuppression caused by zidovudine. The combination has an increased risk of neutropenia and anemia. Foscarnet has anti-CMV activity, but it does not cause myelosuppression. The other drugs are not effective against CMV.

38.4 A 25-year-old man is diagnosed with HIV, and therapy is initiated. After the first week of therapy, the patient complains of headaches, irritability, and nightmares. Which one of the following antiretroviral drugs is most likely to be causing these symptoms?

   A. Efavirenz.
   B. Indinavir.
   C. Lamivudine.
   D. Nevirapine.
   E. Stavudine.

> Correct answer = A. CNS symptoms are characteristic of efavirenz, especially at the beginning of therapy, and occur in nearly 50 percent of patients. These adverse effects abate with continued administration of efavirenz. The other drugs are unlikely to cause CNS side effects.

Anticancer Drugs

39

I. OVERVIEW

It is estimated that 25 percent of the population of the United States will face a diagnosis of cancer during their lifetime, with 1.3 million new cancer patients diagnosed each year. Less than a quarter of these patients will be cured solely by surgery and/or local radiation. Most of the remainder will receive systemic chemotherapy at some time during their illness. In a small fraction (approximately 10 percent) of patients with cancer representing selected neoplasms, the chemotherapy will result in a cure or a prolonged remission. However, in most cases, the drug therapy will produce only a regression of the disease, and complications and/or relapse may eventually lead to death. Thus, the overall 5-year survival rate for cancer patients is about 65 percent, ranking cancer second only to cardiovascular disease as a cause of mortality. (See Figure 39.1 for a list of the anticancer agents discussed in this chapter.)

II. PRINCIPLES OF CANCER CHEMOTHERAPY

Cancer chemotherapy strives to cause a lethal cytotoxic event or apoptosis in the cancer cell that can arrest a tumor's progression. The attack is generally directed toward DNA or against metabolic sites essential to cell replication—for example, the availability of purines and pyrimidines that are the building blocks for DNA or RNA synthesis (Figure 39.2). Ideally, these anticancer drugs should interfere only with cellular processes that are unique to malignant cells. Unfortunately, most currently available anticancer drugs do not specifically recognize neoplastic cells but, rather, affect all kinds of proliferating cells—both normal and abnormal. Therefore, almost all antitumor agents have a steep dose-response curve for both toxic and therapeutic effects.

A. Treatment strategies

1. **Goal of treatment:** The ultimate goal of chemotherapy is a cure (that is, long-term, disease-free survival). A true cure requires the eradication of every neoplastic cell. If a cure is not attainable, then the goal becomes control of the disease (stop the cancer from enlarging and spreading) to extend survival and maintain the best quality of life. This allows the individual to maintain a "normal" existence, with the cancer thus being treated as a chronic disease. In either case, the neoplastic cell burden is initially reduced (debulked), either by surgery and/or by radiation, followed by chemotherapy, immunotherapy, or a combination of these treatment

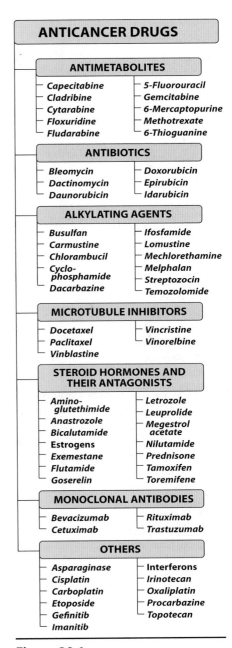

ANTICANCER DRUGS

ANTIMETABOLITES
- Capecitabine
- Cladribine
- Cytarabine
- Floxuridine
- Fludarabine
- 5-Fluorouracil
- Gemcitabine
- 6-Mercaptopurine
- Methotrexate
- 6-Thioguanine

ANTIBIOTICS
- Bleomycin
- Dactinomycin
- Daunorubicin
- Doxorubicin
- Epirubicin
- Idarubicin

ALKYLATING AGENTS
- Busulfan
- Carmustine
- Chlorambucil
- Cyclo-phosphamide
- Dacarbazine
- Ifosfamide
- Lomustine
- Mechlorethamine
- Melphalan
- Streptozocin
- Temozolomide

MICROTUBULE INHIBITORS
- Docetaxel
- Paclitaxel
- Vinblastine
- Vincristine
- Vinorelbine

STEROID HORMONES AND THEIR ANTAGONISTS
- Amino-glutethimide
- Anastrozole
- Bicalutamide
- Estrogens
- Exemestane
- Flutamide
- Goserelin
- Letrozole
- Leuprolide
- Megestrol acetate
- Nilutamide
- Prednisone
- Tamoxifen
- Toremifene

MONOCLONAL ANTIBODIES
- Bevacizumab
- Cetuximab
- Rituximab
- Trastuzumab

OTHERS
- Asparaginase
- Cisplatin
- Carboplatin
- Etoposide
- Gefinitib
- Imanitib
- Interferons
- Irinotecan
- Oxaliplatin
- Procarbazine
- Topotecan

Figure 39.1
Summary of chemotherapeutic agents.

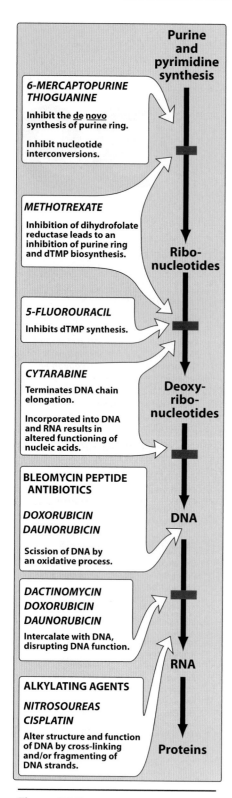

Figure 39.2
Examples of chemotherapeutic agents affecting the availability of RNA and DNA precursors. dTMP = deoxythymidine monophosphate.

modalities (Figure 39.3). In advanced stages of cancer, the likelihood of controlling the cancer is far from reality and the goal is palliation (that is, alleviation of symptoms and avoidance of life-threatening toxicity). This means that chemotherapeutic drugs may be used to relieve symptoms caused by the cancer and improve the quality of life, even though the drugs may not lengthen life.

2. **Indications for treatment:** Chemotherapy is indicated when neoplasms are disseminated and are not amenable to surgery. Chemotherapy is also used as a supplemental treatment, to attack micrometastases following surgery and radiation treatment in which case it is called adjuvant chemotherapy. Chemotherapy given prior to the surgical procedure in an attempt to shrink the cancer is referred as neoadjuvant chemotherapy, and chemotherapy given in lower doses to assist in prolonging a remission is known as maintenance chemotherapy.

3. **Tumor susceptibility and the growth cycle:** The fraction of tumor cells that are in the replicative cycle ("growth fraction") influences their susceptibility to most cancer chemotherapeutic agents. Rapidly dividing cells are generally more sensitive to anticancer drugs, whereas slowly proliferating cells are less sensitive to chemotherapy. In general, nonproliferating cells (those in the G_0 phase; Figure 39.4) usually survive the toxic effects of many of these agents.

   a. **Cell-cycle specificity of drugs:** Both normal cells and tumor cells go through growth cycles (see Figure 39.4). However, the number of cells that are in various stages of the cycle may differ in normal and neoplastic tissues. Chemotherapeutic agents that are effective only against replicating cells—that is, those cells that are cycling—are said to be cell-cycle specific (see Figure 39.4), whereas other agents are said to be cell-cycle nonspecific. The nonspecific drugs, although having generally more toxicity in cycling cells, are also useful against tumors that have a low percentage of replicating cells.

   b. **Tumor growth rate:** The growth rate of most solid tumors in vivo is initially rapid, but growth rate usually decreases as the tumor size increases (see Figure 39.3). This is due to the unavailability of nutrients and oxygen caused by inadequate vascularization and lack of blood circulation. Reducing the tumor burden through surgery or radiation often promotes the recruitment of the remaining cells into active proliferation and increases their susceptibility to chemotherapeutic agents.

B. **Treatment regimens and scheduling**

Drugs are usually administered on the basis of body surface area, with an effort being made to tailor the medications to each patient.

1. **Log kill:** Destruction of cancer cells by chemotherapeutic agents follows first-order kinetics; that is, a given dose of drug destroys a constant fraction of cells. The term log kill is used to describe this phenomenon. For example, a diagnosis of leukemia is generally made when there are about 10^9 (total) leukemic cells. Consequently, if treatment leads to a 99.999-percent kill, then 0.001 percent of 10^9 cells (or 10^4 cells) would remain. This is defined as a five-log kill (reduction of 10^5 cells). At this point, the patient will become asymp-

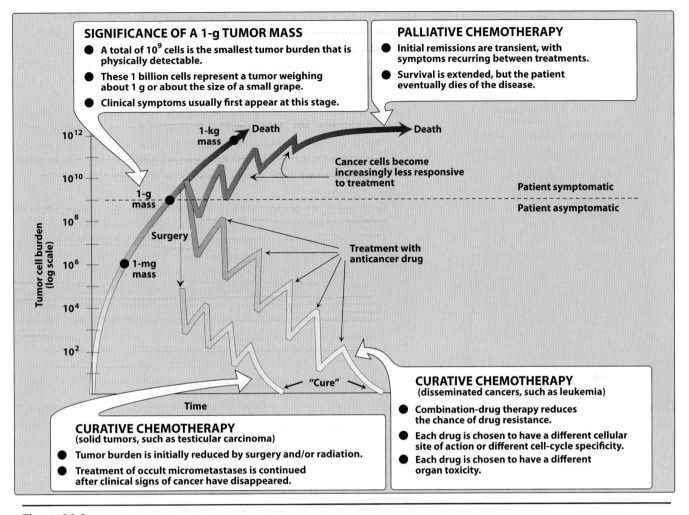

SIGNIFICANCE OF A 1-g TUMOR MASS
- A total of 10^9 cells is the smallest tumor burden that is physically detectable.
- These 1 billion cells represent a tumor weighing about 1 g or about the size of a small grape.
- Clinical symptoms usually first appear at this stage.

PALLIATIVE CHEMOTHERAPY
- Initial remissions are transient, with symptoms recurring between treatments.
- Survival is extended, but the patient eventually dies of the disease.

CURATIVE CHEMOTHERAPY
(solid tumors, such as testicular carcinoma)
- Tumor burden is initially reduced by surgery and/or radiation.
- Treatment of occult micrometastases is continued after clinical signs of cancer have disappeared.

CURATIVE CHEMOTHERAPY
(disseminated cancers, such as leukemia)
- Combination-drug therapy reduces the chance of drug resistance.
- Each drug is chosen to have a different cellular site of action or different cell-cycle specificity.
- Each drug is chosen to have a different organ toxicity.

Figure 39.3
Effects of various treatments on the cancer cell burden in a hypothetical patient.

tomatic; that is, the patient is in remission (see Figure 39.3). For most bacterial infections, a five-log (100,000-fold) reduction in the number of microorganisms results in a cure, because the immune system can destroy the remaining bacterial cells. However, tumor cells are not as readily eliminated, and additional treatment is required to totally eradicate the leukemic cell population.

2. **Pharmacologic sanctuaries:** Leukemic or other tumor cells find sanctuary in tissues such as the central nervous system (CNS), where transport constraints prevent certain chemotherapeutic agents from entering. Therefore, a patient may require irradiation of the craniospinal axis or intrathecal administration of drugs to eliminate the leukemic cells at that site. Similarly, drugs may be unable to penetrate certain areas of solid tumors.

3. **Treatment protocols:** Combination-drug chemotherapy is more successful than single-drug treatment in most of the cancers for which chemotherapy is effective.

   a. **Combinations of drugs:** Cytotoxic agents with qualitatively different toxicities, and with different molecular sites and mechanisms of action, are usually combined at full doses.

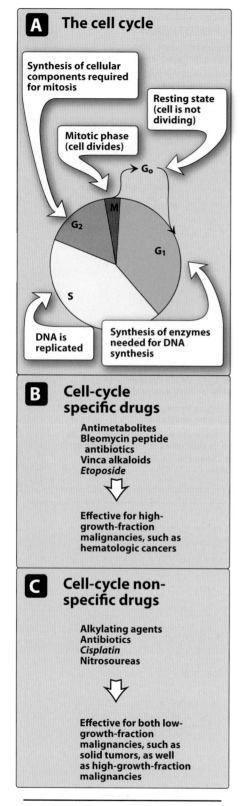

A The cell cycle

Synthesis of cellular components required for mitosis

Resting state (cell is not dividing)

Mitotic phase (cell divides)

G_0

M

G_2

G_1

S

DNA is replicated

Synthesis of enzymes needed for DNA synthesis

B Cell-cycle specific drugs

Antimetabolites
Bleomycin peptide antibiotics
Vinca alkaloids
Etoposide

Effective for high-growth-fraction malignancies, such as hematologic cancers

C Cell-cycle non-specific drugs

Alkylating agents
Antibiotics
Cisplatin
Nitrosoureas

Effective for both low-growth-fraction malignancies, such as solid tumors, as well as high-growth-fraction malignancies

Figure 39.4
Effects of chemotherapeutic agents on the growth cycle of mammalian cells.

This results in higher response rates, due to additive and/or potentiated cytotoxic effects, and nonoverlapping host toxicities. In contrast, agents with similar dose-limiting toxicities, such as myelosuppression, nephrotoxicity, or cardiotoxicity can be combined safely only by reducing the doses of each.

b. **Advantages of drug combinations**: The advantages of such drug combinations are that they 1) provide maximal cell killing within the range of tolerated toxicity, 2) are effective against a broader range of cell lines in the heterogeneous tumor population, and 3) may delay or prevent the development of resistant cell lines.

c. **Treatment protocols:** Many cancer treatment protocols have been developed, and each one is applicable to a particular neoplastic state. They are usually identified by an acronym; for example, a common regimen called POMP—used for the treatment of acute lymphocytic leukemia—consists of **p**rednisone, **o**ncovin (*vincristine*), **m**ethotrexate, and **p**urinethol (*mercapto-purine*). Therapy is scheduled intermittently (approximately 21 days apart) to allow recovery of the patient's immune system, which is also affected by the chemotherapeutic agent, thus reducing the risk of serious infection.

C. Problems associated with chemotherapy

Cancer drugs are toxins that present a lethal threat to the cells. It is therefore not surprising that cells have evolved elaborate defense mechanisms to protect themselves from chemical toxins, including chemotherapeutic agents.

1. **Resistance:** Some neoplastic cells (for example, melanoma) are inherently resistant to most anticancer drugs. Other tumor types may acquire resistance to the cytotoxic effects of a medication by mutating, particularly after prolonged administration of suboptimal drug doses. The development of drug resistance is minimized by short-term, intensive, intermittent therapy with combinations of drugs. Drug combinations are also effective against a broader range of resistant cells in the tumor population. A variety of mechanisms are responsible for drug resistance, each of which is considered separately in the discussion of a particular drug.

2. **Multidrug resistance:** Stepwise selection of an amplified gene that codes for a transmembrane protein (P-glycoprotein for "permeability" glycoprotein; Figure 39.5) is responsible for multidrug resistance. This resistance is due to adenosine triphosphate–dependent pumping of drugs out of the cell in the presence of P-glycoprotein. Cross-resistance following the use of structurally unrelated agents also occurs. For example, cells that are resistant to the cytotoxic effects of the vinca alkaloids are also resistant to *dactinomycin*, to the anthracycline antibiotics, as well as to *colchicine*, and vice versa. These drugs are all naturally occurring substances, each of which has a hydrophobic aromatic ring and a positive charge at neutral pH. [Note: P-glycoprotein is normally expressed at low levels in most cell types, but higher levels are found in the kidney, liver, pancreas, small intestine, colon, and adrenal gland. It has been suggested that the presence of P-glycoprotein may account for the intrinsic resistance to chemotherapy observed with adenocarcinomas.] Certain drugs at high concentrations (for example,

verapamil) can inhibit the pump and, thus, interfere with the efflux of the anticancer agent. However, these drugs are undesirable because of adverse pharmacologic actions of their own. Pharmacologically inert pump blockers are being sought.

3. **Toxicity:** Therapy aimed at killing rapidly dividing cancer cells also affects normal cells undergoing rapid proliferation (for example, cells of the buccal mucosa, bone marrow, gastrointestinal (GI) mucosa, and hair), contributing to the toxic manifestations of chemotherapy.

   a. **Common adverse effects:** Most chemotherapeutic agents have a narrow therapeutic index. Severe vomiting, stomatitis, bone marrow suppression, and alopecia occur to a lesser or greater extent during therapy with all antineoplastic agents. Vomiting is often controlled by administration of antiemetic drugs. Some toxicities, such as myelosuppression that predisposes to infection, are common to many chemotherapeutic agents (Figure 39.6), whereas other adverse reactions are confined to specific agents, such as, cardiotoxicity with doxorubicin and pulmonary fibrosis with *bleomycin*. The duration of the side effects varies widely. For example, alopecia is transient, but the cardiac, pulmonary, and bladder toxicities are irreversible.

   b. **Minimizing adverse effects:** Some toxic reactions may be ameliorated by interventions, such as the use of cytoprotectant drugs, perfusing the tumor locally (for example, a sarcoma of the arm), removing some of the patient's marrow prior to intensive treatment and then reimplanting it, or promoting intensive diuresis to prevent bladder toxicities. The megaloblastic anemia that occurs with *methotrexate* can be effectively counteracted by administering *folinic acid* (*leucovorin*, 5-formyltetrahydrofolic acid; see below). With the availability of human granulocyte colony-stimulating factor (*filgrastim*), the neutropenia associated with treatment of cancer by many drugs can be partially reversed.

4. **Treatment-induced tumors:** Because most antineoplastic agents are mutagens, neoplasms (for example, acute nonlymphocytic leukemia) may arise 10 or more years after the original cancer was cured. [Note: Treatment-induced neoplasms are especially a problem after therapy with alkylating agents.]

III. ANTIMETABOLITES

Antimetabolites are structurally related to normal compounds that exist within the cell. They generally interfere with the availability of normal purine or pyrimidine nucleotide precursors, either by inhibiting their synthesis or by competing with them in DNA or RNA synthesis. Their maximal cytotoxic effects are in S-phase (and, therefore, cell-cycle) specific.

A. Methotrexate

The vitamin folic acid plays a central role in a variety of metabolic reactions involving the transfer of one-carbon units[1] and is essential for

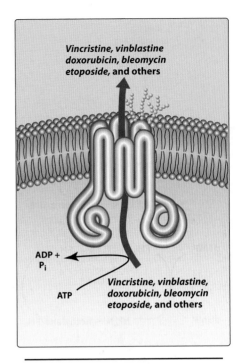

Figure 39.5
The six membrane-spanning loops of the P-glycoprotein form a central channel for the ATP-dependent pumping of drugs from the cell.

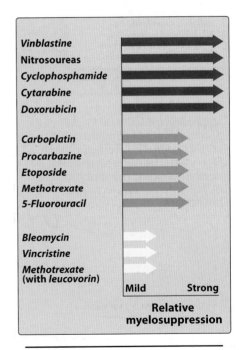

Figure 39.6
Comparison of myelosuppressive potential of chemotherapeutic drugs.

[1]See p. 267 in *Lippincott's Illustrated Reviews: Biochemistry* (4th ed.) for a discussion of the one-carbon pool.

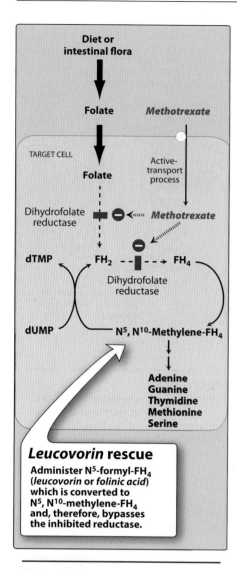

Figure 39.7
Mechanism of action of *methotrexate* and the effect of administration of *leucovorin*. FH_2 = dihydrofolate; FH_4 = tetrahydrofolate; dTMP = deoxythymidine monophosphate; dUMP = deoxyuridine mono phosphate.

cell replication. *Methotrexate* [meth-oh-TREK-sate] (*MTX*) is structurally related to folic acid and acts as an antagonist of that vitamin by inhibiting dihydrofolate reductase[2] (DHFR)—the enzyme that converts folic acid to its active, coenzyme form, tetrahydrofolic acid (FH_4).

1. **Mechanism of action:** Folic acid is obtained from dietary sources or from that produced by intestinal flora. It undergoes reduction to the tetrahydrofolate form (FH_4) via a reaction catalyzed by intracellular nicotinamide-adenine dinucleotide phosphate–dependent DHFR (Figure 39.7). *MTX* enters the cell by active-transport processes that normally mediate the entry of N^5-methyl-FH_4. At high concentrations, the drug can also diffuse into the cell. *MTX* has an unusually strong affinity for DHFR and effectively inhibits the enzyme. Like tetrahydrofolate itself, *MTX* becomes polyglutamated within the cell—a process that favors intracellular retention of the compound due to increased negative charge. *MTX* polyglutamates also potently inhibit DHFR. This inhibition deprives the cell of folate coenzymes and leads to decreased production of compounds that depend on these coenzymes for their biosynthesis. Although these molecules include the nucleotides adenine, guanine and thymidine and the amino acids methionine and serine, depletion of thymidine is the most prominent effect. This leads to depressed DNA, RNA, and protein synthesis and, ultimately, to cell death (see Figure 39.7). The inhibition of DHFR can only be reversed by a 1000-fold excess of the natural substrate, dihydrofolate (FH_2; see Figure 39.7), or by administration of *leucovorin*, which bypasses the blocked enzyme and replenishes the folate pool. [Note: *Leucovorin*, or *folinic acid*, is the N^5-formyl group–carrying form of FH_4.] MTX is specific for the S phase of the cell cycle.

2. **Resistance:** Nonproliferating cells are resistant to *MTX*, probably because of a relative lack of DHFR, thymidylate synthase, and/or the glutamylating enzyme. Decreased levels of the *MTX* polyglutamate have been reported in resistant cells and may be due to its decreased formation or increased breakdown. Resistance in neoplastic cells can be due to amplification (production of additional copies) of the gene that codes for DHFR, resulting in increased levels of this enzyme. The enzyme affinity for *MTX* may also be diminished. Resistance can also occur from a reduced influx of *MTX*, apparently caused by a change in the carrier-mediated transport responsible for pumping the drug into the cell.

3. **Therapeutic uses:** *MTX*, usually in combination with other drugs, is effective against acute lymphocytic leukemia, choriocarcinoma, Burkitt's lymphoma in children, breast cancer, and head and neck carcinomas. In addition, low-dose *MTX* is effective as a single agent against certain inflammatory diseases, such as severe psoriasis and rheumatoid arthritis as well as Crohn's disease. All patients receiving *MTX* require close monitoring for possible toxic effects.

[2]See p. 267 in Lippincott's Illustrated Reviews: Biochemistry (4th ed.) for a discussion of dihydrofolate reductase.

4. Pharmacokinetics:

a. **Administration and distribution:** *MTX* is variably absorbed at low doses from the GI tract, but it can also be administered by intramuscular, intravenous (IV), and intrathecal routes (Figure 39.8). [Note: Because *MTX* does not penetrate the blood-brain barrier, it is administered intrathecally to destroy neoplastic cells that are thriving in the central sanctuary sites.] High concentrations of the drug are found in the intestinal epithelium, liver, and kidney as well as in ascites and pleural effusions. *MTX* is also distributed to the skin.

b. **Fate:** As previously mentioned, *MTX* is metabolized to poly-glutamate derivatives. This property is important, because the polyglutamates, which also inhibit DHFR, remain within the cell even in the absence of extracellular drug. This is in contrast to *MTX* per se, which rapidly leaves the cell as the extracellular drug levels fall. High doses of *MTX* undergo hydroxylation at the 7-position and becomes 7-hyroxymethotrexate. This derivative is much less active as an antimetabolite. It is less water soluble than *MTX* and may lead to crystalluria. Therefore, it is important to keep the urine alkaline and the patient well hydrated to avoid renal toxicity. Excretion of the parent drug and the 7-OH metabolite occurs primarily via the urine, although some of the drug and its metabolite appear in the feces due to enterohepatic excretion.

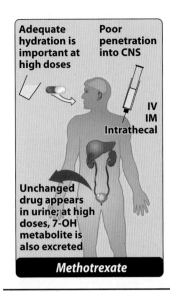

Figure 39.8
Administration and fate of *methotrexate*.

5. Adverse effects:

a. **Commonly observed toxicities:** In addition to nausea, vomiting, and diarrhea, the most frequent toxicities occur in tissues that are constantly renewing. Thus, *MTX* causes stomatitis, myelosuppression, erythema, rash, urticaria, and alopecia. Some of these adverse effects can be prevented or reversed by administering *leucovorin* (see Figure 39.7), which is taken up more readily by normal cells than by tumor cells. Doses of *leucovorin* must be kept minimal to avoid possible interference with the antitumor action of *MTX*.

b. **Renal damage:** Although uncommon during conventional therapy, renal damage is a complication of high-dose *MTX* and its 7-OH metabolite, which can precipitate in the tubules. Alkalinization of the urine and hydration help to prevent this problem.

c. **Hepatic function:** Hepatic function should be monitored. Long-term use of *MTX* may lead to cirrhosis.

d. **Pulmonary toxicity:** This is a rare complication. Children who are being maintained on *MTX* may develop cough, dyspnea, fever, and cyanosis. Infiltrates are seen on radiographs. This toxicity is reversible on suspension of the drug.

e. **Neurologic toxicities:** These are associated with intrathecal administration of *MTX* and include subacute meningeal irritation, stiff neck, headache, and fever. Rarely, seizures, encephalopathy, or paraplegia occur. Long-lasting effects, such as learning

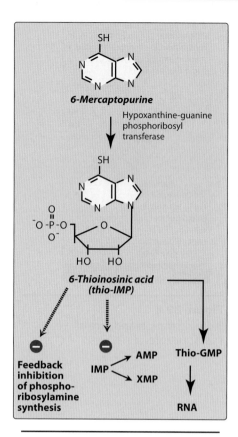

Figure 39.9
Actions of *6-mercaptopurine*.

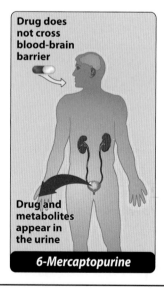

Figure 39.10
Administration and fate of
6-mercaptopurine.

disabilities, have been seen in children who received the drug by this route.

f. Contraindications: Because *MTX* is teratogenic in experimental animals and is an abortifacient, it should be avoided in pregnancy. [Note: *MTX* is used with *misoprostol* to induce abortion.]

B. 6-Mercaptopurine

The drug *6-mercaptopurine* [mer-kap-toe-PYOOR-een] (*6-MP*) is the thiol analog of hypoxanthine. *6-MP* and *6-thioguanine* were the first purine analogs to prove beneficial for treating neoplastic disease. [Note: *Azathioprine*, an immunosuppressant, exerts its cytotoxic effects after conversion to *6-MP*.] *6-MP* is used principally in the maintenance of remission in acute lymphoblastic leukemia. *6-MP* and its analog, *azathioprine*, are also beneficial in the treatment of Crohn's disease.

1. **Mechanism of action:**

   a. Nucleotide formation: To exert its antileukemic effect, *6-MP* must penetrate target cells and be converted to the nucleotide analog, *6-MP*-ribose phosphate (better known as 6-thioinosinic acid, or TIMP; Figure 39.9). The addition of the ribose phosphate is catalyzed by the salvage pathway enzyme, hypoxanthine-guanine phosphoribosyl transferase (HGPRT).[3]

   b. Inhibition of purine synthesis: A number of metabolic processes involving purine biosynthesis and interconversions are affected by the nucleotide analog, TIMP. Like adenosine monophosphate (AMP), guanosine monophosphate (GMP), and inosine monophosphate (IMP), TIMP can inhibit the first step of de novo purine-ring biosynthesis (catalyzed by glutamine phosphoribosyl pyrophosphate amidotransferase). TIMP also blocks the formation of AMP and xanthinuric acid from inosinic acid.[4]

   c. Incorporation into nucleic acids: TIMP is converted to thioguanine monophosphate (TGMP), which after phosphorylation to di- and triphosphates can be incorporated into RNA. The deoxyribonucleotide analogs that are also formed are incorporated into DNA. This results in nonfunctional RNA and DNA.

2. **Resistance:** Resistance is associated with 1) an inability to biotransform *6-MP* to the corresponding nucleotide because of decreased levels of HGPRT (for example, in Lesch-Nyhan syndrome, in which patients lack this enzyme), 2) increased dephosphorylation, or 3) increased metabolism of the drug to thiouric acid or other metabolites.

3. **Pharmacokinetics:** Absorption by the oral route is erratic and incomplete. Once it enters the blood circulation, the drug is widely distributed throughout the body, except for the cerebrospinal fluid (CSF; Figure 39.10). The bioavailability of *6-MP* can be reduced by the first-

[3]See p. 296 in *Lippincott's Illustrated Reviews: Biochemistry* (4th ed.) for a discussion of hypoxanthine-guanine phosphoribosyl transferase.
[4]See p. 295 in *Lippincott's Illustrated Reviews: Biochemistry* (4th ed.) for a discussion of the conversion of IMP to other purine nucleotides.

pass metabolism in the liver; while undergoing metabolism in the liver, *6-MP* is converted to to the 6-methylmercaptopurine derivative or to thiouric acid (an inactive metabolite). [Note: The latter reaction is catalyzed by xanthine oxidase.[5]] Because the xanthine oxidase inhibitor, *allopurinol*, is frequently used to reduce hyperuricemia in cancer patients receiving chemotherapy, it is important to decrease the dose of *6-MP* by 75 percent in these individuals to avoid accumulation of the drug and exacerbation of toxicities (Figure 39.11). The parent drug and its metabolites are excreted by the kidney.

4. **Adverse effects:** Bone marrow depression is the principal toxicity. Side effects also include anorexia, nausea, vomiting, and diarrhea. Occurrance of hepatotoxicity in the form of jaundice has been reported in about one-third of adult patients.

C. 6-Thioguanine

6-Thioguanine [thye-oh-GWAH-neen] (*6-TG*), a purine analog, is primarily used in the treatment of acute nonlymphocytic leukemia in combination with *daunorubicin* and *cytarabine*. Like *6-MP*, *6-TG* is converted intracellularly to TGMP (also called 6-thioguanylic acid) by the enzyme HGPRT. TGMP is further converted to the di- and triphosphates, thioguanosine diphosphate and thioguanosine triphosphate, which then inhibit the biosynthesis of purines and also the phosphorylation of GMP to guanosine diphosphate. The nucleotide form of *6-TG* is incorporated into DNA that leads to cell-cycle arrest.

1. **Pharmacokinetics:** Similar to *6-MP*, the absorption of oral *6-TG* is also incomplete and erratic. The peak concentration in the plasma is reached in 2 to 4 hours after ingestion. When *6-TG* is administered, it is converted the S-methylation product, 2-amino-6-methylthiopurine by thiopurine methyltransferase (TPMT), which appears in the urine. Patients with low or intermediate TPMT activity accumulate higher concentrations of thioguanine cytotoxic metabolites compared to patients with normal TPMT activity. This results in unexpectedly high myelosuppression and has also been associated with the occurrence of secondary malignancies. Approximately three percent of whites and blacks express either a homozygous deletion or mutation of the TPMT gene. An estimated 10 percent of patients may be at increased risk for toxicity because of a heterozygous deletion or mutation of TPMT; therefore, TPMT genotyping is recommended before therapy. To a lesser extent, 6-thioxanthine and 6-thiouric acid are also formed by the action of guanase. Because the deamination product 6-thioanthine is an inactive metabolite, *6-TG* may be administered along with *allopurinol* without any dose reduction.

2. **Adverse effects:** Bone marrow depression is the dose-related adverse effect. *6-TG* is not recommended for maintenance therapy or continuous long-term treatments due to the risk of liver toxicity.

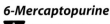

6-Mercaptopurine

CAUTION

Allopurinol

Figure 39.11
Potential drug interaction between *allopurinol* and *6-mercaptopurine*.

*6-TG
not long term*

*6-MP
long term*

[5]See p. 299 in *Lippincott's Illustrated Reviews: Biochemistry* (4th ed.) for a discussion of xanthine oxidase.

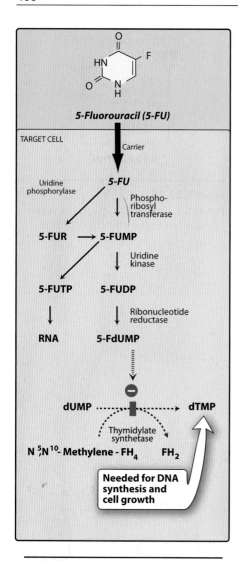

Figure 39.12
Mechanism of the cytotoxic action of *5-FU*. *5-FU* is converted to 5-FdUMP, which competes with deoxyuridine monophosphate (dUMP) for the enzyme thymidylate synthetase. 5-FU = 5-fluorouracil; 5-FUR = 5-fluorouridine; 5-FUMP = 5-fluorouridine monophosphate; 5-FUDP = 5-fluorouridine diphosphate; 5-FUTP = 5-fluoro-uridine triphosphate; dUMP = deoxyuridine monophosphate; dTMP = deoxythymidine mono-phosphate. 5-FdUMP = 5-fluoro-deoxyuridine monophosphate.

D. Fludarabine

Fludarabine [floo-DARE-a-been] is the 5′-phosphate of 2-fluoroadenine arabinoside—a purine nucleotide analog. It is useful in the treatment of chronic lymphocytic leukemia and may replace *chlorambucil*, the present drug of choice. *Fludarabine* is also effective against hairy-cell leukemia and indolent non-Hodgkin's lymphoma. *Fludarabine* is a prodrug, the phosphate being removed in the plasma to form 2-F-araA, which is taken up into cells and again phosphorylated (initially by deoxycytidine kinase). Although the exact cytotoxic mechanism is uncertain, the triphosphate is incorporated into both DNA and RNA. This decreases their synthesis in the S phase and affects their function. Resistance is associated with reduced uptake into cells, lack of deoxycytidine kinase, and decreased affinity for DNA polymerase plus other mechanisms. *Fludarabine* is administered IV rather than orally, because intestinal bacteria split off the sugar to yield the very toxic metabolite, fluoroadenine. Urinary excretion accounts for partial elimination. In addition to nausea, vomiting, and diarrhea, myelosuppression is the dose-limiting toxicity. Fever, edema, and severe neurologic toxicity also occur. At high doses, progressive encephalopathy, blindness, and death have been reported.

E. Cladribine

Another purine analog, *2-chlorodeoxyadenosine*, or *cladribine* [KLA-dri-been], undergoes reactions similar to those of *fludarabine*; that is, it must be converted to a nucleotide to be cytotoxic. It becomes incorporated at the 3′-terminus of DNA and, thus, hinders elongation. It also affects DNA repair and is a potent inhibitor of ribonucleotide reductase.[6] Resistance may be due to mechanisms analogous to those that affect *fludarabine*, although cross-resistance is not a problem. *Cladribine* is effective against hairy-cell leukemia, chronic lymphocytic leukemia, and non-Hodgkin's lymphoma. It also has some activity versus multiple sclerosis. The drug is given as a single, continuous infusion. *Cladribine* distributes throughout the body, including into the CSF. Severe bone marrow suppression is a common adverse effect, as is fever. Peripheral neuropathy has also been reported. The drug is teratogenic.

F. 5-Fluorouracil

5-Fluorouracil [flure-oh-YOOR-ah-sil] (*5-FU*), a pyrimidine analog, has a stable fluorine atom in place of a hydrogen atom at position 5 of the uracil ring. The fluorine interferes with the conversion of deoxyuridylic acid to thymidylic acid, thus depriving the cell of thymidine, one of the essential precursors for DNA synthesis. *5-FU* is employed primarily in the treatment of slowly growing solid tumors (for example, colorectal, breast, ovarian, pancreatic, and gastric carcinomas). Adjuvant therapy with *levamisole*—a veterinary anthelmintic agent—improves the survival of some patients with colon cancer. When applied topically, *5-FU* is also effective for the treatment of superficial basal cell carcinomas.

1. **Mechanism of action:** *5-FU* per se is devoid of antineoplastic activity. It enters the cell through a carrier-mediated transport system and is converted to the corresponding deoxynucleotide (5-fluro-deoxyuridine monophosphate (5-FdUMP) Figure 39.12), which competes with deoxyuridine monophosphate for thymidylate syn-

[6]See p. 297 in ***Lippincott's Illustrated Reviews: Biochemistry*** (4th ed.) for a discussion of ribonucleotide reductase.

thase.[7] 5-FdUMP acts as a pseudosubstrate and is trapped with the enzyme and its coenzyme N^5,N^{10}-methylene tetrahydrofolic acid (*leucovorin*), in a ternary complex that cannot proceed to release products. DNA synthesis decreases due to lack of thymidine, leading to imbalanced cell growth and "thymidine-less death" of rapidly dividing cells. [Note: *Leucovorin* is administered with *5-FU*, because the reduced folate coenzyme is required in the thymidylate synthase inhibition. Addition of the coenzyme increases the effectiveness of the 5-FU to form a ternary complex and produce an antipyrimidine effect. For example, the standard regimen for advanced colorectal cancer today is *irinotecan* plus *5-FU/leucovorin*.] *5-FU* is also incorporated into RNA, and low levels have been detected in DNA. In the latter case, a glycosylase excises the *5-FU*, damaging the DNA. *5-FU* produces the anticancer effect in the S phase of the cell cycle.

2. **Resistance:** Resistance is encountered when the cells have lost their ability to convert *5-FU* into its active form (5-FdUMP) or when they have altered or increased thymidylate synthase levels.

3. **Pharmacokinetics:** Because of its severe toxicity to the GI tract, *5-FU* is given IV or, in the case of skin cancer, topically (Figure 39.13). The drug penetrates well into all tissues, including the CNS. *5-FU* is rapidly metabolized in the liver, lung, and kidney. It is eventually converted to fluoro-β-alanine, which is removed in the urine, and to CO_2, which is exhaled. The dose of *5-FU* must be adjusted in the case of impaired hepatic function. Increased rate of *5-FU* catabolism through elevated levels of dihydropyrimidine dehydrogenase (DPD) can decrease the bioavailability of *5-FU*. The DPD level varies from individual to individual, that may differ by as much as six-fold in the general population. Knowledge about an individual's DPD activity should allow more appropriate dosing of 5-FU.

4. **Adverse effects:** In addition to nausea, vomiting, diarrhea, and alopecia, severe ulceration of the oral and GI mucosa, bone marrow depression (with bolus injection), and anorexia are frequently encountered. An *allopurinol* mouthwash has been shown to reduce oral toxicity. A dermopathy (erythematous desquamation of the palms and soles) called the "hand-foot syndrome" is seen after extended infusions.

G. Capecitabine

Capecitabine [cape-SITE-a-been] is a novel, oral fluoropyrimidine carbamate. It is approved for the treatment of metastatic breast cancer that is resistant to first-line drugs (for example, *paclitaxel* and anthracyclines) and is currently also used for treatment of colorectal cancer.

1. **Mechanism of action:** After being absorbed, *capecitabine*, which is itself nontoxic, undergoes a series of enzymatic reactions, the last of which is hydrolysis to *5-FU*. This step is catalyzed by thymidine phosphorylase—an enzyme that is concentrated primarily in tumors (Figure 39.14). Thus, the cytotoxic activity of *capecitabine* is the same as that of *5-FU* and is tumor specific. The most important enzyme inhibited by *5-FU* (and, thus, *capecitabine*) is thymidylate synthase.

[7]See p. 303 in ***Lippincott's Illustrated Reviews: Biochemistry*** (4th ed.) for a discussion of thymidylate synthase.

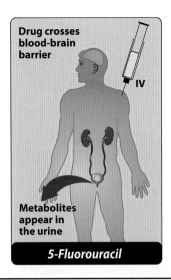

Figure 39.13
Administration and fate of *5-fluorouracil*.

Floxuridine/
Capecitabine →
5-FU

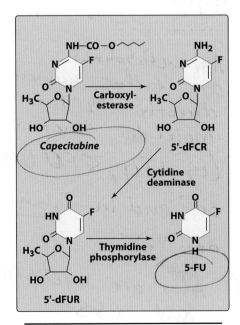

Figure 39.14
Metabolic pathway of *capecitabine* to 5-fluorouracil (5-FU). 5'-dFCR = 5'-deoxy-5-fluorocytidine; 5'-dFUR = 5'-deoxy-5-fluorouridine.

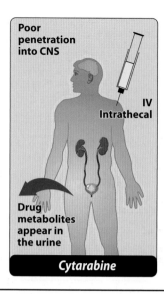

Poor penetration into CNS

IV Intrathecal

Drug metabolites appear in the urine

Cytarabine

Figure 39.15
Administration and fate of *cytarabine*.

2. Pharmacokinetics: *Capecitabine* has the advantage of being well absorbed following oral administration. It is extensively metabolized to *5-FU* (as described above) and is eventually biotransformed into fluoro-β-alanine and CO_2. Metabolites are primarily eliminated in the urine or, in the case of CO_2, it is exhaled.

3. Adverse effects: These are similar to those with *5-FU*, with the toxicity occurring primarily in the GI tract. *Capecitabine* should be used cautiously in patients with hepatic or renal impairment. The drug is contraindicated in individuals who are pregnant or are lactating. Patients taking *coumarin* anticoagulants or *phenytoin* should be monitored for coagulation parameters and drug levels, respectively.

H. Floxuridine   *Fluorylated uridine*

Floxuridine [floks-YOOR-ih-deen] is an analog (floxuridine is 2′-deoxy-5-fluorouridine) of *5-FU*. When given by rapid intra-arterial injection, *floxuridine* is rapidly catabolized in the liver to *5-FU* and produces antimetabolite effects. The primary effect is to interfere with the synthesis of DNA and to a lesser extent inhibit the formation of RNA. The drug is excreted intact and as fluorouracil, urea, and α-fluoro-β-alanine in the urine. Floxuridine is effective in the palliative management of GI adenocarcinoma that has metastasized to the liver. The common adverse effects are nausea, vomiting, diarrhea, enteritis, stomatitis, and localized erythema.

I. Cytarabine   *Cyt - analogue*

Cytarabine [sye-TARE-ah-been] (*cytosine arabinoside*, or *ara-C*) is an analog of 2′-deoxycytidine in which the natural ribose residue is replaced by D-arabinose. *Ara-C* acts as a pyrimidine antagonist. The major clinical use of *ara-C* is in acute nonlymphocytic (myelogenous) leukemia in combination with *6-TG* and *daunorubicin.* → *AL*

1. Mechanism of action: *Ara-C* enters the cell by a carrier-mediated process and, like the other purine and pyrimidine antagonists, must be sequentially phosphorylated by deoxycytidine kinase and other nucleotide kinases to the nucleotide form (cytosine arabinoside triphosphate, or ara-CTP) to be cytotoxic. Ara-CTP is an effective inhibitor of DNA polymerase. The nucleotide is also incorporated into nuclear DNA and can retard chain elongation. It is therefore S-phase (and, hence, cell-cycle) specific.

2. Resistance: Resistance to *ara-C* may result from a defect in the transport process, a change in phosphorylating enzymes activity (especially deoxycytidine kinase), or an increased pool of the natural dCTP nucleotide. Increased deamination of the drug to ara-U can also cause resistance.

3. Pharmacokinetics: *Ara-C* is not effective when given orally, because of its deamination to the noncytotoxic uracil arabinoside (ara-U) by cytidine deaminase in the intestinal mucosa and liver. Given IV, it distributes throughout the body but does not penetrate the CNS in sufficient amounts to be effective against meningeal leukemia (Figure 39.15). However, it may be injected intrathecally. A new preparation that provides slow release into the CSF is also available. *Ara-C* undergoes extensive oxidative deamination in the body to ara-U—a pharmacologically inactive metabolite. Both *ara-C* and ara-U are excreted in the urine.

Antimetabolites are either named directly by their molecular structure (eg 6TG, 5FU, 6MP) or end in "ibine" or "abine".

(All are myelosupressive and CSS

✓

except "Methotrexate"

4. Adverse effects: Nausea, vomiting, diarrhea, and severe myelosuppression (primarily granulocytopenia) are the major toxicities associated with *ara-C*. Hepatic dysfunction is also occasionally encountered. At high doses or with intrathecal injection, *ara-C* may cause leukoencephalopathy or paralysis.

J. Gemcitabine

"cit" → cytidine [handwritten]

Gemcitabine [jem-SITE-ah-been] is an analog of the nucleoside deoxycytidine. It is used for the first-line treatment of locally advanced or metastatic adenocarcinoma of the pancreas. It also is effective against non–small cell lung cancer and several other tumors.

1. Mechanism of action: *Gemcitabine* is a substrate for deoxycytidine kinase, which phosphorylates the drug to 2′,2′-difluorodeoxycytidine triphosphate (Figure 39.16). The latter compound inhibits DNA synthesis by being incorporated into sites in the growing strand that ordinarily would contain cytosine. Evidence suggests that DNA repair does not readily occur. Levels of the natural nucleotide, dCTP, are lowered, because *gemcitabine* competes with the normal nucleoside substrate for deoxycytidine kinase. Gemcitabine diphosphate inhibits ribonucleotide reductase, which is responsible for the generation of deoxynucleoside triphosphates required for DNA synthesis.

2. Resistance: Resistance to the drug is probably due to its inability to be converted to a nucleotide, caused by an alteration in deoxycytidine kinase. In addition, the tumor cell can produce increased levels of endogenous deoxycytidine that compete for the kinase, thus overcoming the inhibition.

3. Pharmacokinetics: *Gemcitabine* is infused IV. It is deaminated to difluorodeoxyuridine, which is not cytotoxic, and is excreted in the urine.

4. Adverse effects: Myelosuppression is the dose-limiting toxicity of *gemcitabine*. Other toxicities include nausea, vomiting, alopecia, rash, and a flu-like syndrome. Transient elevations of serum transaminases, proteinuria, and hematuria are common.

IV. ANTIBIOTICS

The antitumor antibiotics owe their cytotoxic action primarily to their interactions with DNA, leading to disruption of DNA function. In addition to intercalation, their abilities to inhibit topoisomerases (I and II) and produce free radicals also play a major role in their cytotoxic effect. They are cell-cycle nonspecific.

A. Dactinomycin

Dactinomycin [dak-ti-noe-MYE-sin], known to biochemists as *actinomycin D*, was the first antibiotic to find therapeutic application in tumor chemotherapy. *Dactinomycin* is used in combination with surgery and *vincristine* for the treatment of Wilms' tumor. In combination with *MTX*, *dactinomycin* is effective in the treatment of gestational choriocarcinoma. Some soft-tissue sarcomas also respond.

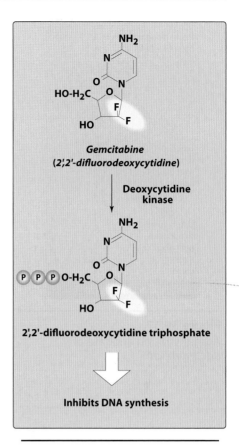

Figure 39.16
Mechanism of action of *gemcitabine*.

[handwritten note]
Antimetabolites
Methotrexate
6-Mercaptopurine
6-Thioguanine
5-Fluorouracil
Fludarabine
Cladribine
Capecitabine
Floxuridine
Gemcitabine

Dactinomycin

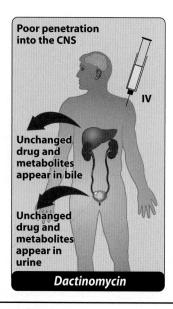

Poor penetration into the CNS

IV

Unchanged drug and metabolites appear in bile

Unchanged drug and metabolites appear in urine

Dactinomycin

Figure 39.17
Administration and fate of *dactinomycin*.

Antibiotics end in "mycin" or "micin" and are not cell-cycle Dependent (except Bleomycin)

1. Mechanism of action: The drug intercalates into the minor groove of the double helix between guanine-cytosine base pairs of DNA,[8] forming a stable *dactinomycin*-DNA complex. The complex interferes primarily with DNA-dependent RNA polymerase, although at high doses, *dactinomycin* also hinders DNA synthesis. The drug also causes single-strand breaks, possibly due to action on topoisomerase II or by generation of free radicals.

2. Resistance: Resistance is due to an increased efflux of the antibiotic from the cell via P-glycoprotein. DNA repair may also play a role.

3. Pharmacokinetics: The drug, administered IV, distributes to many tissues but does not enter the CSF (Figure 39.17). The drug is minimally metabolized in the liver. Most of the parent drug and its metabolites are excreted via the bile, and the remainder are excreted via the urine.

4. Adverse effects: The major dose-limiting toxicity is bone marrow depression. The drug is immunosuppressive. Other adverse reactions include nausea, vomiting, diarrhea, stomatitis, and alopecia. Extravasation during injection produces serious problems. *Dactinomycin* sensitizes to radiation, and inflammation at sites of prior radiation therapy may occur.

B. Doxorubicin and daunorubicin

Doxorubicin [dox-oh-ROO-bi-sin] and *daunorubicin* [daw-noe-ROO-bi-sin] are classified as anthracycline antibiotics. *Doxorubicin* is the hydroxylated analog of *daunorubicin*. *Idarubicin* [eye-da-RUE-bi-sin], the 4-demethoxy analog of *daunorubicin*, and *epirubicin* [eh-pee-ROO bih-sin] are also available. Applications for these agents differ despite their structural similarity and their apparently similar mechanisms of action. *Doxorubicin* is one of the most important and widely used anticancer drugs. It is used in combination with other agents for treatment of sarcomas and a variety of carcinomas, including breast and lung, as well as for treatment of acute lymphocytic leukemia and lymphomas. *Daunorubicin* and *idarubicin* are used in the treatment of acute leukemias.

1. Mechanism of action: The anthracyclines have three major activities that may vary with the type of cell. All three are effective in the S and G_2 phases.

a. Intercalation in the DNA: The drugs insert nonspecifically between adjacent base pairs and bind to the sugar-phosphate backbone of DNA. This causes local uncoiling and, thus, blocks DNA and RNA synthesis. Intercalation can interfere with the topoisomerase II–catalyzed breakage/reunion reaction of supercoiled DNA strands, causing irreparable breaks.

b. Binding to cell membranes: This action alters the function of transport processes coupled to phosphatidylinositol activation.[9]

[8]See p. 396 in *Lippincott's Illustrated Reviews: Biochemistry* (4th ed.) for a discussion of DNA structure.
[9]See p. 205 in *Lippincott's Illustrated Reviews: Biochemistry* (4th ed.) for a discussion of phosphatidylinositol activation.

c. Generation of oxygen radicals: Cytochrome P450 reductase (present in cell nuclear membranes) catalyzes reduction of the anthracyclines to semiquinone free radicals. These in turn reduce molecular O_2, producing superoxide ions and hydrogen peroxide, which mediate single-strand scission of DNA (Figure 39.18). Tissues with ample superoxide dismutase or glutathione peroxidase activity are protected.[10] Tumors and heart tissue are generally low in SOD. In addition, cardiac tissue lacks catalase and, thus, cannot effectively scavenge hydrogen peroxide. Lipid peroxidation therefore may explain the cardiotoxicity of anthracyclines.

2. **Pharmacokinetics:** All these drugs must be administered IV, because they are inactivated in the GI tract. Extravasation is a serious problem that can lead to tissue necrosis. The anthracycline antibiotics bind to plasma proteins as well as to other tissue components, where they are widely distributed. They do not penetrate the blood-brain barrier or the testes. All these drugs undergo extensive hepatic metabolism. The bile is the major route of excretion, and the drug dose must be modified in patients with impaired hepatic function (Figure 39.19). Some renal excretion also occurs, but the dose generally need not be adjusted in patients with renal failure. Because of the dark red color of the anthracycline drugs, the veins may become visible surrounding the site of infusion, and the drugs also impart a red color to the urine.

3. **Adverse effects:** Irreversible, dose-dependent cardiotoxicity, apparently a result of the generation of free radicals and lipid peroxidation, is the most serious adverse reaction and is more common with *daunorubicin* and *doxorubicin* than with *idarubicin* or *epirubicin*. Irradiation of the thorax increases the risk of cardiotoxicity. Addition of *trastuzumab* to protocols with *doxorubicin* or *epirubicin* increases congestive heart failure. There has been some success with the iron-chelator *dexrazone* in protecting against the cardiotoxicity of *doxorubicin*. [Note: A new liposomal-encapsulated *doxorubicin* has been reported to be less cardiotoxic than the usual formulation.] As with *dactinomycin*, both *doxorubicin* and *daunorubicin* also cause transient bone marrow suppression, stomatitis, and GI tract disturbances. Increased skin pigmentation is also seen. Alopecia is usually severe. Occurrence of multidrug resistance is common; however, it is less frequent than with plant alkaloids.

C. Bleomycin

Bleomycin [blee-oh-MYE-sin] is a mixture of different copper-chelating glycopeptides that, like the anthracycline antibiotics, cause scission of DNA by an oxidative process. *Bleomycin* is cell-cycle specific and causes cells to accumulate in the G_2 phase. It is primarily employed in the treatment of testicular cancers in combination with *vinblastine* or *etoposide*. Response rates are close to 100 percent if *cisplatin* is added to the regimen. *Bleomycin* is also effective, although not curative, for squamous cell carcinomas and lymphomas.

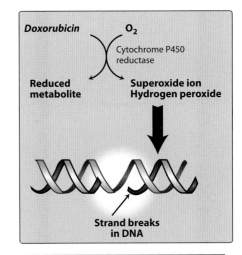

Figure 39.18
Doxorubicin interacts with molecular oxygen, producing superoxide ions and hydrogen peroxide, which cause single-strand breaks in DNA.

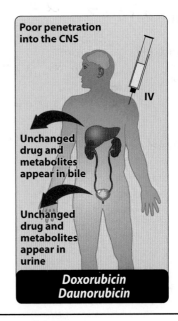

Figure 39.19
Administration and fate of *doxorubicin* and *daunorubicin*.

[10]See p. 148 in **Lippincott's Illustrated Reviews: Biochemistry** (4th ed.) for a discussion of super oxide dismutase and glutathione.

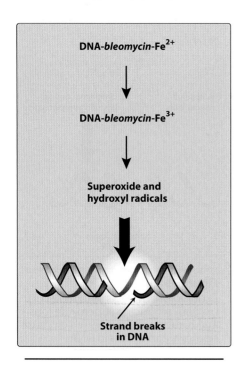

Figure 39.20
Bleomycin causes breaks in DNA by an oxidative process.

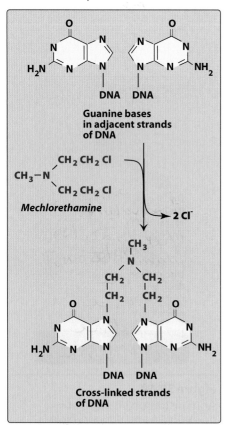

Figure 39.21
Alkylation of guanine bases in DNA is responsible for the cytotoxic effect of *mechlorethamine*.

1. **Mechanism of action**: A DNA-*bleomycin*-Fe^{2+} complex appears to undergo oxidation to *bleomycin*-Fe^{3+}. The liberated electrons react with oxygen to form superoxide or hydroxyl radicals, which in turn attack the phosphodiester bonds of DNA, resulting in strand breakage and chromosomal aberrations (Figure 39.20).

2. **Resistance:** Although the mechanisms of resistance have not been elucidated, experimental systems have implicated increased levels of *bleomycin* hydrolase (or deamidase), glutathione-S-transferase, and possibly, increased efflux of the drug. DNA repair also may contribute.

3. **Pharmacokinetics:** *Bleomycin* is administered by a number of routes, including subcutaneous, intramuscular, IV, and intracavitary. The *bleomycin*-inactivating enzyme (a hydrolase) is high in a number of tissues (for example, liver and spleen) but is low in lung and is absent in skin (accounting for the drug's toxicity in those tissues). Most of the parent drug is excreted unchanged into the urine by glomerular filtration, necessitating dose adjustment in patients with renal failure.

4. **Adverse effects:** Pulmonary toxicity is the most serious adverse effect, progressing from rales, cough, and infiltrate to potentially fatal fibrosis. The pulmonary fibrosis that is caused by *bleomycin* is often referred as "*bleomycin* lung." Mucocutaneous reactions and alopecia are common. Hypertrophic skin changes and hyperpigmentation of the hands are prevalent. There is a high incidence of fever and chills and a low incidence of serious anaphylactoid reactions. *Bleomycin* is unusual in that myelosuppression is rare.

V. ALKYLATING AGENTS

Alkylating agents exert their cytotoxic effects by covalently binding to nucleophilic groups on various cell constituents. Alkylation of DNA is probably the crucial cytotoxic reaction that is lethal to the tumor cells. Alkylating agents do not discriminate between cycling and resting cells, but they are most toxic for rapidly dividing cells. They are used in combination with other agents to treat a wide variety of lymphatic and solid cancers. In addition to being cytotoxic, all are mutagenic and carcinogenic and can lead to second malignancies, such as acute leukemia.

A. Mechlorethamine

Mechlorethamine [mek-lor-ETH-ah-meen] was developed as a vesicant (nitrogen mustard) during World War I. Its ability to cause lymphocytopenia led to its use in lymphatic cancers. Because it can covalently attach to two separate nucleotides, such as guanine on the DNA molecules, it is called a "bifunctional agent." *Mechlorethamine* was used primarily in the treatment of Hodgkin's disease and may find use in the treatment of some solid tumors.

1. **Mechanism of action:** *Mechlorethamine* is transported into the cell, where the drug forms a reactive intermediate that alkylates the N^7 nitrogen of a guanine residue in one or both strands of a DNA molecule (Figure 39.21). This alkylation leads to cross-linkages between guanine residues in the DNA chains and/or depurination, thus facilitating DNA strand breakage. Alkylation can also cause miscoding mutations. Although alkylation can occur in both cycling and resting

cells (and, therefore, is cell-cycle nonspecific), proliferating cells are more sensitive to the drug, especially those in the G₁ and S phases.

2. **Resistance:** Resistance has been ascribed to decreased permeability of the drug, increased conjugation with thiols such as glutathione, and possibly, increased DNA repair.

3. **Pharmacokinetics:** *Mechlorethamine* is very unstable, and solutions must be made up just prior to administration. *Mechlorethamine* is also a powerful vesicant (blistering agent) and is only administered IV. Because of its reactivity, scarcely any drug is excreted.

4. **Adverse effects:** The adverse effects caused by *mechlorethamine* include severe nausea and vomiting (centrally mediated). [Note: These effects can be diminished by pretreatment with *ondansetron, granisetron,* or *palonosetron* with *dexamethasone.*] Severe bone marrow depression limits extensive use. Latent viral infections (for example, herpes zoster) may appear because of immunosuppression. Extravasation is a serious problem. If it occurs, the area should be infiltrated with isotonic *sodium thiosulfite* to inactivate the drug.

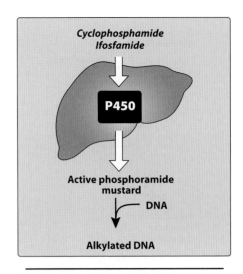

Figure 39.22
Activation of *cyclophosphamide* and *ifosfamide* by hepatic cytochrome P450.

B. Cyclophosphamide and ifosfamide

These drugs are very closely related mustard agents that share most of the same primary mechanisms and toxicities. They are unique in that they can be taken orally and are cytotoxic only after generation of their alkylating species, which are produced through hydroxylation by cytochrome P450. These agents have a broad clinical spectrum, being used either singly or as part of a regimen in the treatment of a wide variety of neoplastic diseases, such as Burkitt's lymphoma and breast cancer. Non-neoplastic disease entities, such as nephrotic syndrome and intractable rheumatoid arthritis, are also effectively treated with low doses of *cyclophosphamide*.

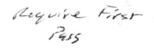

1. **Mechanism of action:** *Cyclophosphamide* [sye-kloe-FOSS-fah-mide] is the most commonly used alkylating agent. Both *cyclophosphamide* and *ifosfamide* [eye-FOSS-fah-mide] are first biotransformed to hydroxylated intermediates primarily in the liver by the cytochrome P450 system (Figure 39.22). The hydroxylated intermediates then undergo breakdown to form the active compounds, phosphoramide mustard and acrolein. Reaction of the phosphoramide mustard with DNA is considered to be the cytotoxic step.

2. **Resistance:** Resistance results from increased DNA repair, decreased drug permeability, and reaction of the drug with thiols (for example, glutathione). Cross-resistance does not always occur.

3. **Pharmacokinetics:** Unlike most of the alkylating agents, *cyclophosphamide* and *ifosfamide* can be administered by the oral route (Figure 39.23). After oral administration, minimal amounts of the parent drug are excreted into the feces (after biliary transport) or into the urine by glomerular filtration.

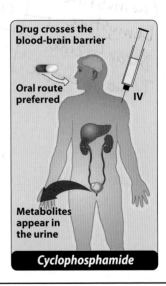

Figure 39.23
Administration and fate of *cyclophosphamide*.

4. **Adverse effects:** The most prominent toxicities of both drugs (after alopecia, nausea, vomiting, and diarrhea) are bone marrow depression, especially leukocytosis, and hemorrhagic cystitis, which can lead to fibrosis of the bladder. The latter toxicity has been attributed to acrolein in the urine in the case of *cyclophosphamide* and to toxic

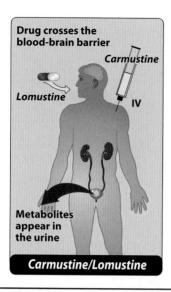

Figure 39.24
Administration and fate of *carmustine/lomustine*.

[Handwritten notes:]
Alkylating Agents

Mecka
Mechlorethamine
Ifosfamide
⊕ Cyclophosphamide] –450

Carmustine
Lomustine   ] Cellular enzymes
Dacarbazine   –450
Temozolomide

metabolites of *ifosfamide*. [Note: Adequate hydration as well as IV injection of MESNA (sodium 2-mercaptoethane sulfonate), which neutralizes the toxic metabolites, minimizes this problem.] Other toxicities include effects on the germ cells, resulting in amenorrhea, testicular atrophy, aspermia, and sterility. Veno-occlusive disease of the liver is seen in about 25 percent of the patients. A fairly high incidence of neurotoxicity has been reported in patients on high-dose *ifosfamide*, probably due to the metabolite, chloroacetaldehyde. Secondary malignancies may appear years after therapy.

C. Nitrosoureas

Carmustine [KAR-mus-teen] and *Lomustine* [LOE-mus-teen] are closely related nitrosoureas. Because of their ability to penetrate into the CNS, the nitrosoureas are primarily employed in the treatment of brain tumors. They find limited use in the treatment of other cancers. [Note: *Streptozocin* [STREP-toe-zoe-sin] is another nitrosourea that is specifically toxic to the β cells of the islets of Langerhans, hence its use in the treatment of insulinomas.]

1. **Mechanism of action:** The nitrosoureas exert cytotoxic effects by an alkylation that inhibits replication and, eventually, RNA and protein synthesis. Although they alkylate DNA in resting cells, cytotoxicity is expressed primarily on cells that are actively dividing. Therefore, nondividing cells can escape death if DNA repair occurs. Nitrosoureas also inhibit several key enzymatic processes by carbamoylation of amino acids in proteins in the targeted cells.

2. **Resistance:** Although the true nature of resistance to nitrosoureas is unknown, it probably results from DNA repair and reaction of the drugs with thiols.

3. **Pharmacokinetics:** In spite of the similarities in their structures, *carmustine* is administered IV, whereas *lomustine* is given orally. Because of their lipophilicity, they distribute widely in the body to many tissues, but their most striking property is their ability to readily penetrate into the CNS. The drugs undergo extensive metabolism. *Lomustine* is metabolized to active products. The kidney is the major excretory route for the nitrosoureas (Figure 39.24).

4. **Adverse effects:** These include delayed hematopoietic depression, which may be due to metabolic products. An aplastic marrow may develop on prolonged use. Renal toxicity and pulmonary fibrosis related to duration of therapy is also encountered. [Note: *Streptozotocin* is also diabetogenic.]

D. Dacarbazine

Dacarbazine [dah-KAR-bah-zeen]—an agent that has found use in the treatment of melanoma, is an alkylating agent that must undergo biotransformation to an active metabolite, methyltriazenoimidazole carboxamide (MTIC). This metabolite is responsible for the drug's activity as an alkylating agent by forming methylcarbonium ions that can attack the nucleophilic groups in the DNA molecule. Thus, similar to other alkylating agents, the cytotoxic action of dacarbazine has been attributed to the ability of its metabolite to methylate DNA on the O^6 position of guanine. *Dacarbazine is administered by IV*. Its major adverse effects are nausea and vomiting. Myelosuppression (thrombocytopenia and neutropenia) occur later in the treatment cycle. Hepatotoxicity with hepatic vascular occlusion may also occur in long-term treatments.

E. Temozolomide

The treatment of tumors in the brain is particularly difficult. Recently, *temozolomide* [te-moe-ZOE-loe-mide], a triazene agent, has been approved for use against treatment-resistant gliomas and anaplastic astrocytomas. *Temozolomide* is related to *dacarbazine*, because both must undergo biotransformation to an active metabolite, MTIC, which probably is responsible for the methylation of DNA on the 6 position of guanine. Unlike *dacarbazine*, *tomozolomide* does not require cytochrome P450 system for metabolic transformation; it undergoes chemical transformation under normal physiological pH. *Temozolomide* also has the property of inhibiting the repair enzyme, O^6-guanine-DNA-alkyltransferase. A property that distinguishes *temozolomide* from *dacarbazine* is the former's ability to cross the blood-brain barrier. *Temozolomide* is taken orally and has excellent oral bioavailability. The parent drug and metabolites are excreted in the urine (Figure 39.25). *Temozolomide* is taken for five consecutive days and repeated every 28 days. Similar to *dacarbazine*, its major initial toxicities are nausea and vomiting. Myelosuppression (thrombocytopenia and neutropenia) occur later in the treatment cycle.

F. Other alkylating agents

Melphalan [MEL-fah-lan], a phenylalanine derivative of nitrogen mustard, is used in the treatment of multiple myeloma. This is a bifunctional alkylating agent that can be given orally. Although *melphalan* can be given orally, the plasma concentration differs from patient to patient due to variation in intestinal absorbtion and metabolism. The dose of *melphalan* is carefully adjusted by monitoring the platelet and white blood cell counts. *Chlorambucil* [clor-AM-byoo-sil] is another bifunctional alkylating agent that is used in the treatment of chronic lymphocytic leukemia. Both *melphalan* and *chlorombucil* have moderate hematologic toxicities and upset the GI tract. *Busulfan* [byoo-SUL-fan] is another oral agent that is effective against chronic granulocytic leukemia. *Busulfan* is also a bifunctional alkylating agent that can cause myelosuppression. In aged patients, *busulfan* can cause pulmonary fibrosis. Like other alkylating agents, all these agents are leukemogenic.

VI. MICROTUBULE INHIBITORS *(Plants)*

The mitotic spindle is part of a larger, intracellular skeleton (cytoskeleton) that is essential for the movements of structures occurring in the cytoplasm of all eukaryotic cells. The mitotic spindle consists of chromatin plus a system of microtubules composed of the protein tubulin. The mitotic spindle is essential for the equal partitioning of DNA into the two daughter cells that are formed when a eukaryotic cell divides. Several plant-derived substances used as anticancer drugs disrupt this process by affecting the equilibrium between the polymerized and depolymerized forms of the microtubules, thereby causing cytotoxicity.

A. Vincristine and vinblastine

Vincristine [vin-KRIS-teen] (*VX*) and *vinblastine* [vin-BLAS-teen] (*VBL*) are structurally related compounds derived from the periwinkle plant, *Vinca rosea*. They are therefore referred to as the vinca alkaloids. A structurally

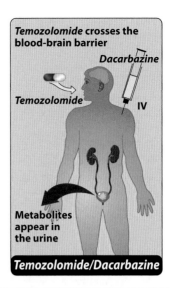

Figure 39.25
Administration and fate of *temozolomide/dacarbazine*.

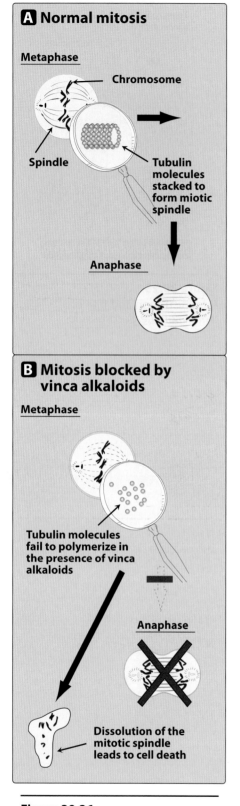

A Normal mitosis

Metaphase

Chromosome

Spindle

Tubulin molecules stacked to form miotic spindle

Anaphase

B Mitosis blocked by vinca alkaloids

Metaphase

Tubulin molecules fail to polymerize in the presence of vinca alkaloids

Anaphase

Dissolution of the mitotic spindle leads to cell death

Figure 39.26
Mechanism of action of the microtubule inhibitors.

related, new (and less toxic) agent is *vinorelbine* [vye-NOR-el-been] (*VRB*). Although the vinca alkaloids are structurally very similar to each other, their therapeutic indications are different. They are generally administered in combination with other drugs. *VX* is used in the treatment of acute lymphoblastic leukemia in children, Wilms' tumor, Ewing's soft-tissue sarcoma, Hodgkin's and non-Hodgkin's lymphomas, as well as some other rapidly proliferating neoplasms. [Note: *VX* (trade name, *Oncovin*) is the "O" in the POMP regimen for leukemia and the MOPP regimen for Hodgkin's lymphoma. Due to relatively milder bone-suppressing ability, *VX* is used in a number of other protocols.] *VBL* is administered with *bleomycin* and *cisplatin* for the treatment of metastatic testicular carcinoma. It is also used in the treatment of systemic Hodgkin's and non-Hodgkin's lymphomas. *VRB* is beneficial in the treatment of advanced non–small cell lung cancer, either as a single agent or with *cisplatin*.

1. **Mechanism of action:** *VX* and *VBL* are both cell-cycle specific and phase specific, because they block mitosis in metaphase (M phase). Their binding to the microtubular protein, tubulin, is GTP dependent and blocks the ability of tubulin to polymerize to form microtubules. Instead, paracrystalline aggregates consisting of tubulin dimers and the alkaloid drug are formed. The resulting dysfunctional spindle apparatus, frozen in metaphase, prevents chromosomal segregation and cell proliferation (Figure 39.26).

2. **Resistance:** Resistant cells have been shown to have an enhanced efflux of *VX*, *VBL*, and *VRB* via P-glycoprotein in the cell membrane. Alterations in tubulin structure may also affect binding of the vinca alkaloids.

3. **Pharmacokinetics:** Intravenous injection of these agents leads to rapid cytotoxic effects and cell destruction. This in turn can cause hyperuricemia due to the oxidation of purines that are released from fragmenting DNA molecules, producing uric acid. The hyperuricemia is ameliorated by administration of the xanthine oxidase–inhibitor *allopurinol*. The vinca alkaloids are concentrated and metabolized in the liver by the cytochrome P450 pathway. They are excreted into bile and feces. Doses must be modified in patients with impaired hepatic function or biliary obstruction.

4. **Adverse effects:** Both *VX* and *VBL* have certain toxicities in common. These include phlebitis or cellulitis, if the drugs extravasate during injection, as well as nausea, vomiting, diarrhea, and alopecia. However, the adverse effects of *VX* and *VBL* are not identical. *VBL* is a more potent myelosuppressant than *VX*, whereas peripheral neuropathy (paresthesias, loss of reflexes, foot drop, and ataxia) is associated with *VX*. Constipation is more frequently encountered with *VX*, which can also cause inappropriate antidiuretic hormone secretion. The anticonvulsants *phenytoin*, *phenobarbital*, and *carbamazepine* can accelerate the metabolism of *VX*, whereas the azole antifungal drugs can slow its metabolism. Granulocytopenia is dose limiting for *VRB*.

B. Paclitaxel and docetaxel

½ the dose, twice the effect

Better known as *Taxol*, *paclitaxel* [PAK-li-tax-el] is the first member of the taxane family to be used in cancer chemotherapy. A semisynthetic *paclitaxel* is now available through chemical modification of a precursor found in the needles of Pacific yew species. Substitution of a side chain has resulted in *docetaxel* [doe-see-TAX-el], which is the more potent of the two drugs. *Paclitaxel* has shown good activity against advanced ovarian cancer and metastatic breast cancer. Favorable results have been obtained in non–small cell lung cancer when administered with *cisplatin*. *Docetaxel* is showing impressive benefits, with fewer side effects, in these conditions.

1. **Mechanism of action:** Both drugs are active in the G_2/M phase of the cell cycle. They bind reversibly to the β-tubulin subunit, but unlike the vinca alkaloids, they promote polymerization and stabilization of the polymer rather than disassembly (Figure 39.27). Thus, they shift the depolymerization-polymerization process to accumulation of microtubules. The overly stable microtubules formed are nonfunctional, and chromosome desegregation does not occur. This results in death of the cell.

2. **Resistance:** Like the vinca alkaloids, resistance has been associated with the presence of amplified P-glycoprotein or a mutation in the tubulin structure.

3. **Pharmacokinetics:** These agents are infused and have similar pharmacokinetics. Both have a large volume of distribution, but neither enters the CNS. Hepatic metabolism by the cytochrome P450 system and biliary excretion are responsible for their elimination into the stool. Thus, dose modification is not required in patients with renal impairment, but doses should be reduced in patients with hepatic dysfunction.

4. **Adverse effects:** The dose-limiting toxicity of *paclitaxel* and *docetaxel* is neutropenia. [Note: Patients with fewer than 1500 neutrophils/mm³ should not be given these agents.] Treatment with granulocyte colony-stimulating factor (*Filgrastim*®) can help to reverse neutropenia and prevent the problems associated with this condition. Peripheral neuropathy can develop with either of these drugs. A transient, asymptomatic bradycardia is sometimes observed with *paclitaxel*, and fluid retention is seen with *docetaxel*. The latter drug is contraindicated in patients with cardiac disease. Alopecia occurs, but vomiting and diarrhea are uncommon. Because of serious hypersensitivity reactions (including dyspnea, urticaria, and hypotension), a patient who is to be treated with *paclitaxel* is premedicated with *dexamethasone* and *diphenhydramine* as well as with an H_2 blocker.

VII. STEROID HORMONES AND THEIR ANTAGONISTS

Tumors that are steroid hormone–sensitive may be either 1) hormone responsive, in which the tumor regresses following treatment with a specific hormone; 2) hormone dependent, in which removal of a hormonal stimulus causes tumor regression; or 3) both. Hormone treatment of responsive tumors usually is only palliative, except in the case of the cytotoxic effect of glucocorticoids at higher doses (for example, *prednisone*) on lymphomas. Removal of hormonal stimuli from hormone-dependent tumors can be accomplished by surgery (for example, in the case of orchiectomy for patients with advanced prostate cancer) or by drugs (for example, in breast cancer, for which treatment with the antiestrogen *tamoxifen* is used to prevent estrogen stimulation of breast cancer cells). For a steroid hormone to influence a cell, that cell must have intracellular (cytosolic) receptors that are specific for that hormone (Figure 39.28A).

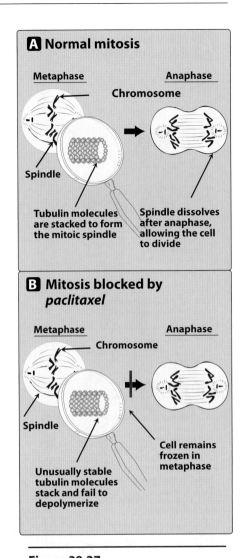

Figure 39.27
Paclitaxel stabilizes microtubules, rendering them nonfunctional.

Plant alkyloids

Vincristin
Vinblustin
Paclitaxel
docetaxel

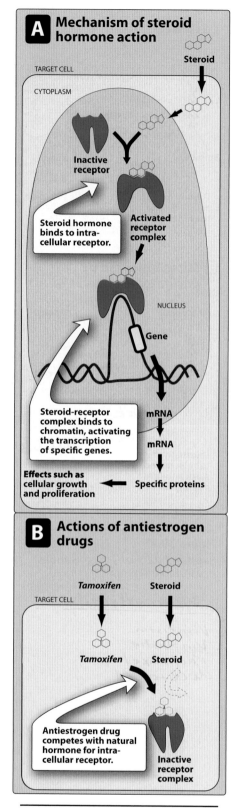

A **Mechanism of steroid hormone action**

TARGET CELL

CYTOPLASM

Steroid

Inactive receptor

Steroid hormone binds to intra-cellular receptor.

Activated receptor complex

NUCLEUS

Gene

Steroid-receptor complex binds to chromatin, activating the transcription of specific genes.

mRNA

mRNA

Effects such as cellular growth and proliferation ← Specific proteins

B **Actions of antiestrogen drugs**

Tamoxifen   Steroid

TARGET CELL

Tamoxifen   Steroid

Antiestrogen drug competes with natural hormone for intra-cellular receptor.

Inactive receptor complex

Figure 39.28
Action of steroid hormones and antiestrogen agents.

A. Prednisone

Prednisone [PRED-ni-sone] is a potent, synthetic, anti-inflammatory cor-ticosteroid with less mineralocorticoid activity than *cortisol*. The use of this compound in the treatment of lymphomas arose when it was observed that patients with Cushing's syndrome, which is associated with hypersecretion of cortisol, have lymphocytopenia and decreased lymphoid mass. [Note: At high doses, *cortisol* is also lymphocytolytic and leads to hyperuricemia due to the breakdown of lymphocytes.] *Prednisone* is primarily employed to induce remission in patients with acute lymphocytic leukemia and in the treatment of both Hodgkin's and non-Hodgkin's lymphomas.

1. **Mechanism of action:** *Prednisone* itself is inactive and must first be reduced to *prednisolone* by 11-β-hydroxysteroid dehydrogenase.[11] This steroid then binds to a receptor that triggers the production of specific proteins (see Figure 39.28A).

2. **Resistance:** Resistance is associated with an absence of the receptor protein or a mutation that lowers receptor affinity for the hormone. However, in some resistant cells, a receptor-hormone complex is formed, although a stage of gene expression is apparently affected.

3. **Pharmacokinetics:** *Prednisone* is readily absorbed orally. Like other glucocorticoids, it is bound to plasma albumin and transcor-tin. It undergoes 11-β-hydroxylation to *prednisolone* in the liver. *Prednisolone* is the active drug. The latter is glucuronidated and excreted into the urine along with the parent compound.

4. **Adverse effects:** *Prednisone* has many of the adverse effects asso-ciated with glucocorticoids. It can predispose to infection (due to its immunosuppressant action) and to ulcers and pancreatitis. Other effects include hyperglycemia, cataract formation, glaucoma, osteo-porosis, and change in mood (euphoria or psychosis).

B. Tamoxifen

Tamoxifen [tah-MOX-ih-fen] is an estrogen antagonist. It is structurally related to the synthetic estrogen *diethylstilbestrol* and is used for first-line therapy in the treatment of estrogen receptor–positive breast can-cer. *Tamoxifen* has weak estrogenic activity, and it is classified as a selec-tive estrogen-receptor modulator (SERM). Another SERM that has been approved for advanced breast cancer in postmenopausal women is *toremifene* [tore-EM-ih-feen]. It also finds use prophylactically in reduc-ing breast cancer occurrence in women who are at high risk. However, because of possible effects stimulating premalignant lesions due to its estrogenic properties, *tamoxifen* is presently approved only for 5 years of use.

1. **Mechanism of action:** *Tamoxifen* binds to the estrogen receptor, but the complex is transcriptionally not productive. That is, the complex fails to induce estrogen-responsive genes, and RNA synthesis does not ensue (Figure 39.28B). The result is a depletion (down-regula-tion) of estrogen receptors, and the growth-promoting effects of the

[11] See p. 238 in *Lippincott's Illustrated Reviews: Biochemistry* (4th ed.) for the reaction catalyzed by 11-β-hydroxysteroid dehydrogenase.

natural hormone and other growth factors are suppressed. [Note: Estrogen competes with *tamoxifen*. Therefore, in premenopausal women, the drug is used with a gonadotropin-releasing hormone (GnRH) analog such as *leuprolide*, which lowers estrogen levels.] The action of *tamoxifen* is not related to any specific phase of the cell cycle.

2. **Resistance:** Resistance is associated with a decreased affinity for the receptor or the presence of a dysfunctional receptor.

3. **Pharmacokinetics:** *Tamoxifen* is effective on oral administration. It is partially metabolized by the liver. Some metabolites possess antagonist activity, whereas others have agonist activity. Unchanged drug and its metabolites are excreted predominantly through the bile into the feces (Figure 39.29).

4. **Adverse effects:** Side effects caused by *tamoxifen* are similar to the effects of natural estrogen, including hot flashes, nausea, vomiting, skin rash, vaginal bleeding, and discharge (due to some slight estrogenic activity of the drug and some of its metabolites). Hypercalcemia requiring cessation of the drug may occur. *Tamoxifen* can also lead to increased pain if the tumor has metastasized to bone. *Tamoxifen* has the potential to cause endometrial cancer. Other toxicities include thromboembolism and effects on vision. [Note: Because of a more favorable adverse effect profile, aromatase inhibitors are making an impact in the treatment of breast cancer.]

C. Aromatase inhibitors

The aromatase reaction is responsible for the extra-adrenal synthesis of estrogen from androstenedione, which takes place in liver, fat, muscle, skin, and breast tissue, including breast malignancies. Peripheral aromatization is an important source of estrogen in postmenopausal women. Aromatase inhibitors decrease the production of estrogen in these women.

1. **Aminoglutethimide:** *Aminoglutethimide* [ah-mee-noe-glue-TETH-ih-mide] was the first aromatase inhibitor to be identified for the treatment of metastatic breast cancer in postmenopausal women. *Aminoglutethimide* was shown to inhibit both the adrenal synthesis of pregnenolone (a precursor of estrogen) from cholesterol as well as the extra-adrenal synthesis. Because the drug also inhibits hydrocortisone synthesis, which evokes a compensatory rise in adrenocorticotropic hormone secretion sufficient to overwhelm the blockade of the adrenal, the drug is usually taken with *hydrocortisone*. Due to its nonselective properties and unfavorable side effects, as well as the need to concomitantly administer *hydrocortisone* (*cortisol*), newer aromatase inhibitors (described below) have been developed.

2. **Anastrozole and letrozole:** The imidazole aromatase inhibitors, such as *anastrozole* [an-AS-troe-zole] and *letrozole* [LE-troe-zole], are nonsteroidal. They have gained favor in the treatment of breast cancer because 1) they are more potent (they inhibit aromatization by greater than 96 percent, compared to less than 90 percent with *aminoglutethimide*), 2) they are more selective than *aminoglutethimide*, 3) they do not need to be supplemented with hydrocortisone, 4) they do not predispose to endometrial cancer, and 5) they are devoid of the androgenic side effects that occur with the steroidal

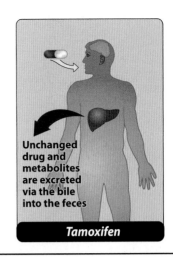

Unchanged drug and metabolites are excreted via the bile into the feces

Tamoxifen

Figure 39.29
Administration and fate of *tamoxifen*.

Estrogen stimulates Osteoblasts
ao stimulate osteoclasts

↓
Block estrogen, block Osteoblasts

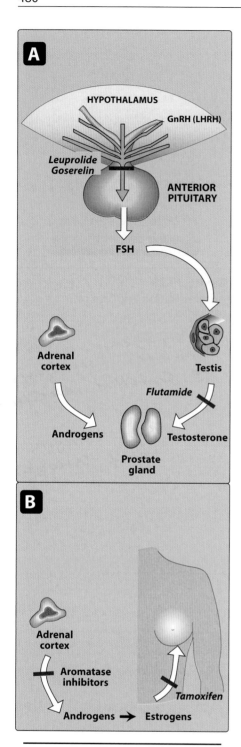

Figure 39.30
Effects of some anticancer drugs on the endocrine system. A. In therapy for prostatic cancer. B. In therapy of postmenopausal breast cancer. FSH = follicle-stimulating hormone; GnRH (LHRH) = gonadotropin-releasing hormone (luteinizing hormone-releasing hormone).

aromatase inhibitors. Although *anastrozole* and *letrozole* are considered to be second-line therapy after *tamoxifen* for hormone-dependent breast cancer in the United States, they have become first-line drugs in other countries for the treatment of breast cancer in postmenopausal women. They are orally active and cause almost a total suppression of estrogen synthesis. They are cleared primarily by liver metabolism.

3. **Exemestane:** A steroidal, irreversible inhibitor of aromatase, *exemestane* [ex-uh-MES-tane], is orally well absorbed and widely distributed. Hepatic metabolism is by the CYP3A4 isozyme, but to date, no interactions have been reported. Because the metabolites are excreted into the urine, doses of the drug must be adjusted in patients with renal failure. Its major toxicities are nausea, fatigue, and hot flashes. Acne and hair changes also occur.

D. Progestins

Megestrol [me-JESS-trole] *acetate* was formerly the progestin used most widely in treating metastatic hormone-responsive breast and endometrial neoplasms. It is orally effective. Other agents are usually compared to it in clinical trials. However, the aromatase inhibitors are replacing it in therapy.

E. Leuprolide and goserelin — GnRH agonists

Gonadotropin-releasing hormone is normally secreted by the hypothalamus and stimulates the anterior pituitary to secrete the gonadotropic hormones, luteinizing hormone (LH; the primary stimulus for the secretion of testosterone by the testes), and follicle-stimulating hormone (FSH; which stimulates the secretion of estrogen). The synthetic nonapeptides, *leuprolide* [loo-PROE-lide] and *goserelin* [GOE-se-rel-in], are analogs of GnRH. As GnRH agonists, they occupy the GnRH receptor in the pituitary, which leads to its desensitization and, consequently, inhibition of release of FSH and LH. Thus, both androgen and estrogen syntheses are reduced (Figure 39.30). Response to *leuprolide* in prostatic cancer is equivalent to that of orchiectomy (surgical removal of one or both testes), with regression of tumor and relief of bone pain. These drugs have some benefit in premenopausal women with advanced breast cancer and have largely replaced estrogens in therapy for prostate cancer. *Leuprolide* is available 1) as a sustained-release preparation, 2) subcutaneous, or 3) as a depot intramuscular injection to treat metastatic carcinoma of the prostate. *Goserelin acetate* is implanted intramuscularly. Levels of androgen may initially rise but then fall to castration levels. The adverse effects of these drugs, including impotence, hot flashes, and tumor flare, are minimal compared to those experienced with estrogen treatment.

F. Estrogens

Estrogens, such as *ethinyl estradiol* or *diethylstilbestrol*, had been used in the treatment of prostatic cancer. However, they have been largely replaced by the GnRH analogs because of fewer adverse effects. Estrogens inhibit the growth of prostatic tissue by blocking the production of LH, thereby decreasing the synthesis of androgens in the testis. Thus, tumors that are dependent on androgens are affected. Estrogen treatment can cause serious complications, such as thromboemboli, myocardial infarction, strokes, and hypercalcemia. Men who are taking estrogens may experience gynecomastia and impotence.

G. Flutamide, nilutamide, and bicalutamide

Flutamide [FLOO-tah-mide], *nilutamide* [nye-LOO-ta-mide], and *bicalutamide* [bye-ka-LOO-ta-mide] are synthetic, nonsteroidal antiandrogens used in the treatment of prostate cancer. They compete with the natural hormone for binding to the androgen receptor and prevent its translocation into the nucleus (see Figure 39.30). *Flutamide* is metabolized to an active hydroxy derivative that binds to the androgen receptor. *Flutamide* blocks the inhibitory effects of testosterone on gonadotropin secretion, causing an increase in serum LH and testosterone levels. Therefore, *flutamide* is always administered in combination with *leuprolide* or *goserelin* which can desensitize the hypothalamus-pituitary axis. These antiandrogens are taken orally. [Note: *Flutamide* requires dosing three times a day and the others once a day.] These agents are cleared through the kidney. Side effects include gynecomastia and GI distress and, in the case of *flutamide*, liver failure could occur. *Nilutamide* can cause visual problems.

VIII. MONOCLONAL ANTIBODIES

Monoclonal antibodies have become an active area of drug development for anticancer therapy and other nonneoplastic diseases, because they are directed at specific targets and often have fewer adverse effects. They are created from B lymphocytes (from immunized mice or hamsters) fused with "immortal" B-lymphocyte tumor cells. The resulting hybrid cells can be individually cloned, and each clone will produce antibodies directed against a single antigen type. Recombinant technology has led to the creation of "humanized" antibodies that overcome the immunologic problems previously observed following administration of mouse (murine) antibodies. Currently, several monoclonal antibodies are available in the United States for the treatment of cancer. *Trastuzumab, rituximab, bevacizumab,* and *cetuximab* are described below. Others include *gemtuzumab ozogamicin,* which is a monoclonal antibody conjugated with a plant toxin that binds to CD33—a cell-surface receptor that is present on the leukemia cells of 80 percent of patients with acute myelocytic leukemia; *alemtuzumab,* which is effective in treatment of B-cell chronic lymphocytic leukemia that no longer responds to other agents; and I^{131}-*tositumomab,* which is used in relapsed non-Hodgkin's lymphoma.

A. Trastuzumab

In patients with metastatic breast cancer, overexpression of transmembrane human epidermal growth factor–receptor protein 2 (HER2) is seen in 25 to 30 percent of patients. *Trastuzumab* [tra-STEW-zoo-mab], a recombinant DNA–produced, humanized monoclonal antibody, specifically targets the extracellular domain of the HER2 growth receptor that has intrinsic tyrosine kinase activity. The drug, usually administered with *paclitaxel,* can cause regression of breast cancer and metastases in a small percentage of these individuals. [Note: At least 50 tyrosine kinases mediate cell growth or division by phosphorylating signaling proteins. They have been implicated in the development of many neoplasms by an unknown mechanism.] *Trastuzumab* binds to HER2 sites in breast cancer tissue and inhibits the proliferation of cells that overexpress the HER2 protein, thereby decreasing the number of cells in the S phase.

1. **Mechanism of action:** How the antibody causes its anticancer effect remains to be elucidated. Several mechanisms have been proposed—for example, down-regulation of HER2-receptor expression, an induction of antibody-dependent cytotoxicity, or a decrease in angiogenesis due to an effect on vascular endothelial growth factor. Efforts are being directed toward identifying those patients with tumors that are sensitive to the drug.

2. **Pharmacokinetics:** *Trastuzumab* is administered IV. *Trastuzumab* does not penetrate the blood-brain barrier.

3. **Adverse effects:** The most serious toxicity associated with the use of *trastuzumab* is congestive heart failure. The toxicity is worsened if given in combination with *anthracycline*. Extreme caution should be exercised when giving the drugs to patients with preexisting cardiac dysfunction. Other adverse effects include infusion-related fever and chills, headache, dizziness, nausea, vomiting, abdominal pain, and back pain, but these effects are well tolerated. Cautious use of the drug is recommended in patients who are hypersensitive to the Chinese hamster ovary (CHO) cell components of the proteins or to benzyl alcohol (in which case sterile water can be used in place of the bacteriostatic solution provided for preparation of the injection).

B. Rituximab

Rituximab (ri-TUCX-ih-mab) was the first monoclonal antibody to be approved for the treatment of cancer. It is a genetically engineered, chimeric monoclonal antibody directed against the CD20 antigen that is found on the surfaces of normal and malignant B lymphocytes. CD20 plays a role in the activation process for cell-cycle initiation and differentiation. The CD20 antigen is expressed on nearly all B-cell non-Hodgkin's lymphomas, but not in other bone marrow cells. *Rituximab* has proven to be effective in the treatment of posttransplant lymphoma and in chronic lymphocytic leukemia.

Rituximab—
Leukemias
(Lymphocytic)

1. **Mechanism of action:** The Fab domain of *rituximab* binds to the CD20 antigen on the B lymphocytes, and its Fc domain recruits immune effector functions, inducing complement and antibody-dependent, cell-mediated cytotoxicity of the B cells. The antibody is commonly used with other combinations of anticancer agents, such as *cyclophosphamide, doxorubicin, vincristine (Oncovin),* and *prednisone* (CHOP).

2. **Pharmacokinetics:** *Rituximab* is infused IV and causes a rapid depletion of B cells (both normal and malignant). The fate of the antibody has not been described.

3. **Adverse effects:** Severe adverse reactions have been fatal. It is important to infuse *rituximab* slowly. Hypotension, bronchospasm, and angioedema may occur. Chills and fever frequently accompany the first infusion, especially in patients with high circulating levels of neoplastic cells, because of rapid activation of complement, which results in the release of tumor necrosis factor α and interleukins. Pretreatment with *diphenhydramine, acetaminophen,* and bronchodilators can ameliorate these problems. Cardiac arrhythmias can also occur. Tumor lysis syndrome has been reported within 24 hours of the first dose of *rituximab*. This syndrome consists of acute renal

failure that may require dialysis, hyperkalemia, hypocalcemia, hyperuricemia, and hyperphosphatasemia (an abnormally high content of alkaline phosphatase in the blood). Leukopenia, thrombocytopenia, and neutropenia have been reported in less than 10 percent of patients.

C. Bevacizumab

The monoclonal antibody, *bevacizumab* [be-vah-SEE-zoo-mab] is the first in a new class of anticancer drugs called antiangiogenesis agents. *Bevacizumab* is approved for use as a first-line drug against metastatic colorectal cancer and is given with *5-FU based chemotherapy*. *Bevacizumab* is infused IV. It attaches to and stops vascular endothelial growth factor from stimulating the formation of new blood vessels. Without new blood vessels, tumors do not receive oxygen and essential nutrients necessary for growth and proliferation. The most common adverse effects of this treatment are hypertension, stomatitis, and diarrhea. Less common are bleeding in the intestines, protein in the urine, and heart failure. Among the rare serious side effects are bowel perforation, opening of healed wounds, and stroke.

Bevacizumab
↓
Vascular antibodies for colorectal cancer

D. Cetuximab

Cetuximab [see-TUX-i-mab] is another chimeric monoclonal antibody that has recently been approved to treat colorectal cancer. It is believed to exert its antineoplastic effect by targeting the epidermal growth factor receptor on the surface of cancer cells and interfering with their growth. It is usually combined with *irinotecan* during treatment. Like other antibodies, it is administered IV. *Cetuximab* has caused difficulty breathing and low blood pressure during the first treatment, and interstitial lung disease has been reported. Other side effects include rash, fever, constipation, and abdominal pain.

Cetuximab — colorectal cancer

IX. OTHER CHEMOTHERAPEUTIC AGENTS

A. Platinum coordination complexes

Cisplatin [SIS-pla-tin] was the first member of the platinum coordination complex class of anticancer drugs, but because of its severe toxicity, *carboplatin* [KAR-boe-pla-tin] was developed. The mechanisms of action of the two drugs are similar, but their potency, pharmacokinetics, patterns of distribution, and dose-limiting toxicities differ significantly. *Cisplatin* has synergistic cytotoxicity with radiation and other chemotherapeutic agents. *Oxaliplatin* [ox-AL-ih-pla-tin], a new member of this class of drugs, is a closely related analog of *carboplatin*. *Cisplatin* has found wide application in the treatment of solid tumors, such as metastatic testicular carcinoma in combination with *VBL* and *bleomycin*, ovarian carcinoma in combination with *cyclophosphamide*, or alone for bladder carcinoma. *Carboplatin* is employed when patients cannot be vigorously hydrated, as is required for *cisplatin* treatment, or if they suffer from kidney dysfunction or are prone to neuro- or ototoxicity. *Oxaliplatin* is showing excellent activity against advanced colorectal cancer.

1. **Mechanism of action:** The mechanism of action for this class of drugs is similar to that of the alkylating agents. In the high-chloride milieu of the plasma, *cisplatin* persists as the neutral species, which enters the cell and loses its chlorides in the low-chloride milieu. It then binds to the N^7 of guanine in DNA, forming inter- and intra-

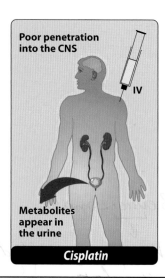

Figure 39.31
Administration and fate of *cisplatin*.

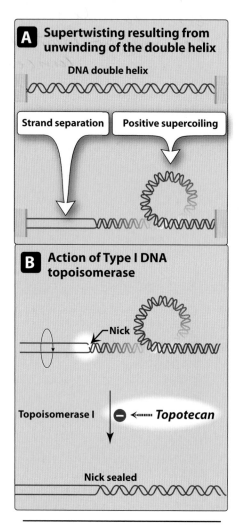

Figure 39.32
Action of Type I DNA topoisomerases.

strand cross-links. The resulting cytotoxic lesion inhibits both DNA replication and RNA synthesis. Similarly, the chemical moieties that replace the chlorides in the *carboplatin* structure are removed hydrolytically to form the active drug. Cytotoxicity can occur at any stage of the cell cycle, but cells are most vulnerable to the actions of these drugs in the G_1 and S phases. Both drugs can also bind proteins and other compounds containing thiol (–SH) groups.

2. **Resistance:** Sensitivity to these agents is decreased if cells have elevated glutathione levels or increased DNA repair or if metallothionein (a protein rich in –SH groups) is induced. Decreased cellular uptake has also been implicated. Cross-resistance between *cisplatin* and *carboplatin* is not invariable. However, there is none with *oxaliplatin*.

3. **Pharmacokinetics:** These agents are administered IV in saline solution. They can also be given intraperitoneally for ovarian cancer and intra-arterially to perfuse other organs. More than 90 percent of *cisplatin* is covalently bound to plasma proteins, but the binding of *carboplatin* to plasma proteins is very low. The highest concentrations of the drugs are found in the liver, kidney, and intestinal, testicular, and ovarian cells, but little penetrates into the CSF. The renal route is the main avenue for excretion (Figure 39.31).

4. **Adverse effects:** Severe, persistent vomiting occurs for at least 1 hour after administration of *cisplatin* and may continue for as long as 5 days. Premedication with antiemetic agents is usually helpful. The major limiting toxicity is dose-related nephrotoxicity, involving the distal convoluted tubule and collecting ducts. This can be ameliorated by aggressive hydration and diuresis. Hypomagnesemia and hypocalcemia usually occur concurrently. [Note: It is important to correct calcium levels before correcting magnesium levels.] Other toxicities include ototoxicity with high-frequency hearing loss and tinnitus, mild bone marrow suppression, some neurotoxicity characterized by paresthesia and loss of proprioception, and hypersensitivity reactions ranging from skin rashes to anaphylaxis. Patients concomitantly receiving aminoglycosides are at greater risk for nephrotoxicity and ototoxicity. Unlike *cisplatin*, *carboplatin* causes only mild nausea and vomiting, and it is not nephro-, neuro-, or ototoxic. Its dose-limiting toxicity is myelosuppression.

B. Irinotecan and topotecan

Irinotecan [eye-rin-oh-TEE-kan] and *topotecan* [toe-poe-TEE-kan] are semisynthetic derivatives of an earlier, more toxic drug, *camptothecin* [camp-toe-THEE-sin]. They have a complicated multiring structure containing a lactone ring that is essential for activity. *Topotecan* is employed in metastatic ovarian cancer when primary therapy has failed and also in the treatment of small-cell lung cancer. *Irinotecan* is used as a first-line drug together with *5-FU* and *leucovorin* for the treatment of colon or rectal carcinoma.

1. **Mechanism of action:** These drugs are S-phase specific. They inhibit topoisomerase I, which is essential for the replication of DNA in human cells (Figure 39.32). Unlike *etoposide*, which inhibits the related enzyme topoisomerase II (see below), *topotecan* was the first clinically useful topoisomerase I inhibitor. SN-38 (the active metabolite of *irinotecan*) is formed from *irinotecan* by carboxylesterase-

mediated cleavage of the carbamate bond between the camptoth-ecin moiety and the dipiperidino side chain. SN-38 is approximately 1000 times as potent as *irinotecan* as an inhibitor of topoisomerase I. The topoisomerases relieve torsional strain in DNA by causing revers-ible, single-strand breaks. By binding to the enzyme-DNA complex, *topotecan* or SN-38 prevent religation of the single-strand breaks.

2. **Resistance:** Several mechanisms may explain resistance. Among them are the ability to transport the drugs out of the cell, decreased ability to convert *irinotecan* to the active SN-38 metabolite, or a down-regulation or mutation in topoisomerase I.

3. **Pharmacokinetics:** *Topotecan* and *irinotecan* are infused IV. Hydrolysis of the lactone ring destroys the activity of these drugs. Both the drugs and their metabolites are eliminated in the urine. Therefore, the dose may have to be modified in patients with impaired kidney function.

4. **Adverse effects:** Bone marrow suppression—particularly neutro-penia—is the dose-limiting toxicity for *topotecan*. Frequent periph-eral blood counts should be performed on patients taking this drug. [Note: *Topotecan* should not be used in patients with a baseline neu-trophil count of less than 1500 cells/mm^3. Doing so could result in infection and death.] Other hematologic complications, including thrombocytopenia and anemia, may also occur. Nonhematologic effects include diarrhea, nausea, vomiting, alopecia, and headache. Myelosuppression is also seen with *irinotecan*, and delayed diarrhea may be severe and require treatment with *loperamide*.

C. Etoposide (VP-16)

Etoposide [e-toe-POE-side] and its analog, *teniposide* [ten-i-POE-side], are semisynthetic derivatives of the plant alkaloid, podophyllotoxin. They block cells in the late S to G$_2$ phase of the cell cycle. Their major target is topoisomerase II. Binding of the drugs to the enzyme-DNA complex results in persistence of the transient, cleavable form of the complex and, thus, renders it susceptible to irreversible double-strand breaks (Figure 39.33). Resistance to topoisomerase inhibitors is con-ferred either by presence of the multidrug-resistant P-glycoprotein or by mutation of the enzyme. *Etoposide* finds its major clinical use in the treatment of oat-cell carcinoma of the lung and in combination with *bleomycin* and *cisplatin* for testicular carcinoma. *Teniposide* is used as a second-line agent in the treatment of acute lymphocytic leukemia. *Etoposide* may be administered either IV or orally, whereas *teniposide* is only administered IV. They are highly bound to plasma proteins and distribute throughout the body, but they enter the CSF poorly. Despite this, *teniposide* has shown effectiveness against gliomas and neuroblastomas. Metabolites are converted to glucuronide and sulfate conjugates and are excreted in the urine. Drugs that induce the cyto-chrome P450 system lead to an acceleration of *teniposide* metabolism. Dose-limiting myelosuppression (primarily leukopenia) is the major toxicity for both drugs. Leukemia may develop in patients who were treated with *etoposide*. Other toxicities are alopecia, anaphylactic reac-tions, nausea, and vomiting.

D. Imatinib

Imatinib [i-MAT-in-ib] *mesylate* is used for the treatment of chronic myel-oid leukemia in blast crisis, as well as GI stromal tumor. It acts as a signal

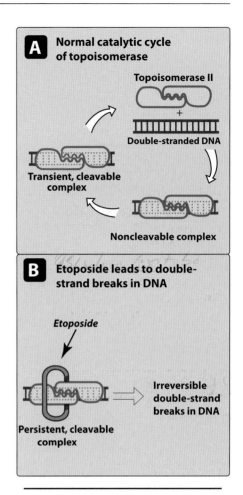

Figure 39.33
Mechanism of action of *etoposide*.

transduction inhibitor, used specifically to inhibit tumor tyrosine kinase activity. A deregulated BCR-ABL kinase is present in the leukemia cells of almost every patient with chronic myeloid leukemia. In the case of GI stromal tumor, an unregulated expression of tyrosine kinase is associated with a growth factor. The ability of *imatinib* to occupy the "kinase pocket" prevents the phosphorylation of tyrosine on the substrate molecule and, hence, inhibits subsequent steps that lead to cell proliferation. *Imatinib* has the advantage over *interferon-α* in that it can be given orally. It also has a more rapid hematologic response than *interferon-α* plus *cytarabine*. Studies of cell lines indicate that resistance may occur by amplification of the BCR-ABL gene and/or by increased efflux due to increased multidrug-resistance protein. The drug is very well absorbed orally. It undergoes metabolism by the cytochrome P450 system to several compounds, of which the N-demethyl derivative is active. Excretion is predominantly through the feces. Adverse effects include fluid retention and edema, hepatotoxicity, thrombocytopenia or neutropenia, as well as nausea and vomiting.

E. Gefitinib (Iressa)

Gefitinib [ge-FIN-ih-tib] targets the epidermal growth factor receptor. It is approved for the treatment of non–small cell lung cancer that has failed to respond to other therapy, and it is effective in 10 to 20 percent of patients with this cancer. *Gefitinib* is usually used as a single agent. *Gefitinib* is absorbed after oral administration and undergoes extensive metabolism in the liver by the cytochrome P450 enzyme CYP3A4. At least five metabolites have been identified, only one of which has significant antitumor activity. The major route of excretion of the drug and its metabolites is the feces. The most common adverse effects are diarrhea, nausea, and acne-like skin rashes. A rare but potentially fatal adverse effect is interstitial lung disease, which presents as acute dyspnea with cough.

F. Procarbazine

Procarbazine [proe-KAR-ba-zeen] is used in the treatment of Hodgkin's disease and other cancers. *Procarbazine* rapidly equilibrates between the plasma and the CSF after oral or parenteral administration. It must undergo a series of oxidative reactions to exert its cytotoxic action that causes inhibition of DNA, RNA, and protein synthesis. Metabolites and the parent drug are excreted via the kidney. Bone marrow depression is the major toxicity, and nausea, vomiting, and diarrhea are common. The drug is also neurotoxic, causing symptoms ranging from drowsiness to hallucinations to paresthesias. Because it inhibits monoamine oxidase, patients should be warned against ingesting foods that contain tyramine (for example, aged cheeses, beer, and wine). Ingestion of alcohol leads to a disulfiram-type reaction). *Procarbazine* is both mutagenic and teratogenic. Nonlymphocytic leukemia has developed in patients treated with the drug.

G. L-Asparaginase

L-Asparaginase [ah-SPAR-a-gi-nase] catalyzes the deamination of asparagine to aspartic acid and ammonia. The form of the enzyme used chemotherapeutically is derived from bacteria. *L-Asparaginase* is used to treat childhood acute lymphocytic leukemia in combination with *VX and *prednisone*. Its mechanism of action is based on the fact that some neoplastic cells require an external source of asparagine because of their limited capacity to synthesize sufficient amounts of that amino acid to support growth and function. *L-Asparaginase* hydrolyzes blood asparagine and, thus, deprives the tumor cells of this amino acid, which is needed for protein synthesis (Figure 39.34). Resistance to the drug is due to increased capacity of tumor cells to synthesize asparagine. The enzyme must be administered either IV or intramuscularly, because it is destroyed by gastric enzymes. Toxicities include a range of hypersensitivity reactions (because it is a foreign protein), a decrease in clotting factors, liver abnormalities, pancreatitis, seizures, and coma due to ammonia toxicity.

H. Interferons

Human interferons have been classified into three types—α, β, and γ—on the basis of their antigenicity. The α interferons are primarily leukocytic, whereas the β and γ interferons are produced by connective tissue fibroblasts and T lymphocytes, respectively. Recombinant DNA techniques in bacteria have made it possible to produce large quantities of pure interferons, including two species designated *interferon-α-2a* and *-2b* that are employed in treating neoplastic diseases. *Interferon-α-2a* is presently approved for the management of hairy-cell leukemia, chronic myeloid leukemia, and acquired immunodeficiency syndrome (AIDS)–related Kaposi sarcoma. *Interferon-α-2b* is approved for the treatment of hairy-cell leukemia, melanoma, AIDS-related Kaposi's sarcoma, and follicular lymphoma.

1. **Mechanism of action:** Interferons secreted from producing cells interact with surface receptors on other cells, at which site they exert their effects. Bound interferons are neither internalized nor degraded. The α and β interferons compete with each other for binding and, therefore, presumably bind at the same receptor or in close proximity; the γ interferons bind at different receptors. As a consequence of the binding of interferon, a series of complex intracellular reactions take place. These include synthesis of enzymes, suppression of cell proliferation, activation of macrophages, and increased cytotoxicity of lymphocytes. However, the exact mechanism by which the interferons are cytotoxic is unknown

2. **Pharmacokinetics:** Interferons are well absorbed after intramuscular or subcutaneous injections. An IV form of *interferon-α-2b* is also available. Interferons undergo glomerular filtration and are degraded during reabsorption, but liver metabolism is minimal.

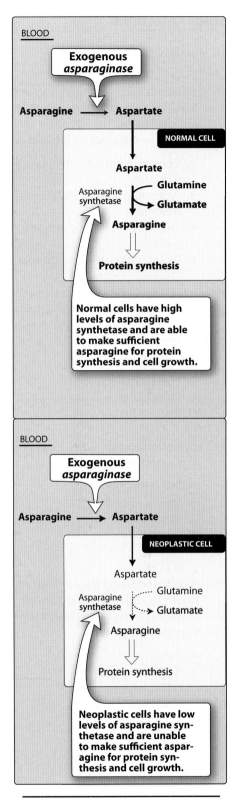

Figure 39.34
Activity of asparagine synthetase in normal and neoplastic cells.

Study Questions

Choose the ONE best answer.

39.1 A patient with colonic cancer is being treated with 5-FU as well as leucovorin (N^5,N^{10}-methylene tetrahydrofolate). The rationale for administering the coenzyme depends on it being essential for:

    A. Conversion of 5-FU to fluorodeoxyuridylic acid (FdUMP).

    B. Protection against the anemia caused by 5-FU treatment.

    C. The inhibition of thymidylate synthase by FdUMP.

    D. Prolongation of the antitumor effect of 5-FU.

> Correct answer = C. Thymidylate synthase forms a ternary complex with thymidine and N^5,N^{10}-methylene tetrahydrofolic acid. Consequently, the coenzyme is required for 5-FU to be effective, albeit as the mononucleotide metabolite (FdUMP). It plays no role in the conversion of 5-FU to FdUMP. 5-FU does not cause megaloblastic anemia. The coenzyme does not affect the pharmacokinetics of 5-FU.

39.2 Neutropenia develops in a patient undergoing cancer chemotherapy. Administration of which one of the following agents would accelerate recovery of neutrophil counts?

    A. Leucovorin.
    B. Filgrastim.
    C. Prednisone.
    D. Vitamin B_{12}.

> Correct answer = B. Filgrastim is a a human granulocyte colony-stimulating factor that can act on hematopoietic cells to stimulate proliferation. It regulates production of neutrophils in the bone marrow and, thus, is effective in reversing neutropenia in patients undergoing cancer chemotherapy. Leucovorin, the N^5,N^{10}-derivative of tetrahydrofolic acid, and vitamin B12, although they would be effective in the treatment of anemias, would not increase neutrophil counts. The glucocorticoid, prednisone, is also ineffective.

39.3 Hydration and/or diuresis can prevent the renal toxicity associated with:

    A. Cisplatin.
    B. Chlorambucil.
    C. Tamoxifen.
    D. Gemcitabine.
    E. MTX.

> Correct answer = A. In the list above, only cisplatin causes renal toxicity.

39.4 A patient is being treated with allopurinol to control hyperuricemia resulting from chemotherapy. Which of the following would have to have its dose reduced to prevent toxicity?

    A. 5-FU.
    B. 6-MP.
    C. 6-TG.
    D. Fludarabine.
    E. Cytarabine.

> Correct answer = B. Mercaptopurine is metabolized to 6-thiouric acid by xanthine oxidase. Prevention of this reaction by allopurinol would divert more of the antimetabolite to cytotoxic pathways. 6-TG undergoes minimal metabolism by the xanthine oxidase pathway and, thus, is not affected by allopurinol. Nor is fludarabine metabolized by this pathway, because it does not undergo deamination by adenosine deaminase, which would be required for metabolization by xanthine oxidase. The other two agents are pyrimidine compounds and, thus, are not biotransformed to uric acid.

Immunosuppressants

40

I. OVERVIEW

The importance of the immune system in protecting the body against harmful foreign molecules is well recognized. However, in some instances, this protection can result in serious problems. For example, the introduction of an allograft (that is, the graft of an organ or tissue from one individual to another who is not genetically identical) can elicit a damaging immune response, causing rejection of the transplanted tissue. Transplantation of organs and tissues (for example, kidney, heart, or bone marrow) has become routine due to improved surgical techniques and better tissue typing. Also, drugs are now available that more selectively inhibit rejection of transplanted tissues while preventing the patient from becoming immunologically compromised (Figure 40.1). Earlier drugs were nonselective, and patients frequently succumbed to infection due to suppression of both the antibody-mediated (humoral) and cell-mediated arms of the immune system. Today, the principal approach to immunosuppressive therapy is to alter lymphocyte function using drugs or antibodies against immune proteins. Because of their severe toxicities when used as monotherapy, a combination of immunosuppressive agents, usually at lower doses, is generally employed. [Note: Immunosuppressive therapy is also used in the treatment of autoimmune diseases; for example, corticosteroids can control acute glomerulonephritis.] Immunosuppressive drug regimens usually consist of anywhere from two to four agents with different mechanisms of action that disrupt various levels of T-cell activation. The immune activation cascade can be described as a three-signal model. Signal 1 constitutes T-cell triggering at the CD3 receptor complex by an antigen on the surface of an antigen-presenting cell (APC). Signal 2, also referred to as costimulation, occurs when CD80 and CD86 on the surface of APCs engage CD28 on T cells. Both Signals 1 and 2 activate several intracellular signal transduction pathways, one of which is the calcium-calcineurin pathway, which is targeted by *cyclosporine* and *tacrolimus*. These pathways trigger the production of cytokines such as interleukin (IL)-2, IL-15, CD154, and CD25. IL-2 then binds to CD25 (also known as the IL-2 receptor) on the surface of other T cells to activate mammalian target of *rapamycin* (mTOR), providing Signal 3, the stimulus for T-cell proliferation. Immunosuppressive drugs can be categorized according to their mechanisms of action: 1) Some agents interfere with cytokine production or action; 2) others disrupt cell metabolism, preventing lymphocyte proliferation; and 3) mono- and polyclonal antibodies block T-cell surface molecules.

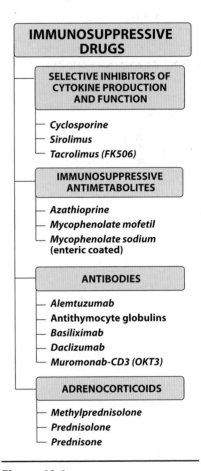

Figure 40.1
Immunosuppressant drugs.

Cytokine	Actions
IL-1	• Enhances activity of NK cells • Attracts neutrophils and macrophages
IL-2	• Induces proliferation of antigen-primed T cells • Enhances activity of NK cells
IFN-γ	• Enhances activity of macrophages and NK cells • Increases expression of MHC molecules • Enhances production of IgG$_{2a}$
TNF-α	• Cytotoxic effect on tumor cells • Induces cytokine secretion in the inflammatory response

Figure 40.2
Summary of selected cytokines.

II. SELECTIVE INHIBITORS OF CYTOKINE PRODUCTION AND FUNCTION

Cytokines are soluble, antigen-nonspecific, signaling proteins that bind to cell surface receptors on a variety of cells. The term cytokine includes the molecules known as ILs, interferons (IFNs), tumor necrosis factors (TNFs), transforming growth factors, and colony-stimulating factors. Of particular interest when discussing immunosuppressive drugs is IL-2—a growth factor that stimulates the proliferation of antigen-primed (helper) T cells, which subsequently produce more IL-2, IFN-γ, and TNF-β (Figure 40.2). These cytokines collectively activate natural killer cells, macrophages, and cytotoxic T lymphocytes. Clearly, drugs that interfere with the production or activity of IL-2, such as *cyclosporine*, will significantly dampen the immune response and, thereby, decrease graft rejection.

A. Cyclosporine

Cyclosporine [sye-kloe-SPOR-een] (*CsA*) is a lipophillic cyclic polypeptide composed of 11 amino acids (several are methylated on the peptidyl nitrogen). The drug is extracted from a soil fungus. *CsA* is used to prevent rejection of kidney, liver, and cardiac allogeneic transplants. *CsA* is most effective in preventing acute rejection of transplanted organs when combined in a double-drug or triple-drug regimen with corticosteroids and an antimetabolite such as *mycophenolate mofetil*. *CsA* is an alternative to *methotrexate* for the treatment of severe, active rheumatoid arthritis. It can also be used for patients with recalcitrant psoriasis that does not respond to other therapies.

1. **Mechanism of action:** *Cyclosporine* preferentially suppresses cell-mediated immune reactions, whereas humoral immunity is affected to a far lesser extent. After diffusing into the T cell, *CsA* binds to a cyclophilin (more generally called an immunophilin) to form a complex that binds to calcineurin (Figure 40.3). The latter is responsible for dephosphorylating NFATc (**c**ytosolic **N**uclear **F**actor of **A**ctivated **T** cells). The *CsA*-calcineurin complex cannot perform this reaction; thus, NFATc cannot enter the nucleus to promote the reactions that are required for the synthesis of a number of cytokines, including IL-2. The end result is a decrease in IL-2—the primary chemical stimulus for increasing the number of T lymphocytes.

2. **Pharmacokinetics:** *Cyclosporine* may be given either orally or by intravenous infusion. Oral absorption is variable. Interpatient variability may be due to metabolism by a cytochrome P450 (CYP3A4) in the gastrointestinal tract, where the drug is metabolized. About 50 percent of the drug is associated with the blood fraction. Half of this is in the erythrocytes, and less than one-tenth is bound to the lymphocytes. *CsA* is extensively metabolized, primarily by hepatic CYP3A4. [Note: When other drug substrates for this enzyme are given concomitantly, many drug interactions have been reported.] It is not clear whether any of the 25 or more metabolites have any activity. Excretion of the metabolites is through the biliary route, with only a small fraction of the parent drug appearing in the urine.

3. **Adverse effects:** Many of the adverse effects caused by *CsA* are dose dependent; therefore, it is important to monitor blood levels of the drug. Nephrotoxicity is the most common and important adverse effect of *CsA*. It is therefore critical to monitor kidney function. Reduction of

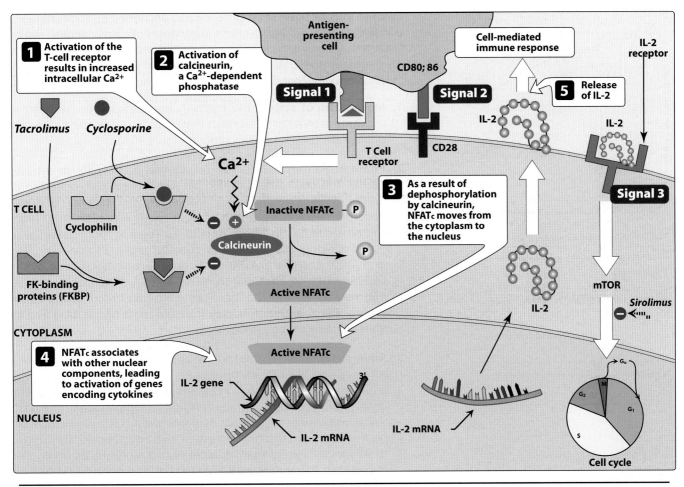

Figure 40.3

Mechanism of action of *cyclosporine* and *tacrolimus*. Il-2 = interleukin-2; mTOR = mammalian target of rapamycin; NFATc = cytosolic nuclear factor of activated T cells.

the *CsA* dosage can result in reversal of nephrotoxicity in most cases, although nephrotoxicity may be irreversible in 15% of patients. [Note: Coadministration of drugs that also can cause kidney dysfunction (for example, the aminoglycoside antibiotics) and anti-inflammatories, such as *diclofenac*, *naproxen*, or *sulindac*, can potentiate the nephro-toxicity of *CsA*.] Hepatotoxicity can also occur; therefore, liver function should be periodically assessed.] Infections in patients taking *CsA* are common and may be life-threatening. Viral infections due to herpes group and cytomegalovirus (CMV) are prevalent. Lymphoma may occur in all transplanted patients due to the net level of immunosuppression and has not been linked to any one particular agent. Anaphylactic reactions can occur on parenteral administration. Other toxicities include hypertension, hyperlipidemia, hyperkalemia (it is important not to use K+-sparing diuretics in these patients), tremor, hirsutism, glucose intolerance, and gum hyperplasia.

B. Tacrolimus

Tacrolimus [ta-CRAW-lih-mus] (*TAC*, originally called *FK506*) is a macrolide that is isolated from a soil fungus. *TAC* is approved for the prevention of rejection of liver and kidney transplants and is given with a corticosteroids and/or an antimetabolite. This drug has found favor over

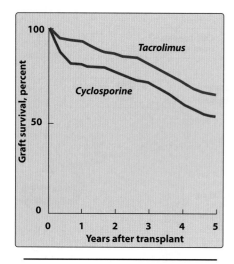

Figure 40.4
Five-year renal allograft survival in patients treated with *cyclosporine* or *tacrolimus*.

CsA, not only because of its potency and decreased episodes of rejection (Figure 40.4) but also because lower doses of corticosteroids can be used, thus reducing the likelihood of steroid-associated adverse effects. An ointment preparation has been approved for moderate to severe atopic dermatitis that does not respond to conventional therapies.

1. **Mechanism of action:** *TAC* exerts its immunosuppressive effect in the same manner as *CsA*, except that it binds to a different immunophilin, FKBP-12 (FK-**b**inding **p**rotein; Figure 40.5).

2. **Pharmacokinetics:** *TAC* may be administered orally or intravenously. The oral route is preferable, but as with *CsA*, oral absorption of *TAC* is incomplete and variable, requiring tailoring of doses. Absorption is decreased if the drug is taken with high-fat or high-carbohydrate meals. *TAC* is from 10- to 100-fold more potent than *CsA*. It is highly bound to serum proteins and is also concentrated in erythrocytes. Like *CsA*, *TAC* undergoes hepatic metabolism by the CYP3A4 isozyme; thus, the same drug interactions occur. At least one metabolite of *TAC* has been shown to have immunosuppressive activity. Renal excretion is very low, and most of the drug and its metabolites are found in the feces.

3. **Adverse effects:** Nephrotoxicity and neurotoxicity (tremor, seizures, and hallucinations) tend to be more severe in patients who are treated with *TAC* than in patients treated with *CsA*, but careful dose adjustment can minimize this problem. Development of posttransplant, insulin-dependent diabetes mellitus is a problem, especially in black and Hispanic patients. Other toxicities are the same as those for *CsA*, except that *TAC* does not cause hirsutism or gingival hyperplasia. Compared with *CsA*, *TAC* has also been found to have a lower incidence of cardiovascular toxicities such as hypertension and hyperlipidemia, both of which are common disease states found in kidney transplant recipients. Anaphylactoid reactions to the injection vehicle have been reported. The drug interactions are the same as those described for *CsA*.

C. Sirolimus

Sirolimus [sih-ROW-lih-mus] (*SRL*) is a recently approved macrolide obtained from fermentations of a soil mold. The earlier name—and one that is sometimes still used—is *rapamycin*. *SRL* is approved for use in renal transplantation, to be used together with *CsA* and corticosteroids, thereby allowing lower doses of those medications to be employed and, thus, lowering their toxic potential. The combination of *SRL* and *CsA* is apparently synergistic because *SRL* works later in the immune activation cascade. To limit the long-term side effects of the calcineurin inhibitor, *SRL* is often utilized in calcineurin inhibitor withdrawal protocols in patients who remain rejection free during the first 3 months posttransplant. The antiproliferative action of *SRL* has found use in cardiology. *SRL*-coated stents inserted into the cardiac vasculature inhibit restenosis of the blood vessels by reducing proliferation of the endothelial cells. In addition to its immunosuppressive effects, *SRL* also inhibits proliferation of cells in the graft intimal areas and, thus, is effective in halting graft vascular disease.

1. **Mechanism of action:** *SRL* and *TAC* bind to the same cytoplasmic FK-binding protein, but instead of forming a complex with calcineurin, *SRL* binds to mTOR interfering with Signal 3). The latter is a serine-

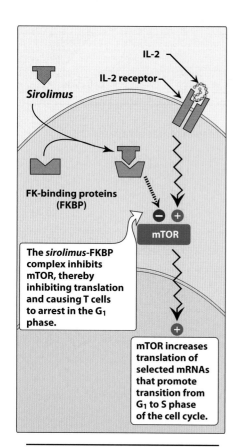

Figure 40.5
Mechanism of action of *sirolimus*. mTOR = molecular target of *rapamycin* (*sirolimus*).

threonine kinase. [Note: TOR proteins are essential for many cellular functions, such as cell-cycle progression, DNA repair, and as regulators involved in protein translation.] Binding of *SRL* to mTOR blocks the progression of activated T cells from the G_1 to the S phase of the cell cycle and, consequently, the proliferation of these cells (see Figure 40.5). Unlike *CsA* and *TAC*, *SRL* does not owe its effect to lowering IL-2 production but, rather, to inhibiting the cellular responses to IL-2.

2. **Pharmacokinetics:** The drug is available only as oral preparations. Although it is readily absorbed, high-fat meals can decrease the drug's absorption. *SRL* has a long half-life compared to those of *CsA* and *TAC*, and a loading dose is required at the time of initiation of therapy. Like both *CsA* and *TAC*, *SRL* is metabolized by the CYP3A4 isozyme and interacts with the same drugs as do *CsA* and *TAC*. *SRL* also increases the drug concentrations of *CsA*, and careful blood level monitoring of both agents must be employed to avoid harmful drug toxicities. The parent drug and its metabolites are predominantly eliminated in the feces.

3. **Adverse effects:** A frequent side effect of *SRL* is hyperlipidemia (elevated cholesterol and triglycerides), which can require treatment. The combination of *CsA* and *SRL* is more nephrotoxic than *CsA* alone due to the drug interaction between the two; therefore, lower doses are initiated. Although the administration of *SRL* and *TAC* appears to be less nephrotoxic, *SRL* can still potentiate the nephrotoxicity of *TAC*, and drug levels of both must be monitored closely. Other untoward problems are headache, nausea and diarrhea, leukopenia, and thrombocytopenia. Impaired wound healing has been noted with *SRL* in obese patients and those with diabetes; this can be especially problematic immediately following the transplant surgery and in patients receiving corticosteroids.

III. IMMUNOSUPPRESSIVE ANTIMETABOLITES

Immunosuppressive antimetabolite agents are generally used in combination with corticosteroids, and the calcineurin inhibitors, *CsA* and *TAC*.

A. Azathioprine

Azathioprine [ay-za-THYE-oh-preen] was the first agent to achieve widespread use in organ transplantation. It is a prodrug that is converted first to *6-mercaptopurine (6-MP)* and then to the corresponding nucleotide, thioinosinic acid. The immunosuppressive effects of *azathioprine* are due to this nucleotide analog. Because of their rapid proliferation in the immune response and their dependence on the de novo synthesis of purines required for cell division, lymphocytes are predominantly affected by the cytotoxic effects of *azathioprine*. [Note: The drug has little effect on suppressing a chronic immune response.] Its major nonimmune toxicity is bone marrow suppression. Concomitant use with angiotensin-converting enzyme inhibitors or *cotrimoxazole* in renal transplant patients can lead to an exaggerated leukopenic response. *Allopurinol*, an agent used to treat gout, significantly inhibits the metabolism of *azatihioprine*; therefore, the dose of *azathioprine* must be reduced by 60 to 75 percent. Nausea and vomiting are also encountered. (See p. 464 for a discussion of the mechanism of action, resistance, and pharmacokinetics of *6-MP*.)

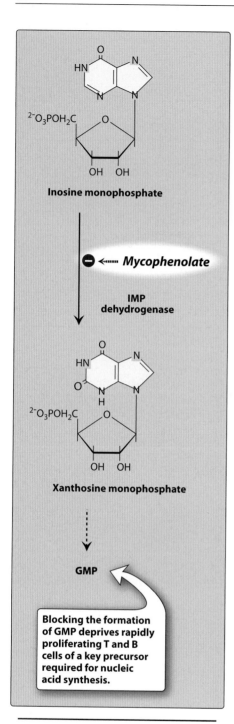

Figure 40.6
Mechanism of action of
mycophenolate.

Within the figure:

Inosine monophosphate

$^{2-}O_3POH_2C$

OH   OH

Mycophenolate

IMP
dehydrogenase

Xanthosine monophosphate

$^{2-}O_3POH_2C$

OH   OH

GMP

Blocking the formation
of GMP deprives rapidly
proliferating T and B
cells of a key precursor
required for nucleic
acid synthesis.

B. Mycophenolate mofetil (MMF)

Azathioprine has for the most part been replaced by *mycophenolate mofetil* [mye-koe-FEN-oh-late MAW-feh-til] (MMF) because of the latter's safety and efficacy in prolonging graft survival. It has been successfully used in heart, kidney, and liver transplants. As an ester, it is rapidly hydrolyzed in the gastrointestinal tract to mycophenolic acid (MPA), which is a potent, reversible, uncompetitive inhibitor of inosine monophosphate dehydrogenase, blocking the de novo formation of guanosine phosphate. Thus, like *6-MP*, it deprives the rapidly proliferating T and B cells of a key component of nucleic acids (Figure 40.6). [Note: Lymphocytes lack the salvage pathway for purine synthesis and, therefore, are dependent on de novo purine production.] MPA is quickly and almost completely absorbed after oral administration. Both MPA and its glucuronidated metabolite are highly bound (greater than 90 percent) to plasma albumin, but no displacement-type interactions have been reported. The glucuronide is excreted predominantly in the urine. The most common adverse effects include diarrhea, nausea, vomiting, abdominal pain, leukopenia, and anemia. Higher doses of *MMF* (3 g/day) were associated with a higher risk of CMV infection. [Note: MPA is less mutagenic or carcinogenic than *azathioprine*.] Concomitant administration with antacids containing magnesium or aluminum, or with *cholestyramine*, can decrease absorption of the drug.

C. Enteric-coated mycophenolate sodium

In an effort to minimize the gastrointestinal effects associated with *MMF*, enteric-coated mycophenolate sodium (EC-*MPS*) was developed. The active drug (MPA) is contained within a delayed-release formulation designed to release in the neutral pH of the small intestine. EC-MPS at 720 mg and *MMF* at 1000 mg contain equivalent amounts of MPA. In Phase III studies, the new formulation was found to be equivalent to MMF in the prevention of acute rejection episodes in kidney transplant recipients. However, the rate of gastrointestinal adverse events was similar to that with MMF.

IV. ANTIBODIES

The use of antibodies plays a central role in prolonging allograft survival. They are prepared either by immunization of rabbits or horses with human lymphoid cells (producing a mixture of polyclonal antibodies directed against a number of lymphocyte antigens), or by hybridoma technology (producing antigen-specific, monoclonal antibodies). [Note: Hybridomas are produced by fusing mouse antibody-producing cells with immortal, malignant plasma cells (Figure 40.7). Hybrid cells are selected and cloned, and the antibody specificity of the clones is determined. Clones of interest can be cultured in large quantities to produce clinically useful amounts of the desired antibody. Recombinant DNA technology can also be used to replace part of the mouse gene sequence with human genetic material, thus "humanizing" the antibodies produced, making them less antigenic.] The names of monoclonal antibodies conventionally contain "muro" if they are from a murine (mouse) source and "xi" or "iz" if they are humanized (see Figure 40.7). The suffix "mab" (monoclonal antibody) identifies the category of drug. The polyclonal antibodies, although relatively inexpensive to produce, are variable and less specific, which is in contrast to monoclonal antibodies, which are homogeneous and specific.

A. Antithymocyte globulins

Thymocytes are cells that develop in the thymus and serve as T-cell precursors. The antibodies developed against them are prepared by immunization of large rabbits or horses with human lymphoid cells and, thus, are polyclonal. They are primarily employed, together with other immunosuppressive agents, at the time of transplantation to prevent early allograft rejection, or they may be used to treat severe rejection episodes or corticosteroid-resistant acute rejection. Rabbit formulations of polyclonal antithymocyte globulin are more commonly used over the horse preparation due to greater potency. The antibodies bind to the surface of circulating T lymphocytes, which then undergo various reactions, such as complement-mediated destruction, antibody-dependent cytotoxicity, apoptosis, and opsonization. The antibody-bound cells are phagocytosed in the liver and spleen, resulting in lymphopenia and impaired T-cell responses. The antibodies are slowly infused intravenously, and their half-life extends from 3 to 9 days. Because the humoral antibody mechanism remains active, antibodies can be formed against these foreign proteins. [Note: This is less of a problem with the humanized antibodies.] Other adverse effects include chills and fever, leukopenia and thrombocytopenia, infections due to CMV or other viruses, and skin rashes.

B. Muromonab-CD3 (OKT3)

Muromonab-CD3 [myoo-roe-MOE-nab] is a murine monoclonal antibody that is synthesized by hybridoma technology and directed against the glycoprotein CD3 antigen of human T cells. *Muromonab-CD3* is used for treatment of acute rejection of renal allografts as well as for corticosteroid-resistant acute allograft rejection in cardiac and hepatic transplant patients. It is also used to deplete T cells from donor bone marrow prior to transplantation.

1. **Mechanism of action:** Binding to the CD3 protein results in a disruption of T-lymphocyte function, because access of antigen to the recognition site is blocked. Circulating T cells are depleted; thus, their participation in the immune response is decreased. Because *muromonab-CD3* recognizes only one antigenic site, the immunosuppression is less broad than that seen with the polyclonal antibodies. T cells usually return to normal within 48 hours of discontinuation of therapy.

2. **Pharmacokinetics:** The antibody is administered intravenously. Initial binding of *muromonab-CD3* to the antigen transiently activates the T cell and results in cytokine release (cytokine storm). It is therefore customary to premedicate the patient with *methylprednisolone, diphenhydramine,* and *acetaminophen* to alleviate the cytokine release syndrome.

3. **Adverse effects:** Anaphylactoid reactions may occur. Cytokine release syndrome may follow the first dose. The symptoms can range from a mild, flu-like illness to a life-threatening, shock-like reaction. High fever is common. Central nervous system effects, such as seizures, encephalopathy, cerebral edema, aseptic meningitis, and headache, may occur. Infections can increase, including some due to CMV. *Muromonab-CD3* is contraindicated in patients with a history of seizures, in those with uncompensated heart failure, in pregnant women, and in those who are breast-feeding. Because of these adverse effects and the improved tolerability of thymoglobulin and the IL-2 receptor antagonists, *muromonab-CD3* is rarely used today.

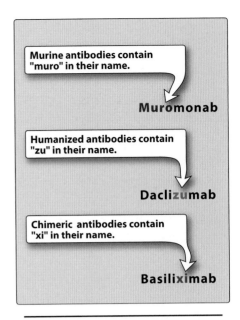

Murine antibodies contain "muro" in their name.

Muromonab

Humanized antibodies contain "zu" in their name.

Daclizumab

Chimeric antibodies contain "xi" in their name.

Basiliximab

Figure 40.7
Conventions for naming monoclonal antibodies. [Note: *Muromonab* was named before the convention was adopted to make the last three letters in their names *mab*.]

C. IL-2-receptor antagonists

The antigenicity and short serum half-life of the murine monoclonal antibody have been averted by replacing most of the murine amino acid sequences with human ones by genetic engineering. *Basiliximab* [bah-si-LIK-si-mab] is said to be "chimerized" because it consists of 25 percent murine and 75 percent human protein. *Daclizumab* [dah-KLIZ-yoo-mab] is 90 percent human protein, and is designated "humanized." Both agents have been approved for prophylaxis of acute rejection in renal transplantation in combination with *CsA* and corticosteroids. They are not used for the treatment of ongoing rejection.

1. **Mechanism of action:** Both compounds are anti-CD25 antibodies and bind to the α chain of the IL-2 receptor on activated T cells. They thus interfere with the proliferation of these cells. *Basiliximab* is about 10-fold more potent than *daclizumab* as a blocker of IL-2 stimulated T-cell replication. Blockade of this receptor foils the ability of any antigenic stimulus to activate the T cell–response system.

2. **Pharmacokinetics:** Both antibodies are given intravenously. The serum half-life of *daclizumab* is about 20 days, and the blockade of the receptor is 120 days. Five doses of *daclizumab* are usually administered—the first at 24 hours before transplantation, and the next four doses at 14-day intervals. The serum half-life of *basiliximab* is about 7 days. Usually, two doses of this drug are administered—the first at 2 hours prior to transplantation, and the second at 4 days after the surgery.

3. **Adverse effects:** Both *daclizumab* and *basiliximab* are well tolerated. Their major toxicity is gastrointestinal. No clinically relevant antibodies to the drugs have been detected, and malignancy does not appear to be a problem.

D. Alemtuzumab

Alemtuzumab [al-em-TOOZ-oo-mab], a humanized monoclonal antibody directed against CD52, exerts its effects by causing profound depletion of T cells from the peripheral circulation. This effect may last for up to 1 year. *Alemtuzumab* is currently approved for the treatment of refractory B-cell chronic lymphocytic leukemia. Although it is not currently approved for use in organ transplantation, it is being utilized in combination with *SRL* and low-dose calcineurin inhibitors in corticosteroid avoidance protocols at many transplant centers. Preliminary results are promising, with low rates of rejection with a *prednisone*-free regimen. Side effects include first-dose cytokine-release syndrome, requiring premedication with *acetaminophen*, *diphenhydramine*, and corticosteroids. Adverse effects include neutropenia, anemia, and rarely, pancytopenia. Early results have not shown an increase in opportunistic infections or lymphomas with *alemtuzumab* despite its potent immunosuppressive activity. A summary of the major immunosuppressive drugs is presented in Figure 40.8

V. CORTICOSTEROIDS

The corticosteroids were the first pharmacologic agents to be used as immunosuppressives both in transplantation and in various autoimmune disorders. They are still one of the mainstays for attenuating rejection episodes. For transplantation, the most common agents are *prednisone* or

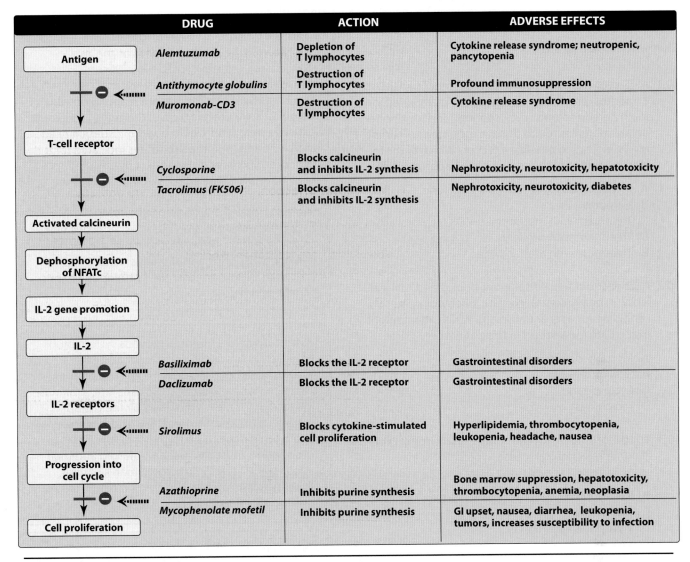

	DRUG	ACTION	ADVERSE EFFECTS
Antigen	*Alemtuzumab*	Depletion of T lymphocytes	Cytokine release syndrome; neutropenic, pancytopenia
	Antithymocyte globulins	Destruction of T lymphocytes	Profound immunosuppression
T-cell receptor	*Muromonab-CD3*	Destruction of T lymphocytes	Cytokine release syndrome
	Cyclosporine	Blocks calcineurin and inhibits IL-2 synthesis	Nephrotoxicity, neurotoxicity, hepatotoxicity
Activated calcineurin	*Tacrolimus (FK506)*	Blocks calcineurin and inhibits IL-2 synthesis	Nephrotoxicity, neurotoxicity, diabetes
Dephosphorylation of NFATc			
IL-2 gene promotion			
IL-2	*Basiliximab*	Blocks the IL-2 receptor	Gastrointestinal disorders
	Daclizumab	Blocks the IL-2 receptor	Gastrointestinal disorders
IL-2 receptors	*Sirolimus*	Blocks cytokine-stimulated cell proliferation	Hyperlipidemia, thrombocytopenia, leukopenia, headache, nausea
Progression into cell cycle	*Azathioprine*	Inhibits purine synthesis	Bone marrow suppression, hepatotoxicity, thrombocytopenia, anemia, neoplasia
Cell proliferation	*Mycophenolate mofetil*	Inhibits purine synthesis	GI upset, nausea, diarrhea, leukopenia, tumors, increases susceptibility to infection

Figure 40.8
Sites of action of immunosuppressants. Il-2 = interleukin-2. NFATc = cytosolic nuclear factor of activated T cells.

methylprednisolone, whereas *prednisone* or *prednisolone* are employed for autoimmune conditions. [Note: In transplantation, they are used in combination with agents described previously in this chapter.] The steroids are used to suppress acute rejection of solid organ allografts and in chronic graft-versus-host disease. In addition, they are effective against a wide variety of autoimmune conditions, including refractory rheumatoid arthritis, systemic lupus erythematosus, temporal arthritis, and asthma. The exact mechanism responsible for the immunosuppressive action of the corticosteroids is unclear. The T lymphocytes are affected most. The steroids are able to rapidly reduce lymphocyte populations by lysis or redistribution. On entering cells, they bind to the glucocorticoid receptor. The complex passes into the nucleus and regulates the translation of DNA. Among the genes affected are those involved in inflammatory responses. The use of these agents is associated with numerous adverse effects. For example, they are diabetogenic, and they can cause hypercholesterolemia, cataracts, osteoporosis, and hypertension on prolonged use. Consequently, efforts are being directed toward reducing or eliminating the use of steroids in the maintenance of allografts.

Study Questions

Choose the ONE best answer.

40.1 A 45-year-old male who received a renal transplant 3 months previously and is being maintained on methylprednisolone, cyclosporine, and mycophenolate mofetil is found to have increased creatinine levels, indicating possible rejection. Which of the following courses of therapy would be appropriate?

A. Increased dose of methylprednisolone.
B. Hemodialysis.
C. Treatment with muromonab-CD3.
D. Treatment with sirolimus.
E. Treatment with azathioprine.

40.2 A 23-year-old female suffering from grand mal epilepsy is being controlled with phenytoin. She is a candidate for a renal transplant. Which agent might exacerbate the seizures in this patient?

A. Mycophenolate mofetil.
B. Sirolimus.
C. Cyclosporine.
D. Tacrolimus.

40.3 Which of the following drugs used to prevent allograft rejection can cause hyperlipidemia?

A. Azathioprine.
B. Basiliximab.
C. Tacrolimus.
D. Mycophenolate mofetil.
E. Sirolimus.

40.4 Which of the following drugs specifically inhibit calcineurin in the activated T lymphocytes?

A. Daclizumab.
B. Tacrolimus.
C. Prednisone.
D. Sirolimus.
E. Mycophenolate mofetil.

Correct answer = C. This patient is apparently undergoing an acute rejection of the kidney. The most effective treatment would be administration of an antibody, and muromonab-CD3 is indicated for this condition. Increasing the dose of methylprednisolone may have some effect, but this exposes the patient to the adverse effects of glucocorticoids. Sirolimus is used prophylactically with cyclosporine to prevent renal rejection but is less effective when an episode is occurring. Furthermore, the combination of cyclosporine and sirolimus is more nephrotoxic than cyclosporine alone. Azathioprine has no benefit over mycophenolate.

Correct answer = D. Central nervous system problems such as headache and tremor as well as seizures are among the adverse effects commonly associated with tacrolimus. Cyclosporine, sirolimus, and tacrolimus are metabolized by the CYP3A4 isozyme of the cytochrome P450 oxidases. Phenytoin can induce this enzyme; thus, the doses of these agents must be carefully adjusted and their blood levels carefully monitored in this patient. Mycophenolate mofetil has predominantly gastrointestinal side effects.

Correct answer = E. Patients who are receiving sirolimus can develop elevated cholesterol and triacylglycerol levels, which can be controlled by statin therapy. None of the other agents has this adverse effect.

Correct answer = B. Tacrolimus binds to FKBP-12, which in turn inhibits calcineurin and interferes in the cascade of reactions that synthesize IL-2 and lead to T-lymphocyte proliferation. Although daclizumab also interferes with T-lymphocyte proliferation, it does so by binding to the CD25 site on the IL-2 receptor. Prednisone can affect not only T-cell proliferation but also that of B cells; therefore, it is not specific. Sirolimus, while also binding to FKBP-12, does not inhibit calcineurin. Mycophenolate mofetil exerts its immunosuppressive action by inhibiting inosine monophosphate dehydrogenase, thus depriving the cells of guanosine—a key component of nucleic acids.

Anti-inflammatory Drugs

41

I. OVERVIEW

Inflammation is a normal, protective response to tissue injury caused by physical trauma, noxious chemicals, or microbiologic agents. Inflammation is the body's effort to inactivate or destroy invading organisms, remove irritants, and set the stage for tissue repair. When healing is complete, the inflammatory process usually subsides. However, inappropriate activation of our immune system can result in inflammation leading to rheumatoid arthritis (RA). Normally, our immune system can differentiate between self and nonself. In RA, white blood cells (WBC) view the synovium (tissue that nourishes cartilage and bone) as nonself and initiates an inflammatory attack. WBC activation leads to activation of T lymphocytes (the cell-mediated part of our immune system), which will recruit and activate monocytes and macrophages. These will secrete proinflammatory cytokines, including tumor necrosis factor (TNF)-α and interleukin (IL)-1 into the synovial cavity. These cytokines will then cause 1) increased cellular infiltration into the endothelium due to release of histamines, kinins, and vasodilatory prostaglandins; 2) increased production of C-reactive protein by hepatocytes (a marker for inflammation); 3) increased production and release of proteolytic enzymes (collagenases and metalloproteinases) by chondrocytes (cells that maintain cartilage), leading to degradation of cartilage and joint space narrowing; 4) increased osteoclast activity (osteoclasts regulate bone breakdown), resulting in focal bone erosions and bone demineralization around joints; and 5) systemic manifestations in which organs such as the heart, lungs, and liver are adversely affected. In addition to T-lymphocyte activation, B lymphocytes are also involved and will produce rheumatoid factor (inflammatory marker) and other autoantibodies with the purpose of maintaining inflammation. These defensive reactions will cause progressive tissue injury, resulting in joint damage and erosions, functional disability, and significant pain and reduction in quality of life. Pharmacotherapy in the management of RA includes anti-inflammatory and/or immunosuppressive agents that will modulate/reduce the inflammatory process with the goals of reducing inflammation and pain and halting (or at least slowing) the progression of the disease. The agents to be discussed include nonsteroidal anti-inflammatory drugs (NSAIDs) and *celecoxib* (cyclooxygenase-2 inhibitor), *acetaminophen*, and disease-modifying antirheumatic drugs. Additionally, agents used for the treatment of gout will be reviewed (Figure 41.1).

ANTI-INFLAMMATORY DRUGS

NSAIDs

- *Aspirin*
- *Diflunisal*
- *Diclofenac*
- *Etodolac*
- *Fenamates*
- *Fenoprofen*
- *Flurbiprofen*
- *Ibuprofen*
- *Indomethacin*
- *Ketorolac*
- *Ketoprofen*
- *Meloxicam*
- *Methyl salicylate*
- *Nabumetone*
- *Naproxen*
- *Oxaprozin*
- *Piroxicam*
- *Sulindac*
- *Tolmetin*

COX-2 INHIBITORS

- *Celecoxib*

OTHER ANALGESICS

- *Acetaminophen*

Figure 41.1
Summary of anti-inflammatory drugs. NSAIDs = nonsteroidal anti-inflammatory drugs; COX = cyclo-oxygenase.
(Continued on next page.)

ANTI-INFLAMMATORY DRUGS (continued)

DRUGS FOR ARTHRITIS

— *Abatacept*
— *Adalimumab*
— *Anakinra*
— *Chloroquine*
— *Etanercept*
— *Gold salts*
— *Infliximab*
— *Leflunomide*
— *Methotrexate*
— *D-Penicillamine*
— *Rituximab*

DRUGS FOR GOUT

— *Allopurinol*
— *Colchicine*
— *Probenecid*
— *Sulfinpyrazone*

Figure 41.1 (continued)
Summary of anti-inflammatory drugs.

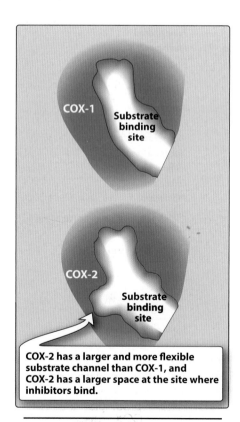

COX-2 has a larger and more flexible substrate channel than COX-1, and COX-2 has a larger space at the site where inhibitors bind.

Figure 41.2
Structural differences in active sites of cyclooxygenase (COX)-1 and COX-2.

II. PROSTAGLANDINS

All of the NSAIDs act by inhibiting the synthesis of prostaglandins. Thus, an understanding of NSAIDs requires comprehension of the actions and biosynthesis of prostaglandins—unsaturated fatty acid derivatives containing 20 carbons that include a cyclic ring structure. [Note: These compounds are sometimes referred to as eicosanoids; "eicosa" refers to the 20 carbon atoms.]

A. Role of prostaglandins as local mediators

Prostaglandins and related compounds are produced in minute quantities by virtually all tissues. They generally act locally on the tissues in which they are synthesized, and they are rapidly metabolized to inactive products at their sites of action. Therefore, the prostaglandins do not circulate in the blood in significant concentrations. Thromboxanes, leukotrienes, and the hydroperoxyeicosatetraenoic and hydroxyeicosatetraenoic acids (HPETEs and HETEs, respectively) are related lipids, synthesized from the same precursors as the prostaglandins, and use interrelated pathways.

B. Synthesis of prostaglandins

Arachidonic acid, a 20-carbon fatty acid, is the primary precursor of the prostaglandins and related compounds. Arachidonic acid is present as a component of the phospholipids of cell membranes—primarily phosphatidylinositol and other complex lipids.[1] Free arachidonic acid is released from tissue phospholipids by the action of phospholipase A_2 and other acyl hydrolases via a process controlled by hormones and other stimuli. There are two major pathways in the synthesis of the eicosanoids from arachidonic acid.

1. **Cyclooxygenase pathway:** All eicosanoids with ring structures—that is, the prostaglandins, thromboxanes, and prostacyclins—are synthesized via the cyclooxygenase pathway. Two related isoforms of the cyclooxygenase enzymes have been described. Cyclooxygenase-1 (COX-1) is responsible for the physiologic production of prostanoids, whereas cyclooxygenase-2 (COX-2) causes the elevated production of prostanoids that occurs in sites of disease and inflammation. COX-1 is described as a "housekeeping enzyme" that regulates normal cellular processes, such as gastric cytoprotection, vascular homeostasis, platelet aggregation, and kidney function. COX-2 is constitutively expressed in tissues such as the brain, kidney, and bone. Its expression at other sites is increased during states of inflammation. The two enzymes share 60 percent homology in amino acid sequence. However, the conformation for the substrate-binding sites and catalytic regions are slightly different. For example, COX-2 has a larger and more flexible substrate channel than COX-1 has, and COX-2 has a large space at the site where inhibitors bind (Figure 41.2). [Note: The structural differences between COX-1 and COX-2 permitted the development of COX-2 selective inhibitors.] Another distinguishing characteristic of COX-2 is that its expression is inhibited by glucocorticoids (Figure 41.3), which may contribute to the significant anti-inflammatory effects of these drugs.

[1]See p. 182 in *Lippincott's Illustrated Reviews: Biochemistry* (4th ed.) for a discussion of the chemistry of arachidonic acid.

2. Lipoxygenase pathway: Alternatively, several lipoxygenases can act on arachidonic acid to form 5-HPETE, 12-HPETE, and 15-HPETE, which are unstable peroxidated derivatives that are converted to the corresponding hydroxylated derivatives (the HETEs) or to leukotrienes or lipoxins, depending on the tissue (see Figure 41.3).[2] Antileukotriene drugs, such as *zileuton*, *zafirlukast*, and *montelukast*, are useful for the treatment of moderate to severe allergic asthma (see p. 324).

C. Actions of prostaglandins

Many of the actions of prostaglandins are mediated by their binding to a wide variety of distinct cell membrane receptors that operate via G proteins, which subsequently activate or inhibit adenylyl cyclase or stimulate phospholipase C.[3] This causes an enhanced formation of diacylglycerol and inositol 1,4,5-trisphosphate. Prostaglandin $F_{2\alpha}$ ($PGF_{2\alpha}$), the leukotrienes, and thromboxane A_2 (TXA_2) mediate certain actions by activating phosphatidyl inositol metabolism, causing an increase of intracellular Ca^{2+}.

D. Functions in the body

Prostaglandins and their metabolites produced endogenously in tissues act as local signals that fine-tune the response of a specific cell type. Their functions vary widely, depending on the tissue. For example, the release of TXA_2 from platelets triggers the recruitment of new platelets for aggregation (the first step in clot formation). However, in other tissues, elevated levels of TXA_2 convey a different signal; for example, in certain smooth muscles, this compound induces contraction. Prostaglandins are also among the chemical mediators that are released in allergic and inflammatory processes.

III. NONSTEROIDAL ANTI-INFLAMMATORY DRUGS

The NSAIDs are a group of chemically dissimilar agents that differ in their antipyretic, analgesic, and anti-inflammatory activities. They act primarily by inhibiting the cyclooxygenase enzymes that catalyze the first step in prostanoid biosynthesis. This leads to decreased prostaglandin synthesis with both beneficial and unwanted effects. Detection of serious cardiovascular events associated with COX-2 inhibitors have led to withdrawal of *rofecoxib* and *valdecoxib* from the market (*celecoxib* is still available for use in patients with RA). Additionally, the U.S. Food and Drug Administration (FDA) has required that the labeling of the traditional NSAIDs and *celecoxib* be updated to include the following: 1) a warning of the potential risks of serious cardiovascular thrombotic events, myocardial infarction, and stroke, which can be fatal; additionally, a warning that the risk may increase with duration of use and that patients with cardiovascular disease or risk factors may be at greater risk; 2) a warning that use is contraindicated for the treatment of perioperative pain in the setting of coronary artery bypass graft surgery; and 3) a notice that there is increased risk of serious gastrointestinal (GI) adverse events, including bleeding, ulceration, and perforation of the stomach or intestines, which can be fatal. These events can occur at any time during use and without warning symptoms. Elderly patients are at greater risk for seri-

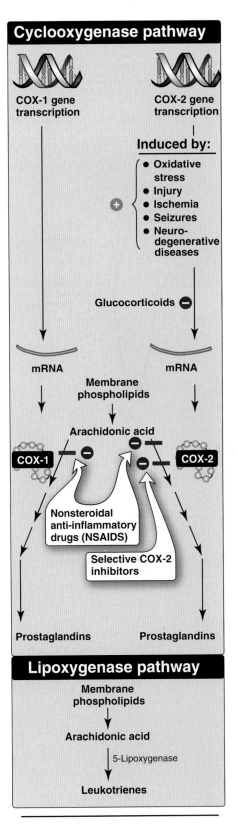

Figure 41.3
Synthesis of prostaglandins and leukotrienes. COX = cyclooxygenase.

[2]See p. 213 in *Lippincott's Illustrated Reviews: Biochemistry* (4th ed.) for a discussion of prostaglandin synthesis.
[3]See p. 205 in *Lippincott's Illustrated Reviews: Biochemistry* (4th ed.) for a discussion of the role of phospholipase C in signal transmission.

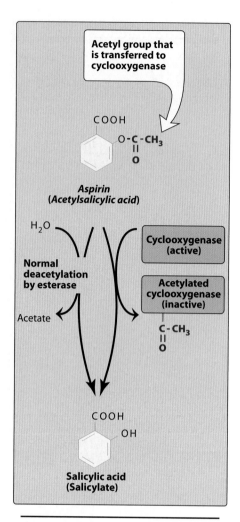

Figure 41.4
Metabolism of *aspirin* and
acetylation of cyclooxygenase
by *aspirin*.

ous GI events. *Aspirin*, however, has proven to be beneficial in patients for the primary and secondary prevention of cardiovascular events and is most commonly used for this purpose rather than for pain control.

A. Aspirin and other salicylic acid derivatives

Aspirin [AS-pir-in] is the prototype of traditional NSAIDs and was officially approved by the FDA in 1939. It is the most commonly used and is the drug to which all other anti-inflammatory agents are compared.

1. **Mechanism of action:** *Aspirin* is a weak organic acid that is unique among the NSAIDs in that it irreversibly acetylates (and, thus, inactivates) cyclooxygenase (Figure 41.4). The other NSAIDs, including salicylate, are all reversible inhibitors of cyclooxygenase. *Aspirin* is rapidly deacetylated by esterases in the body producing salicylate, which has anti-inflammatory, antipyretic, and analgesic effects. The antipyretic and anti-inflammatory effects of salicylate are due primarily to the blockade of prostaglandin synthesis at the thermoregulatory centers in the hypothalamus and at peripheral target sites. Furthermore, by decreasing prostaglandin synthesis, salicylate also prevents the sensitization of pain receptors to both mechanical and chemical stimuli. *Aspirin* may also depress pain stimuli at subcortical sites (that is, the thalamus and hypothalamus).

2. **Actions:** The NSAIDs, including *aspirin*, have three major therapeutic actions—namely, they reduce inflammation (anti-inflammation), pain (analgesia), and fever (antipyrexia; Figure 41.5). However, as described later in this section, not all NSAIDs are equally potent in each of these actions.

   a. **Anti-inflammatory actions:** Because *aspirin* inhibits cyclooxygenase activity, it diminishes the formation of prostaglandins and, thus, modulates those aspects of inflammation in which prostaglandins act as mediators. *Aspirin* inhibits inflammation in arthritis, but it neither arrests the progress of the disease nor induces remission.

   b. **Analgesic action:** Prostaglandin E_2 (PGE_2) is thought to sensitize nerve endings to the action of bradykinin, histamine, and other chemical mediators released locally by the inflammatory process. Thus, by decreasing PGE_2 synthesis, *aspirin* and other NSAIDs repress the sensation of pain. The salicylates are used mainly for the management of pain of low to moderate intensity arising from musculoskeletal disorders rather than that arising from the viscera. Combinations of opioids and NSAIDs are effective in treating pain caused by malignancy. *Diflunisal* [dre-flu-NI-sal] is three- to four-fold more potent than *aspirin* as an analgesic and an anti-inflammatory agent, but it has no antipyretic properties.

   c. **Antipyretic action:** Fever occurs when the set-point of the anterior hypothalamic thermoregulatory center is elevated. This can be caused by PGE_2 synthesis, which is stimulated when an endogenous fever-producing agent (pyrogen), such as a cytokine, is released from white cells that are activated by infection, hypersensitivity, malignancy, or inflammation. The salicylates lower body temperature in patients with fever by impeding PGE_2 synthesis and release. *Aspirin* resets the "thermostat" toward normal, and it rapidly lowers the body temperature of febrile patients by increasing heat dissipation as a result of peripheral vasodilation and sweating. *Aspirin* has no effect on normal body temperature. *Diflunisal* does not reduce fever, because it does not cross the blood-brain barrier.

d. Respiratory actions: At therapeutic doses, *aspirin* increases alveolar ventilation. [Note: Salicylates uncouple oxidative phosphorylation, which leads to elevated CO_2 and increased respiration.] Higher doses work directly on the respiratory center in the medulla, resulting in hyperventilation and respiratory alkalosis that usually is adequately compensated for by the kidney. At toxic levels, central respiratory paralysis occurs, and respiratory acidosis ensues due to continued production of CO_2.

e. Gastrointestinal effects: Normally, prostacyclin (PGI_2) inhibits gastric acid secretion, whereas PGE_2 and $PGF_{2\alpha}$ stimulate synthesis of protective mucus in both the stomach and small intestine. In the presence of *aspirin*, these prostanoids are not formed, resulting in increased gastric acid secretion and diminished mucus protection. This may cause epigastric distress, ulceration, hemorrhage, and iron-deficiency anemia. *Aspirin* doses of 1 to 4.5 g/day can produce loss of 2 to 8 mL of blood in the feces per day. Buffered and enteric-coated preparations are only marginally helpful in dealing with this problem. Agents used for the prevention of gastric and/or duodenal ulcers include the PGE_1-derivative *misoprostol* and the proton-pump inhibitors (PPIs); *esomeprazole, lansoprazole, omeprazole, pantoprazole,* and *rabeprazole*); PPIs can also be used for the treatment of an NSAID-induced ulcer and are especially appropriate if the patient will need to continue NSAID treatment. H_2-antihistamines (*cimetidine, famotidine, nizatidine,* and *ranitidine*) relieve dyspepsia due to NSAIDS, but they may mask serious GI complaints and may not be as effective as PPIs for healing and preventing ulcer formation.

f. Effect on platelets: TXA_2 enhances platelet aggregation, whereas PGI_2 decreases it. Low doses (60–81 mg daily) of *aspirin* can irreversibly inhibit thromboxane production in platelets via acetylation of cyclooxygenase. Because platelets lack nuclei, they cannot synthesize new enzyme, and the lack of thromboxane persists for the lifetime of the platelet (3–7 days). As a result of the decrease in TXA_2, platelet aggregation (the first step in thrombus formation) is reduced, producing an anticoagulant effect with a prolonged bleeding time. Finally, *aspirin* also inhibits cyclooxygenase in endothelial cells, resulting in reduced PGI_2 formation; however, endothelial cells possess nuclei able to re-synthesize new cyclooxygenase. Therefore, PGI_2 is available for antiplatelet action.

g. Actions on the kidney: Cyclooxygenase inhibitors prevent the synthesis of PGE_2 and PGI_2—prostaglandins that are responsible for maintaining renal blood flow, particularly in the presence of circulating vasoconstrictors (Figure 41.6). Decreased synthesis of prostaglandins can result in retention of sodium and water and may cause edema and hyperkalemia in some patients. Interstitial nephritis can also occur with all NSAIDs except *aspirin*.

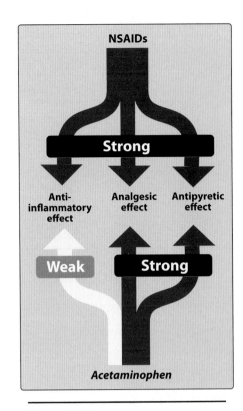

Figure 41.5
Actions of nonsteroidal anti-inflammatory drugs (NSAIDs) and *acetaminophen*.

misoprostol: chemical abortion and gastric protection
-PGE_1

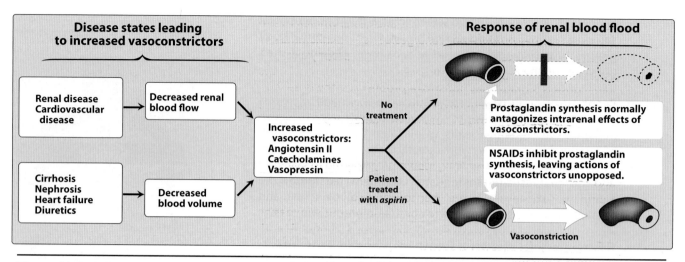

Figure 41.6
Renal effect of *aspirin* inhibition of prostaglandin synthesis. NSAIDs = nonsteroidal anti-inflammatory drugs.

3. **Therapeutic uses:**

   a. **Anti-inflammatory, antipyretic, and analgesic uses:** *The salicylic acid derivatives* are used in the treatment of gout, rheumatic fever, osteoarthritis, and RA. Commonly treated conditions requiring analgesia include headache, arthralgia, and myalgia.

   b. **External applications:** *Salicylic acid* is used topically to treat corns, calluses, and warts. *Methyl salicylate* ("oil of wintergreen") is used externally as a cutaneous counterirritant in liniments.

   c. **Cardiovascular applications:** Aspirin is used to inhibit platelet aggregation. Low doses are used prophylactically to 1) reduce the risk of recurring transient ischemic attacks (TIAs) and stroke or death in those who have had single or multiple episodes of TIA or stroke; 2) reduce the risk of death in those having an acute myocardial infarction; 3) reduce the risk of recurrent nonfatal myocardial infarction and/or death in patients with previous myocardial infarction or unstable angina pectoris; 4) reduce the risk of myocardial infarction and sudden death in patients with chronic stable angina pectoris; 5) reduce the cardiovascular risk in patients undergoing certain revascularization procedures.

4. **Pharmacokinetics:**

   a. **Administration and distribution:** After oral administration, the un-ionized salicylates are passively absorbed from the stomach and the small intestine (dissolution of the tablets is favored at the higher pH of the gut). Rectal absorption of the salicylates is slow and unreliable, but it is a useful route for administration to vomiting children. Salicylates must be avoided in children and teenagers (<15 years old) with varicella (chickenpox) or influenza to prevent Reye's syndrome. Salicylates (except for *diflunisal*) cross both the blood-brain barrier and the placenta and are absorbed through intact skin (especially *methyl salicylate*).

   b. **Dosage:** The salicylates exhibit analgesic activity at low doses; only at higher doses do these drugs show anti-inflammatory activity (Figure 41.7). For example, two 325-mg *aspirin* tablets administered four times daily produce analgesia, whereas 12 to 20 tablets per day produce both analgesic and anti-inflammatory activity. For long-term myocardial infarction prophylaxis, the dose is 81 to 162 mg/day; for those with RA or osteoarthritis, the initial dose is 3 grams/day; for stroke prophylaxis, the dose is 50 to 325 mg/day; in a patient having an acute mycardial infarction, the dose is 162 to 325 mg of nonenteric coated aspirin chewed and swallowed immediately.

c. **Fate:** At dosages of 650 mg/day, *aspirin* is hydrolyzed to salicylate and acetic acid by esterases in tissues and blood (see Figure 41.4). Salicylate is converted by the liver to water-soluble conjugates that are rapidly cleared by the kidney, resulting in elimination with first-order kinetics and a serum half-life of 3.5 hours. At anti-inflammatory dosages (>4 g/day), the hepatic metabolic pathway becomes saturated, and zero-order kinetics are observed, with the drug having a half-life of 15 hours or more (Figure 41.8). Saturation of the hepatic enzymes requires treatment for several days to 1 week. Being an organic acid, salicylate is secreted into the urine and can affect uric acid excretion—namely, at low doses of *aspirin*, uric acid secretion is decreased, whereas at high doses, uric acid secretion is increased. Both hepatic and renal function should be monitored periodically in those receiving long-term, high-dose *aspirin* therapy, and *aspirin* should be avoided in patients with a creatinine clearance of less than 10 mL/min.

5. **Adverse effects:**

a. **Gastrointestinal:** The most common GI effects of the salicylates are epigastric distress, nausea, and vomiting. Microscopic GI bleeding is almost universal in patients treated with salicylates. [Note: *Aspirin* is an acid. At stomach pH, *aspirin* is uncharged; consequently, it readily crosses into mucosal cells, where it ionizes (becomes negatively charged) and becomes trapped, thus potentially causing direct damage to the cells. *Aspirin* should be taken with food and large volumes of fluids to diminish dyspepsia. Additionally, *misoprostol* or a *PPI* may be taken concurrently.]

b. **Blood:** The irreversible acetylation of platelet cyclooxygenase reduces the level of platelet TXA_2, resulting in inhibition of platelet aggregation and a prolonged bleeding time. For this reason, *aspirin* should not be taken for at least 1 week prior to surgery. When salicylates are administered, anticoagulants may have to be given in reduced dosage, and careful monitoring and counseling of patients are necessary.

c. **Respiration:** In toxic doses, salicylates cause respiratory depression and a combination of uncompensated respiratory and metabolic acidosis.

d. **Metabolic processes:** Large doses of salicylates uncouple oxidative phosphorylation.[4] The energy normally used for the production of adenosine triphosphate is dissipated as heat, which explains the hyperthermia caused by salicylates when taken in toxic quantities.

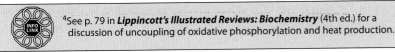

[4]See p. 79 in *Lippincott's Illustrated Reviews: Biochemistry* (4th ed.) for a discussion of uncoupling of oxidative phosphorylation and heat production.

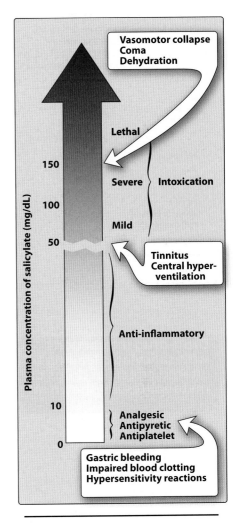

Figure 41.7
Dose-dependent effects of salicylate.

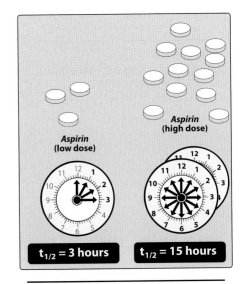

Figure 41.8
Effect of dose on the half-life of *aspirin*.

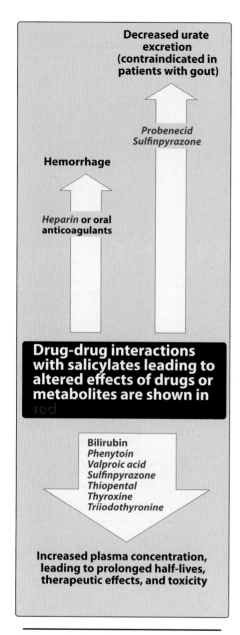

Figure 41.9
Drugs interacting with salicylates.

e. Hypersensitivity: Approximately 15 percent of patients taking *aspirin* experience hypersensitivity reactions. Symptoms of true allergy include urticaria, bronchoconstriction, or angioedema. Fatal anaphylactic shock is rare.

f. Reye's syndrome: *Aspirin* and other salicylates given during viral infections has been associated with an increased incidence of Reye's syndrome, which is an often fatal, fulminating hepatitis with cerebral edema. This is especially encountered in children, who therefore should be given *acetaminophen* instead of *aspirin* when such medication is required to reduce fever. *Ibuprofen* is also appropriate.

g. Drug interactions: Concomitant administration of salicylates with many classes of drugs may produce undesirable side effects. Because *aspirin* is found in many over-the-counter agents, patients should be counseled to read labels to verify *aspirin* content to avoid overdose. Salicylate is 90 to 95 percent protein bound and can be displaced from its protein-binding sites, resulting in increased concentration of free salicylate; alternatively, *aspirin* could displace other highly protein-bound drugs, such as *warfarin, phenytoin,* or *valproic acid,* resulting in higher free concentrations of the other agent (Figure 41.9). Chronic *aspirin* use should be avoided in patients receiving *probenecid* or *sulfinpyrazone,* because these agents cause increased renal excretion of uric acid whereas aspirin (<2 g/day) cause reduced clearance of uric acid. Concomitant use of *ketorolac* and *aspirin* is contraindicated because of increased risk of GI bleeding and platelet aggregation inhibition. Children who have received live varicella virus vaccine should avoid *aspirin* for at least 6 weeks after vaccination to prevent Reye's syndrome.

h. In pregnancy: *Aspirin* is classified as FDA pregnancy category C risk during Trimesters 1 and 2 and category D during Trimester 3. Because salicylates are excreted in breast milk, *aspirin* should be avoided during pregnancy and while breast-feeding.

6. Toxicity: Salicylate intoxication may be mild or severe. The mild form is called salicylism and is characterized by nausea, vomiting, marked hyperventilation, headache, mental confusion, dizziness, and tinnitus (ringing or roaring in the ears). When large doses of salicylate are administered, severe salicylate intoxication may result (see Figure 41.7). The symptoms listed above are followed by restlessness, delirium, hallucinations, convulsions, coma, respiratory and metabolic acidosis, and death from respiratory failure. Children are particularly prone to salicylate intoxication. Ingestion of as little as 10 g of *aspirin* (or 5 ml of *methyl salicylate,* with the latter being used as a counterirritant in liniments) can cause death in children. Treatment of salicylism should include measurement of serum salicylate concentrations and of pH to determine the best form of therapy. In mild cases, symptomatic treatment is usually sufficient. Increasing the urinary pH enhances the elimination of salicylate. In serious cases, mandatory measures include the intravenous administration of fluid, dialysis (hemodialysis or peritoneal dialysis), and the frequent assessment and correction of acid-base and electrolyte balances. [Note: *Diflunisal* does not cause salicylism.]

B. Propionic acid derivatives

Ibuprofen [eye-byoo-PROE-fen] was the first in this class of agents to become available in the United States. It has been joined by *naproxen* [nah-PROX-en], *fenoprofen* [fen-oh-PROE-fen], *ketoprofen* [key-toe-PROE-fen], *flurbiprofen* [flur-bye-PROE-fen], and *oxaprozin* [ox-ah-PROE-zin]. All these drugs possess anti-inflammatory, analgesic, and antipyretic activity; additionally, they can can alter platelet function and prolong bleeding time. They have gained wide acceptance in the chronic treatment of RA and osteoarthritis, because their GI effects are generally less intense than those of *aspirin*. These drugs are reversible inhibitors of the cyclooxygenases and, thus, like *aspirin*, inhibit the synthesis of prostaglandins but not of leukotrienes. All are well absorbed on oral administration and are almost totally bound to serum albumin. [Note: *Oxaprozin* has the longest half-life and is administered once daily.] They undergo hepatic metabolism and are excreted by the kidney. The most common adverse effects are GI, ranging from dyspepsia to bleeding. Side effects involving the central nervous system (CNS), such as headache, tinnitus, and dizziness, have also been reported.

C. Acetic acid derivatives

This group of drugs includes *indomethacin* [in-doe-METH-a-sin], *sulindac* [sul-IN-dak], and *etodolac* [eh-TOE-doh-lak]. All have anti-inflammatory, analgesic, and antipyretic activity. They act by reversibly inhibiting cyclooxygenase. They are generally not used to lower fever. Despite its potency as an anti-inflammatory agent, the toxicity of *indomethacin* limits its use to the treatment of acute gouty arthritis, ankylosing spondylitis, and osteoarthritis of the hip. *Sulindac* is an inactive prodrug that is closely related to *indomethacin*. Although the drug is less potent than *indomethacin*, it is useful in the treatment of RA, ankylosing spondylitis, osteoarthritis, and acute gout. The adverse reactions caused by *sulindac* are similar to, but less severe than, those of the other NSAIDs, including *indomethacin*. *Etodolac* has effects similar to those of the other NSAIDs. GI problems are less common.

D. Oxicam derivatives

Piroxicam [peer-OX-i-kam] and *meloxicam* [mel-OX-i-kam] are used to treat RA, ankylosing spondylitis, and osteoarthritis. They have long half-lives, which permit once-daily administration, and the parent drug as well as its metabolites are renally excreted in the urine. GI disturbances are encountered in approximately 20 percent of patients treated with *piroxicam*. *Meloxicam* inhibits both COX-1 and COX-2, with preferential binding for COX-2, and at low to moderate doses shows less GI irritation than *piroxicam*. However, at high doses, *meloxicam* is a nonselective NSAID, inhibiting both COX-1 and COX-2. *Meloxicam* excretion is predominantly in the form of metabolites and occurs equally in the urine and feces.

E. Fenamates

Mefenamic [meh-FEN-a-mick] *acid* and *meclofenamate* [meh-KLO-fen-a-mate] have no advantages over other NSAIDs as anti-inflammatory agents. Their side effects, such as diarrhea, can be severe, and they are associated with inflammation of the bowel. Cases of hemolytic anemia have been reported.

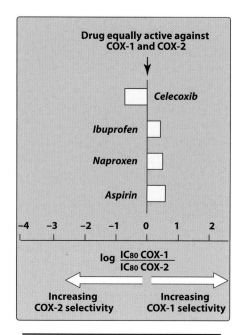

Figure 41.10
Relative selectivity of some commonly used NSAIDs. Data shown as the logarithm of their ratio of IC_{80} (drug concentration to achieve 80 percent inhibition of cyclooxygenase).

F. Heteroaryl acetic acids

Diclofenac [dye-KLO-feh-nak] and *tolmetin* [tole-MEN-tin] are approved for long-term use in the treatment of RA, osteoarthritis, and ankylosing spondylitis. *Diclofenac* is more potent than *indomethacin* or *naproxen*. An ophthalmic preparation is also available. *Diclofenac* accumulates in synovial fluid, and the primary route of excretion for the drug and its metabolites is the kidney. *Tolmetin* is an effective anti-inflammatory, antipyretic, and analgesic agent with a half-life of 5 hours. It is 99 percent bound to plasma proteins, and metabolites can be found in the urine. Toxicities of these two agents are similar to those of the other NSAIDs. *Ketorolac* [key-toe-ROLE-ak] is a potent analgesic but has moderate anti-inflammatory effects. It is available for oral administration, for intramuscular use in the treatment of postoperative pain, and for topical use for allergic conjunctivitis. *Ketorolac* undergoes hepatic metabolism, and the drug and its metabolites are eliminated via the urine. *Ketorolac* is indicated for short-term relief of moderate to severe pain for up to 5 days after the first dose is administered via IV or intramuscular dosing at the doctor's office or in a hospital. This agent is to be avoided in pediatric patients; patients with mild pain, and those with chronic conditions, the dose should not exceed 40 mg/day. *Ketorolac* can cause fatal peptic ulcers as well as GI bleeding and/or perforation of the stomach or intestines.

G. Nabumetone

Nabumetone [na-BYOO-meh-tone] is indicated for the treatment of RA and osteoarthritis and is associated with a low incidence of adverse effects. *Nabumetone* is hepatically metabolized by the liver to the active metabolite, which displays the anti-inflammatory, antipyretic, and analgesic activity. The active metabolite is then hepatically metabolized to inactive metabolites with subsequent renal elimination. Therefore, cautious use of this agent in patients with hepatic impairment is warranted; additionally, the dose should be adjusted in those with creatinine clearance of less than 50 mL/min.

H. Celecoxib

Celecoxib [sel-eh-COCKS-ib] is significantly more selective for inhibition of COX-2 than of COX-1 (Figure 41.10). In fact, at concentrations achieved in vivo, *celecoxib* does not block COX-1. Unlike the inhibition of COX-1 by *aspirin* (which is rapid and irreversible), the inhibition of COX-2 is time dependent and reversible. *Celecoxib* is approved for treatment of RA, osteoarthritis, and pain. Unlike *aspirin*, *celecoxib* does not inhibit platelet aggregation and does not increase bleeding time. *Celecoxib* has similar efficacy to NSAIDs in the treatment of pain and the risk for cardiovascular events. *Celecoxib*, when used without concomitant *aspirin* therapy, has been shown to be associated with less GI bleeding and dyspepsia; however, this benefit is lost when *aspirin* is added to *celecoxib* therapy. In patients at high risk for ulcers (that is, history of peptic ulcer disease), use of PPIs with *celecoxib* and *aspirin* may be necessary to avoid gastric ulcers.

1. **Pharmacokinetics:** *Celecoxib* is readily absorbed, reaching a peak concentration in about 3 hours. It is extensively metabolized in the liver by cytochrome P450 (CYP2C9) and is excreted in the feces and urine. Its half-life is about 11 hours; thus, the drug is usually taken once a day but can be administered as divided doses twice daily. The daily recommended dose should be reduced by 50 percent in those with moderate hepatic impairment, and *celecoxib* should be avoided in patients with severe hepatic and renal disease.

2. **Adverse effects:** Headache, dyspepsia, diarrhea, and abdominal pain are the most common adverse effects. *Celecoxib* is contraindicated in patients who are allergic to sulfonamides. [Note: If there is a history of sulfonamide drug allergy, then use of a nonselective NSAID along with a PPI is recommended.] As with other NSAIDs, kidney toxicity may occur. *Celecoxib* should be avoided in patients with chronic renal insufficiency, severe heart disease, volume depletion, and/or hepatic failure. Patients who have had anaphylactoid reactions to *aspirin* or nonselective NSAIDs may be at risk for similar effects when challenged with *celecoxib*. Inhibitors of CYP2C9, such as *fluconazole*, *fluvastatin*, and *zafirlukast*, may increase serum levels of *celecoxib*. *Celecoxib* has the ability to inhibit CYP2D6 and, thus, could lead to elevated levels of some β-blockers, antidepressants, and antipsychotic drugs.

Figure 41.11 summarizes some of the therapeutic advantages and disadvantages of members of the NSAID family.

IV. ACETAMINOPHEN

Acetaminophen [a-SEAT-a-MIN-oh-fen] inhibits prostaglandin synthesis in the CNS. This explains its antipyretic and analgesic properties. *Acetaminophen* has less effect on cyclooxygenase in peripheral tissues, which accounts for its weak anti-inflammatory activity. *Acetaminophen* does not affect platelet function or increase blood clotting time.

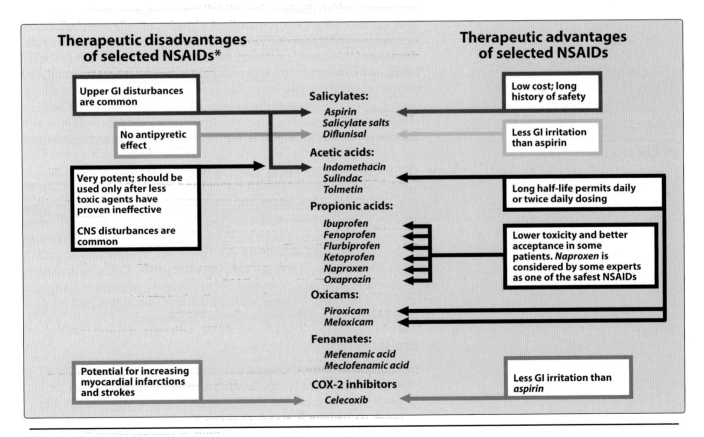

Figure 41.11
Summary of nonsteroidal anti-inflammatory agents (NSAIDs). *As a group, with the exception of *aspirin*, these drugs may have the potential to increase myocardial infarctions and strokes.

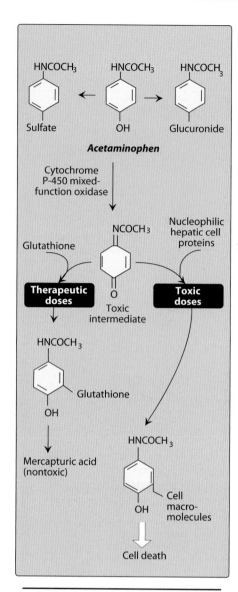

Figure 41.12
Metabolism of *acetaminophen*.

A. Therapeutic uses: *Acetaminophen* is a suitable substitute for the analgesic and antipyretic effects of *aspirin* for those patients with gastric complaints, those in whom prolongation of bleeding time would be a disadvantage, or those who do not require the anti-inflammatory action of *aspirin*. *Acetaminophen* is the analgesic/antipyretic of choice for children with viral infections or chickenpox (recall that *aspirin* increases the risk of Reye's syndrome). *Acetaminophen* does not antagonize the uricosuric agents *probenecid or sulfinpyrazone* and, therefore, may be used in patients with gout who are taking these drugs.

B. Pharmacokinetics: *Acetaminophen* is rapidly absorbed from the GI tract. A significant first-pass metabolism occurs in the luminal cells of the intestine and in the hepatocytes. Under normal circumstances, *acetaminophen* is conjugated in the liver to form inactive glucuronidated or sulfated metabolites. A portion of *acetaminophen* is hydroxylated to form N-acetylbenzoiminoquinone—a highly reactive and potentially dangerous metabolite that reacts with sulfhydryl groups. At normal doses of *acetaminophen*, the N-acetylbenzoiminoquinone reacts with the sulfhydryl group of glutathione, forming a nontoxic substance (Figure 41.12). *Acetaminophen* and its metabolites are excreted in the urine.

C. Adverse effects: With normal therapeutic doses, *acetaminophen* is virtually free of any significant adverse effects. Skin rash and minor allergic reactions occur infrequently. There may be minor alterations in the leukocyte count, but these are generally transient. Renal tubular necrosis and hypoglycemic coma are rare complications of prolonged, large-dose therapy. With large doses of *acetaminophen*, the available glutathione in the liver becomes depleted, and N-acetylbenzoiminoquinone reacts with the sulfhydryl groups of hepatic proteins, forming covalent bonds (see Figure 41.12). Hepatic necrosis, a very serious and potentially life-threatening condition, can result. Renal tubular necrosis may also occur. [Note: Administration of N-acetylcysteine, which contains sulfhydryl groups to which the toxic metabolite can bind, can be lifesaving if administered within 10 hours of the overdose.] This agent should be avoided in patients with severe hepatic impairment. Periodic monitoring of liver enzymes tests is recommended for those on high-dose *acetaminophen*.

V. DISEASE-MODIFYING ANTIRHEUMATIC AGENTS

Disease-modifying antirheumatic drugs (DMARDs) are used in the treatment of RA and have been shown to slow the course of the disease, induce remission, and prevent further destruction of the joints and involved tissues. When a patient is diagnosed with RA, the American College of Rheumatology recommends initiation of therapy with DMARDs within 3 months of diagnosis (in addition to NSAIDs, low-dose corticosteroids, physical therapy, and occupational therapy). Therapy with DMARDs is initiated rapidly to help stop the progression of the disease at the earlier stages.

A. Choice of drug

No one DMARD is efficacious and safe in every patient, and trials of several different drugs may be necessary. Most experts begin DMARD therapy with one of the traditional drugs, such as *methotrexate* or *hydroxychloroquine*. These agents are efficacious and are generally well tolerated, with well-known side-effect profiles. Inadequate response to the traditional agents may be followed by use of newer DMARDs, such as *leflunomide, anakinra,* and TNF-inhibitors (*adalimumab, etanercept,* and *infliximab)*. Combination therapies are both safe and efficacious. In most cases, *methotrexate* is combined with one of the other DMARDs. In patients who do not respond to combination therapy with *methotrexate* plus TNF inhibitors, or other combinations, treatment with *rituximab* or *abatacept* may be tried. Most of these agents are contraindicated for use in pregnant women.

B. Methotrexate

Methotrexate [meth-oh-TREX-ate], used alone or in combination therapy, has become the mainstay of treatment in patients with rheumatoid or psoriatic arthritis. *Methotrexate* slows the appearance of new erosions within involved joints on radiographs. Response to *methotrexate* occurs within 3 to 6 weeks of starting treatment. It is an immunosuppressant, and this may account for its effectiveness in an autoimmune disease. The other DMARDs can be added to *methotrexate* therapy if there is partial or no response to maximum doses of *methotrexate*. Doses of *methotrexate* required for this treatment are much lower than those needed in cancer chemotherapy and are given once a week; therefore, the adverse effects are minimized. The most common side effects observed after *methotrexate* treatment of RA are mucosal ulceration and nausea. Cytopenias (particularly depression of the WBC count), cirrhosis of the liver, and an acute pneumonia-like syndrome may occur on chronic administration. [Note: Taking *leucovorin* once daily after *methotrexate* reduces the severity of the adverse effects.] Contrary to early concerns, there have been minimal unexpected side effects after more than 20 years of surveillance, but periodic monitoring for signs of infections, complete blood counts, and liver enzymes tests are recommended.

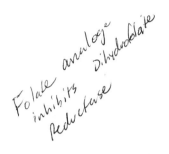
(handwritten note: Folate analog inhibits Dihydrofolate Reductase)

C. Leflunomide

Leflunomide (le-FLOO-no-mide) is an immunomodulatory agent that preferentially causes cell arrest of the autoimmune lymphocytes through its action on dihydroorotate dehydrogenase (DHODH). Activated proliferating lymphocytes require constant DNA synthesis to proliferate. Pyrimidines and purines are the building blocks of DNA, and DHODH is necessary for pyrimidine synthesis. After biotransformation, *leflunomide* becomes a reversible inhibitor of DHODH (Figure 41.13). *Leflunomide* has been approved for the treatment of RA. It not only reduces pain and inflammation associated with the disease but also appears to slow the progression of structural damage. *Leflunomide* can be used in monotherapy as an alternative to *methotrexate* or as an addition to *methotrexate* in combination therapy.

1. **Pharmacokinetics:** *Leflunomide* is well absorbed after oral administration. It is extensively bound to albumin (>90 percent) and has a half-life of 14 to 18 days. [Note: Because of its long half-life, loading doses are necessary.] *Leflunomide* is rapidly converted to the active metabolite. The metabolites are excreted in the urine and the feces. The active metabolite undergoes biliary recycling.

2. **Adverse effects:** The most common of these are headache, diarrhea, and nausea. Other untoward effects are weight loss, allergic reactions including a flu-like syndrome, skin rash, alopecia, and hypokalemia. *Leflunomide* is teratogenic in experimental animals and, therefore, is contraindicated in pregnancy and in women of child-bearing potential. It should be used with caution in patients who have liver disease, because it is cleared by both biliary and renal

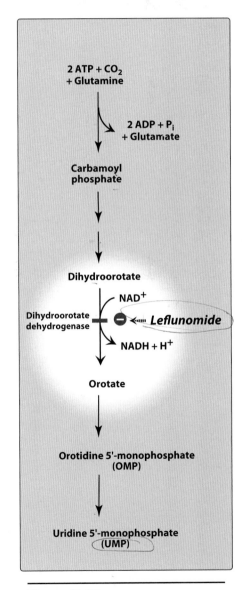

Figure 41.13
Site of action of *leflunomide*.

excretion. Monitoring parameters include signs of infections, complete blood counts, and liver enzymes tests.

D. Hydroxychloroquine *- effects mimic steroids*

This agent is also used in the treatment of malaria. It is used for early, mild RA and has relatively few side effects. When used alone, it does not slow joint damage, therefore, it is often used in combination with *methotrexate*. Its mechanism of action may include inhibition of phospholipase A_2 and platelet aggregation, membrane stabilization, effects on the immune system, and antioxidant activity. It may cause renal toxicity

E. Sulfasalazine

sulfa drug (Folate)

Sulfasalazine [sull-fa-SAH-la-zeen] is also used for early, mild RA in combination with *hydroxychloroquine* and *methotrexate*. Onset of activity is 1 to 3 months, and it is associated with leukopenia.

F. D-Penicillamine

D-Penicillamine [pen-ih-SILL-a-meen], an analog of the amino acid cysteine, slows the progression of bone destruction and RA. This agent is used as add-on therapy to existing NSAID/glucocorticoid therapy, but use in patients on DMARD therapy is avoided due to serious adverse events (for example, blood dyscrasias or renal impairment). Prolonged treatment with *penicillamine* has serious side effects, ranging from dermatologic problems to nephritis and aplastic anemia. [Note: *D-Penicillamine* is used as a chelating agent in the treatment of poisoning by heavy metals. It is also of benefit in treating cystinuria.]

G. Gold salts

(stop phagocytosis)

Gold compounds, like the other drugs in this group, cannot repair existing damage. They can only prevent further injury. The currently available gold preparation is *auranofin* for oral administration. This agent is taken up by macrophages and will suppress phagocytosis and lysosomal enzyme activity. This mechanism retards the progression of bone and articular destruction, and beneficial effects may be seen in 3 to 6 months. The gold compounds are being used infrequently by rheumatologists because of the need for meticulous monitoring for serious toxicity (for example, myelosuppression) and the costs of monitoring.

VI. BIOLOGIC THERAPIES IN RHEUMATOID ARTHRITIS

Interleukin-1b and TNF-α are proinflammatory cytokines involved in the pathogenesis of RA. When secreted by synovial macrophages, IL-1b and TNF-α stimulate synovial cells to proliferate and synthesize collagenase, thereby degrading cartilage, stimulating bone resorption, and inhibiting proteoglycan synthesis. The TNF inhibitors (*etanercept, adalimumab,* and *infliximab*) have been shown to decrease signs and symptoms of RA, reduce progression of structural damage, and improve physical function; clinical response can be seen within 2 weeks of therapy. If a patient has failed therapy with one TNF inhibitor, a trial with a different TNF inhibitor is appropriate. Many experts propose that a TNF inhibitor plus *methotrexate* be considered as standard therapy for patients with rheumatoid and psoriatic arthritis. Indeed, TNF inhibitors can be administered with any of the other DMARDs, except for *anakinra*, an IL-1 receptor antagonist. Patients receiving TNF inhibitors are at increased risk for infections (tuberculosis, and sepsis), fungal opportunistic infections, and pancytopenia. Live vaccinations should not be administered while on TNF-inhibitor therapy. These agents should be used very cautiously in those with heart failure, because these agents can cause and worsen preexisting heart failure.

A. Etanercept

Etanercept [ee-TAN-er-cept] is a genetically engineered fusion protein that binds to TNF-α, thereby blocking its interaction with cell surface TNF receptors. This agent is approved for use in patients with moderate to severe RA, either alone or in combination with *methotrexate*. It is also approved for use in patients with polyarticular-course juvenile RA, psoriatic arthritis, ankylosing spondylitis, and psoriasis. The combination of *etanercept* and *methotrexate* is more effective than *methotrexate* or *etanercept* alone in retarding the disease process, improving function, and achieving remission (Figure 41.14). Upon discontinuation of *etanercept*, the symptoms of arthritis generally return within a month.

1. **Pharmacokinetics:** *Etanercept* is given subcutaneously twice a week. The time to maximum serum concentration after a single injection is about 72 hours. Its median half-life is 115 hours.

2. **Adverse effects:** *Etanercept* is well tolerated. No toxicities or antibodies have been reported. However, it can produce local inflammation at the site of injection.

B. Infliximab

Infliximab (in-FLIX-i-mab) is a chimeric IgGκ monoclonal antibody composed of human and murine regions. The antibody binds specifically to human TNF-α, thereby neutralizing that cytokine. *Infliximab* is approved for use in combination with *methotrexate* in patients with RA who have had inadequate response to *methotrexate* monotherapy. This agent is not indicated for use alone, because monotherapy allows the body to develop anti-*infliximab* antibodies, with a reduction in efficacy. Additional indications include plaque psoriasis, psoriatic arthritis, ulcerative colitis, ankylosing spondylitis, and Crohn's disease for both fistulizing and nonfistulizing disease. [Note: Increased levels of TNF-α are found in fecal samples of patients with Crohn's disease].

1. **Pharmacokinetics:** *Infliximab* is infused IV over at least 2 hours. It distributes in the vascular compartment and has a half-life of 9.5 days. Its metabolism and elimination have not been described.

2. **Adverse effects:** Infusion reactions, such as fever, chills, pruritus, or urticaria, have occurred. Infections leading to pneumonia, cellulitis, and other conditions have also been reported. Leukopenia, neutropenia, thrombocytopenia, and pancytopenia have occurred. Whether treatment with *infliximab* predisposes to lymphoma, a condition that occurs with immunosuppressive or immune-altering drugs, remains to be established. [Note: *Infliximab* treatment does predispose to infections, which may be life-threatening.]

C. Adalimumab

Adalimumab [a-dal-AYE-mu-mab] is a recombinant monoclonal antibody that binds to human TNF-α receptor sites, thereby interfering with endogenous TNF-α activity. This agent is indicated for treatment of moderate to severe RA, either as monotherapy or in combination with *methotrexate*. It is also indicated for psoriatic arthritis, ankylosing

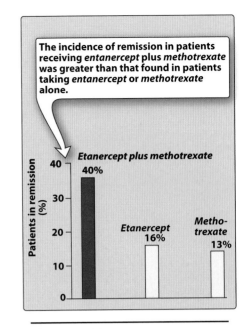

> The incidence of remission in patients receiving *entanercept* plus *methotrexate* was greater than that found in patients taking *entanercept* or *methotrexate* alone.

Figure 41.14
Incidence of remission from the symptoms of rheumatoid arthritis after 1 year of therapy.

[handwritten margin note: → Also used c̄ methotrexate for UC and Chron's]

[handwritten margin note: combination therapy only (methotrexate)]

[handwritten margin note: mono or combo therapy]

spondylitis, and Crohn's disease. *Adalimumab* is administered subcutaneously weekly or every other week. It may cause headache, nausea, rash, reaction at the injection site or increased risk of infection.

D. Anakinra

Interleukin-1 is induced by inflammatory stimuli and mediates a variety of immunologic responses, including degradation of cartilage and stimulation of bone resorption. *Anakinra* [an-a-KIN-ra] is an IL-1 receptor antagonist because it binds to the IL-1 receptor, thus preventing actions of IL-1. *Anakinra* treatment leads to a modest reduction in the signs and symptoms of moderately to severely active RA in adult patients who have failed one or more DMARDs. The drug may be used alone or in combination with DMARDs (other than TNF inhibitors). Patients should be monitored for signs of infection (tuberculosis and opportunistic infections have not been reported with this agent) and undergo absolute neutrophil counts, because this agent is associated with neutropenia. This agent is administered subcutaneously once a day if renal function is normal, and every other day in those with moderate to severe renal impairment.

E. Abatacept

T lymphocytes need two interactions to become activated: 1) the antigen-presenting cell (that is, macrophages or B cells) must interact with the receptor on the T cell, and 2) the CD80/CD86 protein on the antigen-presenting cell must interact with the CD28 protein on the T cell. The result is activated T lymphocytes responsible for the release of proinflammatory cytokines and maintenance of inflammation in RA. However, T lymphocytes contain another protein, CTLA4, which can bind to the CD80/86 protein found on the antigen-presenting cell; in fact, CTLA4 has higher binding affinity for CD80/86 than does CD28. Binding of CTLA4 to CD80/86 results in deactivation of the T lymphocyte. *Abatacept* [a-BAT-ah-cept] (CTLA-4Ig) is a soluble recombinant fusion protein made up of the extracellular domain of human CTLA4, and it competes with CD28 for binding on CD80/CD86 protein, thereby preventing full T-cell activation. This agent is indicated for reducing signs and symptoms, inducing major clinical response, slowing the progression of structural damage, and improving physical function in adult patients with moderate to severe RA who have had an inadequate response to DMARDs such as *methotrexate* or TNF inhibitors. *Abatacept* can be used alone or with DMARDs other than TNF inhibitors or *anakinra*.

1. **Pharmacokinetics:** The recommended dose is based upon weight and is administered as an IV infusion over 30 minutes at Weeks 2 and 4 after the first infusion and every 4 weeks thereafter with monitoring for infusion reactions. The terminal half-life in RA patients administered multiple doses of 10 mg/kg is 13 days (range, 8–25 days).

2. **Adverse effects:** The most commonly reported adverse effects include headache, upper respiratory infections, nasopharyngitis, and nausea. Concurrent use with TNF inhibitors and *anakinra* is not recommended due to increased risk of serious infections.

F. Rituximab

B lymphocytes are derived from the bone marrow and are necessary for efficient immune response; however, in RA, B cells can perpetuate the inflammatory process in the synovium by 1) activating T lymphocytes, 2) producing autoantibodies such as anti-CCP (anti–cyclic citrullinated peptide antibody) and rheumatoid factor, and 3) producing pro-inflammatory cytokines such as TNF-α and IL-1. *Rituximab* [ri-TUK-si-mab]is a genetically engineered chimeric murine/human monoclonal antibody directed against the CD20 antigen found on the surface of normal and malignant B lymphocytes, resulting in B-cell depletion. This agent is indicated for use in combination with *methotrexate* to reduce signs and symptoms in adult patients with moderate to severe RA who have had an inadequate response to one or more TNF-inhibitors. *Rituximab* has been shown to reduce joint erosion and joint space narrowing in these patients.

1. **Pharmacokinetics:** *Rituximab* is administered as two 1000-mg IV infusions separated by 2 weeks. To reduce the severity of infusion reactions, *methylprednisolone* at 100 mg IV or its equivalent is administered 30 minutes prior to each infusion. The mean terminal elimination half-life after the second dose is 19 days.

2. **Adverse effects:** Infusion reactions (that is, urticaria, hypotension, or angioedema) are the most common complaints with this agent and typically occur during the first infusion. The infusion may be interrupted and the patient treated with vasopressors, antihistamines, and fluids. If the infusion is to be continued, then the rate of infusion should be reduced by 50 percent after symptoms have completely resolved.

VII. DRUGS EMPLOYED IN THE TREATMENT OF GOUT

Gout is a metabolic disorder characterized by high levels of uric acid in the blood. Hyperuricemia can lead to deposition of sodium urate crystals in tissues, especially the joints and kidney. Hyperuricemia does not always lead to gout, but gout is always preceded by hyperuricemia. In humans, sodium urate is the end product of purine metabolism.[5] The deposition of urate crystals initiates an inflammatory process involving the infiltration of granulocytes that phagocytize the urate crystals (Figure 41.15). This process generates oxygen metabolites, which damage tissues, resulting in the release of lysosomal enzymes that evoke an inflammatory response. In addition, there is increased production of lactate in the synovial tissues. The resulting local decrease in pH fosters further deposition of urate crystals. The cause of hyperuricemia is an overproduction of uric acid relative to the patient's ability to excrete it. Most therapeutic strategies for gout involve lowering the uric acid level below the saturation point (<6 mg/dL), thus preventing the deposition of urate crystals. This can be accomplished by 1) interfering with uric acid synthesis with *allopurinol*, 2) increasing uric acid excretion with *probenecid* or *sulfinpyrazone*, 3) inhibiting leukocyte entry into the affected joint with *colchicine*, or 4) administration of NSAIDs.

A. Treating acute gout → *Diclofenac + Ketorolac*

Acute gouty attacks can result from a number of conditions, including excessive alcohol consumption, a diet rich in purines, or kidney disease. Acute attacks are treated with *indomethacin* to decrease movement of granulocytes into the affected area; NSAIDs other than *indomethacin*

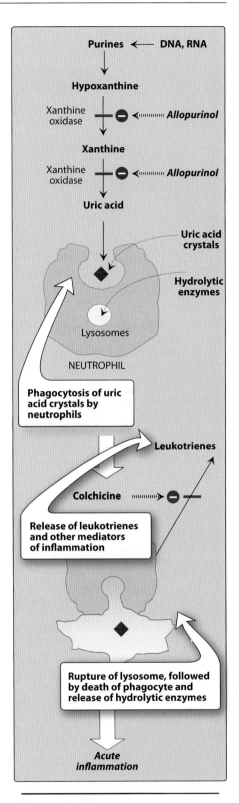

Figure 41.15
Role of uric acid in the inflammation of gout.

[5]See p. 298 in **Lippincott's Illustrated Reviews: Biochemistry** (4th ed.) for a discussion of purine metabolism.

are also effective at decreasing pain and inflammation. [Note: *Aspirin* is contraindicated, because it competes with uric acid for the organic acid secretion mechanism in the proximal tubule of the kidney.] The initial NSAID dose should be doubled within the first 24 to 48 hours (maintain recommended dosing interval per specific NSAID) and then reduced over the next few days. Intra-articular administration of glucocorticoids (when only one or two joints are affected) is also appropriate in the acute setting. Patients are candidates for prophylactic therapy if they have had more than two attacks per year, the first attack is severe or complicated with kidney stones, serum urate is greater than 10 mg/dL, or urinary urate excretion exceeds 1000 mg per 24 hours.

B. Treating chronic gout

Chronic gout can be caused by 1) a genetic defect, such as one resulting in an increase in the rate of purine synthesis; 2) renal deficiency; 3) Lesch-Nyhan syndrome;[6] or 4) excessive productionof uric acid associated with cancer chemotherapy. Treatment strategies for chronic gout include the use of uricosuric drugs that increase the excretion of uric acid, thereby reducing its concentration in plasma, and the use of *allopurinol*, which is a selective inhibitor of the terminal steps in the biosynthesis of uric acid. Uricosuric agents are first-line agents for patients with gout associated with reduced urinary excretion of uric acid. *Allopurinol* is preferred in patients with excessive uric acid synthesis, with previous histories of uric acid stones, or with renal insufficiency.

C. Colchicine

Colchicine [KOL-chi-seen], a plant alkaloid, has been used for the treatment of acute gouty attacks as well as chronic gout. It is neither a uricosuric nor an analgesic agent, although it relieves pain in acute attacks of gout. *Colchicine* does not prevent the progression of gout to acute gouty arthritis, but it does have a suppressive, prophylactic effect that reduces the frequency of acute attacks and relieves pain.

1. **Mechanism of action:** *Colchicine* binds to tubulin, a microtubular protein, causing its depolymerization. This disrupts cellular functions, such as the mobility of granulocytes, thus decreasing their migration into the affected area. Furthermore, *colchicine* blocks cell division by binding to mitotic spindles. *Colchicine* also inhibits the synthesis and release of the leukotrienes (see Figure 41.15).

2. **Therapeutic uses:** The anti-inflammatory activity of *colchicine* is specific for gout, usually alleviating the pain of acute gout within 12 hours. (Note: *Colchicine* must be administered within 24 to 48 hours of onset of attack to be effective). NSAIDs have largely replaced *colchicine* in the treatment of acute gouty attacks. *Colchicine* is currently used for prophylaxis of recurrent attacks and will prevent attacks in more than 80 percent of patients.

3. **Pharmacokinetics:** *Colchicine* is administered orally, followed by rapid absorption from the GI tract. It is also available combined with *probenecid* (see below). *Colchicine* is recycled in the bile and is excreted unchanged in the feces or urine. Use should be avoided in patients with a creatinine clearance of less than 50 mL/min.

[6]See p. 296 in *Lippincott's Illustrated Reviews: Biochemistry* (4th ed.) for a discussion of Lesch-Nyhan syndrome.

4. **Adverse effects:** *Colchicine* treatment may cause nausea, vomiting, abdominal pain, and diarrhea (Figure 41.16). Chronic administration may lead to myopathy, neutropenia, aplastic anemia, and alopecia. The drug should not be used in pregnancy, and it should be used with caution in patients with hepatic, renal, or cardiovascular disease. The fatal dose has been reprted as low as 7 to 10 mg.

D. Allopurinol

Allopurinol [al-oh-PURE-i-nole] is a purine analog. It reduces the production of uric acid by competitively inhibiting the last two steps in uric acid biosynthesis that are catalyzed by xanthine oxidase (see Figure 41.15). [Note: Uric acid is less water soluble than its precursors. When xanthine oxidase is inhibited, the circulating purine derivatives (xanthine and hypoxanthine) are more soluble and, therefore, are less likely to precipitate.]

1. **Therapeutic uses:** *Allopurinol* is effective in the treatment of primary hyperuricemia of gout and hyperuricemia secondary to other conditions, such as that associated with certain malignancies (those in which large amounts of purines are produced, particularly after treatment with chemotherapeutic agents) or in renal disease. This agent is the drug of choice in those with a history of kidney stones or if the creatinine clearance is less than 50 mL/day.

2. **Pharmacokinetics:** *Allopurinol* is completely absorbed after oral administration. The primary metabolite is alloxanthine (oxypurinol), which is also a xanthine oxidase inhibitor with a half-life of 15 to 18 hours; the half-life of *allopurinol* is 2 hours. Thus, effective inhibition of xanthine oxidase can be maintained with once-daily dosage. The drug and its active metabolite are excreted in the feces and urine.

3. **Adverse effects:** *Allopurinol* is well tolerated by most patients. Hypersensitivity reactions, especially skin rashes, are the most common adverse reactions, occurring in approximately three percent of patients. The reactions may occur even after months or years of chronic administration, and *allopurinol* therapy should be discontinued. Acute attacks of gout may occur more frequently during the first several weeks of therapy; therefore, *colchicine* or NSAIDs should be administered concurrently. GI side effects, such as nausea and diarrhea, are common. *Allopurinol* interferes with the metabolism of the anticancer agent *6-mercaptopurine* and the immunosuppressant *azathioprine*, requiring a reduction in dosage of these drugs.

E. Uricosuric agents: Probenecid and sulfinpyrazone

The uricosuric drugs are weak organic acids that promote renal clearance of uric acid by inhibiting the urate-anion exchanger in the proximal tubule that mediates urate reabsorption. *Probenecid* [proe-BEN-e-sid], a general inhibitor of the tubular secretion of organic acids, and *sulfinpyrazone* [sul-fin-PEER-a-zone], a derivative of *phenylbutazone*, are the two most commonly used uricosuric agents. At therapeutic doses, they block proximal tubular resorption of uric acid. [Note: At low dosage, these agents block proximal tubular secretion of uric acid.] These drugs have few adverse effects, although gastric distress may force discontinuance of *sulfinpyrazone*. *Probenecid* blocks the tubular secretion of *penicillin* and is sometimes used to increase levels of the antibiotic. It also inhibits excretion of *naproxen, ketoprofen,* and *indomethacin*. These agents are appropriate for patients who have a creatinine clearance of less than 60 mL/min, undersecrete uric acid (<700 mg/day), and do not have a history of kidney stones.

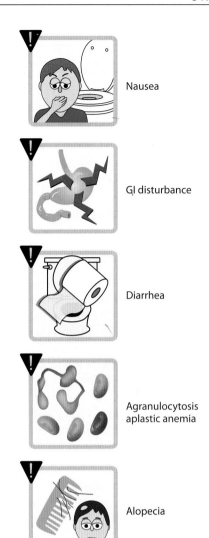

Nausea

GI disturbance

Diarrhea

Agranulocytosis aplastic anemia

Alopecia

Figure 41.16
Some adverse effects of *colchicine*.

Study Questions

Choose the ONE best answer.

41.1 In which one of the following conditions would aspirin be contraindicated?

   A. Myalgia.
   B. Fever.
   C. Peptic ulcer.
   D. RA.
   E. Unstable angina.

Correct answer = C. Among the NSAIDs, aspirin is one of the worst for causing gastric irritation. Aspirin is an effective analgesic and is used to reduce muscle pain. It also has antipyretic actions, so it can be used to treat fever. Because of its anti-inflammatory properties, aspirin is used to treat pain related to the inflammatory process—for example, in the treatment of RA. Low doses of aspirin also decrease the incidence of TIAs.

41.2 Which one of the following statements concerning COX-2 inhibitors is correct?

   A. The COX-2 inhibitors show greater analgesic activity than traditional NSAIDs.
   B. The COX-2 inhibitors decrease platelet function.
   C. The COX-2 inhibitors do not affect the kidney.
   D. The COX-2 inhibitors show anti-inflammatory activity similar to that of the traditional NSAIDs.
   E. The COX-2 inhibitors are cardioprotective.

Correct answer = D. The COX-2 inhibitors show similar analgesic and anti-inflammatory activity compared to traditional NSAIDs. They do not affect platelets. Like NSAIDs, COX-2 inhibitors may cause the development of acute renal failure due to renal vasoconstriction. COX-2 inhibitors have the potential for increasing the risk of myocardial infarction.

41.3 An 8-year-old girl has a fever and muscle aches from a presumptive viral infection. Which one of the following drugs would be most appropriate to treat her symptoms?

   A. Acetaminophen.
   B. Aspirin.
   C. Celecoxib.
   D. Codeine.
   E. Indomethacin.

Correct answer = A. Aspirin should be avoided in children because of an association with Reye's syndrome. Indomethacin has antipyretic activity but is too toxic for use in these circumstances. Celecoxib is indicated for alleviation of pain, and codeine has no antipyretic effects.

41.4 A 70-year-old man has a history of ulcer disease. He has recently experienced swelling and pain in the joints of his hands. His physician wants to begin therapy with an NSAID. Which one of the following drugs might also be prescribed along with the NSAID to reduce the risk of activating this patient's ulcer disease?

   A. Allopurinol.
   B. Colchicine.
   C. Misoprostol.
   D. Probenecid.
   E. Sulindac.

Correct answer = C. Misoprostol is a prostaglandin analog that can reduce gastric acid and pepsin secretion and promote the formation of mucus in the stomach. It is indicated for the purpose of decreasing the risk of ulcer activation in patients taking NSAIDs. The other choices are not appropriate for alleviating the gastric irritation caused by NSAIDs.

Autacoids and Autacoid Antagonists

42

I. OVERVIEW

Prostaglandins, histamine, and serotonin belong to a group of compounds called autacoids. These heterogeneous substances have widely differing structures and pharmacologic activities. They all have the common feature of being formed by the tissues on which they act; thus, they function as local hormones. [Note: The word autacoid comes from the Greek: <u>autos</u> (self) and <u>akos</u> (medicinal agent, or remedy).] The autacoids also differ from circulating hormones in that they are produced by many tissues rather than in specific endocrine glands. The drugs described in this chapter (Figure 42.1) are either autacoids or autacoid antagonists (compounds that inhibit the synthesis of certain autacoids or that interfere with their interactions with receptors).

II. PROSTAGLANDINS

Prostaglandins are unsaturated fatty acid derivatives that act on the tissues in which they are synthesized and are rapidly metabolized to inactive products at the site of action.[1]

A. Therapeutic uses of prostaglandins

Systemic administration of prostaglandins evokes a bewildering array of effects—a fact that limits the therapeutic usefulness of these agents.

1. **Abortion:** Several of the prostaglandins find use as abortifacients (agents causing abortions). The most effective option available involves oral administration *mifepristone* [mi-FEP-ri-stone] (RU-486, a synthetic steroid with antiprogestational effects) followed at least 24 hours later by the synthetic prostaglandin E_1 analog *misoprostol* [mye-so-PROST-ole] administered vaginally (Figure 42.2). Women can self-administer this regimen with complete abortion rates exceeding 95 percent. The overall case-fatality rate for abortion is less than one death per 100,000 procedures. Infection, hemorrhage, and retained tissue are among the more common complications.

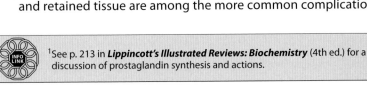

[1]See p. 213 in *Lippincott's Illustrated Reviews: Biochemistry* (4th ed.) for a discussion of prostaglandin synthesis and actions.

AUTACOIDS

PROSTAGLANDINS
- *Misoprostol*

H₁ ANTIHISTAMINES
- *Acrivastine*
- *Cetirizine*
- *Chlorpheniramine*
- *Cyclizine*
- *Desloratadine*
- *Diphenhydramine*
- *Dimenhydrinate*
- *Doxepin*
- *Doxylamine*
- *Fexofenadine*
- *Hydroxyzine*
- *Levocetirizine*
- *Loratadine*
- *Meclizine*
- *Promethazine*

DRUGS USED TO TREAT MIGRAINE HEADACHE
- *Almotriptan*
- *Dihydroergotamine*
- *Eletriptan*
- *Frovatriptan*
- *Naratriptan*
- *Rizatriptan*
- *Sumatriptan*
- *Zolmitriptan*

Figure 42.1
Summary of drugs affecting the autacoids.

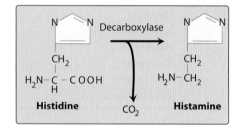

Figure 42.2
Therapeutic applications of *misoprostol*.

Handwritten notes:
Decarboxylase
Histidine → Histamine ↓ Stored ā heparin

2. Peptic ulcers: *Misoprostol* is sometimes used to inhibit the secretion of gastric acid and to enhance mucosal resistance to injury in patients with gastric ulcer who are chronically taking nonsteroidal anti-inflammatory agents. Proton-pump inhibitors, such as *omeprazole*, and H_2 antihistamines also reduce the risk of gastric ulcer and are better tolerated than *misoprostol*, which induces intestinal disorders.

III. HISTAMINE

Histamine is a chemical messenger that mediates a wide range of cellular responses, including allergic and inflammatory reactions, gastric acid secretion, and neurotransmission in parts of the brain. Histamine has no clinical applications, but agents that interfere with the action of histamine (antihistamines) have important therapeutic applications.

A. Location, synthesis, and release

1. **Location:** Histamine occurs in practically all tissues, but it is unevenly distributed, with high amounts found in lung, skin, and the gastrointestinal tract (sites where the "inside" of the body meets the "outside"). It is found at high concentration in mast cells or basophils. Histamine also occurs as a component of venoms and in secretions from insect stings.

2. **Synthesis:** Histamine is an amine formed by the decarboxylation of the amino acid histidine by histidine decarboxylase,[2] an enzyme that is expressed in cells throughout the body, including central nervous system (CNS) neurons, gastric mucosa parietal cells, mast cells, and basophils (Figure 42.3). In mast cells, histamine is stored in granules as an inactive complex composed of histamine and the polysulfated anion, heparin, along with an anionic protein. If histamine is not stored, it is rapidly inactivated by amine oxidase enzymes.

3. **Release of histamine:** The release of histamine may be the primary response to some stimuli, but most often, histamine is just one of several chemical mediators released. Stimuli causing the release of histamine from tissues include the destruction of cells as a result of cold, bacterial toxins, bee sting venoms, or trauma. Allergies and anaphylaxis can also trigger release of histamine.

B. Mechanism of action

Handwritten note: Histamine acts through a G-protein

Histamine released in response to various stimuli exerts its effects by binding to one or more of four types of histamine receptors—H_1, H_2, H_3, and H_4 receptors. H_1 and H_2 receptors are widely expressed and are the targets of clinically useful drugs. H_3 and H_4 receptors are expressed in only a few cell types, and their roles in drug action are unclear. All types of histamine receptors have seven transmembrane helical domains and transduce extracellular signals by way of G protein–mediated second-messenger systems. Some of histamine's wide range of pharmacologic effects are mediated by both H_1 and H_2 receptors, whereas

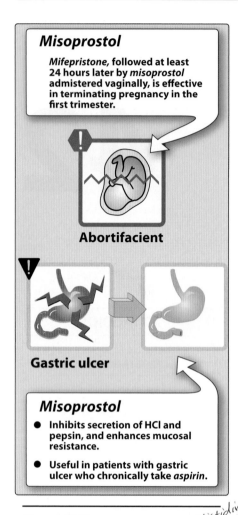

Figure 42.3
Biosynthesis of histamine.

[2] See p. 287 in *Lippincott's Illustrated Reviews: Biochemistry* (4th ed.) for a discussion of histamine.

others are mediated by only one class. For example, the H_1 receptors are important in producing smooth muscle contraction and increasing capillary permeability (Figure 42.4). Histamine promotes vasodilation by causing vascular endothelium to release nitric oxide.[3] This chemical signal diffuses to the vascular smooth muscle, where it stimulates cyclic guanosine monophosphate production, causing vasodilation. Histamine H_2 receptors mediate gastric acid secretion. The two most common histamine receptors exert their effects by different second-messenger pathways. The actions of H_1 antihistamines occur through at least two mechanisms. Antiallergic activities of H_1 antihistamines, such as inhibition of the release of mediators from mast cells and basophils, involves stimulation of the intracellular activity of the polyphosphatidylinositol pathway.[4] Other actions of H_1 antihistamines involve the down-regulation of nuclear transcription factors that regulate the production of proinflammatory cytokines and adhesion proteins. In contrast, stimulation of H_2 receptors enhances the production of cyclic adenosine monophosphate (cAMP) by adenylyl cyclase.

(H₁ mast cells: G protein → PIP
H₂ : cAMP)

C. Role in allergy and anaphylaxis

The symptoms resulting from intravenous injection of histamine are similar to those associated with anaphylactic shock and allergic reactions. These include contraction of smooth muscle, stimulation of secretions, dilation and increased permeability of the capillaries, and stimulation of sensory nerve endings.

1. **Role of mediators:** Symptoms associated with allergy and anaphylactic shock result from the release of certain mediators from their storage sites. Such mediators include histamine, serotonin, leukotrienes, and the eosinophil chemotactic factor of anaphylaxis. In some cases, these cause a localized allergic reaction, producing, for example, actions on the skin or respiratory tract. Under other conditions, these mediators may cause a full-blown anaphylactic response. It is thought that the difference between these two situations results from differences in the sites from which mediators are released and in their rates of release. For example, if the release of histamine is slow enough to permit its inactivation before it enters the bloodstream, a local allergic reaction results. However, if histamine release is too fast for inactivation to be efficient, a full-blown anaphylactic reaction occurs.

IV. H₁ ANTIHISTAMINES

The term antihistamine, without a modifying adjective, refers to the classic H_1-receptor blockers. These compounds do not influence the formation or release of histamine; rather, they block the receptor-mediated response of a target tissue. [Note: This contrasts with the action of *cromolyn* and *nedocromil*, which inhibit the release of histamine from mast cells and are useful in the treatment of asthma.] The H_1-receptor blockers can be divided into first- and second-generation drugs (Figure 42.5). The older first-generation drugs are still widely used because they are effective and inexpensive. However, most of these drugs penetrate the CNS and cause sedation. Furthermore, they tend to interact with other receptors, producing a vari-

---

H₁ Receptors

EXOCRINE EXCRETION

Increased production of nasal and bronchial mucus, resulting in respiratory symptoms.

BRONCHIAL SMOOTH MUSCLE

Constriction of bronchioles results in symptoms of asthma and decreased lung capacity.

INTESTINAL SMOOTH MUSCLE

Constriction results in intestinal cramps and diarrhea.

SENSORY NERVE ENDINGS

Causes itching and pain.

Skin

H₁ and H₂ Receptors

CARDIOVASCULAR SYSTEM

Lowers systemic blood pressure by reducing peripheral resistance. Causes positive chronotropism (mediated by H_2 receptors) and a positive inotropism (mediated by both H_1 and H_2 receptors).

SKIN

Dilation and increased permeability of the capillaries results in leakage of proteins and fluid into the tissues. In the skin, this results in the classic "triple response": wheal formation, reddening due to local vasodilation, and flare ("halo").

H₂ Receptors

← cimetidine

Stomach

Stimulation of gastric hydrochloric acid secretion.

Figure 42.4
Actions of histamine.

---

[3] See p. 150 in *Lippincott's Illustrated Reviews: Biochemistry* (4th ed.) for a discussion of nitric oxide.
[4] See p. 205 in *Lippincott's Illustrated Reviews: Biochemistry* (4th ed.) for a discussion of the polyphosphatidylinositol pathway.

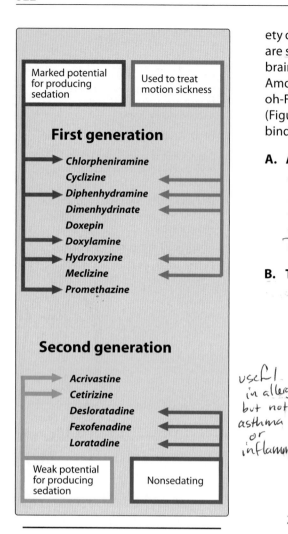

Figure 42.5
Summary of therapeutic advantages and disadvantages of some H₁ histamine–receptor blocking agents.

[Handwritten notes:]
useful in allergies, but not asthma or inflammation

H1 blockers
diphenhydramine
diphenhydrinate
cyclizine
meclizine
hydroxyzine
useful in treating motion sickness

diphenhydramine and doxylamine sedate

ety of unwanted adverse effects. By contrast, the second-generation agents are specific for H₁ receptors, and because they do not penetrate the blood-brain barrier, they show less CNS toxicity than the first-generation drugs. Among these agents *desloratadine* [des-lor-AH-tahdeen], *fexofenadine* [fex-oh-FEN-a-deen], and *loratadine* [lor-AT-a-deen] show the least sedation (Figure 42.6). [Note: The histamine receptors are distinct from those that bind serotonin, acetylcholine, and the catecholamines.]

A. Actions

The action of all the H₁-receptor blockers is qualitatively similar. However, most of these blockers have additional effects unrelated to their blocking of H₁ receptors; these effects probably reflect binding of the H₁ antagonists to cholinergic, adrenergic, or serotonin receptors (Figure 42.7).

B. Therapeutic uses

1. **Allergic and inflammatory conditions:** H₁-receptor blockers are useful in treating allergies caused by antigens acting on immunoglobulin E antibody–sensitized mast cells. For example, antihistamines are the drugs of choice in controlling the symptoms of allergic rhinitis and urticaria, because histamine is the principal mediator. However, the H₁-receptor blockers are ineffective in treating bronchial asthma, because histamine is only one of several mediators of that condition. [Note: *Epinephrine* has actions on smooth muscle that are opposite to those of histamine, and it acts at different receptors. Therefore, *epinephrine* is the drug of choice in treating systemic anaphylaxis and other conditions that involve massive release of histamine.] Glucocorticoids show greater anti-inflammatory effects than the H₁ antihistamines.

2. **Motion sickness and nausea:** Along with the antimuscarinic agent *scopolamine*, certain H₁-receptor blockers, such as *diphenhydramine* [dye-fen-HYE-dra-meen], *dimenhydrinate* [dye-men-HYE-dri-nate], *cyclizine* [SYE-kli-zeen], *meclizine* [MEK-li-zeen], and *hydroxyzine* [hye-DROX-ee-zeen] (see Figure 42.5), are the most effective agents for prevention of the symptoms of motion sickness. The antihistamines prevent or diminish vomiting and nausea mediated by both the chemoreceptor and vestibular pathways. The antiemetic action of these medications seems to be due to their blockade of central H₁ and muscarinic receptors.

3. **Somnifacients:** Although they are not the medication of choice, many first-generation antihistamines, such as *diphenhydramine* and *doxylamine* [dox-IL-a-meen], have strong sedative properties and are used in the treatment of insomnia (see Figure 42.5). The use of first-generation H₁ antihistamines is contraindicated in the treatment of individuals working in jobs where wakefulness is critical.

C. Pharmacokinetics

H₁-receptor blockers are well absorbed after oral administration, with maximum serum levels occurring at 1 to 2 hours. The average plasma half-life is 4 to 6 hours except for *meclizine*, which has a half-life of 12 to 24 hours. H₁-receptor blockers have high bioavailability and are distributed in all tissues, including the CNS. All first-generation H₁ antihistamines and some second-generation H₁ antihistamines, such as *desloratadine* and *loratadine*, are metabolized by the hepatic cytochrome P450 system. *Cetirizine* [seh-TEER-ih-zeen] is excreted largely unchanged in the urine, and *fexofenadine* is excreted largely unchanged in the feces. After a single oral dose, the onset of action occurs within 1 to 3 hours. The duration of action for many oral H₁ antihistamines is at least 24 hours, facilitating once-daily dosing. They are most effective when used prophylactically before allergen exposure rather than as needed. Tolerance to the action of H₁ antihistamines has not been observed.

D. Adverse effects

First-generation H₁-receptor blockers have a low specificity; that is, they interact not only with histamine receptors but also with muscarinic cholinergic receptors, α-adrenergic receptors, and serotonin receptors (see Figure 42.7). The extent of interaction with these receptors and, as a result, the nature of the side effects vary with the structure of the drug. Some side effects may be undesirable, and others may have therapeutic value. Furthermore, the incidence and severity of adverse reactions for a given drug varies between individual subjects.

1. **Sedation:** First-generation H₁ antihistamines, such as *chlorpheniramine* [klor-fen-IR-a-meen], *diphenhydramine*, *hydroxyzine*, and *promethazine* [proe-METH-a-zeen], bind to H₁ receptors and block the neurotransmitter effect of histamine in the CNS. The most frequently observed adverse reaction is sedation (Figure 42.8). Other central actions include tinnitus, fatigue, dizziness, lassitude (a sense of weariness), uncoordination, blurred vision, and tremors. Sedation is less common with the second-generation drugs, which do not readily enter the CNS. Second-generation H₁ antihistamines are specific for H₁ receptors and penetrate the CNS poorly. They show less sedation and other CNS effects.

2. **Dry mouth:** Oral antihistamines also exert weak anticholinergic effects, leading not only to a drying of the nasal passage but also to a tendency to dry the oral cavity. Blurred vision can occur as well with some drugs.

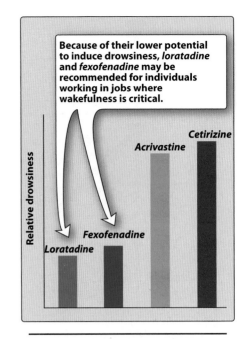

Figure 42.6
Relative potential for causing drowsiness in patients receiving second-generation H₁ antihistamines.

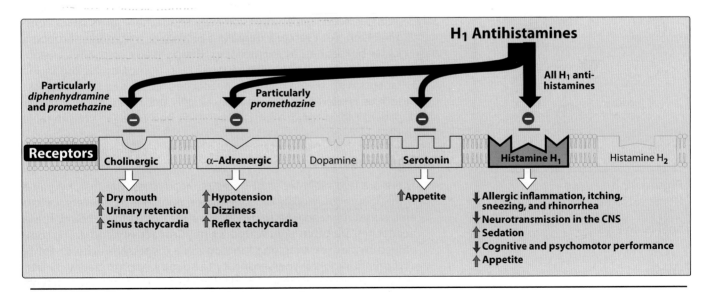

Figure 42.7
Effects of H₁ antihistamines at histamine, adrenergic, cholinergic, and serotonin-binding receptors. Many second-generation antihistamines do not enter the brain and, therefore, show minimal CNS effects.

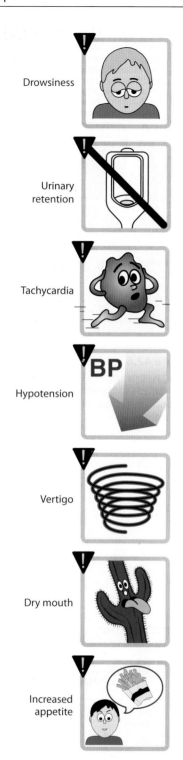

Drowsiness

Urinary retention

Tachycardia

Hypotension

Vertigo

Dry mouth

Increased appetite

Figure 42.8
Some adverse effects observed with first-generation H$_1$ antihistamines.

3. **Drug interactions:** Interaction of H$_1$-receptor blockers with other drugs can cause serious consequences, such as potentiation of the effects of all other CNS depressants, including alcohol. Persons taking monoamine oxidase (MAO) inhibitors should not take antihistamines, because the MAO inhibitors can exacerbate the anticholinergic effects of the antihistamines. In addition, the first-generation antihistamines (*diphenhydramine* and others) have considerable anticholinergic (antimuscarinic) actions. These actions would decrease the effectiveness of cholinesterase inhibitors (*donepezil*, *rivastigmine*, and *galantamine*) in the treatment of Alzheimer's disease.

4. **Overdoses:** Although the margin of safety of H$_1$-receptor blockers is relatively high and chronic toxicity is rare, acute poisoning is relatively common, especially in young children. The most common and dangerous effects of acute poisoning are those on the CNS, including hallucinations, excitement, ataxia, and convulsions. If untreated, the patient may experience a deepening coma and collapse of the cardiorespiratory system.

V. HISTAMINE H$_2$-RECEPTOR BLOCKERS

Histamine H$_2$-receptor blockers have little, if any, affinity for H$_1$ receptors. Although antagonists of the histamine H$_2$ receptor (H$_2$ antagonists) block the actions of histamine at all H$_2$ receptors, their chief clinical use is as inhibitors of gastric acid secretion in the treatment of ulcers and heartburn. By competitively blocking the binding of histamine to H$_2$ receptors, these agents reduce intracellular concentrations of cAMP and, thereby, secretion of gastric acid. The four drugs used in the United States—*cimetidine*, *ranitidine*, *famotidine*, and *nizatidine*—are discussed in Chapter 28.

VI. DRUGS USED TO TREAT MIGRAINE HEADACHE

It has been estimated that 18 million women and 6 million men in the United States suffer from severe migraine headaches. Migraine can usually be distinguished clinically from the two other common types of headaches—cluster headache and tension-type headache—by its characteristics (Figure 42.9). For example, migraines present as a pulsatile, throbbing pain; cluster headaches, as excruciating, sharp, steady pain; and tension-type headaches, as dull pain, with a persistent, tightening feeling in the head. Patients with severe migraine headaches report one to five attacks per month of moderate to severe pain, usually unilateral. The headaches affect patients for a major part of their lives and result in considerable health costs.

A. Types of migraine

There are two main types of migraine headaches. The first, migraine without aura (previously called common migraine), is a severe, unilateral, pulsating headache that typically lasts from 2 to 72 hours. These headaches are often aggravated by physical activity and are accompanied by nausea, vomiting, photophobia (hypersensitivity to light), and phonophobia (hypersensitivity to sound). Approximately 85 percent of patients with migraine do not have aura. In the second type, migraine with aura (previously called classic migraine), the headache is preceded by neurologic symptoms called auras, which can be visual, sensory, and/or cause speech or motor disturbances. Most commonly,

	MIGRAINE	CLUSTER	TENSION TYPE
Family history	Yes	No	Yes
Sex	Females more often than males	Males more often than females	Females more often than males
Onset	Variable	During sleep	Under stress
Location	Usually unilateral	Behind or around one eye	Bilateral in band around head
Character and severity	Pulsating, throbbing	Excruciating, sharp, steady	Dull, persistent, tightening
Duration	2–72 hours per episode	15–90 minutes per episode	30 minutes to 7 days per episode
Associated symptoms	Visual auras, sensitivity to light and sound, pale facial appearance, nausea and vomiting	Unilateral or bilateral sweating, facial flushing, nasal congestion, lacrimation, pupillary changes	Mild intolerance to light and noise, anorexia

Figure 42.9
Characteristics of migraine, cluster, and tension-type headaches.

these prodromal symptoms are visual, occurring approximately 20 to 40 minutes before headache pain begins. In the 15 percent of migraine patients whose headache is preceded by an aura, the aura itself allows diagnosis. The headache itself in migraines with or without auras is similar. For both types of migraines, women are three-fold more likely than men to experience either type of migraine.

B. Biologic basis of migraine headaches

The first manifestation of migraine with aura is a spreading depression of neuronal activity accompanied by reduced blood flow in the most posterior part of the cerebral hemisphere. This hypoperfusion gradually spreads forward over the surface of the cortex to other contiguous areas of the brain. The vascular alteration is accompanied by functional changes; for example, the hypoperfused regions show an abnormal response to changes in arterial partial pressure of CO_2. The hypoperfusion persists throughout the aura and well into the headache phase, after which hyperperfusion occurs. Patients who have migraine without aura do not show hypoperfusion. However, the pain of both types of migraine may be due to extracranial and intracranial arterial dilation. This stretching leads to release of neuroactive molecules, such as substance P.

C. Symptomatic treatment of acute migraine

Acute treatments can be classified as nonspecific (symptomatic) or migraine specific. Nonspecific treatment includes analgesics, such as nonsteroidal anti-inflammatory drugs, and antiemetics, such as *prochlorperazine*, to control vomiting. Opioids are reserved as rescue medication when other treatments of a severe migraine attack are not successful. Specific migraine therapy includes triptans and *dihydroergotamine*, both of which are 5-HT$_{1D}$ receptor agonists. It has been proposed that activation of 5-HT$_{1D}$ receptors by these agents leads either to vasoconstriction or to inhibition of the release of proinflammatory neuropeptides. Despite their high cost, most patients prefer triptans over ergot derivatives.

1. **Triptans:** This class of drugs includes *sumatriptan* [SOO-ma-trip-tan], *naratriptan* [NAR-a-trip-tan], *rizatriptan* [rye-za-TRIP-tan], *eletriptan* [EH-leh-trip-tan], *almotriptan* [AL-moh-trip-tan], *frovatriptan* (frova-TRIP-tan), and *zolmitriptan* [zole-ma-TRIP-tan]. These agents rapidly and effectively abort or markedly reduce the severity of migraine headaches in about 70 percent of patients. The triptans are serotonin agonists, acting at a subgroup of serotonin receptors found on small, peripheral nerves that innervate the intracranial vasculature. The nausea that occurs with *dihydroergotamine* and the vasoconstriction caused by *ergotamine* (see below) are much less pronounced with the triptans, particularly *rizatriptan* and *zolmitriptan*. *Sumatriptan* is given subcutaneously, intranasally, or orally. [Note: All other agents are taken orally.] The onset of the parenteral drug (which is indicated for treatment of cluster headaches) is about 20 minutes, compared with 1 to 2 hours when the drug is administered orally. The drug has a short duration of action, with an elimination half-life of 2 hours. Headache commonly recurs within 24 to 48 hours after a single dose of drug, but in most patients, a second dose is effective in aborting the headache. *Rizatriptan* and *eletriptan* are modestly more effective than *sumatriptan*, the prototype drug, whereas *naratriptan* and *almotriptan* are better tolerated. *Frovatriptan* is the longest-acting triptan, with a half-life of more than 24 hours. Individual responses to triptans vary, and more than one drug trial may be necessary before treatment is successful. Significant elevation of blood pressure and cardiac events have been reported with triptan use. Therefore, triptans should not be administered to patients with risk factors for coronary artery disease without performing a cardiac evaluation prior to administration.

2. **Dihydroergotamine:** *Dihydroergotamine* [dye-hye-droe-er-GOT-a-meen], a derivative of *ergotamine*, is administered intravenously and has an efficacy similar to that of *sumatriptan*, but nausea is a common adverse effect.

D. Prophylaxis

Therapy to prevent migraine is indicated if the attacks occur two or more times a month and if the headaches are severe or complicated by serious neurologic signs. *Propranolol* is the drug of choice, but other β-blockers, particularly *nadolol*, have been shown to be effective. Other drugs that are effective for prevention of recurrent, refractory, severe migraine are shown in Figure 42.10.

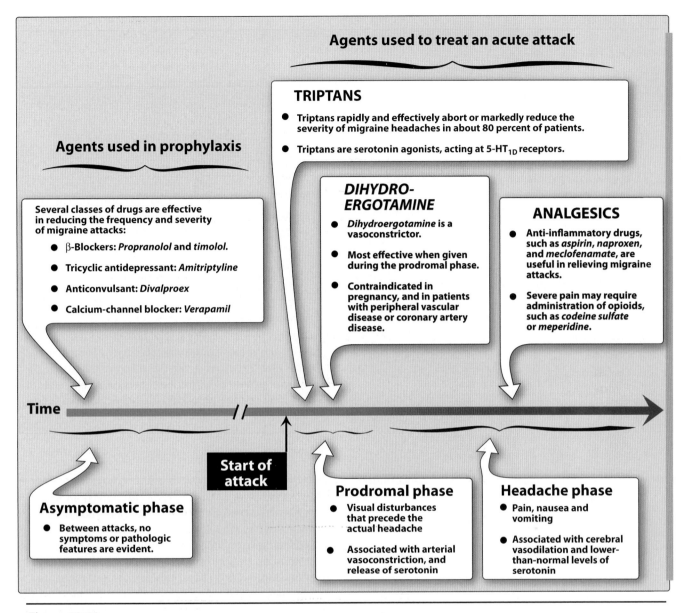

Agents used to treat an acute attack

TRIPTANS

- Triptans rapidly and effectively abort or markedly reduce the severity of migraine headaches in about 80 percent of patients.

- Triptans are serotonin agonists, acting at 5-HT$_{1D}$ receptors.

Agents used in prophylaxis

Several classes of drugs are effective in reducing the frequency and severity of migraine attacks:

- β-Blockers: *Propranolol* and *timolol*.

- Tricyclic antidepressant: *Amitriptyline*

- Anticonvulsant: *Divalproex*

- Calcium-channel blocker: *Verapamil*

DIHYDRO-ERGOTAMINE

- *Dihydroergotamine* is a vasoconstrictor.

- Most effective when given during the prodromal phase.

- Contraindicated in pregnancy, and in patients with peripheral vascular disease or coronary artery disease.

ANALGESICS

- Anti-inflammatory drugs, such as *aspirin, naproxen,* and *meclofenamate*, are useful in relieving migraine attacks.

- Severe pain may require administration of opioids, such as *codeine sulfate* or *meperidine*.

Time

Start of attack

Asymptomatic phase

- Between attacks, no symptoms or pathologic features are evident.

Prodromal phase

- Visual disturbances that precede the actual headache

- Associated with arterial vasoconstriction, and release of serotonin

Headache phase

- Pain, nausea and vomiting

- Associated with cerebral vasodilation and lower-than-normal levels of serotonin

Figure 42.10
Drugs useful in the treatment and prophylaxis of migraine headaches.

Study Questions

Choose the ONE best answer.

42.1 Dihydroergotamine:

    A. Causes vasodilation.
    B. Exerts its actions by binding to specific ergot-amine receptors.
    C. Is useful in treating acute migraine headaches.
    D. Is useful for maintaining uterine muscle tone during pregnancy.
    E. Has actions similar to those of nitroprusside.

Correct answer = C. Ergotamines act to counteract cerebral vasodilation which plays a role in migraine headaches. Vasoconstriction leading to tissue ischemia is one of the toxic complications associated with an overdose of these drugs. The ergot alkaloids interact with adrenergic, dopaminergic, and serotonin receptors. They are contraindicated in pregnancy because of their ability to cause uterine contraction and abortion. Nitroprusside is a powerful vasodilator used to treat the vasoconstriction that is characteristic of an overdose with ergot alkaloids.

42.2 A 43-year-old ship's captain complains of seasonal allergies. Which one of the following would be indicated?

    A. Cyclizine.
    B. Doxepin.
    C. Doxylamine.
    D. Hydroxyzine.
    E. Fexofenadine.

Correct answer = E. The use of first-generation H_1 antihistamines is contraindicated in the treatment of pilots and others who must remain alert. Because of its lower potential to induce drowsiness, fexofenadine may be recommended for individuals working in jobs where wakefulness is critical.

42.3 Which one of the following statements concerning H_1 antihistamines is correct?

    A. Second-generation H_1 antihistamines are relatively free of adverse effects.
    B. Because of the established long-term safety of first-generation H_1 antihistamines, they are the first choice for initial therapy.
    C. The motor coordination involved in driving an automobile is not affected by the use of first-generation H_1 antihistamines.
    D. H_1 antihistamines can be used in the treatment of acute anaphylaxis.
    E. Both first- and second-generation H_1 antihistamines readily penetrate the blood-brain barrier.

Correct answer = A. Second-generation H_1 antihistamines are preferred over first-generation agents because they are relatively free of adverse effects. Driving performance is adversely affected by first-generation H_1 antihistamines. Epinephrine, not antihistamine, is an acceptable treatment for acute anaphylaxis. Second-generation H_1 antihistamines penetrate the blood-brain barrier to a lesser degree than the first-generation drugs.

42.4 Which one of the following drugs could significantly impair the ability to drive an automobile?

    A. Diphenhydramine.
    B. Ergotamine.
    C. Fexofenadine.
    D. Ranitidine.
    E. Sumatriptan.

Correct answer = A. Diphenhydramine can impair operation of an automobile by causing drowsiness and by impairing accommodation. The other agents do not have this restriction.

Toxicology

43

I. OVERVIEW

Toxicology seeks to characterize the potentially adverse effects of foreign chemicals and their dose–response relationships to protect public health. Toxicology is defined as the study of the adverse effects of chemicals on living organisms. The term toxicity is defined as the inherent capacity of a chemical to cause injury. Thus, all chemicals, including drugs, have some degree of toxicity. This was first documented by the physician Paracelsus (1493–1541), who stated "All substances are poisons: There is none which is not a poison. The right dose differentiates a poison from a remedy." The adverse effects of therapeutic drugs have been discussed in previous chapters as the drugs have been presented and, therefore, will not be considered here. Instead, examples of nondrug chemicals and illicit drugs that are of public health concern, along with some basic concepts in toxicology, are presented.

II. TOXIC ACTIONS OF CHEMICALS

Toxic chemicals from the environment may contact the skin and/or be absorbed after ingestion or inhalation. These exogenous chemicals are distributed to various organs, where they may be metabolized to products that may be more or less toxic than the administered chemical (Figure 43.1). The parent compound or its metabolites interact with target macromolecules, resulting in a toxic effect.

A. Common target tissues

Any tissue or organ within the body can potentially be affected by a chemical toxin, and indeed, most chemicals adversely affect more than one tissue. However, the lungs ("portal of entry" for gases, vapors, and particles that can be inhaled), liver ("portal of entry" for ingested chemicals), and tissues with a high blood flow, such as brain and kidney, are particularly vulnerable to the toxic actions of chemicals. In addition the heart is sensitive to any toxin-induced disruption in ionic gradients.

B. Nonselective actions

Exposure to some chemicals, such as corrosive compounds, leads to a local irritation and/or caustic effects that are nonselective in nature and occur wherever the site of application or exposure is located. Examples include exposure to strongly alkaline or acidic substances, which cause injury by denaturation of macromolecules, such as proteins, and cleavage of chemical bonds essential to the function of biomolecules.

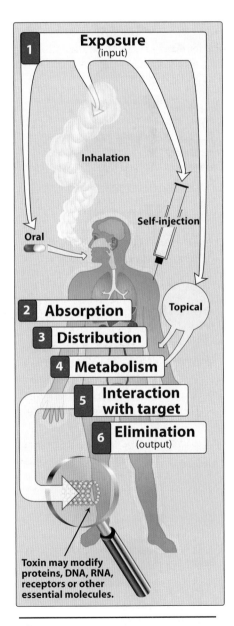

Figure 43.1
Exposure, absorption, distribution, and mode of action of toxins.

C. Selective actions

Many chemicals produce their toxic effects by interfering with the functions of specific biochemical pathways and/or macromolecules within a tissue. For example, the rodenticide *warfarin* inhibits the vitamin K–dependent posttranslational modification of certain clotting factors by the liver (see p. 240). Selective toxic actions of chemicals are usually apparent only after the chemical has been absorbed and distributed within the body, in contrast to nonselective actions, which generally occur at the exposure site.

D. Immediate and delayed actions

Many compounds have toxic actions that will quickly lead to symptoms following exposure. For example, inhibition of acetylcholinesterase by an organophosphate insecticide like malathion will rapidly lead to symptoms of excess acetylcholine at synapses and neuroeffector junctions (see p. 52). However, many chemicals exert effects that have latency periods of as long as several decades—for example, the carcinogen asbestos can lead to formation of significant pulmonary pathology, including cancer, 15 to 30 years after exposure.

III. OCCUPATIONAL AND SPECIFIC ENVIRONMENTAL TOXINS

A. Halogenated hydrocarbons

Halogenated hydrocarbons are usually volatile, and exposure can be through ingestion or inhalation. They are lipid soluble and can pass through the blood-brain barrier. Most will depress the central nervous system (CNS) when acute exposures are high.

1. **Carbon tetrachloride:** Individuals can be exposed to carbon tetrachloride through consumption of contaminated drinking water. Although transient, low-level inhalation of carbon tetrachloride can produce irritation of the eyes and respiratory system. Higher levels, whether inhaled or ingested, can produce nausea, vomiting, stupor, convulsions, coma, and death from CNS depression (Figure 43.2). Carbon tetrachloride undergoes a cytochrome P450–mediated metabolic activation to produce free radicals that are oxidize essential cellular components. A nonlethal acute exposure can occur within a period of several hours to several days and produce liver and kidney damage.

2. **Chloroform:** The adverse effects associated with *chloroform* exposure are similar to those with carbon tetrachloride. Exposures can occur through ingestion or inhalation, and high enough levels will result in nausea, vomiting, dizziness, headaches, and stupor. *Chloroform* can also sensitize the heart to catecholamine-induced arrhythmias. *Chloroform* is hepatotoxic and nephrotoxic as a result of its metabolic activation.

B. Aromatic hydrocarbons

As with the halogenated hydrocarbons, aromatic hydrocarbons tend to be volatile, and exposure can occur through inhalation and ingestion. Large acute exposures can cause CNS depression, and lead to cardiac arrhythmias through sensitization of heart cells to catecholamines. However, other aspects of their toxicological profile can differ significantly from that of the halogenated hydrocarbons.

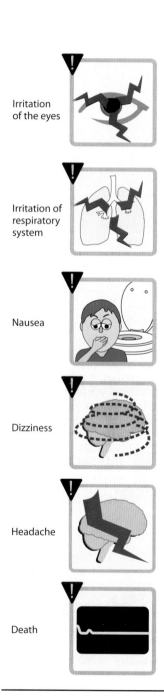

Irritation of the eyes

Irritation of respiratory system

Nausea

Dizziness

Headache

Death

Figure 43.2
Adverse effects of halogenated hydrocarbons.

1. **Benzene:** Approximately half of the national exposure to benzene occurs through tobacco smoke. Chronic benzene exposure in humans produces hematopoietic toxicities, of which the most serious are agranulocytosis and leukemia, particularly acute myelogenous leukemia. Nonoccupational exposures to benzene can occur as a result of combustion of fossil fuels, including automobile gasoline, and by consumption of contaminated water.

2. **Toluene:** Automobile emissions are the principal source of exposure in ambient air, whereas indoors exposure occurs from the use of household products containing toluene-like degreasers, certain paints and primers, and furniture polish. Acute and chronic exposure to toluene can produce CNS depression, with symptoms including drowsiness, ataxia, tremors, impaired speech, hearing, and vision. Chronic exposure may also produce some damage to the liver and kidneys. Deaths have occurred at high levels of exposure.

C. Alcohols

1. **Methanol (wood alcohol) and ethylene glycol:** These primary alcohols are themselves relatively nontoxic and cause mainly CNS sedation. However, methanol and ethylene glycol are oxidized to toxic products—formic acid in the case of methanol, and glycolic, glyoxylic, and oxalic acids in the case of ethylene glycol. *Fomepizole* inhibits this oxidative pathway, preventing the formation of toxic metabolites, and allows the parent alcohols to be excreted by the kidney (Figure 43.3). Coma, seizures, hyperpnea, and hypotension all suggest that a substantial portion of the parent alcohols has been metabolized to toxic acids.

2. **Isopropanol:** This secondary alcohol is metabolized to acetone via alcohol dehydrogenase. Acetone cannot be further oxidized to a carboxylic acids and, therefore, shows only limited acidemia and toxicity.

D. Pesticides

Pesticides are a large class of chemicals designed to kill organisms that society considers to be unhealthy, a nuisance, or destructive. Although their use is often controversial, they have had a significant impact on public health through the reduction of insect-borne diseases, such as yellow fever and malaria, and they have increased crop yields in agriculture. A large variety of different pesticides are currently used throughout the world. Some of the more commonly used compounds are considered here.

1. **Organophosphosphate and carbamate insecticides:** These agents constitute two major classes of insecticides used in the United States and throughout the world. They exert their mammalian toxicity through inhibition of acetylcholinesterase, with subsequent accumulation of excess acetylcholine.

2. **Pyrethroids:** The pyrethroids exert their mammalian and insect toxicity by extending the open time of sodium channels throughout the central and peripheral nervous systems. Symptoms of toxicity include loss of coordination, tremors, convulsions, and burning and itching sensations. Pyrethroids can also act as dermal and respiratory allergens, and exposure can lead to contact dermatitis

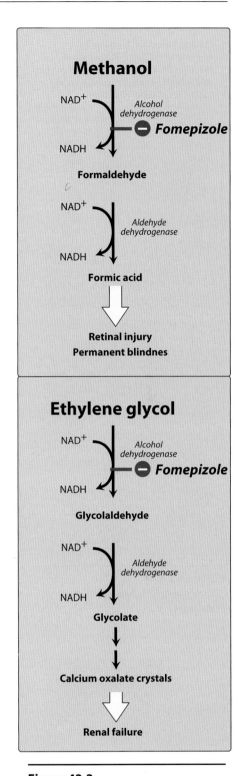

Figure 43.3
Metabolism of methanol and ethyleneglycol.

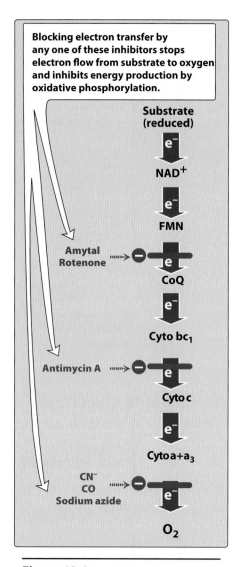

Blocking electron transfer by any one of these inhibitors stops electron flow from substrate to oxygen and inhibits energy production by oxidative phosphorylation.

Figure 43.4
Site-specific inhibitors of electron transport.

or asthma-like symptoms. Death, when it occurs in humans, is usually due to respiratory failure. Fortunately, the pyrethroids are much more toxic to insects due to their limited ability to eliminate these compounds.

3. **Rotenone:** Rotenone is used primarily as an insecticide and is applied to a wide variety of crops. It acts by inhibiting the oxidation of the reduced form of nicotinamide-adenine dinucleotide (Figure 43.4). Symptoms of poisoning include nausea and vomiting, with convulsions and death at very high exposures.

E. Rodenticides

In contrast to insecticides, which are often applied by spraying, the rodenticides are usually used in the form of solid baits ingested by rodents. Consequently, the public health threat posed is usually through the accidental or suicidal ingestion. The most commonly used rodenticides are the anticoagulants, such as *warfarin*.

F. Heavy metals

The heavy metals that are presently of most concern from a public health perspective are lead, mercury, and cadmium. They all exert their toxic effects by binding to certain functional groups on critical macromolecules within the body, thereby inactivating their function. These functional groups include hydroxyl groups, carboxylic acid groups, sulfhydryl groups, and amino groups. Heavy metal intoxication can be treated by drugs termed chelators (see p. 536), which form complexes with the metals and prevent and/or reverse their binding to the endogenous macromolecules. Acute exposures to high levels of heavy metals are rare in the United States and are usually confined to occupational exposures. Such high exposures often result in nonselective corrosive effects. Of much greater public health concern are the more widespread chronic exposures to low levels of these toxic elements.

1. **Lead:** Lead is ubiquitous in the environment, with sources of exposure including old paint, drinking water, industrial pollution, food, and contaminated dust. However, with the elimination of tetraethyl lead in gasoline during the mid-1980s in the United States, environmental exposure to organic lead has been reduced, and most chronic exposure to lead occurs with inorganic lead salts, such as those in paint used in housing constructed prior to 1978. Age-dependent differences in the absorption of ingested lead are known to occur. Adults absorb about 10 percent of an ingested dose, whereas children absorb about 40 percent. Inorganic forms of lead are initially distributed to the soft tissues and more slowly redistribute to bone, teeth, and hair. Most lead will eventually make its way to bone, where it can be detected by x-ray examination. Lead has an apparent blood half life of about 1 to 2 months, whereas its half-life from bone is 20 to 30 years. Chronic exposure to lead can have serious effects on several tissues.

   a. **Central nervous system:** The CNS effects of lead have often been termed lead encephalopathy. Symptoms include headaches, confusion, clumsiness, insomnia, fatigue, and impaired concentration. As the disease progresses, clonic convulsions and coma can occur. Death is rare given the ability to treat lead intoxication with chelation therapy. Children are more susceptible than adults to the CNS effects of lead. Furthermore, blood levels of 5 to 20 μg/dL in children have been shown to lower IQ in the absence of other symptoms. It has been estimated that as many as nine percent of the children in the United States may have blood lead levels greater than 10 μg/dL.

b. **Gastrointestinal system:** The actions of lead on the gastrointestinal tract are varied and often lead subjects to seek medical help. Early symptoms can include discomfort and constipation (and, occasionally, diarrhea), whereas higher exposures can produce painful intestinal spasms (Figure 43.5). Calcium gluconate infusion is effective for relief of pain.

c. **Blood:** Lead has complex effects on the constituents of blood, leading to hypochromic, microcytic anemia as a result of a shortened erythrocyte life span and through disruption of heme synthesis. Lead inhibits several enzymes involved in the synthesis of heme, thereby leading to increased blood levels of protoporphyrin IX and aminolevulinic acid, as well as increased urinary excretion of aminolevulinic acid and coproporphyrinogen (Figure 43.6). Elevated blood and urinary levels of these intermediates can be used diagnostically for lead intoxication, provided that blood lead levels are greater than about 25 μg/dL. Below that, elevated levels of heme intermediates cannot be observed, even though IQ effects can be observed in children.

2. **Mercury:** Potential exposure to mercury constitutes a significant health concern, because various forms of mercury are released into the human environment by industry, by natural release from the oceans and the earth's crust, and through the burning of fossil fuels. Human exposure to three different forms of mercury can occur.

a. **Elemental mercury:** Toxic exposures to elemental mercury are usually occupational, in which the vapors are inhaled. Symptoms of elemental mercury toxicity include tremors, depression, memory loss, decreased verbal skills, and inflammation of the kidneys. High concentrations of elemental mercury are corrosive and cause nonselective toxicity within the pulmonary system.

b. **Inorganic mercury salts:** Exposures to inorganic salts of mercury, such as mercuric chloride, that lead to adverse health effects are usually occupational in nature. Inorganic salts are often corrosive and can destroy the mucosa of the mouth if ingested. Renal damage can also be observed several hours after exposure. Hazardous exposures of the public to inorganic forms of mercury are uncommon.

c. **Organic mercury:** Any form of mercury that contains at least one covalent bond to a carbon atom is considered to be organic mercury. Organic forms of mercury tend to be more lipid soluble than the inorganic salts, as well as much less corrosive. Therefore, significant absorption results after ingestion, which occurs primarily from consumption of foods, particularly fish, contaminated with methylmercury. Symptoms of high levels of organic mercury can appear several days to several weeks after ingestion and are primarily neurologic in nature. These symptoms include visual disturbances, paresthesias, ataxia,

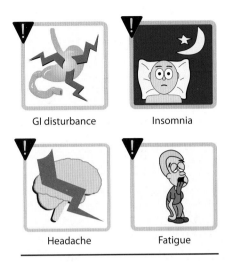

GI disturbance   Insomnia

Headache   Fatigue

Figure 43.5
Adverse effects of lead poisoning.

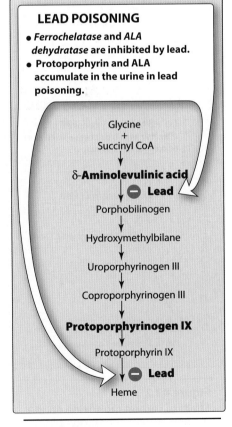

Figure 43.6
Adverse effect of lead poisoning on heme biosynthesis.

hearing loss, mental deterioration, muscle tremors, movement disorders, and with severe exposure, paralysis and death. Organic mercury poisoning in the elderly is sometimes misdiagnosed as Parkinson's disease or Alzheimer's disease. Although all forms of mercury are toxic to the fetus, organic mercury is the most dangerous, because its lipid solubility allows passage through the placenta.

3. **Cadmium:** The most frequent human exposures to cadmium occur through ingestion or inhalation. Widespread exposure to the public can occur through ingestion of food that is contaminated as a result of uptake by plants of cadmium from fertilizers and manure, and through atmospheric deposition. Large inhalational exposures are usually occupational in nature, although low-level exposure occurs from the burning of fossil fuels, which release cadmium into the environment. Cigarette smoke is also a source of cadmium. Cadmium is used heavily by a variety of industries, and environmental contamination from these sources is a major concern. Cadmium absorption upon ingestion is poor, with about five percent bioavailability. Upon inhalation, about 10 to 40 percent of the dose is absorbed. Most of the cadmium in the body will eventually distribute to the liver and kidneys, largely as a result of its binding to metallothionein. The half-life of cadmium is 10 to 30 years. Although cadmium can affect many tissues, its major toxicities are seen in the kidneys and lungs.

G. Gases and inhaled particles

Chemicals can be inhaled as gases, solids, and aerosols. Some chemicals that make their way to the alveoli can be rapidly absorbed and distributed to other tissues. Other particulates can become lodged in the alveoli and exert serious local toxicity without being absorbed into the bloodstream.

1. **Carbon monoxide:** Carbon monoxide is a gas that is colorless, odorless, and tasteless, making it impossible for individuals to detect without a carbon monoxide detector. It is a natural by-product of the combustion of carbonaceous materials, and common sources of this gas include automobiles, poorly vented furnaces, fireplaces, wood-burning stoves, kerosene space heaters, and charcoal grills. Following inhalation, carbon monoxide rapidly binds to hemoglobin to produce carboxyhemoglobin. The binding affinity of carbon monoxide to hemoglobin is 230 to 270 times greater than that of oxygen. Consequently, even low concentrations of carbon monoxide in the air can produce significant levels of carboxyhemoglobin. In addition, bound carbon monoxide increases hemoglobin affinity for oxygen at the other oxygen-binding sites. This high-affinity binding of oxygen prevents the unloading of oxygen at the tissues, further reducing oxygen delivery (Figure 43.7). The symptoms of carbon monoxide intoxication are consistent with hypoxia, with the brain and heart showing the greatest sensitivity. Symptoms include headache, dyspnea, lethargy, confusion, and drowsiness, whereas higher exposure levels can lead to seizures, coma, and death. The management of a carbon monoxide–poisoned patient includes prompt removal from the source of carbon monoxide and institution of 100 percent oxygen by nonrebreathing face mask or endotracheal tube. In patients with severe intoxication, hyperbaric oxygen therapy may be indicated.

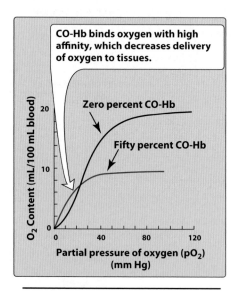

Figure 43.7
Effect of carbon monoxide on the oxygen affinity of hemoglobin. CO-Hb = carbon monoxy-hemoglobin.

2. **Cyanide:** Once absorbed into the body, cyanide quickly binds to many metalloenzymes, thereby rendering them inactive. Its principal toxicity occurs as a result of the inactivation of the enzyme cytochrome oxidase (cytochrome a_3), leading to the inhibition of cellular respiration. Therefore, even in the presence of oxygen, those tissues, such as the brain and heart, which require a high oxygen demand, are adversely affected. Death can occur quickly due to respiratory arrest of central origin. Cyanide poisoning can be treated with specific antidotes (see p. 227) .

3. **Silica:** Workers in mines, foundries, construction sites, and stone cutters are at particular risk for silicosis, perhaps the oldest known occupational disease. Silicosis is a progressive lung disease that results in fibrosis and, often, emphysema. Silicosis is currently incurable, and the prognosis is often poor. However, with lower exposures, silicosis does not always end in death or debilitation.

4. **Asbestos:** The greatest public health threat from asbestos is pulmonary in nature as a result of inhalation of the fibers, some of which stay permanently in the lung alveoli. The three diseases most commonly associated with asbestos exposure are asbestosis, mesothelioma, and lung cancer. Symptoms of these diseases may not be apparent for up to 15 to 30 years following exposure to asbestos. Asbestosis is a chronic pulmonary disease that is characterized by interstitial fibrosis in the lungs and pleural fibrosis or calcification. Initial symptoms include shortness of breath that can eventually develop into severe cough and chest pains. Asbestosis is a progressive disease with no specific treatment, and it can be fatal. Mesothelioma is a rare cancer, usually in the chest wall (although some can appear in the abdominal cavity) which seems to be caused only by asbestos. The first noticeable symptom is usually pain in the vicinity of the lesion, with dyspnea and cough developing with pleural mesothelioma. Patients usually survive no longer than 2 years after diagnosis. With all forms of asbestos-induced treatment, disease is largely symptomatic and supportive.

IV. ANTIDOTES

Specific chemical antidotes for poisonings exist for only a small number of chemicals or classes of chemicals (Figure 43.8). The following are examples of strategies that form the basis for the use of specific chemical antidotes, with an example of how each can be applied.

A. Pharmacologically antagonize toxic action

Atropine is a muscarinic-receptor antagonist that is used as an antidote for intoxication by the anticholinesterases (see p. 55). It works by blocking access of excess acetylcholine to muscarinic receptors.

B. Accelerate detoxification of toxic agent

Acetaminophen at very high doses will produce liver necrosis as a result of its metabolic activation by cytochromes P450. Administration of N-acetylcysteine will serve as a substitute for glutathione by binding to and inactivating the reactive metabolites produced from *acetaminophen*. To be effective, N-acetylcysteine must be given as early as possible (within 8–10 hours of ingestion of acetaminophen).

POISON OR SYNDROME	ANTIDOTE(S)
Acetaminophen	*N-Acetylcysteine*
Anticholinergic agents	*Physostigmine*
Benzodiazepine	*Flumazenil*
Carbon monoxide	*Oxygen (+/– hyperbaric chamber)*
Cyanide	*1) Amyl nitrite pearls 2) Sodium nitrite 3) Sodium thiosulfate*
Digitalis	*Digoxin immune Fab*
Methanol Ethylene glycol	*Fomepizole*
Heparin	*Protamine sulfate*
Lead	*Dimercapto-succinic acid*
Mercury Arsenic Gold	*Dimercaprol*
Methemo-globinemia	*Methylene blue*
Opiates	*Naloxone, nalmefene, or naltrexone*
Organo-phosphates Carbamates Nerve gases	*1) Atropine 2) Pralidoxime*

Figure 43.8
Common antidotes.

C. Provide alternative target

Cyanide poisoning is treated with a two-step process. Sodium nitrite is administered to induce the oxidation of hemoglobin to methemoglobin, which has a high binding affinity for cyanide to produce cyanmethemoglobin. Amyl nitrite can also be used for this purpose. The second step in the antidotal treatment of cyanide intoxication is to accelerate its detoxification. Administration of sodium thiosulfate will accelerate the production of thiocyanate, which is much less toxic than cyanide and is also quickly excreted in the urine. In patients with smoke inhalation and cyanide toxicity, the induction of methemoglobin should be avoided unless the carboxyhemoglobin concentration is less than 10 percent. Otherwise, the oxygen-carrying capacity of blood becomes too low.

D. Reduce metabolic activation

The toxicity of methanol is thought to be mediated by formic acid, which is produced by the metabolism of methanol by alcohol dehydrogenase. *Fomepizole* is considered an antidote to methanol, because it inhibits alcohol dehydrogenase (see Figure 43.xx). Slowing the rate of methanol metabolism reduces the rate of rate formic acid production, thereby protecting the patient from the toxic effects of formic acid.

E. Restore altered target

Acetylcholinesterase that has been inhibited as a result of phosphorylation by organophosphorus compounds often can be reactivated by the antidote *pralidoxime* (see p. 52).

F. Chelators

Chelators are drugs that will form covalent bonds with cationic metals. The chelator-metal complex is then excreted in the urine, thereby greatly facilitating the excretion of the heavy metal. Unfortunately, chelators are not specific to heavy metals, and essential metals, such as zinc, often can also be chelated. Additionally, some chelators have potentially serious adverse effects themselves, and their use in treatment of heavy metal intoxication is undertaken only when the benefits of chelation therapy outweigh the associated risks.

1. **Dimercaprol:** *Dimercaprol*, also known as British Anti-Lewisite, was the first chelator utilized, having been developed during World War II as a chelator for the arsenical war gas Lewisite. *Dimercaprol* is used by itself to chelate mercury and arsenic and in combination with edetate calcium disodium to treat lead intoxication. It is not effective after oral administration and is usually given intramuscularly. Use of *dimercaprol* is often limited by its capacity to increase blood pressure and heart rate.

2. **Succimer:** *Succimer* (dimercaptosuccinic acid) is a derivative of *dimercaprol* that is effective upon oral administration. A second advantage of *succimer* over *dimercaprol* is the lack of increased blood pressure and heart rate during treatment. Some elevation of serum levels of hepatic enzymes can be observed with *succimer* treatment. *Succimer* is currently approved for treatment of lead intoxication, but may be effective in chelation of other metals as well.

3. **Edetate calcium disodium:** Edetate calcium disodium is used primarily for treatment of lead intoxication, but it can also be used for

poisoning by other metals. It is not effective after oral administration and is usually given intravenously or intramuscularly. The calcium disodium salt of EDTA must be the form utilized to prevent chelation of calcium and its depletion from the body. Edetate calcium disodium can cause renal damage that is reversible upon cessation of the drug.

V. DESIGNER AND STREET DRUGS

"Designer drugs" are synthetic derivatives of federally controlled substances, created by slightly altering the molecular structure of existing drugs and produced illegally in clandestine laboratories for illicit use. Most of these drugs have some psychoactive properties and cause visual disturbances, but they are not true hallucinogens like *lysergic acid diethylamide* (*LSD*).

A. Methylenedioxymethamphetamine

Many of the most popular designer drugs on the street today are *amphetamine* analogs. Methylenedioxymethamphetamine (MDMA) is one of the most commonly used designer drugs. Commonly known as Ecstasy, MDMA has central stimulant and psychedelic effects. Its use is popular among those attending late-night "rave" parties, dance clubs, and rock concerts

1. **Mechanism of action:** The main effect of MDMA is on neurons that synthesize and release the neurotransmitter serotonin (5-HT). MDMA causes 5-HT release into the synaptic cleft, inhibits its synthesis, and blocks its reuptake (Figure 43.9). The effect is an increased 5-HT concentration in the synaptic cleft and a depletion of intracellular 5-HT stores. 5-HT regulates mood, appetite, and body temperature. Users of MDMA will therefore manifest more of a serotonergic effect compared with the dopaminergic effects (*amphetamine* toxicity associated with *amphetamines*; see p. 121). MDMA's effects begin within the first hour after ingestion of an oral dose and usually last 3 to 6 hours.

2. **Clinical manifestations:**

   a. **Cardiopulmonary:** Cardiopulmonary manifestations of Ecstasy use include tachycardia, tachypnea, hypertension, vasospasm, pulmonary hypertension, dysrhythmias, valvular disease, and myocardial infarction.

   b. **Neurologic:** symptoms include mydriasis, nystagmus, head jerking, hyperthermia, sexual dysfunction, seizures, cerebral infarction, dopamine and 5-HT depletion in the synapse leading to potential for irreversible neuron destruction, and 5-HT syndrome, especially in combination with other serotonergic drugs.

   c. **Psychologic:** Most users of Ecstasy describe a sense of well-being and social interactivity as well as feelings of empathy, euphoria, agitation, visual and tactile hallucinations, and occasionally, anxiety. Chronic abuse leads to symptoms of psychosis (from dopaminergic affects) and obsessive compulsive behavior.

   d. **Musculoskeletal:** Common signs and symptoms include teeth-grinding (bruxism), jaw clenching (trismus), increased muscular activity resulting in cramping, and rhabdomyolysis.

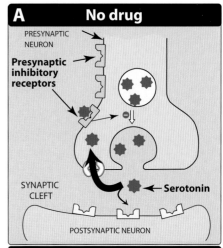

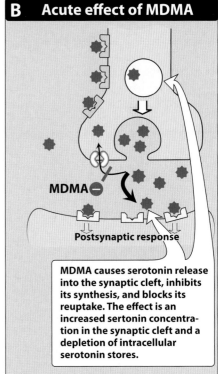

MDMA causes serotonin release into the synaptic cleft, inhibits its synthesis, and blocks its reuptake. The effect is an increased sertonin concentration in the synaptic cleft and a depletion of intracellular serotonin stores.

Figure 43.9
Proposed mechanism of action of methylenedioxymethamphetamine (MDMA).

e. Other manifestations: Dehydration and hyperglycemia are common, as is metabolic acidosis in chronic use and overdose. Hyponatremia is of concern because, as dilution, from increased water intake, in addition to increased diuresis, secondary to inhibition of antidiuretic hormone may reduce sodium, predisposing the patient to seizures and cerebral edema.

3. Treatment: Treatment of isolated MDMA ingestion is supportive. Asymptomatic MDMA-induced hyponatremia is treated with fluid restriction. Refractory hypertension may be treated with *nitroprusside* or *phentolamine*. Hyperthermia is treated by aggressive external cooling with ice water, mist, and fans. Anxiety, agitation, and convulsions are treated with *diazepam*.

B. γ-Hydroxybutyric acid

In the dance and "rave" clubs, γ-hydroxybutyric acid (GHB) has become widely abused due to its ability to rapidly produce a euphoric state. The fast and effective intoxication and the amnestic effect produced by GHB has made the drug attractive to sexual assault perpetrators. GHB is usually administered in an oral form and is rapidly and effectively absorbed by the gastrointestinal tract. The onset of action is quite rapid, with an effect usually being felt within 15 minutes and peaking anywhere between 40 and 120 minutes.

1. Mechanism of action: The actions of exogenous GHB are mediated primarily by the $GABA_B$ receptor. Low doses of the drug stimulate dopamine synthesis but inhibit its release, causing dopamine to concentrate in the nerve terminal. With higher doses of GHB, dopamine release is triggered. GHB also has effects through the endogenous opioid system, which may explain its euphoria-producing properties.

2. Clinical manifestations

a. Cardiopulmonary: Chronic use of GHB can cause severe cardiopulmonary complications, such as hypoxia, bradycardia, hypotension, bradypnea, and dysrhythmia.

b. Central nervous system: CNS effects are common and include euphoria in small doses, deep sleep in moderate doses, and a comatose state in large doses. Amnestic effects and loss of sexual inhibition make GHB a common drug in the commission of sexual battery. Hallucinations, agitation (especially upon arousal), seizures, myoclonus, and slurred speech are also common.

c. Psychologic: Most users describe a sense of well-being and euphoria as well as being socially interactive and empathetic.

d. Other: Other physiologic manifestations include salivation, vomiting, and hypothermia.

3. Treatment: Treatment of isolated GHB ingestion is supportive. In patients with significant CNS depression due to GHB overdose, intubation for airway protection is essential because of the high incidence of emesis. Bradycardia unresponsive to stimulation should be treated with *atropine*. *Pentobarbital* has been used successfully in the treatment of severe GHB withdrawal.

Study Questions

Choose the ONE best answer.

43.1 A 3-year-old male reports to the Emergency Department with, per the mother, continuous crying and "doesn't want to play or eat" for the last few days. The mom also states that the baby has not had regular bowel movements, with mostly constipation and occasional diarrhea, and frequently complains of abdominal pain. This baby now has an altered level of consciousness, is difficult to arouse, and begins to seize. The clinician rules out infection and other medical causes. Upon questioning, the mother states that the house is in an older neighborhood, that her house has not been remodeled or repainted since the 1940s, and that the paint is chipping around the windows and doors. The child is otherwise breathing on his own and urinating normally. Which toxin would you expect to be causing such severe effects in this child?

A. Mercury.
B. Lead.
C. Cadmium.
D. None of the above.

Correct answer = B. Lead poisoning is common among children in older homes painted before lead was removed from paint. Paint chips with lead are easily ingested by toddlers, and excessively high lead levels can lead to the signs and symptoms described plus clumsiness, confusion, headaches, coma, constipation, intestinal spasms, and anemia. Death is rare when chelation therapy is used. Succimer is typically a good chelating agent for lead. Mercury is not typically a concern in this age group. When ingested, elemental mercury is relatively harmless, and children of this age are not typically exposed to occupational mercury salts (mercury chloride) or organic mercury, such as that found in thimerosal. Mercury also has signs and symptoms such as movement disorders and tremors. Cadmium poisoning is typically a result of ingestion through contaminated food and causes kidney and lung damage, which this child does not exhibit.

43.2 A 41-year-old male pocket watch maker reports to the Emergency Department after he was found unconscious on the floor of the shop by a coworker. The coworker states that the patient complained of being cold this morning around 8 AM (the central heat was broken, and the outdoor temperature was 34°F) and that since noon, he had been complaining of headache, drowsiness, confusion, and nausea. The clinician notices that he has cherry red lips and nail beds. What is the most likely toxin causing his signs and symptoms?

A. Asbestos.
B. Cyanide.
C. Chloroform.
D. Carbon monoxide.

Correct answer = D. Although watch makers and other professionals who use electroplating may be at higher risk for cyanide exposure because many plating baths use cyanide-containing ingredients (for example, potassium cyanide), this patients shows classic signs of carbon monoxide poisoning, such as cherry red lips and nail beds, headache, confusion, nausea, and drowsiness leading to unconsciousness. The history also leads us to believe that this person may have been using a Sterno stove or space heater to stay warm, which would be consistent with the description. Asbestos commonly first presents as lung cancer or mesothelioma. Cyanide in low doses from such an occupational exposure can present with loss of consciousness, headache, and confusion. However, cyanide toxicity also typically includes giddiness in the early stages, perceived difficulty breathing, and pink skin (not just lips and nails), and then later rapidly progresses to deep coma and death. Chloroform can cause dizziness, fatigue, and unconsciousness, but these patients do not present with cherry red lips and nails.

Study Questions (continued)

Choose the ONE best answer.

43.3 A 50-year-old migrant worker comes to the Emergency Department from the field he was working in and complains of diarrhea, tearing, nausea and vomiting, and sweating. The clinician notices that he looks generally anxious and has fine fasciculations in the muscles of the upper chest as well as pinpoint pupils. Which antidote should he receive first?

    A. N-Acetylcysteine.
    B. Sodium nitrite.
    C. Edetate calcium disodium.
    D. Atropine.

Correct answer = D. Atropine is appropriate for this patient, who has symptoms consistent with organophosphate (pesticide) poisoning. The mnemonic SLUDGE (salivation, lacrimation, urination, diaphoresis, gastrointestinal motility diarrhea, and emesis) can be used to remember the signs and symptoms of cholinergic toxicity. An anticholinergic antidote like atropine will control these muscarinic symptoms. The antidote pralidoxime can be used to treat the nicotinic symptoms like fasciculations (involuntary muscle quivering or twitching). N-Acetylcysteine is the antidote for acetaminophen overdose and acts as a sulfhydryl donor. Sodium nitrite is one of the antidotes included in the cyanide antidote kit (amyl nitrite, sodium nitrite, and sodium thiosulfate.) Edetate calcium disodium is the chelating agent for heavy metals like lead.

43.4 A 20-year-old female presents to the Emergency Department after being dumped in the ambulance bay with a note that said only that "she was doing ecstasy at a party when she became unconscious." This patient currently remains unconscious, with a heart rate of 140 bpm, temperature of 103.5°F, pin-point pupils, absent bowel sounds, blood pressure of 85/40 mm Hg, profuse sweating, and oxygen saturation of 86 percent on room air. Which of the following would not be a clinical manifestation of an Ecstasy patient?

    A. Tachycardia.
    B. Hyperthermia.
    C. Pinpoint pupils.
    D. Diaphoresis.

Correct answer = C. Tachycardia, hyperthermia, diaphoresis, and unconsciousness are typical signs and symptoms of ecstasy overdose. Pinpoint pupils as well as absent bowel sounds, low oxygen saturation (respiratory depression), and hypotension are good indicators of opioid overdose. This is likely a multidrug overdose.

43.5 A 23-year-old man presents to the Emergency Department unconscious with his girlfriend, who tells the clinician that they were at a rave and a couple who they met gave them what looked like water in a bottle. Her boyfriend drank about one-fourth of the bottle and suddenly collapsed. He currently is hypoxic, bradycardic, hypotensive, bradypnic, and has electrocardiographic changes. She states that they do not do drugs; they just went for the music. The urine drug screen is negative for opioids, marijuana, methadone, benzodiazepines, barbiturates, PCP, amphetamines, and cocaine. The clinician suspects GHB intoxication. GHB ingestions commonly produce which of the following?

    A. Tachycardia.
    B. Hyperthermia.
    C. Hypertension.
    D. Respiratory depression.

Correct answer = D. Respiratory depression is associated with GHB ingestion. This patient has symptoms associated with GHB toxicity. Choices A, B, and C are all associated with an Ecstasy overdose.

POISON CONTROL CENTER : Call the nation-wide toll-free Poison Control Center number: 1-800-222-1222 and follow the instructions give by the center from the area in whch the call is made.

Appendix

I. CONTROLLED SUBSTANCES

Controlled Substances are a special class of prescription drugs. For the sake of regulation, controlled substances are classified into five groups or "schedules" based on 1) whether they have an accepted medical use; 2) their relative potential for abuse; 3) the degree of dependence that may be caused by abuse of the drug. Originally controlled substances referred to narcotic drugs exclusively, hence the term narcotics is a commonly used term. The classification of controlled substances has over the years been broadened to include other dangerous drugs as defined by the US Food and Drug Administration (US FDA). For more information see: http://www.deadiversion.usdoj.gov/schedules/schedules.htm

A. Definition of Schedules for Controlled Substances

1. **Schedule I (CI):** The drug or other substance:

   - has a high potential for abuse,

   - has no currently accepted medical use in treatment in the United States, or

   - has no accepted safe use under medical supervision.

   Examples: heroine, marijuana and a host of designer-drugs

2. **Schedule II (CII):** The drug or other substance:

   - has a high potential for abuse,

     - has a currently accepted medical use in treatment in the United States, or

     - has a currently accepted medical use but with severe restrictions, and

     - abuse of the drug or other substances may lead to severe psychological or physical dependence.

   Examples: morphine, oxycodone, hydromorphone, meperidine, codeine, anabolic steroids

3. **Schedule III (CIII):** The drug or other substance:

   - has a potential for abuse less than the drugs or other substances in schedules I and II,

   - has a currently accepted medical use in treatment in the United States, and

   - abuse of the drug or other substance may lead to moderate or low physical dependence or high psychological dependence.

   Examples: hydrocodone, codeine and others in combination with other drugs

4. **Schedule IV (CIV):** The drug or other substance:

- has a low potential for abuse relative to the drugs or other substances in schedule III,

- has a currently accepted medical use in treatment in the United States, and

- abuse of the drug or other substance may lead to limited physical dependence or psychological dependence relative to the drugs or other substances in schedule III.

  Examples: benzodiazepines (Valium, Ativan, etc), propoxyphene combinations

5. **Schedule V (CV):** The drug or other substance:

- has a low potential for abuse relative to the drugs or other substances in schedule IV,

- has a currently accepted medical use in treatment in the United States, and

- abuse of the drug or other substance may lead to limited physical dependence or psychological dependence relative to the drugs or other substances in schedule IV.

  Examples: Diphenoxylate combination, cough syrups

II. PREGNANCY CATEGORIES

The pregnancy category of a pharmaceutical agent is an assessment of the risk of fetal injury due to the pharmaceutical, if it is used as directed by the mother during pregnancy. It does not include any risks conferred by pharmaceutical agents or their metabolites that are present in breast milk.

Pregnancy Category A: The pregnancy category of a pharmaceutical agent is an assessment of the risk of fetal injury due to the pharmaceutical, if it is used as directed by the mother during pregnancy. It does not include any risks conferred by pharmaceutical agents or their metabolites that are present in breast milk.

Pregnancy Category B: Animal reproduction studies have failed to demonstrate a risk to the fetus and there are no adequate and well-controlled studies in pregnant women OR Animal studies which have shown an adverse effect, but adequate and well-controlled studies in pregnant women have failed to demonstrate a risk to the fetus in any trimester.

Pregnancy Category C: Animal reproduction studies have shown an adverse effect on the fetus and there are no adequate and well-controlled studies in humans, but potential benefits may warrant use of the drug in pregnant women despite potential risks.

Pregnancy Category D: There is positive evidence of human fetal risk based on adverse reaction data from investigational or marketing experience or studies in humans, but potential benefits may warrant use of the drug in pregnant women despite potential risks.

Pregnancy Category X: Studies in animals or humans have demonstrated fetal abnormalities and/or there is positive evidence of human fetal risk based on adverse reaction data from investigational or marketing experience, and the risks involved in use of the drug in pregnant women clearly outweigh potential benefits.

Figure Sources

Figure 1.23 modified from H. P. Range and M. M. Dale, Pharmacology, Churchill Livingstone (1987).

Figures 6.9, 6.11 and 6.11 modified from Allwood, Cobbold and Ginsburg, British Medical Bulletin 19:132 (1963).

Figure 8.14, modified from R. Young, American Family Physician, 59:2155 (1999).

Figure 9.5 modified from A. Kales, Excertpa Medical Congress Series 899:149 (1989).

Figure 9.6 from data of E. C. Dimitrion, A. J. Parashos, J. S. Giouzepas, Drug Invest. 4:316 (1992).

Figure 10.5 modified from N. L. Benowitz, Science 319:1318 (1988).

Figure 16.6 data from Results of the Cooperative North Scandinavian Enalapril Survival Study, N. Engl. J. Med. 316:80 (1988).

Figure 16.7 modified from the Effect of metoprolol CR/XL in chronic heart failure: Metoprolol CR/XL Randomised Intervention Trial in Congestive Heart Failure (MERIT-HF), Lancet 353:2001 (1999).

Figure 16.12 modified from M. Jessup, and S Brozena, N. Engl. J. Med. 348: 2007 (2003).

Figure 16.13 modified from T.B Young, M. Gheorghiade, and B. F. Uretsky, J. Am. Coll Cardiol. 32:686 (1998).

Figure 17.3 modified from J. A. Beven and J. H. Thompson, Essentials of Pharmacology, Harper and Row (1983).

Figure 17.9 modified from J. W. Mason, N. Engl. J. Med., 329:452 (1993).

Figure 19.5 modified from B. J. Materson, Drug Therapy, November p. 157 (1985).

Figure 20.8, modified from D. J. Schneider, P. B. Tracy, and B. E. Sobel, Hospital Practice, May 15, (1998), p. 107.

Figure 20.15, Effects of glycoprotein IIb/IIIa receptor antagonists on the incidence of death or nonfatal myocardial infarction followingpercutaneous transluminal coronary angioplasty. [Note: Data are from several studies; thus reported incidence of complicationswith standard therapy is not the same for each drug.] data from D.A. Vorchheimer, J. J. Badimon, and V. Fuster, Journal American Medical Association 281: 1407 (1999).

Figure 21.6. Modified from M. K. S. Leow, C. L. Addy, and C. S. Mantzoros. J. Clin. Endocrinol. Metab., 88:1961 (2003).

Figure 21.7, modified from Knopp, R. H., N. Engl. J. Med. 341:498 (1999).

Figures 21.10 modified from R. H. Knopp, Hospital Practice 23:22 (1988).

Figures 23.2 modified from B. G. Katzung, Basic and Clinical Pharmacology, Appleton and Lange (1987).

Figure 24.5 modified from M. C. Riddle, Postgraduate Med. 92:89 (1992).

Figure 24.7 modified from I. R. Hirsch, N. Engl. J. Med. 352:174 (2005).

Figure 24.9 modified from O. B Crofford, Ann. Rev. Medicine 46:267 (1995).

Figures 25.6 and 25.7 modified from D. R. Mishell, Jr., N. Engl. J. Med. 320:777 (1989).

Figure 25.8 modified from M. Polaneczky, G. S. Slap, C.F. Forke, A. R. Rappaport, and S. Sondheimer, N. Engl. J. Med 331:1201 (1994).

Figure 25.9 modified from A. S. Dobs, A. W. Meikle, S. Arver, S. W. Sanders, Ki. E. Caramelli and N. A. Mazer. J. Clin Endo & Met: 84:3469 (1999).

Figure 25.10 modified from J. D. McConnell, C. G. Roehrborn, O. M Bautista. N. Engl. J. Med. 349:2387 (2003).

Figure 28.2 modified from D. Cave, Hospital Practice, Sept 30, 1992.

Figure 28.6 modified from F. E. Silverstein, D. Y. Graham, J. R. Senior. Ann. Intern. Med 123:241 (1995).

Figure 28.7 modified from S. M. Grunberg and P. J. Hesketh, N. Engl. J. Med. 329: 1790 (1993).

Figures 28.9, 28.10 from data of S. Bilgrami and B. G. Fallon, Postgraduate Medicine, 94:55 (1993).

Figure 29.5 photo from Jordan, V. C., Scientific American, October, p. 60 (1998).

Figure 34.4 modified from data of D. A. Evans, K. A. Maley and V. A. McRusick, British Medical Journal 2:485 (1960).

Figure 34.5 modified from data of Neuvonen, P. J., Kivisto, K. T., and Lehto, P. Clin. Pharm Therap., 50: 499 (1991).

Figure 38.3 modified from R. Dolin, Science 227:1296 (1985).

Figure 38.15 modified from Balfour, H. H., N. Engl. J. Med. 340:1255 (1999).

Figure 39.5 modified from N. Kartner and V. Ling. Scientific American, March (1989).

Figure 42.9 modified from D. D. Dubose, A. C. Cutlip, and W. D. Cutlip. American Family Medicine 51:1498 (1995).